Classics of Community Psychiatry

Classics of Community Psychiatry

Fifty Years of Public Mental Health Outside the Hospital

Edited by

Michael Rowe

Martha Lawless

Kenneth Thompson

Larry Davidson

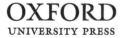

OXFORD
UNIVERSITY PRESS

OXFORD
UNIVERSITY PRESS

Oxford University Press, Inc., publishes works that further
Oxford University's objective of excellence
in research, scholarship, and education.

Oxford   New York
Auckland   Cape Town   Dar es Salaam   Hong Kong   Karachi
Kuala Lumpur   Madrid   Melbourne   Mexico City   Nairobi
New Delhi   Shanghai   Taipei   Toronto

With offices in
Argentina   Austria   Brazil   Chile   Czech Republic   France   Greece
Guatemala   Hungary   Italy   Japan   Poland   Portugal   Singapore
South Korea   Switzerland   Thailand   Turkey   Ukraine   Vietnam

Copyright © 2011 by Oxford University Press

Published by Oxford University Press, Inc.
198 Madison Avenue, New York, New York 10016
www.oup.com

Oxford is a registered trademark of Oxford University Press

Library of Congress Cataloging in Publication Data

Classics of community psychiatry : fifty years of public mental health outside the hospital /
edited by Michael Rowe ... [et al.].
p. ; cm.
Includes bibliographical references and index.
ISBN 978-0-19-532604-8 (alk. paper)
1. Community psychiatry.   2. Community mental health services.   I. Rowe, Michael, 1947–
[DNLM: 1. Community Psychiatry—Collected Works.   2. Community Mental Health Centers—Collected Works.
3. Community Mental Health Services—Collected Works.   4. Deinstitutionalization—Collected Works. WM 30.6]
RC455.C555 2011
362.2'2—dc22   2011001663

Contents

Foreword

How do we, as leaders in behavioral health care, transform old beliefs and ways of doing business so that individuals we serve, providers, administrators, programs, and even whole systems embrace the changes we believe are both necessary and achievable? This is a question I have come back to many times in my career as a mental health leader. In his book *Deep Change*, Robert Quinn writes, "At least one person must recognize that more is possible. Someone must then lead the group toward the collective goal."[i] The authors represented in the pages of this remarkable book are the leaders who have helped us understand that more is possible for individuals living with or at risk for mental health conditions.

From the personal to the political, the programmatic to the pragmatic, the authors collected in this volume have been our guide on a journey that began, not that very long ago, when mental illnesses were believed to be debilitating, lifelong conditions, requiring long-term custodial care. They showed us, in word and deed, through personal struggle and rigorous research, that there is another way. Today, thanks to their vision, courage and commitment, we know that given acceptable and accessible treatment and supports, and a voice in decisions concerning their care, *individuals with mental illnesses can and do recover*. The concept of recovery, and the changes in policy and practice it engenders, is essentially transformative.

I have had the distinct privilege to lead and facilitate both state and federal efforts to help transform the way we organize, deliver, and evaluate mental health services in this country. My thinking about transformation was guided by the writings of the late Vice Admiral Arthur Cebrowski, who headed up the Pentagon's Office of Force Transformation and laid out many of the tenets of transformation we follow today, whether in the government or private sector. Vice Admiral Cebrowski studied the concept in depth by looking at corporations and systems that had been able to recreate themselves successfully, and he identified several common characteristics that define transformation. It is instructive to consider these characteristics as you read the contributions in this volume.

Transformation is meant to create or anticipate the future. Without those visionaries whose works are collected herein, we may not have foreseen the time when individuals with even the most serious mental illnesses and co-occurring substance use disorders would live among us, not only *in* the community, but as members *of* the community. These authors' thinking, their writing, and their practice compelled us to reexamine our beliefs and begin to reshape the way we offer services.

Transformation is accomplished through changes at the core of a system and not at its margins. These fundamental changes result in new behaviors and new competencies. In

---

[i] Quinn, R.E. (1996). *Deep change: Discovering the leader within*. San Francisco: Jossey-Bass.

transformation, we look at what we are able to do now that we were unable to do before. Before we began listening to the intensely personal and powerful stories of mental health recovery, including many that are gathered herein, we offered what we thought individuals needed, rather than what they wanted. We are learning how to offer respectful, culturally competent, trauma-informed services and supports. Today, we ask "what do you want to do/ how do you want to live/what do you need to know to manage your life?" rather than "what is wrong with you?" We understand that individuals with mental health and substance use conditions and their families must drive the system, from the top down and the bottom up.

Transformation is meant to identify, leverage, and even create new underlying principles for the way things are done. New sources of power emerge. Think of the terms we use every day that weren't identified or even imagined when these writings began: recovery oriented, trauma informed, consumer operated, peer support, social inclusion. They reflect new energizing principles but also new sources of power, which reside in the very individuals we used to believe we had to isolate and protect from the rigors of everyday life. Today, individuals living with a mental illness help set the agenda. They establish goals and evaluate outcomes. *We work for them.*

Finally, once the process of transformation begins, a profoundly different organization materializes—changed in structure, culture, policies, and programs. Today, many communities and some states require that providers show evidence of a recovery orientation to be eligible for funds. Consumers, youth, and family members are not just at the table—they are wielding the gavel. Evidence-based programs, including those profiled in these pages, help individuals with even the most serious conditions learn self management, get off the streets, stay out of jail, and live lives of promise and possibilities.

Ultimately, transformation is about newness—new values, new attitudes, and new beliefs that are expressed in new behaviors of individuals and institutions. However, the paradox of this type of change is that what we create today is not the end product. It isn't the end of transformation. If that were the case, we would be back where we started, perpetuating the status quo. *Transformation is a continuous process, without end.* We can review the writings in this book as part history lesson, part roadmap for change, and part success story. But we must never be content to let the story end here.

When the next volume of this type is written, it will have articles about the science, research and practice of mental health promotion and mental illness and substance abuse prevention. It will highlight the public health approach to behavioral health care and the ways in which behavioral health and primary care are integrated and coordinated. It will feature the writings of those who helped us understand that *behavioral health is essential to health* and that we are all diminished when even one of us is excluded from full participation in our own health care, our homes, our schools, our workplaces, and our neighborhoods.

Martin Luther King, Jr. said, "Human progress is neither automatic nor inevitable... Every step toward the goal of justice requires sacrifice, suffering, and struggle; the tireless exertions and passionate concern of dedicated individuals."[ii] I commend each and every one of the writers in this volume for being passionate, dedicated transformational leaders who have shown us that more is possible—not only for individuals living with or at risk for mental health illness, but for all of us.

A. Kathryn Power, M.Ed.
Director of the Center for Mental Health Services,
Substance Abuse and Mental Health Services Administration,
US Department of Health and Human Services

[ii] Washington, J.M. (Ed.). (1990). *A testament of hope: The essential writings and speeches of Martin Luther King, Jr.* New York: HarperOne.

Preface

Michael Rowe

This volume began about five years ago with the thought that the history of community psychiatry, starting with the downsizing of state psychiatric hospitals and deinstitutionalization movement, would be a good topic for an undergraduate course in psychology at our institution, Yale University. To teach that course, though, we needed to become students ourselves to supplement what we had learned in a somewhat scattershot fashion in graduate school and through researching and writing articles and books. With so much study to be undertaken, why not kill two birds with one stone, we thought, by creating a volume of some of the best work in community psychiatry, from its research and theoretical to policy-oriented, legislative, first person, and literary accounts? We—Rowe, Lawless, and Davidson—of the Program for Recovery and Community Health in the Department of Psychiatry, recruited an old friend and colleague, Kenneth Thompson, Medical Director of Recovery Innovations, Inc., faculty member of the Department of Psychiatry at the University of Pittsburgh School of Medicine, and former Medical Director of the Federal Center for Mental Health Services.

We decided to seek experts we knew of, and that they knew of, to ask for their nominations of classics in the field and of other potential nominators. Carol M. Anderson, Carl C. Bell, Paul Carling, Carl I. Cohen, Patrick Corrigan, David L. Cutler, Ronald J. Diamond, Jeffrey Draine, Sue Estroff, Roger D. Fallott, Leonard Roy Frank, Jeffrey Geller, Howard H. Goldman, Ezra Griffith, Gerald Grob, David Healy, Keith Humphreys, Nora Jacobson, Ronald C. Kessler, Arthur Kleinman, H. Richard Lamb, Harriet P. Lefley, Jeffrey Moussaieff Masson, Harold W. Neighbors, Herbert Pardes, Joseph A. Rogers, Alan Rosen, Robert Rosenheck, Andrew Scull, William Sledge, Phyllis Solomon, Leonard I. Stein, John S. Strauss, Thomas S. Szasz, John A. Talbott, Mary Ann Test, Graham Thornicroft, and E. Fuller Torrey suggested, collectively, some 300 possible classics in addition to those we had put on our list. We thank them for their time and expertise. No doubt some of them will wish we had included some texts that we did not and exclude some that we did, but they have helped us mightily.

Six months in and at risk of drowning in a sea of history, potential classics, and the discord of considered opinion about them among experts who weighed in at the time of their publication and afterward, we reached out to colleagues—Luis Añez-Nava, Chyrell Bellamy, Thomas Dinzeo, Christine Dunn, Elizabeth Flanagan, Dietra Hawkins, Nancy Leisa, Rebecca Miller, Allison Ponce, Priscilla Ridgway, and Mary Snyder—and asked them to write commentaries on a number of articles, books, and legislative documents we had collected. Some of these would prove to be introductory commentaries on our classic documents. (Authors are named with their commentaries that introduce those classics; commentaries without a named author were written by Michael Rowe.) Others were to be commentaries for an annotated bibliography of additional reading to be included in the appendix. In the end, we ran out of space for this section. We are grateful to all of these colleagues for their time and expertise.

Work went on apace and we found that we needed to reach out again to our friends and colleagues. Elizabeth Flanagan, Richard Freeman, Francesca Martin, Rebecca Miller, Allison Ponce, and Priscilla Ridgway plunged into the classics and other reference works to co-author the introduction to the volume (Freeman, with Rowe), a "pre-community psychiatry" historical overview (Martin and Flanagan), introductory chapters for the first—1954–1976 (Miller and Ponce, with Thompson)—and second—1977–1997 (Ridgway, with Davidson)—eras of three we chose to mark important shifts in the span of community psychiatry from the first stirrings of deinstitutionalization through our third, from 1998 to the present.

John Strauss, whom we consider to be one of the great psychiatrists and researchers of community psychiatry over the past 50 years and more, encouraged and mentored us, dug up old volumes and articles, suggested new approaches, and cheered us on even as he cautioned us not to forget this topic and that almost forgotten contributor. John, Howard Goldman, and Gerald Grob read various parts of the next-to-final draft of the volume. We are grateful to them for their insights and the breadth and depth of knowledge they shared with us. We are responsible, of course, for any failures to understand or integrate what they taught us.

Marion Osmun, our original editor at Oxford University Press, championed this project at the outset. Shelley Reinhardt took over as editor when Marion moved on to other projects, aiding and advising us as we moved into the middle and final stages of collection, permission seeking, and assemblage. Yvonne Honigsberg briefly took the helm in Shelley's absence, and Catherine Barnes, with Craig Panner's able assistance, steered it home. We thank them all for seeing this complex project through to the end.

Kristine Gallaher provided able in-house assistance with us in contacting nominators, creating tracking documents, and procuring articles and books during the first few months of work on this volume. Megan Alley, Lucas Broster, and Esther Quintana, under Christine Dunn's supervision, helped with copying and related help early on. Kimberly Antunes, PRCH Project Coordinator, scrambled to pull staff from their research interviews for our own studies and countless other day-to-day activities that keep our program running. Daniel Rowe contributed his formidable editing skills toward completion of the final versions of editorial chapters, introductions to individual classics, and other material. Lesley Schwab, a research assistant, in tracking down documents that simply could not be found by normal humans, in creating, revising, and recreating dozens of organizing documents, and in patiently locating again classics she had given us and that we had misplaced (lost), took a place at the center of this project, a trooper and field general at once, and the reason we finished this project. Our hats are off to her. As Lesley had moved on to new challenges at the time of final production work, Ashley Clayton filled in admirably, helping us find missing references and other essential 11th hour editorial activities. Rajashri Ravindranathan and the team at Newgen Imaging Systems Pvt. Ltd. provided thorough editing of the manuscript, exhibiting along the way great patience and good cheer in regard to the errors and omissions in our work that found their way to them. We are grateful for their help in making our text seaworthy as a book.

We hope this volume will contribute to the understanding and advancement of the field of community psychiatry and of recovery for persons with psychiatric disabilities.

Introduction

Richard Freeman and Michael Rowe

Community Psychiatry

Some minds seem to work differently from others, and we have long been intrigued by them. Some seem to fail after working for a long time, some seem never to have worked so well at all. A challenge they pose is to the bounds of our understanding of what is real. A second challenge they pose is how we should relate to the persons who "have" them. That is to say these minds and persons challenge our own minds and persons.

We contain this threat by systems of thought. We make sense of what seems nonsensical by forming new boundaries, constructing new categories of reason and unreason that have been given by more general ways of thinking, including those of religion, art, science, justice, and medicine. Each gives its own account of the source or cause of difference—physical, spiritual, or mental—its implications—positive or negative—and the responsibility for managing or resolving it—privately or in some way publicly. To the extent that we believe in and identify with them, our own mental health turns on the workings of these systems of thought.

We are concerned here with community psychiatry, a particular way of knowing and thinking about mental illness and responding to it. Community psychiatry, for our purposes, refers to all the policies, services, agencies, and staff deployed in treating people with mental health problems who are poor and for whom publicly funded services are the default, if not the only, option. Community psychiatry is public psychiatry.

Our first purpose is educational, to set out for ourselves and others what community psychiatry is and has been, where it has come from, and where it might go. Our immediate aim is to explain how we think of community psychiatry and why we took up this project.

Psychiatry

Some may claim that using "psychiatry" rather than "mental health" to name our field gives too much weight to the role of medicine in general and psychiatry in particular. We have chosen and stuck with it, though, to keep in play a term and a field—psychiatry—the legitimacy and effectiveness of which has consistently been questioned, especially in respect to poor people and its purported collusion in social control of the different. Antipsychiatry, in fact, is part of the story of community psychiatry over the past 50-plus years. We keep psychiatry because we want to keep this questioning of it. Furthermore, the linking of community and psychiatry, rather than community and mental health, has the advantage of keeping in play another tension, that between the social, nonmedical aspects of lives and the wide range of psychotherapeutic, biopsychosocial, and pharmacological interventions that are put into place to address illness in those lives.

Community

"Community" refers here to the place where services are delivered. It has both physical and social status. It is where individuals come together in myriad forms of association for work, trade, pleasure, and ritual and for social needs such as meeting, eating, and caring. It is realized in metropolitan, urban, and rural contexts and consists of public, commercial, charitable, and private organizations as well as chance and purposeful encounters between individuals and among groups of people outside those organizations. It is comprised of many subcommunities identified by ethnicity, belief, neighborhood, and other distinctions.

In psychiatry, "community inclusion" of persons with psychiatric disabilities is a term for efforts to promote the ability of persons with mental illnesses to live satisfying and stable lives in their home communities outside of institutions such as hospitals and nursing homes. It does not mean a world without institutions, though, since institutions of different sorts may be employed to help people regain a level of function that will help them return to or stay in the community.

A critical issue for community psychiatry is who gets to define "community" and for what purpose, since community is a catch-all term with strong emotional content. The term works politically in part because it is seemingly so apolitical, appealing to both liberal and conservative views. Community functions as a kind of collective fantasy, an unarguable "good," a memory or imagination of home. Community is what we imagine remains when both the state and family have gone AWOL. In practice, however, setting community as the gold standard for treating persons with mental illness has often led to removing them from the total institutions[1] of state hospitals to hard-to-negotiate environments in which they are isolated and at high risk of violence and victimization. Or it can lead to their developing so strong a connection to mental health and other social service institutions located in the community that they end by possessing "program citizenship" rather than full democratic citizenship.[2]

Many of us who write about community inclusion do not live it the way we may think of it for persons with psychiatric disabilities. We may write about helping people with psychiatric problems develop relationships with the grocer, the next-door neighbor, and the mailman, yet lack these relationships ourselves. We may live in one town and work in another, and many of our most important personal and professional relationships are with people who live hundreds or thousands of miles away. We may wish we knew our neighbors better, may lament the fact that we are "bowling alone,"[3] but we do not require what we may wish for persons with psychiatric disabilities. Through our jobs and other valued roles, many of us develop what Mark Granovetter calls "weak ties"[4] and Peggy Thoits calls "multiple identities"[5] that prove more important to our sense of community membership than do our relationships with neighbors. We may yet maintain a strong sense of connection to the abstractions of "community" and "society" because we have so many different and meaningful connections with specific others—individuals, groups, associations—that offer us the means for maintaining and building upon our valued roles and resources, including such assets as jobs and home ownership. We maintain our affective sense of entitlement not only through the instrumental use of those roles and resources that enable us to live comfortably, but also because they are widely acknowledged to be worthy of esteem and status.

Community, then, often seems to be what we wish for other people, although we wouldn't dream of being so constrained, so obligated ourselves. This points us to a pair of important features of its use in community psychiatry. First, community has class connotations: it is a place for poor people, since they live in it. In this sense, middle- and upper-class intellectuals, bureaucrats, and legislators can be seen as missionaries who create community for others and determine what it should be for them, dissolving old communities and creating new ones, as with urban renewal programs of the 1970s and beyond. These parties also have the power to structure theories of and approaches to mental illness and treatment and to designate and allocate the functions of authority, sanction, and surveillance associated with them. Second and at the same time, community is an organic thing. Communities are endlessly defeated by artificial attempts to recreate them, yet reconstitute themselves in ever-unexpected ways. Changing conceptions and practices of community may be harbingers of changing eras or paradigms in public psychiatry.

The Instability of Community Psychiatry

We have suggested that community psychiatry not only results from but consists of arguments about psychiatry on one hand and community on the other. Community psychiatry is a category that is inherently unstable, simultaneously a thought system and a space for thinking and acting. What community psychiatry is and what it has been or should be made to be is given by repeated attempts to define it, advocate for it, and act it out.

We know from the sociology of knowledge that every new case added to a category changes the way we think about both case and category.[6] Every new study, program, or initiative that defines itself or is defined by others as community psychiatry, is so. Something as heterogeneous, as derivative, as social as community psychiatry can never be finally described. Definitions are never definitive, and this has important implications for the field and the way it develops. Every use of the term "community psychiatry" is an act of judgment, informed by similar, previous judgments made by others but an act of judgment all the same. Every claimed instance of community psychiatry alters the ground on which later judgments and claims will be made. Thinking about, writing, and doing community psychiatry turn on what others have thought, said, and done in its name but cannot be wholly determined by them. As Harold Garfinkel wrote, each application of a term is made for "another first time."[7]

Going back to our idea of community psychiatry as a thought system, what is system-like about thinking about (and doing) community psychiatry? Community psychiatry is an open, complex, adaptive system. It is built of people, agencies, and programs, and its elements are the relationships among them as played out in meetings, consultations, prescriptions, conferences, initiatives and budget lines. It is remarkably open to newcomers, whether people, ideas, or organizations, and every newcomer changes the field in some way for all the others just as, at a different level, changes in related systems, such as social security, change the context for community psychiatry. In this way, community psychiatry is made up of people drawn from different worlds—from broken homes, military service, chronic illness, and medicine, from social work and criminal justice, and from cities, states, and charities—and consists in parties and elements forming relationships to invent new worlds, parties, and elements. For these reasons we should think of community psychiatry as emerging both from and in the practices of which it is composed.

Educating for Community Psychiatry

Doing community psychiatry is difficult. Understanding what community psychiatry is, is difficult as well. The problem of doing community psychiatry, then, results at least in part from knowing what it is.

The immediate origins of this project lie in teaching. In our efforts to develop courses and programs in community psychiatry we realized that we were not sure what community psychiatry is and how we should represent it to our students. In conceiving this book, we were led by three key ideas. The first is that community psychiatry should speak for itself as much as possible, and that students (and practitioners and policy makers) should confront its claims, arguments and debates as they were first written and presented. In reviewing the field, we were struck by how many seminal texts remain seminal, how they continue to have relevance and force in sometimes different and sometimes all too familiar circumstances.

The second idea is that community psychiatry has a history, and understanding that history is key to understanding what it is and to creating a sense of continuing possibility among those who engage in it. We measure the life of community psychiatry (at least in the United States) at 50 years plus, and think that a good time to take the measure of its achievements, its failures, and its prospects.

The third idea is that community psychiatry is created in practice and that an important part of that practice is writing. Writing is a way of making sense of the world, of sponsoring action and sustaining it over space and time. We thought we could represent best the richness of community psychiatry that spans most of six decades by gathering together the different forms of writing through which, in part, it came into being. So we present here an eclectic sample of policy statements, histories, theories and reflections, research studies, and personal accounts. By juxtaposing and commenting on them, in editorial introductions that sometimes refer to the classics they introduce and sometimes to work not represented in this volume, and by offering brief commentaries on each chosen classic, we hope to convey the interactions among all that characterize the field.

As editors who are scholars and researchers but also have backgrounds as clinicians in or administrators of public mental health programs, we have had an eye to the relation between text and policy, theory and practice. That is, we have been reluctant to let the hundreds of documents we have drawn on stand alone as findings or theories or syntheses of current knowledge. Instead, we have asked the "So what?" question of our potential classics: What is their relationship to the field of community psychiatry? What influence did they have, should they have had, or might have still? What clues did they offer that policy makers and practitioners took up, interpreted by their own lights and needs, or failed to register in their attention to other demands or ways of thinking? Such questions have complicated our task, but this complexity is unavoidable given our intention to bring together a volume that is relevant to contemporary practitioners, policy makers, researchers, scholars, and students. Which leads us to a question.

What is a Classic?

What is a classic of community psychiatry? Dictionary definitions tell us that a classic has recognized value, serves as a standard of excellence, and is regarded as being authentic and authoritative. A classic is a work of enduring excellence. But how does a classic document come to be recognized as such? What is it classic about or in relation to? Does a classic require literary or intellectual brilliance, or might it simply have had a strong influence on its field? Can a text be deemed classic by virtue of its visionary or prophetic elements even if it had a minor influence on its field, perhaps because it was ahead of its time? Should controversy be part of the acid test, based on the thought that no classic is worth its salt if it did not shake up its field? Yet if so, we would have to rule out works that are notable for providing a comprehensive survey or synthesis of a field or subfield. Finally, who gets to decide that a text is or has become a classic?

We take a classic of community psychiatry to be a consummate expression of one or more aspects of the nature, object, and extent of the field. The classic may be descriptive, analytic, or normative. It may be at odds with established conceptions of the field or serve as a critical or summative account of some part of it. In one way or another, it will serve as a reference point for those in the field who are trying to think about what they do. It will be read, re-read, and misread. Like community psychiatry itself, a classic is defined in use, by the reading or practice of it. This means that there is nothing intrinsically "classic" about a classic. A classic is a work that is repeatedly referred to, both in practice—in meetings and conversations among practitioners—and in other writings. Or, in our stretching of its boundaries in this volume, a classic may be a work that, if not repeatedly referred to then or now, should have been, or should be again. The classic lives in a network or system of connections to situations and other texts both like and unlike it, including proposals, reports, minutes of meetings, and books, papers and research studies, or it lives at the margins of these among contrarians who, with a handful of fugitive classics, help to define a field by pointing to the places where its reach exceeds its grasp. The classic's status is made and sustained by the connections it makes and which are made with it.

The classics we have collected here tend to have one or both of two essential purposes, definitive and programmatic. They are concerned with either describing what is or setting out what should be at issue in community psychiatry. They may address *the origin and nature of mental illness*, including whether it is seen as primarily biological or social, linear and determined or complex and contingent; the *nature and logic of scientific or professional interventions*, whether clinical or social, unilateral or multilateral, and whether and how they should be allocated among different subfields such as psychopharmacology, child and adolescent psychiatry, and psychogerontology; *the identity and status of the patient*, including his or her capacity and entitlement to services and position as the object or subject of those services, whether patient, client, consumer, or agent; or *the identity and authority of the practitioner*, whether clinical provider, caretaker, guide, or other; and they may address more than one of these at the same time.

Choosing Classics

We have wanted to take account of a rich, diverse, and voluminous field. Following our precepts about the use of classics, we asked colleagues in the field—researchers, academics, practitioners, and activists—for nominations. We asked them to tell us which texts they thought indispensable to the field and who else they thought we should consult. We expected this process to be a classic exercise in snowball sampling by which we would identify fairly quickly a core set of material on which most of our colleagues would agree. The more new people we asked, the fewer new nominations classics and of nominators we would get. That did not happen. Both lists simply got longer, and we began to wonder why.

The failure of our snowball sampling seemed to testify to the diversity and contested nature of the field. The number and range of backgrounds, disciplines, occupations, and interests of our correspondents led them to recommend an equivalent, if not greater, range of material. It may be that there is no agreed-on core literature of community psychiatry. In Kuhnian terms, we might describe the field and its literature as being "pre-paradigmatic." The crucial consequence of this is that, in the end, our choice of classics is to some degree arbitrary. We have included material others would not have and left out some that others deemed essential. In a few cases, difficulty obtaining permission to reprint a text or the cost to do so was prohibitive. We will be glad if the arguments we provoke contribute to a more general discussion of the field.

Of course, given the limited space a single volume allows, we wanted to be as inclusive as possible. We have also tried to take account of the variety of topics and issues with which practitioners, policy makers, and patients or clients of community psychiatry have been concerned. We have included a range of forms of writing, from policy statements, theoretical papers and empirical studies, to evaluations and personal or literary accounts, attempting to reflect the range of things community psychiatry is and does. And finally, we have tried to present a survey of the field, through some of its most durable texts, which is as comprehensive as possible given limitations of length of the volume and that is comprehensible in historical terms.

Ordering Classics: Texts and Eras

An element always associated with a classic is time. Classics are seen as such in the light of history, as in our sense of enduring excellence. This relationship holds in an equal and opposite way when we speak of an instant classic or when a work is recognized as a classic in its own time. A classic may epitomize, rise above, or look beyond its time. It may come to be seen as possessing a certain timelessness, but its classic quality also refers and is linked to its own time, to the ephemeral and evanescent, if only by contrast to it. In this way, a classic may serve in part as a repository of memory either of its own time or of an era it helped to usher in. A classic is of its time but transcends it, too.

Yet while classics are, arguably, the most alive, most vital works of their era, they may also serve to ossify it, imposing hegemony with explanatory or stylistic power that sweeps away other aspects of their era, which they downplay or dismiss, rightly so in most ways but still tossing out some wheat with the chaff. Meanwhile, and paradoxically, the classic imprimatur that is overlaid on a text may tame what was most new and revelatory about it when readers first encountered it, may confer the status of accepted truth on ideas or findings that were anything but that when it first appeared. Finally, characterizations and understandings of what is a classic, along with the very notion of designating some works as classic and others as ephemeral, are shaped by cultural and intellectual traditions that will themselves change and be superseded by others. There may be nothing in this volume as time-bound as the conception of the volume itself.

The classic stimulates new ways of thinking or brings together systematically a number of ideas that have not been connected before, or summarizes previously articulated ideas in a more complete or elegant way than has been done before. A classic must know its time before it can take issue with and rise above it, and so we can group classics according to the era or time in which they were born and to which they refer. What defines an era, then, in community psychiatry?

In an era, something new is proposed, something old is critiqued, and a new paradigm emerges. There is a kind of organic growth within an era, too, and so the sources of the next era will likely be found somewhere in the current one. But how can we distinguish one era from another in a way that does not seem arbitrary, such as thinking, say, in decades might? We suggest that a given era of community psychiatry will host assumptions or theories about the origin and nature of mental illness, the nature and logic of scientific or professional intervention, the identity and status of the patient, and the identity and authority of the practitioner. It will also touch on the nature of the state, including the role and function of public bodies, the nature of civil society, including the assumed nature, role, charitable, and function of community, of independent, charitable, and other organizations and of the family, or on the relationship between knowledge and action. These different elements are interactive, in that each requires the others in order to have any effective meaning. Change in one element affects the others, which begins to explain how change takes place in community psychiatry and ultimately, how we pass from one era to the next.

There is an evolving relationship between public policy and public opinion throughout the era of community psychiatry. A constant theme is the public's reluctance to pay for the state to take responsibility for persons with mental illness, although the degree of that reluctance has varied over time. This theme and how it plays out at different times is a function of how people think of those with mental illness and the system of agencies and professionals responsible for them—whether as a system of care, a system for containing and isolating stigmatized persons, a mechanism for keeping the community safe, or various combinations of these elements. In addition, much depends in community psychiatry on assumptions, usually implicit, about the relationship of different kinds of knowledge to policy and practice. To what extent is what we do driven by expertise, experience, ideology, morality, or research? Who is an expert, and what should count as expertise? How do we answer this last question in regard to practitioners and patients? In what ways is public action informed by moral or political belief? What counts as research "evidence?" Different conceptions of the relationships among knowledge, policy and practice are expressed in different forms of writing, whether governmental, scientific-academic, epidemiological, literary, journalistic, or autobiographical.

The psychiatry with which we are concerned is a public thing, and thus we may look to government commission reports as one way to locate and bound our eras. This is so in part because government writings and reports are "texts of texts" that synthesize, sum up, restate, redefine, and cite other writings. At bottom, our field is defined in good measure by assumptions about what government makes possible and what it denies, at least since the early 1950s, which we have designated as the starting point of community psychiatry in the U.S.

To summarize, "classics" crystallize or break new ground in prevailing conceptions of community psychiatry. They answer questions in a distinct way or raise questions that have waited to be asked. A classic may crystallize or codify the main elements of a given era, foreshadow the one to come, or give a glimpse of possibilities not yet been acted upon. The eras we have chosen—deinstitutionalization and the community mental health movement from the mid-1950s to the latter 1970s, the Community Support Movement and its demise from the latter 70s to the latter 90s, and the recovery movement from the late 90s to the present—preceded by a century-plus period before these eras and followed by thoughts about the era to come—constitute hypotheses. The classics we have chosen to represent these eras express hypotheses, too, about the interrelationships over time among texts, policies, and practices. Still, even with the establishment of new paradigms and the transition from old to new ones, in and across eras all is fluid. A classic is and must be essentially unstable, dependent on finding new readers who will reinforce or reject its claims to authority. Our classics, that is, are shiftable pillars of an evolving structure.

References

1. Goffman, E. (1961). *Asylums: Essays on the social situation of mental patients and other inmates asylums.* New York: Anchor Books/Random House.
2. Rowe, M. (1999). *Crossing the border: Encounters between homeless people and outreach workers.* Berkeley: University of California Press.
3. Putnam, R. (2000). *Bowling alone: The collapse and revival of American community.* New York: Simon & Schuster.
4. Granovetter, G. (1973). The strength of weak ties. *American Journal of Sociology, 78*(6), 1360–1380.
5. Thoits, P. A. (1986). Multiple identities: Examining gender and marital status differences in distress. *American Sociological Review,* 51(2), 259–272.
6. Barnes, B., Bloor, D., Henry, J. (1996). *Scientific knowledge. A sociological analysis.* London: Athlone Press.
7. Garfinkel, H. (1967). *Studies in ethnomethodology* (p. 9). Englewood Cliffs, NJ: Prentice-Hall.

Contributors

AIKEN, L. H.
University of Pennsylvania

ANDREASEN, N. C.
The University of Iowa

ANTHONY, W. A.
Boston University

ASHIKAGA, T.
National Institute of Mental Health

BACHRACH, L. L.
University of Maryland

BESTMAN, E. W.
North Miami Florida

BLECK, D. S.
no info

BOCKOVEN, J. S.
Harvard Medical School

BRENNER, M. H.
University of North Texas

BRIER, A.
Indiana University

BROOKS, G. W.
University of Vermont

CAPLAN, G.
Deceased, no affiliation info

CHAMBERLIN, J.
National Empowerment Center

CRESSLER, D. L.
Portland State University

DAVIDSON, L.
Yale University

DIXON, L.
University of Maryland

DRAKE, R. E.
Dartmouth University

ESTROFF, S. E.
University of North Carolina
    at Chapel Hill

FAIRWEATHER, G. W.
Michigan State University

FEIGHNER, J. P.
Feighner Research Institute

FRANK, R. B.
Harvard University

GLIED, S. A.
Columbia University

GOERTZEL, V.
University Friends Meeting, WA

GOFFMAN, E.
University of Pennsylvania

GOLDMAN, H. H.
University of Maryland

GREENBERG, J.
Colorado School of Mines

GRIFFITH, E. E. H.
Yale University

GROB, G. N.
Rutgers University

GRONFEIN, W.
Indiana University-Purdue University
   Indiana

GUZE, S. B.
Washington University

HAFEZ, H.
Yale University

HARDING, C. M.
Institute for the Study of Human Relations

HAUGLAND, G.
Nathan S. Kline Institute

HAY, T.
Policy Research Associates

HOGE, M. A.
Yale University

HOLLINGSHEAD, A. B.
Yale University

HOPPER, K.
Nathan S. Kline Institute

HUGHES, C. C.
Medical Superintendent, Aro Hospital
   for Nervous Diseases, Western Region,
   Nigeria (deceased)

JOINT COMMISSION ON MENTAL ILLNESS
   AND HEALTH

JOST, J.
New York University

LAMB, H. R.
University of Southern California

LAMBO, T. A.
World Health Organization

LEETE, E.
Colorado Alliance for the Mentally Ill

LEFF, H. S.
Harvard University

LEFLEY, H. P.
University of Miami

LEHMAN, A. F.
University of Maryland

LEIGHTON, A. H.
Harvard University

LEIGHTON, D. C.
Cornell University

LIBERMAN, R. P.
University of California, Los Angeles

LIEBERMAN, P.
Boston University

LOVELL, A. M.
Santé Mentale, Société, Paris, France

MACKLIN, D. B.
Cornell University Medical College

MARX, A. J.
Mendota State Hospital, Wisconsin

MAYNARD, H.
Portland State University

MCDIARMID, J. S.
Voices in the Night

MECHANIC, D.
Rutgers University

MERRILL, M. E.
Connecticut Mental Health Center

MORRISSEY, J. P.
University of North Carolina at
   Chapel Hill

MOSHER, L. R.
University of California at San Diego

MUESER, K. T.
Dartmouth University

MUNOZ, R.
University of California, San Diego

MURPHY, J. M.
Massachusetts General Hospital

NATIONAL ASSOCIATION OF STATE
   MENTAL HEALTH PROGRAM DIRECTORS

RAKFELDT, J.
Southern Connecticut State University

REDLICH, F. C.
Yale University

ROBINS, E.
Washington University

ROSENHAN, D. L.
Stanford University

ROSENHECK, R.
Yale University

SANDERS, D. J.
Michigan State University

SCHEPER-HUGHES, N.
University of California, Berkeley

SCULL, A. T.
University of California San Diego

SHARFSTEIN, S. S.
Sheppard Pratt Health System

STEIN, L. I.
University of Wisconsin

STRAUSS, J. S.
Yale University

SZASZ, T. S.
State University of New York
  at Syracuse

TALBOTT, J. A.
University of Maryland

TANSELLA, M.
University of Verona, Italy

TEST, M. A.
University of Wisconsin

THORNICROFT, G.
King's College London, UK

TORREY, W. C.
Dartmouth-Hitchcock Psychiatric
  Associates

U.S. GOVERNMENT ACCOUNTABILITY
  OFFICE

WEINER, S.
The Suspicious Humanist

WELBER, S.
Legal Aid Society
Nathan S. Kline Institute

WING, J. K.
Royal College of Psychiatrists, London,
  England

WINOKUR, G.
University of Iowa

WOODRUFF, R. A.
Washington University

I

The Pre–Community Psychiatry Period (1850–1953)

Francesca Martin and Elizabeth H. Flanagan

No part of the subject committed to us has given us more anxiety than that relating to the insane poor ... Circulars were sent to the selectmen of the one hundred and sixty-six towns of the State, and returns have been received from about one hundred of them ... From these returns it appears that there are now ... between four and five hundred of the indigent insane for whom provisions should be made.

At Tarriffville we found about ten who were either insane or imbecile. They ought not to be there; it is no proper place for these feeble persons, and it is an outrage upon humanity, a disgrace to the civilization of the State, and a sad reflection upon our Christianity that they are there at all.

We found in the almshouse at Hartford eight or ten people, who were as comfortably cared for as could be expected at that place.

At the New Haven almshouse there were fifty-four of the insane in the different rooms of the building and in cells in a special department. A few of these were lying upon loose hay, were without much clothing, and were in a very filthy condition.

State of Connecticut, Report of the Governor's Commission on Charities, 1877

The asylum era is widely regarded by historians and scholars of social medicine as contributing both the form and structure to many of our contemporary institutions of psychiatry. These institutions, which began in a spirit of optimism and reform, were created out of a unique joining of diverse interests. Advocates for improved social conditions were among the first who called attention to growing gaps in quality of life among social classes in the United States during the nineteenth century, and who also raised the question of societal responsibility for poor and infirm persons. A new class of professionals—the alienists/superintendents/psychiatrists who would run the asylums—was emerging just as the intersection of economic and social status would largely come to define and determine social participation and access to resources. And the public sector, in the form of state and local governments that organized the allocation of community resources to their citizens, began to take shape at a time when social and political structures were relatively simple, loosely structured, and receptive to influence.

The defining establishment of this era were the asylums—self-sufficient cities that were both a part of, and apart from, mainstream society —that were established to restore disordered citizens who had been relegated, by virtue of their misfit and their family members' incapacity to care for them, to their local poorhouse or jail or sent away to become someone else's problem. The promise of the asylum was not only to offer shelter from the storm but to influence people with mental illness in such a way as to make possible their return to family and productive participation in the community. The asylums were also established to influence the communities from which these distressed persons came, by creating a new model of social relations for a society still in formation. This latter role has been investigated and explored more thoroughly by contemporary social historians, particularly in the work of David Rothman with his focus on the role of the total institution in maintaining the social order.[1] With organized attention to and management of the core components of the daily life experience of inmates, including basic needs of food and shelter, social experiences of interpersonal interaction and leisure activity, and vocational opportunities, asylum superintendents embarked on a unique but short-lived process of planned reform.

Asylums were also unique in being the first institutions to be defined by place as much as by purpose. They took shape in the transformative decades of the nineteenth century and grew as their nearby towns grew, expanding with buildings, farmland, and reservoirs and creating a permanent infrastructure that would supply a growing population of persons deemed unwell, even after the purpose of these institutions changed from cure to care and fewer patients who were place in them returned to their home communities. As perhaps the earliest of planned communities, the asylums were designed according to meticulous standards that were most carefully articulated by Thomas Kirkbride of the first generation of asylum superintendents and promoted through the hospital superintendent trade association.[2] A trove of archival material has survived of Kirkbride's detailed descriptions of building layout, structure, size and layout of rooms, and siting and configuration of asylum grounds, marvels of planning and intentionality.

The historical trajectory of the asylum age can be broken down into three phases:

- *Laying the foundation.*   The first half-century of the newly independent nation saw the creation of the first specialty hospitals for persons deemed insane, bringing private practice and public interest together for perhaps the first time, with the intended goal of improving people's lives through moral treatment.
- *The building blocks.*   At the end of the Civil War, with the violent affirmation of a national state and the accelerated pace of social transformation through industrialization, urbanization, and rapid population growth, asylums could be found in every state and territory as asylum superintendency became the nation's first medical specialty and, over the next few decades, presided over a growing population of putatively incurable patients needing custodial care.
- *The structural collapse.*   The sense of optimism with which the asylums were created—that persons whose lives were disordered could be cured—gave way to disappointment in the latter years of the nineteenth century and early twentieth century. Person-centered moral treatment collapsed under the contradiction caused by conflicting policy decisions that shifted too many people to institutions with too few resources. As a result, asylums became overcrowded warehouses as their mission of social reform was reframed to narrowly focus on the individual, and medical beliefs about curability were set aside, or radically reforumulated, with a new focus on the biology of brain disease. This search for new solutions through physical interventions occurred as societal attitudes affirmed the deficiency of persons deemed insane.

In kind, three critical primary textual sources for understanding the asylum age stand out:

- *The asylum superintendents.*   The first voices of the asylum were the nineteenth century medical superintendents who led the efforts to establish these new social institutions by taking on a unique combination of roles—as medical providers, town planners, and social reformers in one. As such, the superintendents, or alienists, gathered information about and presented an understanding of the problems brought forward by their patients, issued reports to the state government and the public about asylum operations, were attentive to the tone of the hospital–town relationship, and were motivated by a belief in their ability to effect change, both in the individual patient who was sent to them for reform and as agents of collective social change. In taking on these tasks and roles, they came to occupy privileged positions within the social, economic and political structures of their communities. As the asylums began to fall out of favor, the alienists began to redefine their role apart from the institutions, aspsychiatrists. As medical specialists at the pinnacle of their profession's hierarchy, they successfully repositioned themselves to assume leadership roles in areas of policy and practice from that time up to the present.

- *Institutional records and superintendent reports.*   Going back to some of the earliest asylums and overlapping with the writings of the heads of these institutions, we have handwritten admission records; deed books of land transactions (some of which continue in use in at least a handful of towns as the most comprehensive land use records available); and annual reports to the governor and legislature that summarize activities and provide an in-depth view of the accomplishments and challenges of a new type of social institution. While some of these texts have been collected, archived and mined for their rich trove of data, many more remain untouched in boxes in basements or back rooms. Finally, perhaps the most substantive texts that still exist are the institutions themselves—the buildings, fields, stories and memories, records and reports. Some remain as abandoned relics, others have been replaced by high-end real estate, and still others remain as grounds of contention as efforts to preserve and remember are challenged by demands for economic returns in the face of ongoing public sector shortfalls.[3–5]

- *The inmates/patients.*   Just as superintendent reports and other institutional records articulate the point of view of the evolving profession of psychiatry, inmates also emerged as a group with a unique voice and perspective. The deeply personal insider accounts they left behind are part memoir, part social criticism, and part catharsis, relying as they did on the experience of their authors, who variously examined, challenged, and demanded change in the institutions and sometimes even the social structures that allowed them to exist. Clifford Beers' autobiographical *A Mind that Found Itself*[6] is a remarkable example of a tradition of personal accounts from former institutional patients. Beers, who was himself a patient for a number of years at Connecticut Hospital for the Insane, documented his mistreatment while in the hospital as part of his eloquent appeal for a compassionate and patient-responsive approach to caring for persons with mental illness. His writing and advocacy led to the formation of the earliest advocacy movement on behalf of persons with mental illness, the National Committee for Mental Hygiene—today the advocacy and policy organization, Mental Health America.

From Asylum to Psychiatry

By the time the Association of Medical Superintendents of American Institutions of the Insane, founded in 1844 by thirteen of the first twenty-four asylums, changed its name to the American Psychiatric Association in 1922, the profession of psychiatry and the class of people identified as mentally ill were well established within American society. The institution of professional psychiatry began, in many ways, with the institution of the asylum at a time when options for caring for the sick, infirm elderly, and the otherwise economically unsound were determined mainly by local ties. There was no organized system of social or health supports or of income support at that time. For "disordered" persons and others who could not fend for themselves there were only other family members, the almshouse when available, the jail, or the street. Into this void stepped various representatives of what today we would loosely identify as private philanthropy—the merchant barons of Boston who founded McLean Hospital, the Quakers of Philadelphia who established the Pennsylvania Hospital for the Insane using proceeds from the sale of excess farmland, and others. These philanthropists established the first wave of new social institutions that would provide highly organized, well-financed care to persons of means and a fraction of the newly ill among the laboring classes.

Social advocates such as Dorothea Dix framed this new approach as that of society taking responsibility for its least well off members.[7] The speed with which state legislatures adopted the asylum approach and committed resources to their construction and initial operation was also related, according to Rothman and others, to the demand for institutions to help address a rapidly growing social transformation in the United States that was outstripping its social infrastructure.[1] Building on this multistate response, efforts by Dorothea Dix and others in the mid-century to secure federal involvement in affairs of social welfare through the purchase of millions of acres of land to be used for asylums failed at the hands of President Pierce's veto. Over time, however, Dix built alliances with asylum doctors and state legislators, creating a coalition of allies and supporters of the asylum movement. (A century later, Congress' initial funding of community-based mental health centers as the first substantial federal investment in mental health occurred during another time of social transformation in the United States, one punctuated by disruption, turmoil, and violence.)

As important as the asylum itself is the societal context in which it developed. The dominant social institutions of the time were the family and church. Most people lived in small towns or villages with few other organizing institutions. This first institutional effort to respond to the distress of the obviously disordered (and perhaps to mitigate the guilt of the nondisordered) was extraordinarily comprehensive in scope and intention, albeit established through the efforts of small groups of individuals acting privately for the benefit, mainly, of their family and class members. Nineteenth-century asylum hospitals were unlike any other institution or organized community resource of the time, intended not for custodial warehousing or punishment but as places set apart for the purpose of restoring people who were impaired, disordered, distracted, or infirm. They were communities unto themselves, often self-sustaining with working farms, independent sources of water and power, and, as they grew in size and complexity, their own fire and police personnel. They were also the locus of a new approach to solving the problems of individuals so disordered in their daily experience that they were not able to participate in the everyday activities of their families or communities. As such, they also served as the setting within which a new program of social intervention—moral therapy—would be practiced at the exact time when social change was altering the foundational institutions of family and local community.

Moral therapy linked the expectation of personal improvement with the intrinsic value of the social group. Its guiding principles were applied through a set of detailed operating practices, as alluded to in a statement by Dr. Amariah Brigham, one of the earliest asylum superintendents, regarding the moral treatment program at Utica State Hospital in New York:

> The removal of the insane from home and former associations, with respectful and kind treatment under all circumstances, and in most cases manual labor, attendance on religious worship on Sundays, the establishment of regular habits of self-control, diversion of the mind from morbid trains of thought, are now generally considered as essential in the moral treatment of the Insane.[7]

These values and practices, disseminated to other superintendents through the Association of Medical Superintendents of American Institutions of the Insane, laid the foundation for the formation of the new profession of psychiatry, as well as that of other mental health care professions.

Views of Psychiatric Illness in the Asylum

During the asylum period, views of people with mental illness changed dramatically in concert with change in the response to them. In Colonial America, a person with mental illness was seen as suffering from an excess of one of the four humors—blood, yellow bile, black bile, phlegm—and was treated with general nonspecific physical therapies including bleeding and purging. These physical causes of mental illness were in turn related, in Bockoven's words, to "supernatural, religious, astrological, scientific, and medical elements."[7,p.8] Unless they threatened public safety, however, people with mental illness resided in the community and were taken care of, when possible, by their families. With the shift away from a diverse array of causes of insanity starting in the eighteenth century, however, society was charged with the responsibility for identifying the cause of, and prescribing effective responses to, a wide-ranging and shifting set of "problem" behaviors. Science grew in stature to be on a par with religion, as rational philosophy stood on a par with ideals based on faith.

Moral therapy provided, in effect, a bridge between a waning belief in supernatural causes of behavioral aberration and a modern set of beliefs of more controllable causation—that of biological factors within the person or social factors from without. This polarity defines what continues to be an ongoing debate within organized psychiatry, from the first generation of asylum doctors to today's psychiatrists. While acknowledging the presence of physiological effects in the form of brain lesions, the early asylum doctors focused their interventions almost entirely on behavior and the social components of mental illness. Their highly detailed reports and other published and nonpublished documents describe the social environment and attitudes of the time through the patients—not only their age and gender, but also their occupations, nativity (American-born or foreign-born), and causes of illness including intemperance, overexertion, masturbation, or business anxiety, among others. Along with the seeming uniformity of ideas about the cause of mental illness and moral therapy as it was applied through the asylum system, however, a diversity of beliefs, articulated by individual asylum doctors, existed about the underlying manifestations of mental illness.

Treatment in the Asylums

Moral treatment was based on the premise that the person's current environment caused him or her to be unwell. Treatment involved moving people from a stressful to a benign environment in which restoration of health and recovery from mental illness could occur. The person with the mental illness was seen as blameless, and moral treatment involved compassionate treatment for its victims. The international adoption of the model can be attributed, in part, to broad humanitarian concerns that had grown out of the European Enlightenment.[8] The York Retreat in England was founded in 1792 by William Tuke, an English Quaker and merchant, with the intention of developing an environment in which internal self-restraint and discipline replaced external control of behavior.[9] Across the English Channel, Tuke's contemporary in France, Phillipe Pinel, objected to the traditional "treatments" for mental illness such as bleeding, corporal punishment, and confinement and argued for psychologically oriented therapy.[10]

Pinel and Tuke were joined by others, including Benjamin Rush in the United States and Vincenzio Chiarugi in Italy. All concluded that recovery from insanity was possible with enlightened and compassionate treatment and that the asylum was the proper venue for accomplishing this task.[8]

In its initial stages, moral treatment demonstrated remarkable success. From 1833 to 1852 two-thirds of patients at Worcester State Hospital in Massachusetts were discharged within one year as "recovered" from mental illness.[7] The exact interpretation of this percentage is difficult since no information is available about diagnosis or the definition of recovery. The question of how many of these cured persons had repeat admissions, however, was answered by a study at Worcester State Hospital that followed until their deaths about a thousand patients who were discharged as recovered in the mid-nineteenth century. Fifty-four percent were never again institutionalized,[11,12] a percentage similar to contemporary recovery rates.[13]

As the number of asylums began to increase in the mid-nineteenth century, many treated middle-class persons who could not afford the high costs of private care or poor persons of primarily American birth or English ancestry. As immigration increased, however, and people were shifted from almshouses to asylums, non-native, very poor, and non–English-speaking persons came to constitute a higher portion of the patient population. In Massachusetts, Bockoven writes, "these particular foreign-born were usually destitute. Mental hospitals were becoming vast alms-houses."[7,p.179] At Worcester State Hospital between 1844 and 1853, 10% of admitted patients were foreign-born, while between 1893 and 1902, 67% were foreign-born. Wealthier folk went to private facilities, leaving lower-class, primarily foreign-born patients to the state asylums and thus creating a two-class system of psychiatric care.[14]

Demographic changes brought challenges to asylum staff in responding to new cultures and languages, since, as Bockoven notes, moral treatment presupposed shared ethnic, cultural, and religious backgrounds among both patients and staff.[7] When the predominant treatment philosophy of asylums was moral treatment and the asylum patients were upper-class Euro-Americans, helpers were often quite engaged, personally and socially, with patients, and the helper-patient relationship was less hierarchical than it would later become. Helpers and patients ate meals together, worked side-by-side, and engaged in joint recreational activities. As more immigrants and poor people came to the asylum, though, the nature of the helper-patient interaction slowly deteriorated.

Admissions, patient-staff ratios, and costs ballooned over the decades. At Worcester State Hospital, the average yearly admission increased from about 500 people per year in 1883–1892 to 2500 people in 1943–1950. As patient census increased, spending and staffing decreased. Worcester State Hospital had 88 patients per physician from 1833 to 1842 and 230 per physician from 1943 to 1950. In 1833, the per capita weekly patient expenditure was $2.00, similar to the U.S. weekly per capita income of $2.25; in 1943 expenditures were about $9.00 per patient week compared to U.S per capita income of more than $32.00.[7] The Great Depression of the 1930s bankrupted most states and the advent World War II led to a dramatic shortage of personnel. Overcrowding and lack of funds and personnel reached crisis levels as states lacked the funds or the commitment to support their asylums.[8]

As the asylums became overcrowded across the turn of the twentieth century, the individuality of a person was lost, little or no attention was paid to the environment of the asylum, and the goal of the asylums was reduced to that of meeting the basic survival needs of people, not to providing mental health treatment.[7] The dramatic recovery rates attributed to moral treatment disappeared as more and more people were moved from the poor houses to the asylums. These became overcrowded and overwhelmed by "non-curables." Numerous exposés[15] and surveys,[16] along with revealing memoirs of conditions in mental hospitals,[6,17] led to demands for immediate change in the treatment of people with mental illnesses.[7] In 1961 the Joint Commission on Mental Health called for the establishment of the community-based mental health centers, supplemented by general hospitals with short-term units to treat acute problems and state hospitals with a maximum of 1000 beds to treat chronic diseases. The ultimate purpose of these treatment facilities would be to contribute to helping their patients resume stable and normal lives in their communities.[18]

Conclusion: a Tale of Two Publics

For more than a century, asylums were the preeminent social welfare institution in the United States. Built on the premise of a new sense of public sector responsibility, the asylums were established not only to provide refuge and sanctuary to those sent there, but also to restore people to themselves and return them to their families and communities. A century plus later, at the end of World War II, population pressures on such public institutions were enormous. Hospitals were underfunded as state funding was grossly inadequate to the need. Admissions mounted with the closing of the almshouses, an increase of elderly admissions, and conceptualization of dementia as a mental illness. The primary functions of the asylum–state mental hospital had become those of management and control. Elderly patients remained institutionalized until the passage of Medicaid, which shifted responsibility to the federal government for treatment costs and led to substantial discharges of elderly patients to nursing homes.[5]

As American social institutions were being transformed during the decades of the 1950s and 1960s through organized movements pushing for greater participation and equality in economic, political and social life, the longstanding foundations of family and community, were being newly shaken. A new "migration" to be absorbed by American society during this time was the relocation of thousands of former asylum inmates to downtowns and Main Streets across the country. Unlike other migrations, however, these former asylum inmates were not filling a labor market demand for more workers but were being expelled by institutions that needed to reduce their patient populations. Another migration was the movement of psychiatrists and a newly energized mental health industry out of the asylums and into a still-expanding array of practice and policy settings.

The asylum era, among other accomplishments, set the stage for the burgeoning field of community psychiatry in the latter half of the twentieth century. At the peak of the asylum-state mental hospital era in the United States, 350 hospitals across the country contained 559,000 patients. The class of medical professionals they hosted had become the medical specialty of psychiatry. The depopulation of state and county mental hospitals moved hundreds of thousands of patients into communities, creating new classes of mental health professionals in the newly developed community-based treatment centers, yet structural ties established over the past century of asylum activity became foundational elements of the shift of psychiatry from the asylums to the community. Even as the asylums themselves moved into the background of organized mental health care, then, they continue to influence the organization and practice of contemporary public mental health care in the United States.

References

1. Rothman, D. J. (2002). *The discovery of the asylum: Social order and disorder in the new republic.* New Brunswick: Aldine Transaction Books.
2. Shorter, E. (1997). *A history of psychiatry: From the era of the asylum to the age of Prozac.* New York: John Wiley and Sons.
3. Connecticut Hospital for the Insane. (1895). *Reprint of one quarter century of annual reports.* Hartford, CT: Case, Lockwood and Brainard Company.

4. Connecticut Valley Hospital Property Report. (1994). *Table 1: 1994 net acreage, history, and restriction(s) of Connecticut Valley Hospital properties.* Middletown, CT: Connecticut Valley Hospital.

5. Grob, G. (1991). *From asylum to community: Mental health policy in modern America.* Princeton, NJ: Princeton University Press.

6. Beers, C. W. (1908). *A mind that found itself: An autobiography.* New York: Longmans, Green, and Co.

7. Bockoven, J. S. (1956). Moral treatment in American psychiatry (Parts I–IV). *Journal of Nervous and Mental Disease, 124,* 167–194.

8. Grob, G. N. (1994). *The mad among us: A history of the care of America's mentally ill.* New York: The Free Press.

9. Tuke, S. (1813). *Description of the retreat, an institution near York for insane persons of the Society of Friends.* York, England.

10. Pinel, P. (1801). *Traite medico-philosophique sur L'alienation mentale ou la Manie.* Paris.

11. Bockoven, J. S. (1956). Moral treatment in American psychiatry (Parts V–IX). *Journal of Nervous and Mental Disease, 124,* 292–321.

12. Grob, G. N. (1966). *The state and the mentally ill (a history of Worcester State Hospital in Massachusetts, 1830–1920).* Chapel Hill: University of North Carolina Press.

13. Strauss, J. S., Carpenter, W. T. (1977). Prediction of outcome in schizophrenia: III. Five-year outcome and its predictors. *Archives of General Psychiatry, 34,* 159–163.

14. Morrissey, J. P., Goldman, H. H. (1986). Care and treatment of the mentally ill in the United States: Historical developments and reform. *Annals of the American Academy of Political and Social Science, 484,* 12–27.

15. Deutsch, A. (1948). *The Shame of the States.* New York: Arno Press.

16. roup for the Advancement of Psychiatry. (1946). GAP Circular Letter No. 12: *Archives of Psychiatry.*

17. Ward, M. J. (1946). *The snake pit.* New York: Random House.

18. Joint Commission on Mental Illness and Health. (1961). Recommendations for a national mental health program: summary. In: *Action for Mental Health, Final Report of the Joint Commission on Mental Illness and Health.* New York: Basic Books.

II

Deinstitutionalization and the Community Mental Health Center Movement (1954–1976)

Rebecca Miller, Allison N. Ponce,
and Kenneth S. Thompson

If we are to make any substantial progress in promoting mental health and preventing mental and social disorder we must involve ourselves in informed activism to change our national goals and priorities.

Jack R. Ewalt and Patricia L. Ewalt[1]

America, emerging victorious from the trials of the Great Depression and the horrors of World War II, entered the era of postwar era with a renewed optimism and competitiveness, on one hand, and a sense of grave insecurity in the face of the Soviet threat and the hydrogen bomb, on the other. Amid this anxious collective state of mind, the 1940s and 1950s saw a renewed interest in mental health and mental illness and in its chief disciplines, psychology and psychiatry.

Contributors to this new focus on mental health included Freudian analysts from Hitler's Europe, clinicians' wartime experiences with the high prevalence of mental disorders among military recruits, and their treatment of soldiers with combat-related psychiatric disorders.

In the late 1940s, conscientious objectors who worked in psychiatric hospitals as an alternative to military service and exposés such as *The Shame of the States*[2] and *The Snake Pit*[3] brought to light the deplorable conditions for psychiatric patient inmates in state mental hospitals. The Civil Rights movement and growing awareness of the link between poverty and mental illness began to have an impact on mental health policy and practice. These views and approaches, expressed and institutionalized in the postwar establishment of the National Institute for Mental Health (NIMH), were linked with increased federal support for science that was spurred on by Sputnik and the space race, NIMH's expanding service and scientific activities, including support for the newly emergent field and business of psychopharmacology, reinforced a growing faith in science and psychiatry, renewed therapeutic optimism, and a call for dramatic change in mental health care. The stage was set, then, for national action when President Eisenhower launched the Joint Commission on Mental Health and Illness and thus, arguably, initiated the community mental health era.

Initial National Action

While the Community Mental Health Centers (CMHC) Act of 1963 represents to many the turning point in the orientation of mental health service provision, the earlier National Mental Health Act of 1946 and Mental Health Study Act of 1955 were major legislative movements that had already highlighted the need for increased federal funding for research and treatment. The National Mental Health Act of 1946, which funded NIMH to oversee grants focusing on research on neuropsychiatric problems, training of professionals, and establishment of community-based care for those with mental illness, laid the groundwork for larger changes to come in the 1950s and 1960s concerning research, services, and workforce development.[4]

Robert Felix, the first director of the NIMH, mapped out an ambitious agenda for psychiatry as it began to turn its attention away from hospitals and toward the community as the primary locus of mental health care. Psychiatry's task, Felix argued, starts with addressing the needs of people with chronic mental illness in the community, but it goes beyond this to include prevention of mental illness, which involves work with youth and with families. Community psychiatry also would involve liaisons with churches, schools, neighborhood groups, and places of employment where persons at risk of, or suffering from, mental illness would be identified and treated, and research to understand the extent of mental illness in society would be conducted.[5]

The Mental Health Study Act was passed unanimously by the U.S. Congress, in part due to the support of NIMH, the American Medical and American Psychiatric Associations, the National Committee Against Mental Illness, and several key legislators , including then-Senator John F. Kennedy. The Act also called for a Joint Commission on Mental Illness and Health, to be charged with performing a comprehensive review of current mental health practices and resources. The product of this evaluation was a 10-volume series of monographs, *Action for Mental Health*, with a *Final Report* published in 1961.[6] The report's assessments and recommendations were categorized by manpower, facilities, and costs. The Commission recommended significant funding and resources for basic research and long-term projects, along with support for early career investigators and capital investments in geographic regions with underdeveloped scientific institutions. Workforce development recommendations focused on the competency and scope of practice of those delivering services, recruitment of personnel from various disciplines, and support for the education of future mental health workforce members. George Albee's project director report provided much of the ammunition to address these issues of "manpower" through its discussion of the inadequacy of the current supply of professionals to meet the challenges of the new era of community care.[7]

The most dramatic of the Commission's recommendations was that funding for public mental health services be doubled in a 5-year span and tripled over 10 years. The Commission urged a shift in the burden of the cost of services and responsibility for persons with mental illnesses away from the states and to the federal government (assuming individual states' acceptance of this shift). It proposed that public opinion surveys be conducted to assess support for these proposals, that legislative opinion be gauged on the same issues, and that a congressional committee of consultants be appointed to determine the legislation needed to support the Commission's recommendations.

Newly elected President Kennedy, long invested in issues of mental health and disability in part due to his sister Rosemary's long-time institutionalization following a lobotomy, appointed a working group to analyze the Joint Commission's findings. The findings of this group informed his special address to Congress in February 1963, in which he decried the high number of people with mental illness in institutions, the shameful state of these facilities, and the steep cost of this care. Kennedy proposed a National Mental Health Program with funding of $42 million for planning grants to be distributed by NIMH, arguing that community-based supports and community integration of persons with mental illness were possible, given the emergence of new therapies including psychotropic medications. His message emphasized the importance of "community" in the reform of mental health systems, particularly through its joint ownership of comprehensive and coordinated services. Prevention services for adults with serious mental illness and services for children, families, and adults with less disabling psychological problems were also key items on his agenda.

Kennedy's proposal included federal matching grants for construction of comprehensive CMHCs and funding to train personnel, improve the quality of care, and promote research. Despite these promises heralding a turning point in U.S. mental health services, however, little was accomplished before Kennedy's assassination. His matching grants proposal languished in Congress until October 1963, when he signed the CMHC Act into law. At this point, the program had been stripped of all but the construction component. It was not until the CMHC Act Amendments of 1965 under Lyndon B. Johnson that federal funding for personnel materialized.

Snow and Newton note that while two central intentions of the CMHC movement were to develop direct care services and indirect initiatives such as consultation and mental health education, the proposed focus on prevention that might have strengthened community resources and assets was not fully integrated into the plan. Development of indirect services would require effort and initiation, as opposed to direct clinical services that directly address an obvious need and often consume the bulk of the resources in the mental health care system. Due to the lack of effective preventive services and the system's inability to respond to indirect needs, people who otherwise might have been diverted from a path of psychiatric disability found themselves requiring more intensive treatment and rehabilitation. This exacerbated the use of hospital-level care and increased the number of patients among those who left inpatient settings to face an uncoordinated, disjointed,, and underfunded community system, or nonsystem, of care.[8]

Beginning in 1967, a series of amendments reauthorized funding and established additional sites for CMHCs. The Alcoholic and Narcotic Addiction Rehabilitation Amendments expanded treatment for alcoholism and drug addiction in 1968 and in 1970 was expanded to help with staffing. In addition, as a result of the Joint Commission on Mental Health of Children's 1969 study report, the 1970 amendments directed funds to mental health services for children, who had been largely neglected up to this point. Finally, through legislation, the earlier promises of the original CMHC Act began to be realized. However, these acts were essentially gutted by Ronald Reagan's presidency beginning in 1980 as the country took a conservative turn.

The mere existence of CMHCs did not ensure the care of those with serious mental illness who were discharged from state hospitals. In fact, the federal approach to funding and overseeing community mental health purposefully bypassed the states and their unwieldy bureaucracies. Federal monies were given directly to local community mental health care providers, thereby guaranteeing a disconnect between people discharged from state hospitals and CMHCs. Cutler and colleagues describe the multiple ways in which the states and CMHCs failed to cooperate effectively with state hospitals to ensure a smooth transition into the community and provide people discharged with appropriate care.[9] In the late 1960s some innovative programs were developed to improve coordination, including redeployment of some state hospital staff to community centers, but these initiatives were inadequate to address the difficulties that existed in this community-based model of service.

"Deinstitutionalization," starting in 1955 when state mental hospitals reached their peak census nationally at 559,000 patients, involved the movement of people previously warehoused in state mental hospitals back into their communities, with or without community treatment and services. Between 1966 and 1975, over 250,000 people left institutions nationwide.[10] By the end of this era of community psychiatry, the state inpatient hospital census had decreased to 170,000.[11] The decrease in census, however, tells only a small portion of the story of the impact on the lives of formerly hospitalized persons and society as a whole.

Did the deinstitutionalization movement constitute a radical change? Similar to the civil rights movement with its roots in post civil war Reconstruction and cultural movements in the 1920s, most of the new thinking and changes in policy regarding mental health were not so new at all. Many had been proposed at the turn of the century, beginning with Clifford Beers' mental hygiene movement and the development and influence of psychoanalytic theory and practice. The deinstitutionalization and CMHC era did, however, involve a dramatic reconceptualization of psychiatry and the concept of mental illness.[12] Psychiatry's outlook simultaneously shifted toward viewing mental illness as both a social and medical problem, as demonstrated by advances in the sociological study of poverty and mental health and the emergence of psychopharmacology.[1]

Social Radicalization in the 1960s and 1970s

The 1960s in America was a time of intellectual and cultural ferment and of social change. Moving from the conservative Eisenhower era of stricter social mores, new faultlines were opening up and new ideas and movements associated with them were opening up at the time of the President Kennedy's election in 1960 and his vow to "get the country moving again.[13,p4] Kennedy's early efforts regarding civil rights resulted in legislation that was later passed under Johnson—the Civil Rights Act in 1964 and the Voting Rights Act of 1965. Johnson's pursuit of the Vietnam Conflict fueled the counterculture among the young, with the emergence of the antiwar movement initially shifting the cultural tone toward increased social engagement and participatory democracy.

The evolution of these politics and policies was echoed in the mental health world. Authors like Goffman in his work, *Asylums*,[14] and Rosenhan, in his study on pseudopatients,[15] fueled further study of the impact of psychiatric institutions on human development, including learned helplessness, loss of a sense of self-efficacy, and interpretation of behavior as pathological. Greenberg's "social breakdown syndrome"[16] gave a name to some of the negative effects of institutionalization, including the pattern of people who are treated as ill beginning to manifest more psychiatric symptoms, thus matching their behavior to staff formulations and expectations. Knowledge of these social phenomena, along with representations of inhumane hospital conditions in books such as *One Flew Over the Cuckoo's Nest*,[17] became part of the social and professional context that led to the creation of short-term hospital units as alternatives to long-term institutionalization.

Evidence emerged during this era confirming the long-suspected link between mental illness and poverty. Most significant was Hollingshead and Redlich's landmark 1958 sociological study, *Social Class and Mental Illness: A Community Study*, which demonstrated that persons who were poor were twice as likely to be diagnosed with mental illness and were more likely to be given the most serious diagnoses. The authors also found that persons of lower socioeconomic status were the most likely to receive aggressive physical treatments such as insulin coma therapy or electric shock therapy and the least likely to receive psychotherapy.[18] While the exact relationship between poverty and mental illness remains controversial, acknowledgement that a relationship existed led to steps during this era to address factors related to poverty using federal resources. Charitable and state-funded health and mental health care were found to be grossly inadequate, as the newly created CMHCs were given no ongoing funding for services, leaving a gap in services for disadvantaged populations.

When President Johnson declared a War on Poverty and promoted the notion of the Great Society in 1965, Congress worked with him to create the Medicaid program (Title XIX) of the Social Security Act. Medicaid was designed to serve as a federally and state-funded medical safety net for low-income people including elderly, blind, and disabled persons, and those with psychiatry disabilities who were unable to work and used welfare assistance. Passage of Social Security Disability Insurance (SSD or SSDI) and Supplemental Security Income (SSI) legislation in 1956 and 1972, respectively, provided for a subsistence living and regular income for people with disabilities who were living in poverty.

As the War on Poverty and the Civil Rights and New Left movements gained momentum, each met growing resistance from conservative politicians, resulting in budgetary shortfalls for the new social programs. The War on Poverty was scrapped, sacrificed to the war effort, while the Civil Rights movement and the New Left became increasingly outspoken and militant, and increasingly divided. Although born in the Civil Rights and New Left movements, groups such as the Weathermen and the Black Panthers took radical turns toward armed resistance, partly in reaction to the slow progress of their parent movements, frustration with social policies, and outrage and despair at the assassinations of Martin Luther King Jr. and Robert Kennedy in 1968.

The field of community psychiatry mirrored the political and social turmoil of the time, and did not emerge unscathed. As critiques of society grew in intensity, so did the radical critique of psychiatry and community mental health. Many within the field of psychiatry participated in social movements, setting up on-site treatment centers for the marches on Washington of the Civil Rights movement and antiwar groups.[19] Psychiatry and psychology were accused of institutionalized racism, demonstrated in part by their lack of researchers and clinicians of color.[20] While often differing in their approaches, psychiatrists such as Thomas Szasz and R.D. Laing called attention to what they argued was psychiatry's collusion in social oppression. Szasz questioned the existence of mental illness, regarding it as a method of state control of social and political deviance, and promoted a strict separation of psychiatry and the state.[21] Laing, who established Kingsley Hall in 1964 as a therapeutic community where people with mental illness, seen as active agents in their recovery, could regain social relatedness, became a hero to the student movement.[22] In Italy, Franco Basaglia, convinced that therapeutic communities did not go far enough to produce social change beyond the walls of institutions, founded Psychiatria Democratica in 1973. Basaglia's aims were no less ambitious than to change social structures and cultural attitudes in order to break down both the physical walls of the institution and patients' internal barriers to exerting their own freedom and control of their lives.[23]

The mental health consumer movement took root around the same time as the antipsychiatry movement. Psychiatric "survivors"—people who had experienced the conditions of institutions as well as the inadequacies of community-based care—began to organize, also forming alliances with feminist and gay rights activists. The advocacy that these alliances made possible contributed to the removal in 1973 from the *Diagnostic and Statistical Manual* of homosexuality as a mental illness.[24] People with experience of psychiatric hospitalizations formed activist coalitions such as the Insane Liberation Front, the Mental Patients' Liberation Front, and the Network Against Psychiatric Assault, in the early 1970s. These groups encouraged consciousness-raising regarding psychiatric oppression while promoting self-determination and awareness. Many who joined considered themselves survivors of damaging psychiatric systems and held a profound distrust of psychiatric or medically based care for mental distress.

Family members also began to organize, in part in reaction to the concept of the "schizophrenogenic" mother who putatively "created" schizophrenia in her child through cold treatment and mixed messages. Laing had popularized the notion of the "double-bind,"[25] a hypothesis developed by Bateson and colleagues[26] regarding the influence of family members on an individual's development of mental illness. (Simplifications of Bateson's work led, often, to mischaracterizations of it.) The notion of family causality contributed in part to the eventual establishment of the National Alliance on Mental Illness (originally founded as the National Alliance for the Mentally Ill), or NAMI, in 1979 as an advocacy organization of parents of children with mental illness. In the meantime, a Republican-led backlash against psychiatry and the social welfare state weakened the community mental health movement, primarily via funding cuts.

John Talbott has argued that the most important influences on deinstitutionalization were shifts in funding for Medicaid, Medicare, and SSI; the emergence of the community mental health philosophy; the development of new medications; and an assortment of other legal, judicial, and legislative actions.[11] Brenner, in his study of the relationship between mental illness and the economy, demonstrated the impact of unstable economies on discharge rates from mental hospitals, separately from the incidence of mental illness.[27] Regardless of which influence was paramount, the collision of social, political, economic, and other forces marks this era as one of tumultuous change.

Scientific and Technological Changes in Care and Treatment

In terms of psychiatric care, then, the era was defined by the flux of tensions among numerous opposing influences—state and federal government, medical versus social understandings of mental illness, and ideological tensions between freedom and authoritarianism. Against this backdrop, a number of major advances in treatment for mental health problems, including psychotropic medications, therapeutic communities, case management, and community treatment, were developed. Their impact warrants additional consideration.

Psychiatric care and treatment during this era began with a variety of theories and practices, with those with biological and medical approaches gaining ascendancy over time. According to some historians and psychiatrists, the use of chlorpromazine (Thorazine), along with other medications, is *the* story deinstitutionalization, as these, they argued, made it possible for persons with serious mental illnesses to live stably in the community.[28,29] Gronfein, however, found no evidence of a direct connection between the development and use of psychiatric medications and the movement of people from hospitals into the community,[10] and Scull saw the putative advances in technology and community psychiatry as cloaking the driving force of economic necessity. Rising costs, he argued, led states to offer incentives to counties to divert patients from state institutions to nursing homes or board and care homes, a process called "transinstitutionalization." Communities, unprepared to receive people coming out of institutions, protested fiercely, leading to the ghettoization of discharged patients.[30]

Regardless of its impact on deinstitutionalization, psychopharmacology changed both the psychiatric community's and the public's view of mental illness and heavily influenced the directions of research and funding. The introduction of new medications resulted in significantly increased costs for institutions, thus providing an additional incentive to states to find more cost-effective forms of care.[31] Having a medication that alleviated symptoms, although termed by many as a "chemical straitjacket" rather than a targeted treatment, offered hope of a cure and coincided with other major medication discoveries such as the first oral contraceptive and Salk's discovery of the vaccine for polio.

The public's new optimism in the power of science contributed to its embrace of new medications and the hope of conquering a wide range of medical disorders. Introduced in 1952 in Europe and in 1954 in the United States, Thorazine was one of the first pharmacological agents considered to be a treatment specifically for psychotic symptoms. In 1956, psychiatrists added two new antidepressants to their arsenal: imipramine, in the class of tricyclic antidepressants, and iproniazid, a monoamine oxidase inhibitor. In 1949, Australian psychiatrist John Cade discovered the effects of lithium, a naturally occurring element, in controlling the manic phase of bipolar disorder. Although not officially approved by the U.S. Food and Drug Administration until 1970, lithium was used beginning in the 1950s and continues today as a treatment for bipolar disorder.

Treatment with pharmaceuticals cast new light on the cause and nature of mental illness. Instead of considering mental illness to be determined solely by parent or family environment, the psychiatric community began to think of illness as a neurochemical process and determinant. Evidence of medication's impact on community living can be found in studies such as that of Pasamanick and colleagues, who demonstrated that individuals with schizophrenia who received phenothiazines in addition to community care were hospitalized for psychiatric reasons less often than those receiving care and placebo.[32] As one author stated, "[f]inally we were like other doctors in that we had a treatment that actually worked.[33] This belief and view, as Grob writes, reflected the reintegration of psychiatry into mainstream medicine.[34]

The idea that schizophrenia was a brain illness[33] took hold. Neurochemical research pointed to a deficit in dopamine, a neurotransmitter, as the primary cause. While the dopamine hypothesis has been largely discredited as a single explanation, it provided a heuristic for further research and impetus for continued drug development and treatment via pharmaceuticals.[34] Moncrieff points to the changing nature of the description of chlorpromazine's effects, considered to be nonspecific as to symptoms when first introduced but considered to be "antischizophrenic" by 1964, according to NIMH guidance. This shift supported the agency's research goals as psychiatry's continued to strive for medical legitimacy.[35] Much debate occurred over the question as to whether these psychiatric drugs were worth their costs, and whether should be given in place of psychosocial treatment. Some authors and activists contend that medications increase the likelihood of symptom recurrence.[36] Evidence emerged of persons in developing countries diagnosed with serious psychiatric disorders having better outcomes than those in the United States,[37] although these findings have recently been reexamined.[38]

While pharmaceutical treatment influenced thinking on the nature of mental illness, psychoanalytic approaches to treatment continued to dominate the field, particularly for those with private insurance or other means. The successes of psychotherapy, the growing popularity of Freudian theories, and public exposure to new treatments fueled optimism regarding the ability of medicine to treat psychological problems. Books such as *I Never Promised You a Rose Garden*[39] provided firsthand accounts and persuasive anecdotal evidence of the effectiveness of the psychoanalytic approaches and promoted the idea of the "heroic" psychiatrist, able to cure patients with the most difficult problems.

Despite popular culture's representations of the benefits of psychotherapy and psychoanalytic approaches, few studies were conducted to examine effectiveness and practice was not standardized. Behaviorism and cognitive science contributed to the advent of new therapies pioneered by Beck (cognitive therapy)[40] and Ellis (rational emotive therapy). These, in turn led to the development of cognitive-behavioral therapy,[41] now considered by many to be an effective practice for treating schizophrenia. Carl Rogers developed client-centered therapy, promoting empathy and "unconditional positive regard."[42] Outcome studies on psychotherapy's effectiveness were conducted in the 1940s. In 1975, Luborsky and colleagues reported that different modalities of psychotherapy, when compared head to head in clinical trials, showed no discernable differences.[43] The study of psychotherapy then turned to the client–clinician relationship and the "therapeutic alliance."

Other new treatment modalities, reflecting with the increased value placed upon community involvement and integration, were developed and tested during this time. One was Fountain House, established in 1948 as the first clubhouse for people with psychiatric disabilities. The Fountain House model emphasizes ownership and participation by all, staff and persons with mental illness alike. A 1963 article based on an evaluation of the program found low rates of hospitalization for participants during the first 9 months after discharge.[44] The model took hold and was replicated across the country and overseas.

The "therapeutic community," or "milieu therapy," also won passionate adherents. Maxwell Jones in Britain, known for his work in rehabilitating former prisoners of war, recognized the impact of social and environmental influences and extended his ideas to psychiatric institutions.[45] Research confirmed the importance of work and valued social roles, community involvement, and relationships as factors in rehabilitation of people with mental illness as well as other conditions.[46] These ideas influenced a shift toward unlocked hospital wards and encouraged the establishment of day hospitals with expressive arts and other therapies, all geared toward counteracting the pernicious effects of institutionalization and "social breakdown syndrome." Grob argues that the popularity of this approach reflects the ideological struggle in the post–World War II era between democracy and communism, or between freedom and authoritarianism, with a slant toward freedom and democracy directly reflected in the building of organizations such as consumer councils and patient governance in hospitals.[34]

One of the more controversial of approaches was Loren Mosher's Soteria, a community residential treatment program for people with schizophrenia. Mosher's approach to community psychiatry rested on the premise that care should be located within the community, with interactions in a neighborhood and integration with the local area, as opposed to cloistered in mental health centers. The program was also built on the psychoanalytic argument that medications inhibit symptoms the person needs to work through, subduing those signs of mental illness without healing underlying psychological problems. This approach differs from medical models that see disordered thinking as an organic product of an illness in which symptoms express no meaning related to the person. Mosher and colleagues saw psychotic experience as valid and as having a place along the continuum of all human experience. Soteria staff, employing non–mental health professionals and using psychiatric medications sparingly, showed similar outcomes in terms of symptom reduction, better quality of life, and a lower rate of return to hospital rates compared to a control group treated with higher doses of psychotropics in a traditional mental health setting.[47] Despite evidence of *Soteria*'s effectiveness, Mosher's controversial approach and provocative publications led to discontinuation of funding for the project. (It was taken up later in Berne, Switzerland.[48]

Other significant changes in treatment include the development of the assertive community treatment (ACT) model by Stein and Test in Madison, Wisconsin, involving a team approach to helping people live in the community. Initially described as a "hospital without walls," ACT was designed to provide treatment, supervision, and support to people being discharged from state hospitals. The first ACT team (named PACT, for Program for Assertive Community Treatment) was composed of both patients and staff from Mendota State Hospital. The staff, that is, had been "discharged" along with their patients, and their task was to provide the same level of 24-hour, 7-day-a-week care to these former patients. Care provided outside a hospital setting gave staff the opportunity to act as role models for appropriate social behaviors in the community for their clients.[49] The most original contribution of ACT came to be seen as its *in vivo* skills training for clients. This training, previously offered in group rooms in the state hospital, was now offered to individual clients in natural community settings that required the skills being taught.

Growth of the Mental Health Disciplines

The role of the "helper" in the mental health field underwent major shifts during this period. *Action for Mental Health* called on psychiatrists, clinical psychologists, psychiatric social workers, and psychiatric nurses to provide most care to people with mental illnesses. Consistent with an emerging community orientation to care, however, the report encouraged the use of services from "persons with psychological orientation and mental health training and access to expert consultation as needed."[6,p.xxi] Training was to be given to professionals such as teachers, clergy, family physicians, scoutmasters, and others to enable them to provide mental health counseling. The report also suggested the involvement of mental health consultants to support counselors and pediatricians who would receive enough psychiatric training to work with emotionally disturbed children.

While *Action for Mental Health* described how mental health professionals could provide community-based care, its identification of types of services that members of various disciplines were suited or qualified to provide provoked contentious discussion and turf battles. Psychiatry has historically taken the place as the central discipline in hospital-based care as well as in the community movement. Talcott Parsons described the position of the psychiatrist as one that stands at the center of a network of professional groups, including psychologists, sociologists, occupational therapists, social workers, and nurses.[50] Training needs, however, identified by the 1955 and 1961 Joint Commission reports, led to increased funding for teaching that psychologists were trained to provide, and post–World War II developments such as increased recognition of postcombat stress and its sequelae fueled the need for more psychologists. In order to address this demand, many Veterans Administration facilities began training psychologists to attend to the needs of returning veterans. Psychologists lobbied for legitimacy and licensure, a move that psychiatrists opposed, arguing that only those with a medical degree were qualified to practice psychotherapy. After losing this battle, psychiatrists returned to their medical roots and focused more intently on biopsychology and psychopharmacology.

As the community-based care model emerged more prominently, the question of discipline-specific training and practice came under scrutiny. Early CMHC staff frequently referred to themselves as psychotherapists, but many lacked graduate training in the practice. Many of those who *had* received training geared toward treating those with severe mental illness preferred, and were better equipped by their training, to practice office-based psychotherapy for the "worried well." Many psychiatrists and psychologists fled to private practice. The tasks of providing community supports for persons with serious mental illness, closely linked with social work and rehabilitation practice, conflicted with professional identities based on providing medical care and psychotherapy.

Where Did We Get By 1976?

To understand the enormous impact of shifting priorities in mental health during this era, it is helpful to understand the number of people affected by the transition. By 1965, around 58,000 individuals had left state hospitals and gone to communities that often were unprepared with programs to support them. Between 1969 and 1976, the pace of movement out of institutions accelerated to over 10% per year.[51] By 1977, 85,000 people had been transferred from mental hospitals to nursing homes. Most assessments of the deinstitutionalization process, including those conducted by the NIMH, were highly critical. A 1969 report published by NIMH and the American Psychiatric Association reveals the frustration of administrators and policy makers brought together to comment on the state of the CMHC. The interim assessment, reflecting a grim appraisal of progress to date, states that "given the considerable fragmentation of the mental health services in this country, it does indeed seem bold and new to attempt to develop coordinated and comprehensive services."[52,p.31] A review of outcomes of studies on the impact of deinstitutionalization found, unsurprisingly, that people living in the community fared better when provided with care in those communities.[53] Yet with the oil crisis of the early 1970s and continued spending for the war in Vietnam, the money was not forthcoming to support such care.

Broad cultural changes, scientific advances, and societal shifts are reflected in the growth of community psychiatry during the era of deinstitutionalization and the CMHC movement. Legislation promised a new day for those who had lived hopeless lives in the dark back wards of mental institutions. Yet with disjointed systems of care and cost and burden shifting across institutions, the result for many was a movement from "the back ward to the back alley."[54] The great promise of the era, epitomized in the Community Mental Health Act, follows the narrative arc of other movements of this time—that of great hopes thwarted. In the case of mental health, services eroded, or were never implemented, due to lack of attention, funding that never materialized, and poor planning.

During the 1970s, the nation became increasingly socially conservative in both political and cultural arenas. Federal funding faltered, leading, some argue, to the failure of the community mental health movement. This assessment does not do full justice, however, to theoretical, humanistic, programmatic, and scientific advances that were made during this period. The emergence of activists in the psychiatric survivors movement, the beginnings of support groups, ACT teams, social clubs, and other innovative modalities brought new hope and empowerment to people diagnosed with mental illness, albeit waiting for more fertile soil for growth.

Here and in the two eras that follow, we divide our classics into the overlapping categories of (1) government, legislative, and policy texts, (2) first-person and literary texts, (3) clinical and systems theory, conceptual, and historical texts, and (4) practice and research texts. This is not the neatest of schematizations. The individual categories leave room for odd bedfellows, and the overlap among the four categories threatens, at times, to sink the whole arrangement. Clinical and systems theory and/or conceptual and/or historical work is not the happiest of categories for its occupants, for example, because it traverses so wide a swath. Combining classics of research and classics of practice can be problematic, but in most cases, our research classics involve attempts to create better services or interventions for people with mental illness. But then again, those research classics often contain or segue into theoretical formulations, as with Sue Estroff's *Making it Crazy* from our second era, while Goffman's theoretical formulation of "total institutions" from the first era emerged from his ethnographic research. Some theoretical-conceptual classics, such as Graham Thornicroft and Michele Tansela's "Components of a Modern Mental Health Service" and Robert Rosenheck's "Bringing the Community Back In," are so closely attuned to practice that another group of editors might have placed them in that category. Other classics may stand even more ambiguously at the border of two categories. It may be in the nature of community psychiatry, involving as it does the allocation of contested public resources (first category) for interventions (fourth category) that are developed, in part, in relation to testing of and reflection on such interactions (fourth and third categories), and affecting not only populations but individuals with mental illness (second category), to resist the kind of categorization we have imposed here. Nonetheless, we hope these groupings will be useful, at worst breaking up for readers the long stretch of classics in each era, and at best helping them grab the bundle of them in a way that makes sense to them.

References

1. Ewalt, J. R., & Ewalt, P. L. (1969). History of the community psychiatry movement. *American Journal of Psychiatry, 126*(1), 43–52, 51.
2. Deutsch, A. (1948). *The shame of the states.* New York: Harcourt Brace.
3. Ward, M. J. (1946). *The snake pit.* New York: Random House.
4. Rochefort, D. A. (1993). *From poorhouses to homelessness: Policy analysis and mental health care.* Westport, CT: Auburn House.
5. Felix, R. H. (1956). The strategy of community mental health work. In *The elements of a community mental heath program* (pp. 36–46). [Papers presented at the 1955 annual conference of the Milbank Memorial Fund.] New York: Milbank Memorial Fund.
6. Joint Commission on Mental Illness and Health. (1961). Recommendations for a national mental health program. In *Action for Mental Health: Final report of the Joint Commission on Mental illness and Health.* New York: Basic Books.
7. Albee, G. W. (1959). *Mental health manpower trends.* New York: Basic Books.
8. Snow, D. L., & Newton, P. M. (1976). Task, social structure, and social process in the community mental health center movement. *American Psychologist, August,* 582–594.
9. Cutler, D. L., Bevilacqua, J., & McFarland, B. H. (2003). Four decades of community mental health: A symphony in four movements. *Community Mental Health Journal, 39,* 381–398.
10. Gronfein, W. (1985). Psychotropic drugs and the origins of deinstitutionalization. *Social Problems, 32*(5), 437–454.
11. Talbott, J. (1979). Deinstitutionalization: Avoiding the disasters of the past. *Hospital & Community Psychiatry, 30*(55), 621–624.
12. Porter, R. (1987). *A social history of madness: The world through the eyes of the insane.* New York: Weidenfeld & Nicolson.
13. McWilliams, J. C. (2000). *The 1960s cultural revolution.* Westport, CT: Greenwood Press.
14. Goffman, E. (1961). *Asylums: Essays on the Social Situation of Mental Patients and Other Inmates.* New York: Anchor.
15. Rosenhan, D. L. (1973). On being sane in insane places. *Science, 179,* 250–258.
16. Gruenberg, E. M. (1967). The social breakdown syndrome—Some origins. *American Journal of Psychiatry, 123*(12), 1481–1489.
17. Kesey, K. (1962). *One flew over the cuckoo's nest.* New York: Signet,
18. Hollingshead, A. B., & Redlich, F. C. (1958). *Social class and mental illness.* New York: John Wiley and Sons.
19. Strauss, J. S. (2008). Personal communication, New Haven, CT.
20. Thomas, A., & Sillen, S. (1972). *Racism and psychiatry.* New York: Brunner/Mazel.
21. Szasz, T. S. (1960). The myth of mental illness. *American Psychologist, 15,* 115–118.
22. Laing, R. D. (1969). *Self and others.* New York: Pantheon Books.
23. Scheper-Hughes, N., & Lovell, A. M. (1986). Breaking the circuit of social control: Lessons in public psychiatry from Italy and Franco Basaglia. *Social Science & Medicine, 23*(2), 159–178.
24. Rissmiller, D. J., & Rissmiller, J. H. (2006). Evolution of the antipsychiatry movement into mental health consumerism. *Psychiatric Services, 57*(6), 863–866.
25. Laing, R. D. (1960). *The divided self: An existential study in sanity and madness.* Harmondsworth: Penguin.
26. Bateson, G., Jackson, D. D., Haley, J., & Weakland, J. (1956). Toward a theory of schizophrenia. *Behavioral Science, 1,* 251–264.
27. Brenner, M. H. (1973). *Mental illness and the economy.* Cambridge: Harvard University Press.
28. Rosenbloom, M. (2002). Chlorpromazine and the psychopharmacologic revolution. *Journal of the American Medical Association, 287*(14), 1860–1861.

29. Meyer, J. M., & Simpson, G. M. (1997). From chlorpromazine to olanzapine: A brief history of antipsychotics. *Psychiatric Services, 48*(9), 1137–1139.
30. Scull, A. T. (1976). The decarceration of the mentally ill: A critical view. *Politics & Society, 6*(2), 173–212.
31. Geller, J. L. (2000). The last half-century of psychiatry services as reflected in Psychiatric Services. *Psychiatric Services, 51*(1), 41–67.
32. Pasamanick, B., Scarpitti, F. R., & Dinitz, S. (1967). *Schizophrenics in the community: An experimental study in the prevention of hospitalization.* New York: Appleton-Century Crofts.
33. Cancro, R. (2000). The introduction of neuroleptics: A psychiatric revolution. *Psychiatric Services, 51*(3), 333–335.
34. Grob, G. N. (1994). *The mad among us.* Cambridge, MA: Harvard University Press.
35. Baumeister, A. A., & Francis, J. L. (2002). Historical development of the dopamine hypothesis of schizophrenia. *Journal of the History of the Neurosciences, 11*(3), 265–277.
36. Moncrieff, J. (1999). An investigation into the precedents of modern drug treatment in psychiatry. *History of Psychiatry, 10,* 475–490.
37. Whitaker, R. (2002). *Mad in America: Bad science, bad medicine, and the enduring mistreatment of the mentally ill.* Cambridge, MA: Perseus.
38. World Health Organization. (1979). *Schizophrenia: An international follow-up study.* New York: Wiley.
39. Greenberg, J. (1964). *I never promised you a rose garden.* New York: Penguin Books.
40. Beck, A. T., Rush, J., Shaw, B., & Emery, G. (1979). *Cognitive therapy of depression.* New York: Guilford Press.
41. Rachman, S. (1997). The evolution of cognitive behaviour therapy. In D. Clark, C. G. Fairburn, & M. G. Gelder, editors. *Science and practice of cognitive behaviour therapy* (pp. 1–26). Oxford: Oxford University Press.
42. Rogers, C. R. (1951). *Client-centered therapy.* Boston: Houghton Mifflin.
43. Luborsky, L., Singer, B., & Luborsky, L. (1975). Comparative studies of psychotherapies: Is it true that "everyone has won and all must have prizes?" *Archives of General Psychiatry, 32*(8), 995–1008.
44. Beard, J. H., Pitt, R. B., Fisher, S. H., & Goertzel, V. (1963). Evaluating the effectiveness of a psychiatric rehabilitation program. *American Journal of Orthopsychiatry, 33,* 701–712.
45. Jones, M. (1953). *The therapeutic community: A new treatment method in psychiatry.* New York: Basic Books.
46. DeLeon, G. (2000). *The therapeutic community. Theory, model, and method.* New York: Springer.
47. Mosher, L. B., & Menn, A. Z. (1978). Community residential treatment for schizophrenia: Two-year follow-up. *Hospital & Community Psychiatry, 29*(11), 715–723.
48. Ciompi, L., Dauwalder, H. P., Maier, C., et al. (1992). The pilot project 'Soteria Berne': Clinical experiences and results. *British Journal of Psychiatry Supplementum, 18,* 145–153.
49. Stein, L. I., & Test, M. A. (1980). Alternative to mental hospital treatment. I. Conceptual model, treatment program, and clinical evaluation. *Archives of General Psychiatry, 37*(4), 392–397.
50. Parsons, T. (1957). The mental hospital as a type of organization. In M. Greenblatt, D. J. Levinson, & R. H. Williams, editors. *The patient and the mental hospital* (pp. 108–129). Glencoe, IL: The Free Press.
51. Morrissey, J. P., & Goldman, H. H. (1986). Care and treatment of the mentally ill in the United States: Historical developments and reforms. *Annals of the American Academy of Political and Social Science, 484*(The Law and Mental Health: Research and Policy), 12–27.
52. Glasscote, R. M., Sussex, J. N., & Cumming, E. (1969). *The community mental health center: An interim appraisal.* Washington, D.C.: The Joint Information Service of the American Psychiatric Association and the National Association for Mental Health.
53. Braun, P., Kochansky, G., Shapiro, R., et al. (1981). Overview: Deinstitutionalization of psychiatric patients, a critical review of outcome studies. *American Journal of Psychiatry, 138*(6), 736–749.
54. Trotter, S., & Kuttner, B. (1974). The mentally ill: From back wards to back alleys. *The Washington Post,* C1.

Government, Legislative, and Policy Classics

1

Joint Commission on Mental Illness and Health. (1961). Recommendations for a national mental health program. In *Action for Mental Health: Final Report of the Joint Commission on Mental illness and Health.* New York: Basic Books

The Mental Health Study Act of 1955 authorized creation of the Joint Commission on Mental Illness and Health to study the needs of persons with mental illness and make recommendations for a national mental health program. The commission recommended the development of a national plan that would address the key domains of personnel, facilities, and costs. Regarding *personnel*, it recommended that the federal government invest money and resources in research on the causes and characteristics of mental illness. Regarding *facilities*, it recommended that community-based mental health centers be made available for every 50,000 people in the United States, to provide both basic mental health treatment for persons with serious mental illnesses and prevention-related activities. Other facilities that would provide mental health care were to include general hospitals with short-term units for treating acute problems and state hospitals, with restricted bed capacity, for persons with chronic mental illnesses. Regarding *costs*, the commission agreed that the federal government should bear the brunt of funding for the new community mental health centers. It also suggested changes in reimbursement strategies so that treatment in the community could be reimbursed, thus encouraging community-based treatment as an alternative to hospitalization. The report summary, included here, concludes with the assertion that the commission's proposal was the first in American history to address the issue of public support for care of all persons with mental illness. The assertion was true. The optimism it implied proved to be misplaced.

Elizabeth Flanagan

Recommendations for a National Mental Health Program: Summary

The Mental Health Study Act of 1955 directed the Joint Commission on Mental Illness and Health, as chosen by the National Institute of Mental Health, to analyze and evaluate the needs and resources of the mentally ill in the United States and make recommendations for a national mental health program. Our examination of the factors operating at the action level and the supporting level has shown that progress depends on the solution of the same three problems. They are (1) manpower, (2) facilities, and (3) costs. Our recommendations have been so ordered in the following three sections. We present them under the self-explanatory titles of Pursuit of New Knowledge, Better Use of Present Knowledge and Experience, and The Cost:

Pursuit of New Knowledge

The philosophy that the Federal government needs to develop and crystallize is that science and education are resources—like natural resources—and that they deserve conservation through intelligent use and protection and adequate support—period. They can meet an ends test, but not a means test and not a timetable or appeal for a specified result. Science and education operate not for profit but profit everybody; hence, they need adequate support from human society, whether this support comes from wise public philanthropy or private.

What is needed in mental health research is a balanced portfolio. Toward this end we recommend the following:

1. *A much larger proportion of total funds for mental health research should be invested in basic research as contrasted with applied research. Only through a large investment in basic research can we hope ultimately to specify the causes and characteristics sufficiently so that we can predict and therefore prevent various forms of mental illness or disordered behavior through specific knowledge of the defects and their remedies.*
2. *Congress and the State legislatures increasingly should favor long-term research in mental health and mental illness as contrasted with short-term projects.*
3. *Increased emphasis should be placed on, and greater allocations of money be made for, venture, or risk, capital in the support both of persons and of ideas in the mental health research area.*
4. *The National Institute of Mental Health should make new efforts to invest in, provide for, and hold the young scientist in his career choice. The Federal government*

must provide, on a stable base, more salary support for mental health career inves-
tigators, more full-time positions must be established for ten-year periods as well
as some on the basis of lifetime appointments, and, in the case of medical schools
and universities, these latter positions must be awarded on condition that the scien-
tist receive a faculty appointment with tenure.

5. *Support of program research in established scientific and educational institutions,*
as initiated by the National Institutes of Health, should be continued and consider-
ably expanded in the field of mental health.

6. *The Federal government should support the establishment of mental health*
research centers, or research institutes. These centers or institutes may operate in
collaboration with educational institutions and training centers, or may be estab-
lished independently.

7. *Some reasonable portion of total mental health research support should be*
designated as capital investment in building up facilities for research in States or
regions where scientific institutions are lacking or less well developed.

8. *Diversification should be recognized as the guiding principle in the distribution*
of Federal research project, program, or institute grants from the standpoint of
categories of interest, subject matter of research, and the branches of science
involved.

In general, what we propose is an extension and expansion, combined with certain shifts of emphasis, in the research grant program ably administered at present by the National Institute of Mental Health through the wisdom of Congress. No specific sums will be recommended here, as it is felt that the needs, advances, and areas of interest will alter the sums required from year to year. We endorse and support *Federal Support of Medical Research* (Report of the Committee of Consultants on Medical Research to the Subcommittee on Departments of Labor and Health, Education, and Welfare of the Committee on Appropriations, United States Senate, May 1960). This committee, chaired by Boisfeuillet Jones, recommended total Federal expenditures for medical research which appeared to us currently adequate and reasonable. While substantially supported in the 1960 summer session of the Congress, the recommendations of the Jones Report unfortunately were not fully carried out, particularly as they applied to more realistic support of the indirect costs of research to the institutions which make the research possible. We would memorialize the Congress on the urgent need of reviewing this now notoriously sore point. Too many business-minded governing boards of deficit-ridden universities and teaching hospitals now conceive research as being operated at a direct loss to the institution and therefore are reluctant to approve of further expansion of research efforts.

Better use of Present Knowledge and Experience

Manpower, Its Training and Utilization.

1. *Policy.   In the absence of more specific and definitive scientific evidence of the*
causes of mental illnesses, psychiatry and the allied mental health professions
should adopt and practice a broad, liberal philosophy of what constitutes and who
can do treatment within the framework of their hospitals, clinics, or other profes-
sional service agencies, particularly in relation to persons with psychoses or severe

personality or character disorders that incapacitate them for work, family life, and everyday activity. All mental health professions should recognize:

A. *That certain kinds of medical, psychiatric, and neurological examinations and treatments must be carried out by or under the immediate direction of psychiatrists, neurologists, or other physicians specially trained for these procedures.*

B. *That psychoanalysis and allied forms of deeply searching and probing "depth psychotherapy" must be practiced only by those with special training, experience, and competence in handling these techniques without harm to the patient—namely, by physicians trained in psychoanalysis or intensive psychotherapy, plus those psychologists or other professional persons who lack a medical education but have an aptitude for, training in, and demonstrable competence in such techniques of psychotherapy.*

C. *That nonmedical mental health workers with aptitude, sound training, practical experience, and demonstrable competence should be permitted to do general, short-term psychotherapy—namely, treating persons by objective, permissive, nondirective techniques of listening to their troubles and helping them resolve these troubles in an individually insightful and socially useful way. Such therapy, combining some elements of psychiatric treatment, client counseling, "someone to tell one's troubles to," and love for one's fellow man, obviously can be carried out in a variety of settings by institutions, groups, and individuals, but in all cases should be undertaken under the auspices of recognized mental health agencies.*

2. *Recruitment and Training.   The mental health professions need to launch a national manpower recruitment and training program, expanding on and extending present efforts and seeking to stimulate the interest of American youth in mental health work as a career. This program should include all categories of mental health personnel. The program should emphasize not only professional training but also short courses and on-the-job training in the subprofessions and upgrading for partially trained persons.*

3. *Image-Making.   Steps should be taken to create the President's Prizes in the Humane Sciences, large awards to be made each year by the president of the United States to a young scientist and to a science teacher or professor for outstanding scientific or educational contributions in the life sciences, social sciences, or physical sciences of importance to mental health.*

4. *Volunteers.   The volunteer work with mental hospital patients done by college students and many others should be encouraged and extended.*

5. *Support of Education.   Leaders of the mental health professions should actively and aggressively participate in support of constructive legislation in the field of education, general as well as medical and scientific education.*

The Federal government not only should support a student scholarship and loan program but also should foster financial responsibility for education of one's own children wherever possible. The time has come for the Federal government to adopt, and affirm through income tax law amendments permitting deductions from taxable income of direct expenses for higher education, the policy that education is an essential resource of modern life, the same as industrial investment capital, farm products, natural resources, housing, and, of course, medical care. In all these categories, income tax allowances are made, but the demonstrable fact that higher education is a resource and that investment in it increases the future taxable income of the Nation's children has been ignored.

The problems of medical education, the need for expansion of present medical schools, and the need for new medical schools have been impressively set forth in two studies by Federally appointed groups conducted independently o£ the Mental Health Study. These are the Final Report of the Secretary's Consultant on Medical Research and Education (U.S. Department of Health, Education, and Welfare, 1958 [Bayne-Jones Report]), and the Report of the Surgeon General's Consultant Group on Medical Education (U.S. Department of Health, Education, and Welfare, 1959 [Bane Report]). The Joint Commission endorses these reports and favors the recommendations summarized in Chapter VI of the Bane Report.

Services to Mentally Troubled People.

Persons who are emotionally disturbed—that is to say, under psychological stress that they cannot tolerate—should have skilled attention and helpful counseling available to them in their community if the development of more serious mental breakdowns is to be prevented. This is known as secondary prevention, and is concerned with the detection of beginning signs and symptoms of mental illness and their relief; in other words, the earliest possible treatment. In the absence of fully trained psychiatrists, clinical psychologists, psychiatric social workers, and psychiatric nurses, such counseling should be done by persons with some psychological orientation and mental health training and access to expert consultation as needed.

1. *Mental Health Counselors.*   A host of persons untrained or partially trained in mental health principles and practices—clergymen, family physicians, teachers, probation officers, public health nurses, sheriffs, judges, public welfare workers, scoutmasters, county farm agents, and others—are already trying to help and to treat the mentally ill in the absence of professional resources. With a moderate amount of training through short courses and consultation on the job, such persons can be fully equipped with an additional skill as mental health counselors.
2. *Mental Health Consultants.*   Persons fully trained in a mental health profession— psychologists, social workers, nurses, family physicians, pediatricians, or psychiatrists with particular interest in community services—should be available for systematic consultation with mental health counselors. The basic functions of these consultants would be to provide on-the-job training, general professional supervision of subprofessional activities, and the moral support and reassurance found to be essential for most persons working with the emotionally disturbed or mentally ill.
3. *Pediatricians.*   Child specialists offer a considerable potential for helping emotionally disturbed children, but in many cases lack sufficient psychiatric orientation to capitalize on this potential. The National Institute of Mental Health should provide support for resident training programs in pediatrics that make well-designed efforts to incorporate adequate psychiatric information as a part of the pediatrician's graduate training. It also should provide stipends for pediatricians who wish to take postgraduate courses in psychiatry. The aim is not to convert pediatricians into psychiatrists but to increase the mental patient care resources of the community in which the pediatrician practices.
4. *Resident Schools.*   Pilot studies should be undertaken in the development of centers for the re-education of emotionally disturbed children, using different types of personnel than are customary. The schools would be operated by carefully selected teachers working with consultants, from the mental health disciplines.

Immediate Care of Acutely Disturbed Mental Patients.

Immediate professional attention should be provided in the community for persons at the onset of acutely disturbed, socially disruptive, and sometimes personally catastrophic behavior—that is, for persons suffering a major breakdown. The few pilot programs for immediate, or emergency, psychiatric care presently in existence should be expanded and extended as rapidly as personnel becomes available.

Intensive Treatment of Acutely Ill Mental Patients.

A national mental health program should recognize that major mental illness is the core problem and unfinished business of the mental health movement, and that the intensive treatment of patients with critical and prolonged mental breakdowns should have first call on fully trained members of the mental health professions. There is a need for expanding treatment of the acutely ill mental patient in all directions, via community mental health clinics, general hospitals, and mental hospitals, as rapidly as psychiatrists, clinical psychologists, psychiatric nurses, psychiatric social workers, and occupational, physical, and other nonmedical therapists become available in the community. There is a related need for revision of commitment laws to ease the movement of patients through the various treatment facilities.

1. *Community Mental Health Clinics.   Community mental health clinics serving both children and adults, operated as out-patient departments of general or mental hospitals, as part of State or regional systems for mental patient care, or as independent agencies, are a main line of defense in reducing the need of many persons with major mental illness for prolonged or repeated hospitalization. Therefore, a national mental health program should set as an objective one fully staffed, full-time mental health clinic available to each 50,000 of population. Greater efforts should be made to induce more psychiatrists in private practice to devote a substantial part of their working hours to community clinic services, both as consultants and as therapists.*

For Children:

Psychiatric clinics providing intensive psychotherapy for children, plus appropriate medical or social treatment procedures, should be fostered and, where they exist, expanded. Of all categories of psychiatrists, child psychiatrists are in shortest supply—children being especially trying to work with and requiring the close cooperation of the parents and infinite patience on the part of therapists. The present State aid program is insufficient to provide for the needs in this area. It should be expanded.

For Adults:

The principal functions of a mental health clinic serving adults (the majority serve both adults and children) should be (1) to provide treatment by a basic mental health team (usually psychiatrist, psychologist, and social worker) for persons with acute mental illness, (2) to care for incompletely recovered mental patients either short of admission to a hospital or following discharge from the hospital, and (3) to provide a headquarters base for mental health consultants working with mental health counselors. The function of such a clinic as a center of mental health education for the public is of incidental importance, and should preferably be left to other agencies.

2. *General Hospital Psychiatric Units.   No community general hospital should be regarded as rendering a complete service unless it accepts mental patients for short-term hospitalization and therefore provides a psychiatric unit or psychiatric beds. Every community general hospital of 100 or more beds should make this provision. A hospital with such facilities should be regarded as an integral part of a total system of mental patient services in its region.*

It is the consensus of the Mental Health Study that definitive care for patients with major mental illness should be given if possible, or for as long as possible, in a psychiatric unit of a general hospital and then, on a longer-term basis, in a specialized mental hospital organized as an intensive psychiatric treatment center.

3. *Intensive Psychiatric Treatment Centers.   Smaller State hospitals, of 1000 beds or less and suitably located for regional service, should be converted as rapidly as possible into intensive treatment centers for patients with major mental illness in the acute stages or, in the case of a more prolonged illness, those with a good prospect for improvement or recovery. All new State hospital construction should be devoted to these smaller intensive treatment centers.*

<u>The most important requirement for an intensive treatment center is a well-trained and competent staff at least as large in number as the patients served</u>. This staff should have a good-sized complement of skilled psychiatrists who know how to work comfortably with a clinical team including a variety of professional and subprofessional persons who can assist them in the treatment of patients. Such workers would include occupational, recreational, and physical therapists as well as psychologists, social workers, nurses, and attendants. The medical superintendent of such a mental hospital should be a competent psychiatrist, thoroughly aware of and prepared to use modern psychological and social concepts of treatment as well as physical techniques of treatment, and should be trained in hospital administration.

Care of Chronic Mental Patients.

No further State hospitals of more than 1000 beds should be built, and not one patient should be added to any existing mental hospital already housing 1000 or more patients. It is further recommended that all existing State hospitals of more than 1000 beds be gradually and progressively converted into centers for the long-term and combined care of chronic diseases, including mental illness. This conversion should be undertaken in the next ten years.

Special techniques are available for the care of the chronically ill and these techniques of socialization, relearning, group living, and gradual rehabilitation or social improvement should be expanded and extended to more people, including the aged who are sick and in need of care, through conversion of State mental hospitals into combined chronic disease centers.

A chronic disease center could be operated by a trained hospital administrator (layman or physician) with the psychiatrists and other physicians coming in as a visiting staff or functioning as a full-time medical staff. The layman professionally trained in hospital administration could effect a saving in scarce manpower.

It would be necessary to provide the intensive treatment services for the acutely ill, outlined in the preceding section, before large State hospitals could be converted to treat chronic diseases. It also would be necessary to make certain changes in Federal and State Laws.

Many of the facilities needed for the prolonged care of mental patients are identical with those necessary for the prolonged care of any type of chronic physical illness. Therefore, communities should find it practical to care for patients with all types of chronic physical and mental disorders in the same chronic disease hospital.

Aftercare, Intermediate Care, and Rehabilitation Services.

The objective of modern treatment of persons with major mental illness is to enable the patient to maintain himself in the community in a normal manner. To do so, it is necessary (1) to save the patient from the debilitating effects of institutionalization as much as possible, (2) if the patient requires hospitalization, to return him to home and community life as soon as possible, and (3) thereafter to maintain him in the community as long as possible. Therefore, aftercare and rehabilitation are essential parts of all service to mental patients, and the various methods of achieving rehabilitation should be integrated in all forms of services, among them day hospitals, night hospitals, aftercare clinics, public health nursing services, foster family care, convalescent nursing homes, rehabilitation centers, work services, and ex-patient groups. We recommend that demonstration programs for day and night hospitals and the more flexible use of mental hospital facilities, in the treatment of both the acute and the chronic patient, be encouraged and augmented through institutional, program, and project grants.

Aftercare services for the mentally ill are in a primitive stage of development almost everywhere. Where they do exist, services and agencies caring for the former patient tend to split off from mental patient services as a whole and further to approach the patient's problems piecemeal. Rehabilitation agencies should work closely with treatment agencies and preferably have representatives in the latter's institutional settings. It is important that rehabilitation be regarded as a part of a comprehensive program of patient services in which each and every member of the mental health team has a part to play.

Public Information on Mental Illness

A national mental health program should avoid the risk of false promise in "public education for better mental health" and focus on the more modest goal of disseminating such information about mental illness as the public needs and wants in order to recognize psychological forms of sickness and to arrive at an informed opinion in its responsibility toward the mentally ill.

It is possible to make certain general recommendations about dissemination of information concerning mental illness aimed at (1) greater public understanding of the mentally ill person and those who care for him, (2) the avoiding of *mis*understanding in the relations of one professional group with another, and (3) the importance of making sure, in the relations of the mental health professions with the lay public, that others understand what we are driving at.

An important point has been missed in overinsistence that the public recognize that mentally ill persons are sick, the same as if they were physically sick, and should be treated no differently from other sick persons. *Mental illness is different from physical illness in the one fundamental aspect that it tends to disturb and repel others rather than evoke their sympathy and desire to help.*

A sharper focus in a national program against mental illness might be achieved if the information publicly disseminated capitalized on the aspect in which mental differs from physical illness. Such information should have at least four general objectives:

1. *To overcome the general difficulty in thinking about recognizing mental illness as such—that is, a disorder with psychological as well as physiological, emotional as well as organic, social as well as individual causes and effects.*
2. *To overcome society's many-sided pattern of rejecting the mentally ill, by making it clear that the major mentally ill are singularly lacking in appeal, why this is so, and the need consciously to solve the rejection problem.*
3. *To make clear what mental illness is like as it occurs in its various forms and is seen in daily life and what the average person's reactions to it are like, as well as to elucidate means of coping with it in casual or in close contact. As an example, the popular stereotype of the "raving maniac" or "berserk madman" as the only kind of person who goes to mental hospitals needs to be dispelled. We have not made it clear to date that such persons (who are wild and out of control) exist, but in a somewhat similar proportion as airplanes that crash in relation to airplanes that land safely.*
4. *To overcome the pervasive defeatism that stands in the way of effective treatment. While no attempt should be made to gloss over gaps in knowledge of diagnosis and treatment, the fallacies of "total insanity," "hopelessness," and "incurability" should be attacked, and the prospects of recovery or improvement through modern concepts of treatment and rehabilitation emphasized. One aspect of the problem is that hospitalization taking the form of ostracization, incarceration, or punishment increases rather than decreases disability.*

Attention is also needed to the manner in which professional persons and groups approach the public, since winning friends and support for care of the mentally ill depends first and foremost on not giving cause for offense. *We recommend that the American Psychiatric Association make special efforts to explore, understand, and transmit to its members an accurate perception of the public's image of the psychiatrist.* Such efforts could pay a great dividend in "education of the public" if the profession were to be educated, perhaps as a part of its formal training, against overvaluing, overreaching, and overselling itself.

The primary responsibility for preparation of mental health information for dissemination to laymen should rest with "laymen" who are experts in public education and mass communications and who will work in consultation with mental health experts. But the mental health expert and the educator or mass communications expert have the primary problem of fully communicating with one another before communicating with the public. Too often the basis for discussions among mental health professionals and laymen is the easy assumption on both sides that the other fellow doesn't "understand the problem" or "know what he is talking about."

As a matter of policy, *the mental health professions can now assume that the public knows the magnitude if not the nature of the mental illness problem and psychiatry's primary responsibility for care of mental patients. Henceforth the psychiatrist and his teammates should seek ways of sharing this responsibility with others and correcting deficiencies and inadequacies without feeling the need to be overbearing, defensive, seclusive, or evasive. A first principle of honest public relations bears repeating: To win public confidence, first confide in the public.*

The Cost

Expenditures for public mental patient services should be doubled in the next five years—and tripled in the next ten.

Only by this magnitude of expenditure can typical State hospitals be made in fact what they are now in name only—hospitals for mental patients. Only by this magnitude of expenditure can outpatient and ex-patient programs be sufficiently extended outside of the mental hospital, into the community. It is self-evident that the States, for the most part, have defaulted on adequate care for the mentally ill, and have consistently done so for a century. It is likewise evident that the States cannot afford the kind of money needed to catch up with modern standards of care without revolutionary changes in their tax structure.

Therefore, *we recommend that the States and the Federal government work toward a time when a share of the cost of State and local mental patient services will be borne by the Federal government, over and above the present and future program of Federal grants in aid for research and training.* The simple and sufficient reason for this recommendation is that under present tax structure only the Federal government has the financial resources needed to overcome the lag and to achieve a minimum standard of adequacy. The Federal government should be prepared to assume a major part of the responsibility for the mentally ill insofar as the States are agreeable to surrendering it.

For convenience, the Veterans Administration mental hospitals can be taken as financial models of what can be done in the operation of public mental hospitals. *Congress and the National Institute of Mental Health, with the assistance of the intervening administrative branches of government, should develop a Federal subsidy program that will encourage States and local governments to emulate the example set by VA mental hospitals.*

Certain principles should be followed in a Federal program of matching grants to States for the care of the mentally ill:

The *first principle* is that the Federal government on the one side and State and local governments on the other should *share in the costs* of services to the mentally ill.

The *second principle* is that the total Federal share should be arrived at in a *series of graduated steps* over a period of years, the share being determined each year on the basis of State funds spent in a previous year.

The *third principle* is that the grants should be awarded according to *criteria of merit and incentive* to be formulated by an expert advisory committee appointed by the National Institute of Mental Health.

In arriving at a formula, such an expert committee would establish conditions affecting various portions of the available grant, including the following:

1. *Bring about any necessary changes in the laws of the State to make professionally acceptable treatment as well as custody a requirement in mental hospitalization, to differentiate between need of treatment and need of institutionalization, and to provide treatment without hospitalization.*
2. *Bring about any necessary changes in laws of the State to make voluntary admission the preferred method and court commitment the exceptional method of placing patients in a mental hospital or other treatment facilities, and to emphasize ease of patient movement into and out of such facilities.*
3. *Accept any and all persons requiring treatment and/or hospitalization on the same basis as persons holding legal residence within the State.*
4. *Revise laws of the State governing medical responsibility for the patient to distinguish between administrative responsibility for his welfare and safekeeping and responsibility for his professional care.*
5. *Institute suitable differentiation between administrative structure and professional personnel requirements for (1) State mental institutions intended primarily as intensive treatment centers (i.e., true hospitals) and (2) facilities for humane and progressive care of various classes of the chronically ill or disabled, among them the aged.*

6. *Establish State mental health agencies with well-defined powers and sufficient authority to assume overall responsibility for the State's services to the mentally ill, and to coordinate State and local community health services.*

7. *Make reasonable efforts to operate open mental hospitals as mental health centers, i.e., as part of an integrated community service with emphasis on outpatient and aftercare facilities as well as inpatient services.*

8. *Establish in selected State mental hospitals and community mental health programs training for mental health workers, ranging in scope, as appropriate, from professional training in psychiatry through all professional and subprofessional levels, including on-the-job training of attendants and volunteers. Since each mental health center cannot undertake all forms of teaching activity, consideration here must be given to a variety of programs and total effort. States should be required ultimately to spend 2½ per cent of State mental patient service funds for training.*

9. *Establish in selected State mental hospitals and community mental health programs scientific research programs appropriate to the facility, the opportunities for well-designed research, and the research talent and experience of staff members. States should be required ultimately to spend 2½ per cent of State mental patient service funds for research.*

10. *Encourage county, town, and municipal tax participation in the public mental health services of the State as a means of obtaining Federal funds matched against local mental health appropriations.*

11. *Agree that no money will be spent to build mental hospitals of more than 1000 beds, or to add a single patient to mental hospitals presently having 1000 or more patients.*

Our proposal would encourage local responsibility of a degree that has not existed since the State hospital system was founded, while at the same time recognizing that the combined State-local responsibility cannot be fulfilled by the means at hand.

Our proposal is the first one in American history that attempts to encompass the total problem of public support of mental health services and to make minimum standards of adequate care financially possible.

The outstanding characteristics of mental illness as a public health problem are its staggering size, the present limitations in our methods of treatment, and the peculiar nature of mental illness that differentiates its victims from those with other diseases or disabilities. It would follow that *any national program against mental illness adopted by Congress and the States must be scaled to the size of the problem, imaginative in the course it pursues, and energetic in overcoming both psychological and economic resistances to progress in this direction.* We have sought to acquit our assignment in full recognition of these facts and judgments.

First Person and Literary Classics

2

Greenberg, J. (1964). *I never promised you a rose garden.* New York: New American Library

This autobiographical novel written by Joanne Greenberg under the pen name of Hannah Green recounts Greenberg's experiences of mental illness and recovery during a 3-year hospitalization for schizophrenia and intensive therapy with the famed analyst Frieda Fromm-Reichmann. The book, one of the first patient narratives to be widely read by the general public, helped motivate others to tell their stories and inspired many young people to work in the fields of psychiatry and psychology. Deborah Blau, Greenberg's pseudonym in the book, has created a complex world, called Yr, to which she escapes during times of stress and particularly in reaction to the anti-Semitism she experiences at school and summer camp. While at first Yr is a peaceful kingdom of green pastures with its own host of gods, it becomes a place of torture and recriminations where "the Collect" criticizes and "the Pit" resembles Dante's circles of hell. Of additional interest is Greenberg's description of her protagonist's difficulty returning to the community following her discharge from hospitalization. Following the publication of *DSM-III,* Cadoret and North cited *Rose Garden* in a 1981 article in *Archives of General Psychiatry* in an attempt to show that Deborah and others who had written illness narratives could not, in fact, have suffered from schizophrenia, based on the new diagnostic criteria. We include here the penultimate chapter of Greenberg's book.

Rebecca Miller

Chapter 28, pp. 232–242

Deborah spent the next months simply, working on a series of pen-and-ink drawings and cleaving the past in heavy-hours with Dr. Fried. As the world began to gain form, dimension, and color, she started to find the sessions of choir practice and sewing class too fragile a scaffold on which to build hope. No matter how pleasant, sane or cooperative she was, invisible and inaudible was all she would ever be. She would know the Methodist liturgical year and some of the gossip of the Ladies' Altar Club, but she would never penetrate an inch under the politely closed faces whose motions she duplicated in those places. Over the text of John Stainer's "Seven-Fold Amen," she looked out into the congregation on Sunday and wondered if they ever thanked God for the light in their minds, for friends, for cold and pain responsive to the laws of nature, for enough depth of sight into these laws to have expectations, for friends, for the days and nights that follow one another in stately rhythm, for the sparks that fly upward, for friends.... Did they know how beautiful and enviable their lives were? She realized more and more that her few spare-hour pastimes provided too little in which to test or exercise her fragile "yes" to a newborn reality.

Although she read Latin and some Greek, she had never graduated from high school and her memory of it was now almost four years old—the memories of an occasional visitor from a foreign place. She looked in the town papers and was surprised at her feeble knowledge of the world and its requirements. No job, even the simplest, was open to her. The town was small and slow; a waitress or 5 & 10 girl would not be under the pressure of hurrying crowds; these jobs required little intellect; but she did not have enough education to qualify for them.

For a while there was no help from the hospital. The psychiatrists were all themselves strangers to the town and had been long years away from considerations of skilled and unskilled labor. Dr. Fried implied subtly that it might be Deborah's problem to solve, and the outpatient administrator, after saying somewhat the same thing, mentioned offhandedly that he would look into the problem. When he called her back to his office two week later, he seemed a little surprised.

"I've talked to several people," he said, "and apparently you'll have to get through high school, before you can get any job." To her terror-stricken look he said, "Well...think about it for a while... ."

He did not know that Deborah had gone during the day to look at the town high school. It was a great and sudden stand of buildings all the way over on the other side of town. The stone heaps brooded like a great moa, too big to fly. She might have to be one of the students at that school. She had been broken in a school like that, years ago. Certainly the sickness had been building up inside her for years, but the final terrors of it—the missing days, the sudden falls into dark Yr—were all walked through in halls like the ones

38

inside that building, among faces like the ones that would be there. She remembered the struggle before she had given up the pretense of consubstantiality. She thought again of the secret Japanese, bearing untreated the wounds which had led to his capture, secretly dead and bearing unnoticed the pressure-crazing Semblance, secretly a citizen and captive of Anterrabae, the Censor, the Collect, and the Pit.

Even as she had compromised her captors, she had lost the wish for Semblance—to be a picture of belonging at all costs. She knew the costs now; in a tightened, frightened small town where her classmates would be three years younger and light years distant, she knew that at best such a world would be a no man's land. Even if she no longer belonged to Yr, there would still be the awful alienation from Earth that had once made her run to other-ness in pain day after day. Yr or no, it was too late to join students such as these again, too late for the proms, the cliques, the curlers, and the class pins. She had had quite enough of a "special vocabulary of belonging."

"I'm nineteen..." she said to the heap of buildings. "It's too late." She turned shivering
    in the Yri wind that blew over all the miles of a real and unreal separation.
"I can't go back to my merry high-school days again," she said to the out-patient adminis-
    trator, "volleyball in the gym and teeth-teeth at the school dances."
"But unless you have that diploma to show..."
"Non omnia possumus omnes...," she said, and reminded him that it was Virgil, but she
    knew that what he said was true.
"Why don't you make a list of all the things you can do?" he said. She knew that it was
    make-work, "doing something useful," something Deborah felt was nothing more than
    juggling dead-end signs. The administrator wanted to get off the hook, he wanted not
    to be bothered with the world of commerce and livelihood, and Deborah, seeing this,
    was moved out of sympathy to be dutiful and do what he said. Perhaps she would find
    hiding in a word some preference, or talent, or something that could really be used.
    There it was again, the little Maybe, building its compelling heat from a small and
    vulnerable spark.

She went back to her little table at the rooming house, sat down, and ruled a piece of paper down the middle. On one side she wrote Knowledge and on the other, Possible Job.

KNOWLEDGE	POSSIBLE JOB
1. Ride a bicycle	Rural delivery girl
2. Know all of Hamlet by heart from beginning to end	Tutor of Hamlet to kids who are taking it in school
3. Can wake up from dead sleep in full possession of faculties	Night watchman
4. Have a tremendous vocabulary of obscene words	Language consultant
5. Some Greek	(Not enough)
6. Some Latin	Tutor of Latin for kids
7. Have potential for callousness	Professional assassin
8. Artist for 10 years	Not genius — not commercially practical
9. Know the components of most forms of mental illness and could act them realistically from seeing the original	Actress (too dangerous)
10. Don't smoke	Wine taster

She rewrote the list leaving out numbers 4, 5, 7, and 9. She felt a special poignancy at having to leave out "Professional assassin." She realized that she was too poorly coordinated and clumsy, and professional assassins should be very wiry and graceful. She was so lacking in *atumai* that she knew her victims would always fall the wrong way, and picturing herself trying to crawl out from beneath the body of a three-hundred-pound former wrestler, she knew that 7 was a lost cause.

The next day she took the list to the administrator, but did not stay to see him read it. Even Anterrabae was embarrassed by the poor showing of his queen and victim, and the Collect was jubilantly self-righteous. She was frightened by the choices that the world offered her. The possible futures stretched before her like the hall down which she was now walking from the administrative offices: a long road with carefully labeled doors every ten feet of the way—all closed.

"Oh, Miss Blau—" a voice called behind her. It was one of the social workers. (What now? she wondered. I have a room, so I don't need a room-tracker, unless there's one to rescind the other's trackings.) "Doctor Oster was talking to me about you going to the high school." (There it was again, the lock-step-lock of the world; they had reassigned her to her place under the juggernaut.) Redness seethed upward from the tumor until she was hot to the eyes with its pain.

"I should have thought of it right away," the social worker was saying. "There's a place in the city that might be able to prepare you for them."

"For what?" Deborah said.

"For the examinations."

"What examinations?"

"Why, the high-school equivalency. As I was saying, it seems the practical way . . . .' The social worker was looking at her quizzically. Deborah wanted to tell her that it is not possible to hear through a red wash, and that the relief of her news, which had turned her face a chalk white, was also giving her "the bends" from the change in pressure.

"I wouldn't have to go to the town high school?"

"No, as I was just saying, there is a tutorial school in the city—"

"I could choose, then?"

"You could talk to them about the possibilities—"

"Does one call for an appointment?"

"Well, you are still a ward of . . ."

"Could *you* call them for an appointment?"

"Yes, I could do that."

"And will you tell me what they say?"

The social worker said that she would, and Deborah sat down and watched her walk away. The pain in the red wash was fading, but the panic was not withdrawing from her. *Listen to your heart,* Anterrabae said, falling beside her. She heard it slamming like a latchless door in the wind.

What is it? What is it? she called to Yr. *I was real, just here, just before!* Her vision was ragged and distorted and the words came in an odd Yri form, as if even Yri had been coded for secrecy. *Why? Why is this happening?*

Her question broke the earth's silence, and she sensed people near, perhaps Doctor Oster coming out of his office. But her hearing was distorted like her vision, and when she stumbled into someone, she cried, "The senses are not discrete!"

"Is she going to be *violent?"* (or something like that, came in bored annoyance from the blur). Deborah began to answer that violence to a volcano is natural law, but she could no longer communicate at all. Flanked and followed by the handed blurs, she entered the steel patient-elevator and was carried up to D ward—the beginning all over again.

When she cleared—again, all over again, wrapped and restrained yet again—she laughed down at herself looking the length of the case.

"Now I know, you sudden, falling calendars. Now I know, Lactamaeon, you sad god. Now I know why Carla and Doris Rivera were so damned exhausted!" Her throat seemed to be breaking with the hard, hurting laugh.

After a while Quentin Dobshansky came in to take her pulse.

"Hi, ..." he said, trying to figure out if he should be cheerful or grave, "...is the pack helping?"

"Well, I can see again," she said, "and hear, and talk." She looked at him. "Are you still a friend of mine?"

"Well, sure!" he said uncomfortably.

"Then don't do anything to your face, Quentin. Just; leave it hanging there."

He let his face go, and it fell back into disappointment. "Just...well, I liked to think of you being outside and starting along, that's all."

He was beginning to feel an ache of anxiety because this person toward whom he felt kindly was a crazy person (even, though the doctors had told him to call them mentally ill) and he could make her crazier if he said the wrong things. The doctors and all the books he had been reading told him not to be too definite, not to argue or show strong feelings, but to be cheerful and helpful. In spite of these instructions, he knew that he could move her, and this made him try, and the trying made him feel something for her, and his success at this feeling made her a human being to him. She was homely and straggle-haired, but he had been laughed at for his looks, too; and he had been defeated once as she seemed to be now. He had been in an accident which had left him lying on a road all broken, his father beside him. The rescuers had taken him to the hospital tied up in a blanket, as she was tied up now, and he remembered that trip. Before the pain there had been something worse: the awful feeling of being crushed to a pulp—body and soul. It had whispered to him over and over with the turning of the wheel rims: stove-in and broke, stove-in and broke. Of the later pain he was curiously proud. His father's death left a raw, clean sorrow; the broken ribs made each breath-in-breath-out a kick in the face of death, a hurt of being alive. Now he looked at Deborah and heard his mind go again around the rims of the wheels, stove-in and broke, stove-in and broke. It must be what she was feeling now.

"You want a drink?"

"No, thank you."

Suffering, shy with each other, waiting for his disappointment and her fear to make their weights known between them, they looked at each other, and Deborah was suddenly struck that Quentin Dobshansky, her friend, was a man—a sexual man—a passionate man who seemed to be sounding a cry of passion into the echo-places of her emptiness. Only at that moment did she become aware of them as empty. And at the instant she discovered emptiness, she discovered hunger. It was a long, hard hunger, years late and never plumbed before. But the measure of hunger was the measure of capacity. Furii had been right; nuts or not, Deborah could feel.

She looked up at Quentin. He was pausing at the door, waiting to give hope, of which he had less than he wanted to show. "You have another hour," he said.

"It's okay." She knew that she was ugly and she didn't want to hurt his eyes or his mind's eyes, so she turned her head and let him close the door.

Now it was not Anterrabae who mocked, but Lactamaeon, the black god with the icy blue eyes. *The fisherman has won, and the fish is in the net, but it does not die and be dead. It keeps flapping and slapping against the sides of the boat, turning and seeking for its element and suffering the deprivation of the essence by which it lives. This distresses the fisherman. He does not want to think about the death-throes of the fish, which is his prize and his victory. Thus are you to the world and to us also. Re-die, and let things stand as they were.*

Don't you see! she cried out at him, *I don't know* how *any more!*

Back on the ward that afternoon, an attendant left a smoldering cigarette on an ash tray near the nursing station. Deborah picked it up, hid it, and took it to the dormitory where she was staying, now between an Ann and Dowben's Mary. She sat on the floor, hidden by the other beds, and looked at her scarred arm. The tissue would have no feeling, the burn do no good. She began to start a new place, moving the burning cigarette to put it out against undeadened flesh. As it came closer she felt the warmth of it, the heat, the burn. The first singe of hair brought a red-hot stab with it so that she jerked her arm away, astonished.

"It was a reflex!" she said incredulously to the bedrail. She tried again and again, but at every place, a burning hot pain prevailed upon instinct and she had to pull away from the burn before it had even closed upon the flesh. She put out the cigarette against the bed-leg and said aloud in Yri:

"To all gods and Collects of all the worlds: No more burnings and no more fires, for I seem to begin to be bound—" She had begun to cry because of the terror and joy of it, *"I seem to begin to be bound to this world...."*

When it was time *to* see Furii, she ran to her office, terrifying her tracker, and burst in to the beginning of the session. "Hey! You know what happens when you burn yourself? You get burnt, that's what! And it has a hurt called a burn, that's what!"

"You burned yourself again?" Furii asked, drawing away the smile with which she had answered Deborah's.

"I tried to, but I couldn't."

"Oh?"

"Because it *hurt!*"

"Oh, I'm glad!" They smiled at each other. Then Furii saw the tracker behind Deborah and asked her why she was with her and was told. When the nurse left to wait outside, Furii gave the quizzical look that Deborah knew and had winced at long in advance of its coming.

"I always had warnings before—an explanation of why it was going to happen-"

"Maybe 'it' knew that you needed help. You were in calling distance of that help, but you didn't dare ask for it outright, lest it be refused."

"But the oncoming was so sudden and severe. How can I be getting any better at all when it is so sudden and complete?"

"These defenses against getting well and casting with the world are at their last barricades. Of course, there is a desperation to save everything that can be saved of your sickness."

Deborah told her about the school, how frightened she had been and how despairing at the thought of three years inside the town's vast silence, and how she had thought that it was predecided, the lock-step-lock of being a victim. She came to the part about meeting the social worker and hearing her suggestion, the sudden release of forgiveness and hope, and how she had sat down with "the bends" and been overwhelmed without warning. As she described the oncoming of the Pit, it struck her that there had been a change in it. "Something ... funny,"

"What, funny?"

"Well, Yr used to be the logical and understandable place, and the world, the anarchic thing. There were sets of formulas to help in the escape. They got more and more elaborate, but always...they were predictable...."

"Well?"

"Well, when I began to have the world, it was as if Yr said, 'We'll take the other way of it, whatever it is.' When the world was without logic or law, Yr was the place with form and caused effects. When the world began to be the rational one, Yr stopped giving reasons at all."

"Yes," said Furii gently, as she did when she wanted to remonstrate without an overtone of anger. "When will you stop straddling these two worlds?"

"I'm not ready yet!" Deborah shouted.

"All right," Furii said mildly, "but you will never be able to grasp the world really, with all of its advantages, until you relinquish your double allegiance."

The wind of panic beat over Deborah and her heart began to rattle with it. She called silently to Anterrabae and he came, fleet and reassuring to her. *Suffer, Victim.* (The familiar Yri greeting.)

Is it true that you bring me beauty lately only when you are threatened? she asked him, waiting for his sardonic half-smile. He did not give it, but winced instead.

Pity me.

She was thrown by the surprise of this action. *Of what do you suffer?*

Of burning.

But you are not consumed.

When you were exalted and beyond the range of human fire, I was also. Since the flames burn you, they burn me also. He breathed in again, sharply, and she saw the upward planes of his face as they were lit by his fire, shining with sweat and tears. *Oh!* she cried out for him, so that he turned his eyes toward her again.

You see—you endure and share with me. We are of a voice, of a look. Could you ever hope or imagine to be so sharing with anyone of earth? And he made the gesture of turmoil and renunciation that was Yri hand-language for the world.

"Where have you gone?" Furii was asking. "Take me with you."

"I was with Anterrabae. He's right. The world may have law and logic, even if it is dangerous and twisted sometimes. It has challenge, too, and things I don't know to learn, like mathematics, which the gods can't teach me, but where else"—and here her eyes suddenly filled with tears—-"where else is there the sharing that I have with them?'"

"What are those tears?" Furii asked, still very softly. Deborah looked at her and recognized the opening words of their formula, hers and Furii's. She had to smile.

"Of ten units; four self-pity, three what Yr calls 'the Hard Rind' and one desperation."

"That is only eight." (Still the formula.)

"And two miscellaneous."

They smiled again. "You see," Furii said, "it can be as clear between the two of us as with your gods. I never hid my nature, but sometimes you forget that I am and have always been a representative of and a fighter with you for this present world." And she blew her nose as if to show how typical a member of the world she was. "What is that which you call 'the Hard Rind'?"

"Well, when I first came to the hospital I was not unhappy. I didn't care about anything and that had a kind of peace about it. Then you made me care and as soon as I did, Yr punished me and I got desperate with it. When I begged for mercy from Yr, Anterrabae said, 'You have eaten down hope from the red to the rind.' I thought that I would have to live and watch that old rind shrivel up and get hard and be thrown away at last. He used that allusion now and then, and when I realized that I was alive, really alive and of the same substance as the world's inhabitants, I told him that I would chew that dry rind and keep chewing until it gave me nourishment. This time, when I was back and everybody was so disappointed in me, Anterrabae said, 'That hard rind is cracking your teeth—why not spit it out at last?' "

"And what do you feel about doing that?"

"I can't stop chewing now, even if I don't seem to be getting anything much," Deborah said. "Since I have the reflexes and instincts of a world one, I guess I'm stuck with it...," and she smiled sheepishly because it was an admission; it counted and someday she might have to hang from it.

If only I could tell her... , Furii thought. How do you tell someone born and raised in the desert what rich and fertile lands there are, just out of sight? Instead she said, "How is it going for you on the ward?"

"Well, of course the patients are mad at me, and the staff is kind of disappointed. I'm down to see Dr. Halle today."

"Oh, something special?"

"No ... I have to tell him to let the social worker know that it's still on with me, and that if it's okay with the people down at that place she mentioned, I'll be ready whenever they are."

REQUISITION

Date: Sept. 3   *Ward:* D
Patient: Blau, Deborah   *Ward Administrator:* Dr. Halle, H.L.
Items: *Date:*   *Time:*
         Sept. 5   8:30 a.m

     1 dress, suitable for city wear
     1 pr. hose
     1 pr. shoes
27 "clip-type" curlers
     1 coat
     1 tube lipstick
     $.80 suburban bus fare (for social worker and self)
     4 city bus tokens (for social worker and self)
The above to be requisitioned from patient's rooming house.

                 Signed:
                 H. L. Halle

Clinical and Systems Theory, Conceptual, and Historical Texts

3

Grob, G. N. (1991). *From asylum to community: mental health policy in modern America*. Princeton: Princeton University Press

Grob is the preeminent historian of mental illness and mental health in America. In this book, his third volume on "the ways in which American society [has] dealt with the human, social, and economic problems associated with mental illnesses" [p. xiii], he covers the 1940–1970 period of mental health care in the United States. We include an excerpt from Chapter 6, "Care and Treatment," breaking our own rule at the outset, but only this one time, by including an out-of-era classic. Grob's subject matter—the psychodynamic orientation of psychiatry and related developments at and after the end of World War II—is important in charting the transition from the end of our "pre-era" period to our 1954–1976 era of community psychiatry. Grob notes that the psychodynamic approach in psychiatry remained dominant over biological psychiatry at this time even in the face of a lack of evidence of its effectiveness. Psychodynamic psychiatry was absorbing influences from other fields, particularly the social sciences, and changes in the discipline, along with economic concerns over the cost of maintaining state hospitals and other factors, would lead, Grob writes, to a new community orientation for public psychiatry. Among other developments that Grob discusses are Harry Stack Sullivan's concern with the influence of interpersonal patterns and social factors on mental illness; the toxic and deadening atmosphere for patients of mental hospitals as documented by researchers such as H. Warren Dunman, Alfred H. Stanton, and Morris S. Schwartz; Maxwell Jones's therapeutic communities, a response to the dehumanizing environments of traditional mental hospitals (a movement influenced, Grob notes, by democratic concerns and ideals following the defeat of totalitarian enemies in World War II); and the realization that therapeutic communities would fail if the communities to which patients returned did not accept them as full-fledged members.

Care and Treatment

The psychodynamic orientation in the postwar era stood as a counterweight to somatic interpretations and the use of electroshock and psychosurgery—both approaches rested partly on situational differences. Psychodynamic psychiatry was associated with medical schools and private and community practices; somatic (or biological) psychiatry was generally (but not exclusively) linked with traditional mental hospitals. The demarcation line between the two, however, remained indistinct and shifting.

Psychodynamic and psychoanalytic psychiatrists were by no means a singular or unified group. Eclecticism was characteristic, and their interventions ranged from individual psychotherapy to various forms of socio- and environmental therapy. Because of the importance of war-related experiences, the initial emphasis was upon individual psychotherapy. The concept of psychotherapy, of course, was not of recent origin, although it was given concrete form in the twentieth century by such figures as Freud in Europe and Meyer in the United States. By World War II the term had come into common use. In 1938 the Association for the Advancement of Psychotherapy was founded by a group of European-born or trained eclectic psychoanalysts who wanted to expand contacts with other disciplines. Two years later Lewellys F. Barker of Johns Hopkins published a volume on the subject in which he defined psychotherapy as a treatment "that attempts to improve the condition of a human being by means of influences that are brought to bear upon his mind (psyche)." In 1947 the *American Journal of Psychotherapy* made its appearance. Psychotherapy, however, was not incompatible with somatic therapies, for structure and function were inseparable. Indeed, Barker noted that experimental work using mescaline and hashish to induce abnormal states of mind offered the prospect that in the future a part of psychotherapy might give way "to new forms of chemotherapy."[18]

Despite its attractiveness, psychotherapy presented intellectual and practical difficulties. That troubled individuals sought assistance and were often helped with their problems by others—lay as well as professional—was a truism. All human beings, after all, require assurance and assistance at various points in their lives. Given its medical context, however, psychotherapy had to involve more than mere human contact and understanding. To delineate the medical features that distinguished this therapy—either in theory or practice—was a formidable task. Many of those making the effort often employed vague language and concepts. The APA's Committee on Psychotherapy (whose members included Harry Stack Sullivan and Oskar Diethelm) conceded in 1944 that "some of the medical thinking about psychotherapy can scarcely be generalized" but insisted that psychiatry was in the midst of "a progressive simplification of theoretic formulae and corresponding increasingly precise and definable types of interaction of physician and patient."[19]

Wartime experiences seemed to confirm the effectiveness of psychotherapy in dealing with stress-related neuropsychiatric symptoms. Whether or not such experiences were an analogue for its use in alternative settings or with other kinds of patients was problematical. There was virtually no agreement on methods or techniques. Moreover, data demonstrating efficacy were virtually nonexistent. Joseph Wilder, an avowed proponent of psychotherapy, conceded as much in a study published in 1945. "Psychotherapeutic statistics are based on different standards," he observed. Available data ignored such categories as spontaneous remissions, demographic variables like age, the possible presence of organic disease, and duration of treatment. Diagnostic categories were imprecise, and follow-up studies nonexistent. "Shrouded in the mystery of the psychotherapist's office, its evaluation is left to the two parties least suited to express objective judgment: the patient and the psychotherapist." For hospitalized patients the situation was equally murky. Even though many patients received little or no treatment in the usual meaning of the word, there were serious reasons "to believe that for many cases hospitalization in itself represents a treatment." Cognizant of profound methodological difficulties, Wilder nevertheless insisted that "a scientific evaluation of psychotherapeutic results simply must be made."[20]

Psychotherapy, of course, became one of the most widely acclaimed psychiatric interventions of the postwar era. It was offered by a multiplicity of professional groups, including psychiatrists and nonpsychiatric physicians, irregular practitioners such as chiropractors and naturopaths, clinical psychologists, social workers, marriage counselors, rehabilitation and vocational counselors, parole officers, clergymen, and others. Its popularity grew out of a fortuitous combination of circumstances: the rise of private and community practice in psychiatry; the general receptivity toward psychological explanations; an economic prosperity that created a middle-class clientele able to pay for and eager to use psychological services; favorable clinical results; and the general popularization of Freudian theories. Although psychotherapy was widely used in a few select private institutions—notably at the Menninger Foundation and Chestnut Lodge[21]—it was more often employed in the treatment of noninstitutionalized psychoneurotic individuals capable of functioning independently. "The pattern of psycho therapeutic practice in America," wrote Jerome D. Frank, an eminent psychiatrist at Johns Hopkins, "is seriously imbalanced in that too many of the ablest, most experienced psychiatrists spend most of their time with patients who need them least." Affluent and well-educated persons were the most numerous candidates for psychotherapy, whereas "lower class, seriously ill patients" received the least attention even though they constituted "by far the greater challenge."[22] For psychiatrists in private or community practice, psychotherapy was generally the treatment of choice; somatic therapies such as lobotomy or shock were rarely employed.

Beneath the surface, however, lurked elements of doubt. "I...have been trying to get an adequate definition of psychotherapy," Daniel Blain told Marion E. Kenworthy in 1946, "and, in a broad manner of speaking, for the word therapy itself, attempting to combat the tendency to use therapy in terms of every type of influence on the patient." Psychotherapy, admitted Leo Bartemeier in his APA presidential address in 1952, "still remains a rather vague concept." A year later Jules H. Masserman, a distinguished psychoanalyst and psychiatrist, suggested that psychotherapy might be nothing more than the institutionalization of certain delusions that were "so essential in protecting us against harsh reality that existing without them would be as excruciatingly unbearable as existing without our skin." He was especially critical of gross misunderstandings and popularizations of technique even among better-educated groups. Masserman recounted his tongue-in-cheek lecture on "The Psychosomatic Profile of an Ingrown Toe Nail" before a group of internists. The toenail, he told his audience, is the most protuberant part of the body, hard and rounded; in locomotion it describes a most suggestive to-and-fro movement—obviously, then, it is a basic penile symbol displaced, for a change, downward. But let us also remember the anatomic origin of this important little phallus, namely the *nail-bed* ... a region consummately feminine in its conformation, physiology, and import.... . But now consider what happens when this normal functioning is disrupted by frustration and conflict: when, specifically, the erect nail is stubbed and traumatized, or is too long opposed by unyielding reality in the form of a repressive shoe. Clinically and perhaps personally we know the effects all too well: the nail, particularly at the peripheral portions of its individuality (or more technically, its "ego boundaries") turns about and digs its way back into the flesh of its origin.

Masserman was chagrined when he was congratulated for his "clinical and analytic perspicacity" in illuminating "the etiology and possible therapy of that hitherto unexplored psychosomatic disorder—onychocryptosis, or ingrown toenail." Nor were doubts absent among psychologists. At the Conference on Graduate Education in Clinical Psychology in 1949 a facetious but revealing statement was made: "Psychotherapy is an undefined technique applied to unspecified problems with unpredictable outcome. For this technique we recommend rigorous training." The protean nature of the term was evident in its myriad forms, which included brief, depth, multiple, social, and group psychotherapy.[23]

Humorous characterizations notwithstanding, psychotherapy presented formidable intellectual and philosophical problems. At its most basic level it involved complex human relationships that could not be easily disaggregated into smaller and presumably more manageable components. It was possible to describe such emotions as love and hate in purely physiological terms (e.g., blood pressure), but to do so in all probability vitiated, if not destroyed, their holistic meaning. Equally significant, psychotherapy brought together a subject and a therapist, and their interaction introduced a new variable. Psychotherapy, therefore, involved more than technique, and to distinguish among its different forms and to measure their respective effectiveness posed a difficult, if not insoluble, challenge.

The absence of serious evaluative research did not go unnoticed. Lawrence S. Kubie noted that members of the National Research Council's Committee on Neuropsychiatry and Sub-Committee on Psychiatry included respected figures. Few of them, he added, had "experimental experience" in psychotherapy. The indiscriminate admixture of neurologists and psychiatrists inhibited any genuine scientific investigation of the subject. "1 am not bitter about any of this," Kubie told a colleague.

> It should be a sobering thought to you and all medical educators and Foundation directors that in spite of all of the money that has been poured into American psychiatry during the last 50 years, not a single one of the major psychiatric developments has come from this country. We are surrounded by great and expensive monuments to predictable and in many instances predicted failure: the Phipps, the Payne Whitney, the New York Psychiatric Institute, the Institute of Human Relations, the MGH, etc., etc. Must we go on repeating old follies as these two committees seem bent on doing?

A decade later Benjamin Pasamanick, a noted psychiatrist, observed that too many of his colleagues were more interested in the process than the outcome of psychotherapy. Consequently, relatively little was known about its efficacy, which inhibited efforts to improve current practices."[24]

At a more fundamental level the deficiency of outcome studies was but a reflection of the complexity of the therapy itself. Psychotherapy was not a standardized intervention; innumerable variables had the potential to influence the process. Even control-group studies, as Frank—a noted authority—pointed out, necessitated contacts with the control subjects themselves, contacts that vitiated the precise measurement of any outcome. He also emphasized that the effectiveness of psychotherapy was limited by unmodifiable environmental stresses (e.g., serious illness of family member, stresses arising from racism) and internally set limitations (e.g., biological deficiencies, deeply ingrained maladaptive patterns). The clinician's dilemma, Frank noted in his classic study *Persuasion and Healing* (1961), was that the "practice of psychotherapy cannot wait until research has yielded a solid basis for it." He insisted that virtually all psychotherapies involved persuasion and the restoration of hope. Their effectiveness, he concluded, "may be due to those features that all have in common rather than to those that distinguish them from each other."[25]

The deliberations at the first Conference on Research in Psychotherapy in 1958, sponsored by the American Psychological Association, were also revealing. Though much research had been done, noted Morris B. Parloff and Eli A. Rubenstein in their summation comments, "there has been relatively little progress in establishing a firm and substantial body of evidence to support very many research hypotheses." The most sustained criticism came from Hans J. Eysenck, an influential British psychologist. In exhaustive reviews of research during the 1950s, Eysenck insisted that the therapeutic effects of psychotherapy were "small or non-existent, and do not in any demonstrable way increase the rate of recovery over that of a comparable group which receives no treatment at all."[26]

The difficulties of evaluation were dramatically illustrated in the Menninger Foundation's Psychotherapy Research Project, one of the most detailed and sophisticated longitudinal studies ever undertaken. Begun in 1954 and spanning several decades, the project focused on forty-two adult patients who had entered therapy between 1954 and 1958. The conclusions were scarcely revolutionary: the investigators found that a patient's ego was the critical variable in success or failure, and that psychoanalytic therapy was inapplicable to psychotics. Equally significant, project personnel developed an appreciation of the immense complexities involved in developing a methodology to evaluate the psychotherapeutic process. The majority of their publications, as a matter of fact, dealt with the barriers that impeded scientific measurement of psychotherapy.[27]

The psychodynamic orientation of American psychiatrists also heightened interest in environmentally oriented interventions. In brief, many psychiatrists developed a sensitivity to the possible role of environmental modifications as a means of treating mentally ill individuals. Of all the approaches that were popular after 1945, "milieu therapy" had the greatest potential to impact upon the lives of tens, if not hundreds, of thousands of severely mentally ill individuals confined in mental hospitals.

The idea that institutionalization could have serious consequences for the patient was by no means novel. Early nineteenth-century mental hospital superintendents had developed "moral treatment" or "moral management"—a therapeutic system that rested on the belief that the institutional environment could be used to reeducate patients in a proper moral atmosphere. Moral treatment, of course, grew out of an entirely different context: many of its basic tenets were derived from religious sources.[28] The change in the nature of the patient population and the emergence of the mental hospital as an institution providing care for geriatric cases and individuals suffering from organically based disorders—groups with little hope of recovery—had dealt the therapeutic ideal a severe setback; by World War II the custodial character of mental hospitals was self-evident.

After 1945 interest in using the institution as a possible therapeutic tool reemerged. Even before World War II Dexter Billiard experimented with new therapies at Chestnut Lodge Sanitarium (a small private psychoanalytically oriented institution in Maryland). He persuaded Frieda Fromm-Reichmann to join the staff and employ psychoanalytic techniques in working with psychotic patients, and he encouraged Harry Stack Sullivan to continue his work at the hospital.[29] In many respects Sullivan played a key role during the interwar years. He altered the traditional preoccupation of psychiatry with the individual;

his theory of interpersonal relations shifted the focus to interpersonal phenomena, relationships between people, and the social context of behavior. As early as 1930 Sullivan
admitted "that it would be a very difficult proposition to show wherein psychiatry is more
of a medical than a social science." Personality, he wrote in 1938, "is made manifest in
interpersonal situations, and not otherwise." Sullivan's close relationships with members
of the Chicago School of Sociology (which shaped the discipline in these years) ultimately
transformed both psychiatry and the social sciences. More than any other figure, Sullivan
paved the way for the collaboration of psychiatry and social science, and thus facilitated
the emergence of socially oriented therapies after World War II.[30]

Unlike the theory of moral management, the concept of milieu therapy (or therapeutic
community) was overwhelmingly secular in its origins. The concept of the therapeutic
community was partly rooted in psychodynamic psychiatry. If mental disorders had some
environmental etiology, might it not follow logically that environmental modifications
could play a therapeutic role? Certainly the leading psychodynamic psychiatrists of these
years all shared a common belief in the importance of the milieu for therapy.

An equally important contribution came from social and behavioral scientists. Their
long-standing preoccupation with the role and function of institutions, interest in the
mediating influence of culture and social structure on personality, and environmental and
activist ideological orientation were approaches that promoted interest in mental illnesses.
During the 1940s and 1950s the social and behavioral science emphasis on the social
and cultural roots of behavior became even more pronounced. Bruno Bettelheim's classic
analysis of behavior in Nazi concentration camps anticipated a variety of investigations of
other kinds of institutions, including mental hospitals.[31] The impact on American psychiatry was dramatic. Postwar changes within academic disciplines in particular and higher
education in general, together with a confident and expansive psychodynamic psychiatry,
created an environment conducive to cross-disciplinary cooperation between psychiatry
and the social and behavioral sciences—a development that rapidly became the norm
rather than the exception.

The concept of the mental hospital as a potential therapeutic community was given concrete meaning by Maxwell Jones, a British psychiatrist. During World War II Jones worked
with servicemen who had developed neuropsychiatric symptoms during combat as well as
with repatriated prisoners of war. He found that group discussions with mutual feedback
involving patients and staff assisted the former to view their symptoms more objectively,
gain insight, and thus improve sufficiently to return either to their units or to their communities. "In a limited sense," he later recalled, "the treatment was being carried on by the
patients in collaboration with the staff."[32]

These experiences led to the establishment at Belmont Hospital in 1947 of what subsequently became known as the Social Rehabilitation Unit. Belmont was a traditional inpatient institution that admitted neurotic and early psychotic patients. The average stay was
four to six months, although some remained up to one year. In the new unit the multidisciplinary staff and one hundred patients met daily for an hour, and smaller group meetings
were not uncommon. The result was the creation of a "therapeutic culture" that encouraged communication. Patients gained insight and psychiatrists were "taught to speak the
patient's language." The lesson to Jones and his associates was clear. Personality disorders
resulted from adverse environmental factors. Hence a therapeutic community, organized
along democratic and permissive lines, inhibited the reproduction of hostile or repressive
responses from society normally anticipated by patients, who, in turn, altered their behavior. It was thus possible, Jones reported in his influential volume, *Social Psychiatry* (1952),
"to change social attitudes in relatively desocialized patients with severe character disorders, provided they are treated together in a therapeutic community." The work of Jones

and his colleagues, therefore, unerringly led to a heightened appreciation of the impact of the hospital on the individual patient and the possibility of employing the hospital community "as an active force in treatment."[33]

Even as Jones was popularizing the concept of the hospital as a therapeutic community, multidisciplinary teams in the United States were already studying the mental hospital as a social system and the implications for patient care and treatment. One of the earliest was undertaken by H. Warren Dunham, coauthor of an important ecological analysis published in 1935 *(Mental Disorders in Urban Areas)*. Dunham arranged with Ohio officials to launch a detailed analysis of the mental hospital as "a special kind of community experience." Completed in 1948, the full study was not published until 1960. Nevertheless, some early articles indicated its basic thrust. In a brief piece in the *American Journal of Psychiatry* in 1948, Dunham and a psychiatric associate reported that the interpersonal relationships and group dynamics of employees and patients created an institutional culture that only aggravated the latter's "existing personality conflicts." Patient welfare was often subordinated to institutional needs. Only when the existing social organization was broken and reoriented in ways compatible with therapy, they concluded, would the situation change.[34]

By the early 1950s an extensive multidisciplinary literature focusing on the hospital as a social organization had appeared in psychiatric as well as social and behavioral science professional journals. In a comprehensive summary, Charlotte Schwartz identified nearly two hundred items, most of which were published between 1945 and 1952. Their authors emphasized not only the treatment of disease per se, but also the need to employ a holistic approach that took into account all of the relevant social and emotional factors relating to mental illnesses. Psychiatric exclusiveness had clearly begun to give way to a multidisciplinary approach that required the integration of sociological, anthropological, and medical knowledge in order to develop a total treatment program. Such a program recognized the significance of the environment, interpersonal relationships, and the social needs of patients. Irrespective of disciplinary affiliation, virtually every researcher found that the attitudes and outlook of staff and patients played a key role in outcome. Understanding the complex elements that shaped the character of mental hospitals, in turn, led to a search for methods and techniques that were effective in promoting meaningful change. Optimistic that new multidisciplinary findings would illuminate the roots of existing problems, researchers were not unmindful of the substantial barriers that impeded beneficial innovations, including the traditional inertia of established routines within institutions and professional fears, as well as the lack of adequate funding.[35]

The concept of the therapeutic community gained new momentum with the publication of a series of volumes in the mid- and late 1950s that reached a wide audience. Most of these studies resulted from collaborations between two kinds of professionals: psychiatrists familiar with the behavior and outlook of patients, and social scientists sensitive to the complexities of social organizations and better trained in research design and methods. One of the first and most influential was Alfred H. Stanton's and Morris S. Schwartz's *The Mental Hospital,* published in 1954. Stanton, a psychiatrist, and Schwartz, a sociologist, designed an intensive two-year sociopsychiatric study of a disturbed ward at Chestnut Lodge. The administration and psychiatric staff at this small psychoanalytically oriented institution provided sympathetic support. The two investigators found that the hospital successfully protected the public and minimally met patient needs but was less effective in "bringing about lasting improvement." Many of the administrative, therapeutic, and nursing procedures reflected the needs of staff rather than patients. The authors' study of administration and interoccupational conflicts led to the observation that staff procedures and attitudes contributed to the maintenance of chronic patterns of behavior. Stanton and

Schwartz thus posed a direct challenge to the paternalistic character of Chestnut Lodge, for they emphasized that patients were active participants rather than passive observers even though their influence was not always visible or self-evident. Possessing different characteristics, mental hospitals still tended to emulate the authoritarian structure of general hospitals and thus failed to create a therapeutic environment. The proposition that patient-staff interaction shaped outcomes, they insisted, had to be a guiding principle in organizing mental hospitals. Their work pointed in the direction of a more democratically organized and participatory institution.[36]

The Stanton-Schwartz study was quickly followed by the publication of another significant work by Milton Greenblatt and his colleagues. With the support and encouragement of the Russell Sage Foundation, three Bay State institutions—the Boston Psychopathic Hospital, the Bedford VA Hospital, and the Metropolitan State Hospital in Waltham—designed a joint and collaborative experiment to improve institutional care that involved patients as well as the entire staff. Traditional means of control—seclusion, restraint (mechanical and chemical)—virtually disappeared; the physical environment was made more attractive; socialization therapies—games, music, work, entertainment—became common; patient self-government was encouraged; the therapeutic potential of personnel was fostered; teaching and research opened new possibilities; and close relationships with the community were institutionalized. The combination of intensive physiological treatments (shock, lobotomy, and drug) and environmental changes seemed to have dramatic results. Intensive treatment "necessitated longer stays and fewer cases; yet more patients were treated, more improved, and more were discharged than ever before." Equally striking, the discharge rate to the community in all diagnostic categories rose, "suggesting that no diagnostic label necessarily indicated that a patient had a black future." "The prognosis for the future of psychiatric hospitals," concluded Esther L. Brown and Greenblatt, "is hopeful.... With prompt and intensive treatment provided through the somatic therapies, including chemotherapy, individual and group psychotherapy, and the therapeutic use of the social environment, a large proportion of patients admitted to psychiatric hospitals can return to the community within a relatively brief period."[37]

The argument on behalf of such optimism was further elaborated by Otto von Mering, an anthropologist at the University of Pittsburgh School of Medicine. With the support of the Russell Sage Foundation, Mering visited about thirty institutions that were seeking to alter their traditional custodial role. Too many hospitals, Mering reported, casually accepted what he described as "The Legend of Chronicity," which justified therapeutic passivity toward withdrawn, passive, and hostile patients with no hope of recovery. Yet some institutions were in the process of demonstrating that effective alternatives existed. The primary features of what Mering termed "social remotivation" included the acceptance of the patient "as a worthwhile individual, capable of improvement, regardless of the degree of observable deterioration," and able to take an active role in therapy.

> Social mobilization seeks to mobilize the entire ward routine and program for therapeutic ends. Once the patient has been accepted as worthwhile and as having potential for growth, the daily activities of ward life can take on new meaning.... Thus, the social milieu of the ward is mobilized to bring out latent energies toward health, reinforce them through a series of social rewards, looking toward an improved hospital adjustment or eventual return to the community.

In short, improved interpersonal relationships had the potential to alter traditional institutional environments and foster more promising outcomes.[38]

During the latter half of the 1950s multidisciplinary works describing and analyzing the mental hospital in sociological and anthropological terms proliferated. The context and specific subject matter differed, but their underlying methodology and conclusions were remarkably similar. Ivan Belknap's study of a large southern state hospital emphasized the authoritarian and coercive nature of the internal social structure, which militated against effective therapy, William Caudill analyzed the mental hospital in terms of a total social system whose character was shaped by broad historical circumstances over long periods of time. "One of the brightest stars in the social psychiatric firmament," wrote Robert N. Rapoport in 1960, "is the 'therapeutic community idea. According to this approach, the hospital is not seen as a place where patients are classified and stored, nor a place where one group of individuals (the medical staff) gives treatment to another group of individuals (the patients) according to the model of general medical hospitals; but as a place which is organized as a community in which everyone is expected to make some contribution towards the shared goals of creating a social organization that will have healing properties."[39]

Whatever the specifics, it is clear that the concept of the therapeutic community stood as the obverse of the traditional mental hospital. The former was based on the proposition that patients as well as staff had to take active participatory roles in the therapeutic process; the latter reflected an authoritarian ideology that fostered dependency and actually strengthened pathological symptoms characteristic of the mental illnesses. The emphasis on the therapeutic community was in some ways related to the postwar proclivity to interpret social reality in terms of a perennial struggle of democracy and freedom on the one hand and authoritarianism on the other. Indeed, the reaction against authoritarianism was fostered, if not led, by European-born emigre scholars with firsthand knowledge of Nazism, and by their American counterparts who had served in the military or government during the war. Their experiences facilitated the incorporation of an activist democratic ideology into social and behavioral science theory. Postwar social and behavioral science and psychiatric thinking emphasized the proposition that freedom and democracy, when applied in a setting that promoted participation on more or less equal terms, led to responsible and mature behavior, whereas authoritarian patterns simply reinforced apathy and dependency.[40] The ideology of the therapeutic community also drew part of its inspiration from the optimism of these years; its creators and supporters assumed that administrative and organizational change could lead to the creation of an internal environment conducive to patient recovery. It was hardly surprising that the emphasis on the therapeutic community during the 1950s also led to the rediscovery of the early nineteenth-century formulation of moral treatment and insistence that cure was possible.[41]

Advocates of milieu therapy quickly recognized that their efforts would be in vain if communities were unwilling to accept former mental patients. They therefore moved to blur the demarcation between the hospital and community by creating what in the mid-1950s had become known as the open-door hospital, which had been popularized by T. P. Rees and other British psychiatrists. Advocates of the concept in Britain and the United States believed that the isolation and prisonlike antitherapeutic character of traditional mental hospitals could be altered through the elimination of such features as locked doors and fences. The open-door hospital, like the therapeutic community, represented an institutional deviation. Moreover, supporters of the open-door concept also believed that psychiatric services had to be integrated along an unbroken continuum to ease the release of patients into the community; a range of services was required to meet the needs of a diverse population requiring psychiatric and psychological assistance. An open-door policy and experimentation with novel institutional forms (e.g., the day hospital where patients were treated during the day and returned to their homes in the evening, and the night hospital) would allay public suspicions and mistrust and would facilitate the gradual movement of patients between institutions and communities. "Continuity of care," a New York State legislator observed, "is the heart of the open hospital system" and required the complete integration of psychiatric services—"pre-care, hospital care and after-care." In effect, the open-door, day, and night hospitals represented the fusion of the postwar emphasis on community care with the principles of milieu therapy.[42]

References

18. Joseph Wilder, "Twenty-Five Years of the Association for the Advancement of Psychotherapy," *American Journal of Psychotherapy*, 18 (1964): 452–57; "Editorial," ibid., 1 (1947): 125–28; Lewellys F. Barker, *Psychotherapy* (New York, 1940), 2, 181–82. See also Barker's article "Psychotherapy—A Modern Medical Science," *American Scholar*, 11 (1942): 201–7.
19. *AJP*, 101 (1944): 266.
20. Wilder, "Facts and Figures on Psychotherapy," *Journal of Clinical Psychopathology and Psychotherapy*, 7 (1945): 311–47.
21. See Harold Maine, "We Can Save the Mentally Sick," *Saturday Evening Post*, 220 (1947): 20–21, 160, 162, 165–66, and *If a Man Be Mad* (Garden City, N.Y., 1947). Lawrence J. Friedman's *Menninger: The Family and the Clinic* (New York, 1990) provides detailed descriptions and analyses of one of the nation's most important postwar psychiatric institutions.
22. Jerome D. Frank, *Persuasion and Healing: A Comparative Study of Psychotherapy* (Baltimore, 1961), 11–13, 231–32.
23. Daniel Blain to Marion E. Kenworthy, Nov. 12, Kenworthy to Blain, Nov. 12, 1946, Kenworthy Papers, AP; Leo H. Bartemeier, "Presidential Address," *AJP*, 109 (1952): 1–7; D. Ewen Cameron, "Postgraduate Instruction in Psychotherapy in the University," *Journal of the Association of American Medical Colleges*, 25 (1950): 338–44; Jules H. Masserman, "Faith and Delusion in Psychotherapy," *AJP*, 110 (1953): 324–33; Samuel H. Hadden, "Historic Background of Group Psychotherapy," *International Journal of Group Psychotherapy*, 5 (1955): 162–68; American Psychological Association, Conference on Research in Psychotherapy, *Proceedings*, 1 (1958): 292.
24. Kubie to Lewis Weed, Apr. 14, WCM to Kubie, June 20, 1950, WCM Papers, MFA; Albert Deutsch interview with Benjamin Pasamanick, May 10, 1960, Deutsch Papers, APAA.
25. Frank, "Problems of Controls in Psychotherapy as Exemplified by the Psychotherapy Research Project of the Phipps Psychiatric Clinic," in Conference on Research in Psychotherapy, *Proceedings*, 1 (1958): 10–26, and *Persuasion and Healing*, 223, 231–32.
26. Parloff and Rubenstein, "Research Problems in Psychotherapy," Conference on Research in Psychotherapy, *Proceedings*, 1 (1958): 292; Hans J. Eysenck, "The Effects of Psychotherapy: An Evaluation," *Journal of Consulting Psychology*, 16 (1952): 319–23, and "The Effects of Psychotherapy," *International Journal of Psychiatry*, 1 (1965): 99–144 (see also the discussion by various individuals on 144–78); Herbert J. Cross, "The Outcome of Psychotherapy: A Selected Analysis of Research Findings," *Journal of Consulting Psychology*, 28 (1964): 413–17. Eysenck's "The Effects of Psychotherapy," cited above, contains a lengthy bibliography on the subject (138–42). See also American Psychological Association, Conference on Research in Psychotherapy, *Proceedings*, 2–3 (1961–1966).
27. The Menninger Foundation's Psychotherapy Research Project generated numerous publications. The most detailed summary was Robert Wallerstein's *Forty-Two Lives in Treatment: A Study of Psychoanalysis and Psychotherapy* (New York, 1986). For a history of the project, see Friedman, *Menninger*, 287–89.
28. For varying interpretations of moral treatment, see Norman Dain, *Concepts of Insanity in the United States 1789–1865* (New Brunswick, N.J., 1964); David Rothman, *The Discovery of the Asylum: Social Order and Disorder in the New Republic* (Boston, 1971); Gerald N. Grob, *Mental Institutions in America: Social Policy to 1875* (New York, 1973); Nancy Tomes, *A Generous Confidence: Thomas Story Kirkbride and the Art of Asylum-Keeping,*

1840–1883 (New York, 1984); and Constance McGovern, *Masters of Madness: Social Origins of the American Psychiatric Profession* (Hanover, N.H., 1985).

29. Dexter M. Bullard, "The Organization of Psychoanalytic Procedure in the Hospital," *Journal of Nervous and Mental Disease*, 91 (1940): 697–703; Robert A. Cohen, "The Hospital as a Therapeutic Instrument," *Psychiatry*, 21 (1958): 29.

30. Helen S. Perry, *Psychiatrist of America: The Life of Harry Stack Sullivan* (Cambridge, Mass., 1982), 258; Sullivan, "The Data of Psychiatry," *Psychiatry*, 1 (1938): 121, reprinted in *The Fusion of Psychiatry and Social Science* (New York, 1964), 31–55. See especially Sullivan's article, "A Note on the Implications of Psychiatry, the Study of Interpersonal Relations, for Investigations in the Social Sciences," *American Journal of Sociology*, 42 (1937): 848–61, reprinted in *The Fusion of Psychiatry and Social Science*, 15–29.

31. Bruno Bettelheim, "Individual and Mass Behavior in Extreme Situations," *Journal of Abnormal and Social Psychology*, 38 (1943): 417–52. See also Bettelheim and E. Sylvester, "A Therapeutic Milieu," *American Journal of Orthopsychiatry*, 18 (1948): 191–206, and Bettelheim, *Love Is Not Enough* (Glencoe, Ill., 1950).

32. Jones, "The Treatment of Personality Disorders in a Therapeutic Community," *Psychiatry*, 20 (1957): 212–13. See also Milton and M. Silverman, "Asylums without Bars," *Saturday Evening Post*, 231 (Oct. 25, 1958): 110.

33. Jones, "Treatment of Personality Disorders in a Therapeutic Community," 213–17; idem, *The Therapeutic Community: A New Treatment Method in Psychiatry* (New York, 1953), 156–57 (this work was first published in England under the title *Social Psychiatry*). See also Deutsch's interview with Jones and Harry Wilmer, Aug. 29, 1959, Deutsch Papers, APAA.

34. J. Fremont Bateman and H. Warren Dunham, "The State Mental Hospital as a Specialized Community Experience," *AJP*, 105 (1948): 445–48. See also *Bulletin of the Menninger Clinic*, 10 (1946): 65–100, which contains a series of articles by British psychiatrists dealing with what subsequently became known as the therapeutic community concept. The book-length study by Dunham and S. K. Weinberg was based on data collected at Columbus State Hospital in 1946 and completed in 1948. By the time that it was published in 1960, its methodology and conclusions were commonplace, given the appearance of other institutional studies during the 1950s. Essentially, Dunham and Weinberg argued that the employee culture that shaped the institution was directed toward "the complete subjection and control of patients" (249). Patients, on the other hand, created their own culture to facilitate their adjustment to hospital life and their eventual release. Most therapies had meager results precisely because they were interwoven with the institutional culture. A dramatic change in the cultural climate was essential if recovery was to become the hospital's primary goal. Dunham and Weinberg, *The Culture of the State Mental Hospital* (Detroit, 1960), chap. 12.

35. Charlotte G. Schwartz, *Rehabilitation of Mental Hospital Patients: Review of the Literature (Public Health Monograph No. 17*, issued as PHS *Publication* 297: 1953). See also the bibliography in Greenblatt et al., *From Custodial to Therapeutic Patient Care*, 431–84.

36. Alfred H. Stanton and Morris S. Schwartz, *The Mental Hospital: A Study of Institutional Participation in Psychiatric Illness and Treatment* (New York, 1954).

37. Greenblatt et al., *From Custodial to Therapeutic Patient Care*, passim (quotations from 237, 424).

38. Otto von Mering and Stanley H. King, *Remotivating the Mental Patient* (New York, 1957), 51.

39. Ivan Belknap, *Human Problems of a State Mental Hospital* (New York, 1956); William Caudill, *The Psychiatric Hospital as a Small Society* (Cambridge, Mass., 1958); Robert N. Rapoport, *Community as Doctor* (London, 1960), 10; Greenblatt, D. J. Levinson, and R. H. Williams, eds., *The Patient and the Mental Hospital* (Glencoe, Ill., 1957); Morris S. Schwartz and E. L. Shockley, *The Nurse and the Mental Patient: A Study in Interpersonal Relations* (New York, 1956). The literature on the therapeutic community is immense; the above-mentioned examples are only offered as illustrations. For a more extensive

bibliography listing relevant citations through the beginning of 1957, see Mering and King, *Remotivating the Mental Patient*, 201–7.

40. Cf. T. W. Adorno, E. Frenkel-Brunswik, D. J. Levinson, and R. N. Sanford, *The Authoritarian Personality* (New York, 1950).

41. See especially J. Sanbourne Bockoven, "Moral Treatment in American Psychiatry," *Journal of Nervous and Mental Disease*, 124 (1956): 167–94, 292–321; Greenblatt, *From Custodial to Therapeutic Patient Care*, 407–14; Earl D. Bond, "Therapeutic Forces in Early American Hospitals," *AJP*, 113 (1956): 407–8.

42. Bertram Mandelbrote, "An Experiment in the Rapid Conversion of a Closed Mental Hospital into an Open-Door Hospital," *Mental Hygiene*, 42 (1958): 3–16; George R. Metcalf, "The English Open Mental Hospital: Implications for American Psychiatric Services," *Milbank Memorial Fund Quarterly*, 39 (1961): 586; "Observations on the British 'Open' Hospitals," *Mental Hospitals*, 8 (1957): 5–9, 12, 14, 16; "Laying the Foundations for an Open Mental Hospital" and "Legal Implications of the Open Hospital" (discussions at the ninth APA Mental Hospital Institute in 1957), ibid., 9 (1958): 10–12, 24–26; Milbank Memorial Fund, *An Approach to the Prevention of Disability from Chronic Psychoses: The Open Mental Hospital within the Community* (New York, 1958); APA, *Proceedings of the 1958 Day Hospital Conference* (Washington, D.C., 1958).

4

Bockoven, J. S. (1956). Moral treatment in American psychiatry. *Journal of Nervous and Mental Diseases, 124, 167–194, 292–321*

Bockoven provides a historical review of psychiatry, institution-based care, and theory in the "moral treatment" of mental illness in America from the late eighteenth into the mid-nineteenth centuries. Moral treatment was characterized by a conviction that persons with mental illness required human contact and friendship, stimulating physical and intellectual activities, and hope. Bockoven draws upon available statistics and studies from the time to argue that moral treatment was highly successful in facilitating recovery from mental illness. Debate continues over the validity of this argument, including the degree to which the figures represent persons with serious and persistent mental illnesses as understood today. A later period of custodial care, with overcrowding in state hospitals, a loss of belief in the curability of mental illness, and an overreliance on brain disease explanations for mental illness spelled the end of moral treatment, but the approach, Bockoven contends, still has much to offer to mental health care in mid-twentieth century America. Moral psychiatry's emphases on friendship and social relationships, physical activity and meaningful work, and the importance of optimism and hope represent interesting parallels to elements of recovery-oriented approached in contemporary community mental health. It should be noted, though, that consistent with its era, moral treatment was more paternalistic, in the person of the hospital superintendent, than would be tolerated today in recovery-oriented practice. This excerpt from Bockoven's two-part article includes the opening section on the purpose of mental hospitals and historical background on the moral psychiatry era.

Moral Treatment in American Psychiatry

I. Mental Hospitals: The Problem of Fulfilling Their Purpose

What is a mental hospital? Is it a permanent home for the insane and no different from what used to be called an insane asylum? Is it a place where people go for operations or medicines which cure certain kinds of illnesses? Or is it a place where people go to talk with psychiatrists about disturbing personal problems? There is a currently growing volume of literature, both fiction and non-fiction, which seeks to elucidate the problems of individual failure and unhappiness by presenting them as understandable and solvable in terms of modern dynamic psychiatry. Science news reporters, on the other hand, have kept the average citizen up to date on the development of wonder drugs or other medical and surgical treatments which cure mental disorders.

It may well appear to the average citizen that there are many indications that medical science has already conquered or is very near conquering mental illness, but he also knows that from time to time the public press has a great deal to say about bad conditions in mental hospitals. The massive collection of brick buildings, isolated from the rest of the community, several miles from town is still an unknown entity to him. The sheer size and number of the buildings demonstrate that large numbers of people have to be kept locked up. This fact is difficult to reconcile with the indications that modern psychiatry knows how to cure mental illness. It serves to intensify the feeling of dread which has always been associated with the word asylum.

The typical mental hospital as it exists in America today can be better understood if described and discussed in much the same terms that one would use in telling about a place such as a resort hotel, a naval vessel, a military post or a university where he had lived for a period of time.

It is not inaccurate to say that the typical mental hospital impresses a visitor approaching its grounds as having something of the appealing quality of the typical college campus, with the exception that there are almost no people passing to and fro on the walks. The Administration Building, in particular, differs little from that of a college. Its interior has an appearance of good taste and dignity, but again it is strangely quiet, and surprisingly few people are in evidence.

It is not until one enters the wards where the patients live that one feels the impact of what it means to be a patient in a typical mental hospital. Contrary to one's expectations, ward after ward may be passed through without witnessing the violent, the grotesque, or the ridiculous. Instead, one absorbs the heavy atmosphere of hundreds of people doing nothing and showing interest in nothing. Endless lines of people sit on benches along the walls. Some have their eyes closed; others gaze fixedly at the floor or the opposite wall. Occasionally, a head is turned to look out a window or to watch someone coming back from the toilet to take his place on a bench. All and all, it is an innocuous scene characterized by inertness, listlessness, docility and utter hopelessness. Not so bad as might have been expected, one may think. Of course, there are worse wards where people lie on the floor naked and attendants are kept busy mopping up human excreta. Then there are those intrepid ones who approach the visitor and plead pathetically for him to intercede in their behalf to help them get out of the hospital. And then, again someone may pace the floor who mutters to himself and thereby breaks the monotony. Or there may be a sudden chill of excitement when someone breaks into angry shouting for no apparent reason at all.

The visitor may well feel restless and irritated by the apathy of the patients and their willingness to waste these hours of their lives in meaningless tedium. His irritation may lead to his asking questions. If so, he learns that the attendant is proud of the ward because it is quiet and no mishaps have occurred while he was on duty; because the floor is clean; because the patients are prompt and orderly in going to and from meals. The visitor finds that the scene which appalls him with the emptiness and pointlessness of human life is regarded by the attendant as good behavior on the part of the patients. This opinion, voiced by the attendant, introduces the visitor to the outlook of institutional psychiatry as it is practiced today. He may well be puzzled at their outlook, for there is little indication that it has anything to do with the psychiatry of current popular literature with its accent on hope and its accounts of enriching human life and showing the way to individual happiness. He must strain his imagination to see how the surrender of actually thousands of people to abject despair and inertia could possibly represent an improvement in their mental condition. On the contrary, he can envision himself going out of his mind if forced to spend many days in such a setting.

The more intimately acquainted a visitor becomes with the mental hospital, the sooner he reaches the final realization that it is engaged solely in the business of providing the physical needs and preserving the physical health and safety of rudderless, despairing people. He may come to admire the efficiency with which the basic operations of feeding, clothing, bathing and laundering are performed. But he will wonder at the absence not only of treatment in the psychiatric sense but of any regimen whatsoever that the average layman would regard as conducive to mental health. He will learn that every patient is examined by a physician and given a psychiatric diagnosis. He will also learn that some newly admitted patients receive electric shock. But he cannot escape the overwhelming fact that patients numbered in the thousands receive no treatment for their mental disorders.

If the visitor talks with the physician and asks questions, he may be told that no treatment has yet been discovered which will cure the vast majority of the patients. Another physician trained in modern dynamic psychiatry may tell him that most of the patients could be treated with psychotherapy but that there are no psychotherapists available. Still another may tell him that one-third to one-half of the patients no longer need to be in the hospital because their illness has subsided. They remain in the hospital, he says, because there is no place for them to go and no one will give them a job. The superintendent will more than likely tell him that the hospital is crowded with more patients than it was built to care for, and that the hospital is badly understaffed and in need of many more attendants, nurses, social workers and psychiatrists than the State budget provides or can be expected to provide. The visitor is then given to understand from the superintendent that the hospital as it is does not meet the needs of the patients, but the superintendent may also tell him that everything is being done for the patients that can be done in the way of cure of their mental illnesses.

The visitor can see for himself that the facts, as they stand, clearly indicate that the patients are dealt with by the hospital personnel on a collective mass basis and not as individuals. The patients are moved like an army from their sleeping quarters to their sitting places, to their eating places and back to their sitting places. Movement occurs only in connection with getting out of bed, eating, and going back to bed.

There are some exceptions, for a number of patients do work in the various service centers of the hospitals such as the kitchen and the laundry. Others may work on the hospital farm or on the hospital grounds. There may be other patients who are allowed out of doors to take a walk in the fresh air. And there may be a select few patients who go to the occupational therapy department, where they are taught to make something with their hands. But even those patients, who do more than spend their days sitting, show by their expressionless faces and reluctance to speak that they have become accustomed to loneliness.

From observation of the great mass of patients, the visitor cannot help but be impressed with their obedience and conformity to the wishes of the hospital authorities. "But why," he may ask, "would the authorities wish the patients to lead an inactive, uncommunicative, lonely existence?" The answer he finds is that it is necessary to prevent the patients from exciting one another and creating an unmanageable bedlam. The hospital authorities regard their chief objective to be protection of the patient from insane acts harmful to himself or others. All hospital personnel who come into contact with patients are taught to be constantly on the lookout for impending mishaps. They must also be on the alert to prevent the patients from getting hold of any article which might conceivably be used as a tool of destruction. Matches are not allowed, for a patient might set himself afire. Patients are not allowed to shave themselves lest they hide razor blades with which to cut their throats. Belts are not allowed lest patients hang themselves. Checker games are not allowed lest the patients attempt to swallow the checkers and choke. Every effort is made to prevent the recurrence of any dangerous act committed by any patient at any time in the past, and to anticipate any new way of committing one which might be invented in the future. (This might seem to rest on the theory that removal of all opportunity or occasion for insane acts or insane talk will eventually break the patient of insane habits and behavior.) The patients are handled as though their insanity were entirely due to an internal disorder and had nothing to do with the effects of external events on their emotions. Abuse of patients by personnel is strictly forbidden for obvious human reasons and not because it is thought that abuse has any effect on their illness.

There is total absence within the domain of the typical mental hospital of opportunity to participate in or give attention to any of the activities with which the members of any free community occupy themselves in some form or another. Patients have neither the materials nor the freedom of movement to develop their talents or acquire skills, nor to have the experiences of ordinary life. They have nothing in their current lives to exchange with one another, either in the realm of material objects or of observations, which is not a tedious repetition of something that is already known to all. There is also total absence of application of any of the principles of mental hygiene in the day to day program of living in the hospital. There is no work; there is no play; there is no program of living.

The forced non-participation in human affairs of the mentally ill would necessarily seem to be based on certain knowledge that the mentally ill are wholly lacking in social intelligence, are totally incapable of perceiving the rights of others and are completely unable to learn to be members of society. The extreme caution exercised in the control of patients must be based on some such assumptions. These assumptions are, of course, in accord with the concept that mental illnesses are malignant, irradicable diseases which totally destroy the capacity of the individual to behave like a human being or to be a person in any sense of the word.

One who visits the typical mental hospital will not find, however, that the hospital staff holds such a concept of mental illness. On the contrary, he will find that small scale endeavors are made to provide the patients with entertainments and recreational opportunities which recognize their sensibilities as persons. He will learn that the extreme caution and the stringent restrictions placed on the vast majority of the patients are practical necessities resulting from the limited resources of the hospital in terms of personnel and facilities with which to meet the needs of the huge number of patients. The hospital has, in short, barely sufficient resources to discharge the minimal responsibility of preserving the patients from physical injury.

The visitor may detect an enigma in the relation of the hospital to its source of financial support—the citizenry at large—which arises from a serious misunderstanding. The citizenry assumes that the medical specialists in diseases of the mind who operate the public mental hospitals know that the wretched poverty of normal life activities in the hospital is an inevitable consequence of the diseased mind. The medical directors of the hospital, on the other hand, assume that the citizenry is not interested in giving money or time to provide mentally ill patients with a fuller, busier, more worthwhile life. They regard public disinterest in the happiness and welfare of the mentally ill as inevitable, while the public regard their expert opinion to be that the degraded living conditions of patients are an inevitable result of mental disease which cannot be corrected. The result of this impasse and misunderstanding is that patients are seriously demoralized by the disrespect they suffer in being compelled to live sub-human lives. Indeed, it is difficult to find an example of members of lower species being compelled to suffer the indignity of functioning so far beneath their own level.

Changes Which Facilitate Return of the Mentally Ill to Normal Life

The foregoing account of the mental hospital as it is today refers to many of the conditions of life, in the hospital which prevent patients from taking part in practically all the activities engaged in by other people. Removal of these negative conditions constitutes a first and vitally important step toward raising the mental hospital to a level where it can perform the function for which it exists, namely, that of restoring the capacity of its patients to resume life outside the hospital.

The most damaging "negative condition" of the mental hospital is that which derives from what may fittingly be called the "closed door" policy. This policy not only locks patients in and confines them to a seat on a bench, but it also locks out the mentally well members of society whose participation in hospital life can bring the interests and healthful breath of normality of the outside community into the hospital. The mingling of outsiders with patients not only does away with the deteriorating effects of monotony, but it raises patients to their rightful status as human beings by actual demonstration that they are recognized as worthy of being the associates of citizens in good standing.

The mental hospital that welcomes outsiders within its walls and publicizes the need of its patients for normal human contacts has made an important step toward raising its standards of care. Outsiders who become volunteer workers soon recognize the multitudinous needs of patients and communicate them to the rest of the community. Sooner or later there is a flow of good into the hospital in the form of books, magazines, playing cards, checkers, bingo games, sewing materials, pictures, clothing, hot plates, coffee percolators, tea pots, radios, phonographs and pianos. Besides material goods, outsiders will give time as instructors in such activities as dancing, sewing and cooking.

As outsiders become better acquainted with the patients, they come to develop a personal interest in particular individual patients whom they take on shopping trips and invite to their homes.

Outsiders who become active volunteers become motivated to organize as a society which can raise funds for the benefit of patients.

The activities of volunteers in conjunction with patients lead to a great increase in the comings and goings in and out of wards. Increase in traffic, in turn, leads to the discovery that locked doors are not only inconvenient but unnecessary. Patients who would ordinarily try to escape become more interested in the new activities than in running away. Along with the unlocking of doors comes a relaxation of other restrictions and rules which become not only too difficult to administer in a setting of activity, but also unnecessary.

As patients regain contact with the community through their new friends, they not only learn of opportunities for jobs, but experience the advantage of being introduced to a prospective employer by a volunteer.

Adoption of an "open-door" policy is presented as the first step toward raising the standards of care in a mental hospital. Equally important is the adoption of what might be called a policy of self-examination on the part of the administrative staff of the hospital in the interests of learning how the effectiveness of hospital personnel is impeded by traditional functioning as a dictatorship. Serious thought must be given to the advantages to be gained from democratic procedures which facilitate communication from below to above and make the knowledge and experience of those in top positions accessible to those dealing directly with patients. Freedom of expression and participation in policy determination by attendants stimulates their initiative and paves the way for the formation of patient organizations, such as patient government. The inclusion of patient organizations as responsible bodies having a role in the administrative affairs of the hospital is a powerful stimulus in motivating patients to acquire those social and political skills which are indispensable to successful living in the community.

The central theme of mental hospital improvement is removal of barriers to the development of all the positive assets of the mentally ill and provision not only of the maximum possible degree of freedom but also of access to whatever means facilitate their becoming more useful citizens. The improvement of the mental hospital requires what is essentially a social revolution in the management of the mentally ill, for it involves casting off those antiquated asylum methods which were dictated by the ignorance and prejudices of the past and are perpetuated to the present by fear and misunderstanding.

Recent developments in the treatment of the mentally ill which impose minimal obstructions to the patient's participation in society are the establishment of clinics for the treatment of psychoses on an out-patient basis, the establishment of psychiatric wards in general hospitals, and the increase in the number of psychiatrists in private practice who treat patients in their offices.

The purpose of this essay is to give an account of what human endeavor in America has done and can be expected to do toward relief of the severe grades of mental illness which require individuals to be held in mental hospitals. The remaining chapters seek to give accounts of three phases in American psychiatry. The first tells of the understanding care which our society sought to give the mentally ill when democracy was young and inspired with its mission to mankind. The second is an account of the decline in human understanding which accompanied social changes during the course of the nineteenth century, and the damage it has done Americans who have suffered nervous breakdowns. The third tells of the new hope which modern understanding of human thought, feeling, and behavior has for present-day and future victims of nervous breakdowns.

At the present time, the American people are faced with the responsibility of learning what modern psychiatry has to offer the mentally ill and how to bring its benefits to them. Americans have not as yet been fully informed of the most significant aspect of modern scientific knowledge of the hospitalized mentally ill—namely their great need *for psychological aid and moral support which all people in distress need and which our society is already able to give if it is motivated to do so.* Scientific controversy within psychiatry over the validity of particular psychological theories and techniques still obscures from public view the great importance of bringing ordinary psychological and material aids to the mentally ill who are deprived of all contacts in our mental hospitals as they are now constituted.

The condition of the institutionalized mentally ill in America today is a matter of particular interest in this age of experts and specialists in that it can be scrutinized as a result of public opinion being led to adopt and retain a point of view which contradicts the primary value of the individual and harms many citizens. The sobering aspect of the present harmful public attitude toward mental illness is that it was formed under the influence of supposedly scientific authority which pronounced mental illness incurable over three-quarters of a century ago.

The enormous number of man-years of wasted living which attends present day institutional management of the mentally ill is a matter of great importance not only to psychiatrists but also to those citizens who by their participation in social and political activities of the community exercise an influence on the manner of operation of both private and public institutions which effect the general welfare.

II. Moral Treatment—Forgotten Success in History of Psychiatry

Backsliding has time and again followed progress in man's understanding of self and neighbor. Periods of enlightenment at times left an imprint strong enough to survive generations of darkness and inspire progress anew. At other times, the principle on which these periods were based had to be rediscovered. On the whole, progress over the centuries has been substantial. Religion, politics and science have all made their contributions.

The greatest challenge to the capacity of men (individually and collectively) to understand neighbor and self arises when mental illness disrupts their relationship to one another. Society's reaction to the mentally ill has oscillated throughout recorded history between brutality and benevolence. When neither was extreme, pernicious neglect was the rule.

A basis for understanding human behavior was laid by Plato, who wrote, "And indeed it may almost be asserted that all intemperance in any kind of pleasure, *and all disgraceful conduct,* is not properly blamed as the consequence of voluntary guilt. For no one is voluntarily bad; but he who is depraved becomes so through a certain habit of body, and an ill-governed education. All the vicious are vicious through two most involuntary causes, which we shall always ascribe to the planters, than to the things planted, and to the trainers than to those trained" (6).

Hippocrates declared the behavior in psychoses to be due to brain disease and decried belief in demon possession.

These elements of understanding were lost to mankind for several hundred years only to reappear in the writings of *Coelius Aurelianus* and again disappear during the Dark Ages. They were once more brought to light by *Paracelsus* and *John Weyer* in the sixteenth century. They raised their voices against abuses arising from superstition and warped theological interpretation of the symptoms of mental illness. Their influence resulted in partial acceptance of mental disorder as a province of medicine. Consistent humanitarian care and scientific clinical study were not adopted until the eighteenth century. The liberal philosophy and political movements of this century contained the hope that science would enable the achievement of humanitarian ends. The possibility that science could solve the riddle of mental illness captured the imagination. In this endeavor, the goals of science and humanitarianism were undistinguishable. There was no clear-cut dividing line indicating where elimination of abuse ended and scientific therapy began.

Indeed, the humanistic science of the eighteenth century could not interpret human behavior in other than humanitarian terms. The very method of science involved clearing the mind of *a priori* bias in order that it might uncover universal laws. The assumption that laws of science as yet undiscovered were universal in the sense that the "law" of falling bodies was universal carried with it the connotation that human behavior, too, was the result of laws. Hence, human behavior must be influenced greatly by unknown forces over which the individual could not have complete control. This had the effect of emphasizing those qualities which individuals have in common and the impossibility of an absolute standard of individual responsibility. Logically then, from this point of view, all men could be looked upon as equal and forgivable for their evil actions. Democratic government and humanitarian treatment of criminals, paupers and psychotics thus appeared to have their foundations in science.

Humanitarianism favored the view that lunatics had undergone stresses which robbed them of their reason. That such stress could result from disappointment as well as inflammation was a basic assumption. Stresses of a psychological nature were referred to as *moral causes*. Treatment was called *moral treatment,* which meant that the patient was made comfortable, his interest aroused, his friendship invited, and discussion of his troubles encouraged. His time was managed and filled with purposeful activity.

The use of the word "moral" in the terms *moral causes* and *moral treatment* has, at first glance, the capacity to arouse animosity in the well-informed modern who is acquainted with that literature of anthropology and social psychology which demonstrates the relativity of moral standards. Knowledge that the early psychiatrist used the word moral as the equivalent of emotional or psychological serves to allay such animosity. Deeper reflection on the genesis and meaning of the word "moral" discloses the logic of the usage. The term "moral" is intimately related to the word "moral" and carries within it emotional connotations of the words, zeal, hope, spirit and confidence. It also has to do with custom, conduct, way of life and inner meaning. The word moral (and the word ethics, too) has many shades of meaning with respect to interpersonal relations, besides having to do with abstract ideas, right and wrong and good and evil.

The word "moral" in *moral treatment* and *moral causes* bears within it an implication also about moral responsibility; namely, that the mentally ill were not morally responsible for their acts which were assumed to result either from ignorance or incorrect understanding. Indeed, to its founders, moral treatment of the mentally ill was considered to be a moral mandate on those who were more fortunate. Moral treatment was never clearly defined, possibly because its meaning was self-evident during the era in which it was used. In the context of that era it meant compassionate and understanding treatment of innocent sufferers. Indeed even innocence was not a prerequisite to meriting compassion. Compassion was also extended to those whose mental illness was thought due to willful and excessive indulgence in the passions.

Moral treatment is of great significance in the history of psychiatry not only because it was the first practical effort made to provide systematic and responsible care for an appreciable number of the mentally ill; it was also eminently successful in achieving recoveries.

The great step to moral treatment was taken almost simultaneously by a French physician and an English Quaker in the last decade of the eighteenth century. Phillipe Pinel transformed a madhouse into a hospital, and William Tuke built a *retreat* for the mentally ill. Similar reforms were wrought in Italy, Germany and America by Chiarurgi, Reil, and Rush. Man was not only reaching a new height in his understanding, but he was applying it on a wider front than ever before. Pinel has special priority on the debt the world owes for moral treatment.

The reforms of Benjamin Rush in America, though not as extensive as those of Pinel, were based on inspiration derived from the same source. Both were steeped in the liberal writings of the physician-philosopher John Locke. Rush's great influence did much to stimulate the interest of American physicians in mental illness and paved the way for full acceptance of the principles of moral treatment.

Although the mentally ill had for many years been accepted as patients in several hospitals in America (namely, the Pennsylvania Hospital, the New York Hospital, the Eastern State Hospital at Williamsburg, Virginia, and the Maryland Hospital at Baltimore), it was not until 1817, four years after Rush's death, that a hospital was founded in America expressly for the purpose of providing moral treatment. This hospital, patterned after the York Retreat in England, was built by Pennsylvania Quakers and named the Friends' Asylum. Within seven years, three more privately endowed mental hospitals were built: McLean, Bloomingdale, and the Hartford Retreat. Within thirty years, eighteen hospitals had been built for moral treatment of the mentally ill in America.

The high standards of hospitals built by private philanthropy set a good example for the many state-supported institutions which soon came into being. First of these was the Eastern State Hospital at Lexington, Kentucky, built in 1824, the same year as the Hartford Retreat in Connecticut. Within ten more years, four more state hospitals were built, now known as the Manhattan State Hospital (New York), 1825; the Western State Hospital (Staunton, Virginia), 1828; the South Carolina State Hospital (Columbia), 1828; and the Worcester State Hospital (Massachusetts), 1833.

The Worcester State Hospital merits special attention not only because of its prominence in present day psychiatry, but also because of the role it played in the history of moral treatment. The first superintendent at Worcester was Dr. Samuel B. Woodward, who, with Dr. Eli Todd, had persuaded the Connecticut Medical Society to sponsor the founding of the Hartford Retreat. These two physicians were long standing friends who, in the course of their practice of general medicine, shared an abiding interest in the treatment of mental disorders. Both became "specialists" of their day; at least patients with mental diseases were referred to them by other physicians.

These pioneer psychiatrists conducted a survey of mental illness in Connecticut to determine the size of hospital necessary to care for the mentally ill of that state. The elder of the two, Dr. Todd, was appointed superintendent of the Retreat. Nine years later, Dr. Woodward was chosen superintendent of the hospital at Worcester, the first state institution for the mentally ill in New England. This hospital was built largely through the enthusiastic support of Horace Mann, father of the American public school. It might be mentioned in passing that the New Hampshire State Hospital was founded largely through the efforts of Dr. Luther Bell (who later became superintendent of McLean Hospital) and the clergymen of New Hampshire. These are but a few examples of the active support which professional men—clergymen, educators, physicians —gave in behalf of the mentally ill in the early history of American psychiatry.

Table 4.1. Outcome in Patients Admitted to Worcester State Hospital III Less Than One Year Prior to Admission, 1833–1852*

Five-Year Period	Number Admitted	Number Discharged Recovered	Per Cent Discharged Recovered	Number Discharged Improved	Per Cent Discharged Improved
1833–37	300	211	70	39	8.3
1838–42	434	324	74.6	14	3.2
1843–47	742	474	63.9	34	4.6
1848–52	791	485	61.3	37	4.7

* Data for table were derived from the Annual Reports of the Worcester State Hospital.

Worcester State Hospital under the direction of Dr. Woodward served as a proving ground for moral treatment and demonstrated beyond doubt that recovery was the rule! Year after year Dr. Woodward gave the statistics of recovery in the Annual Reports of his hospital.

It was Dr. Todd, however, who first called the attention of the public to the success of moral treatment. He reported recovery in over 90% of patients who had been admitted to the Hartford Retreat with mental illness of less duration than one year. This result was based on relatively few admissions, however, and it remained for Dr. Woodward to demonstrate, on the basis of a large series of cases, that recovery was the rule in recently ill patients.

It is pertinent at this point to present the statistics of the Worcester Hospital during the time moral treatment was still applicable, that is before crowding and expansion beyond optimum size fully disrupted vital interpersonal relationships among patients, attendants and physicians.

Table 4.1 shows the number and per cent discharged recovered and improved of the total number of patients admitted who had been ill less than one year prior to their admission. During the entire 20 years there were 2,267 such admissions, of whom 1,618 were discharged as recovered or improved, or 71% (66% recovered, 5% improved). During this same period the total of all admissions (including those whose illness had lasted longer than one year prior to admission) was 4,119, of whom 2,439 or 59% were discharged recovered or improved (45% recovered, 14% improved).

Such statistical data cannot be ignored. They at least invite attention to the assumptions on which the idea of moral treatment was based and its cultural setting. America in the 1830's and '40's was rapidly developing a new liberal philosophy of the individual. Leading American thinkers of the period turned to nature in search of truth. Societies were formed for the abolition of slavery. Experiments were made in communal living. A spirit of freedom and self-expression was in the air. New England Puritanism was growing milder. The jealous God of Cotton Mather was becoming the loving God of William Channing, and a new intellectual independence was coming to the fore. Emerson encouraged the individual to self-reliance, and in one of his addresses, "The Scholar," he stated, "The world is nothing, the man is all." Historically, in the United States, this period has been referred to by Fisher as "The Rise of the Common Man, 1820–1850."

American thought was at this time in close communion with the romantic movement in Germany. American psychiatry was influenced by the then current psycho-biological trend in German psychiatric literature. In particular, the now forgotten name of von Feuchtersleben was often referred to by American psychiatrists. Indeed his contributions to psychiatric thought have only recently been recognized in modern times by Dr. Gregory Zilboorg who credits von Feuchtersleben's view of mental illness in the 1840's as being much the same as that of present-day psychiatry.

One of the leading spokesmen of early American psychiatry was Dr. Isaac Ray, whose psychiatric career began in the 1830's as superintendent of the Augusta State (Maine) Hospital. Dr. Ray subscribed to the view that the mind includes those qualities which make possible those relations among people which have to do with man's greatest welfare. Love and hate were to him as much manifestations of mind as rational processes. He also contended that every appetite and faculty must have its means of gratification and protested that belief to the contrary was wholly repugnant. He believed in the unity of the individual man and referred specifically to the unity of mind and brain. In his book "Mental Hygiene" (1863) he gave particular attention to the influence of passions, emotions, and temperament on mental health. He strongly recommended, after von Feuchtersleben, that ill-humored individuals be regarded as suffering from disease and advised them to seek every means to rid themselves of it to prevent becoming insane. He also held the view that insanity is but an exaggeration of personality traits which in their less extreme form are regarded as merely disagreeable.

Both Dr. Ray and his colleague, Dr. John S. Butler, superintendent of the Hartford Retreat (Connecticut), were impressed with the importance of child rearing to mental health. Indeed, Dr. Butler categorically stated that he had traced the cause of insanity to the malign influences of childhood in a large proportion of over 3,000 patients he had personally studied. Dr. Butler also voiced a commonly held opinion of the times that all bodily processes are under the influence of the mind.

The psychodynamic and psychosomatic orientation of psychiatry in the early 1800's found its fullest expression in the elaboration of the psychological therapeutic approach known as the moral treatment of insanity. In the language of Dr. Ray, the proper administration of moral treatment required that the physician learn through inquiry and conversation what occupies the minds of his patients. It required further that he investigate the mental make-up of patients' relatives. The greatest requirement of all was that the physician spare no effort in gaining the confidence and good will of his patients and strive to discover their experiences and supply their needs. The recommendation was made that the physician acquire a large fund of knowledge in order to converse with patients on matters interesting to them and thus gain an understanding of their inner life. The physician was strongly reminded that even the most insane patients are sensitive to manifestations of interest and good will. He was warned, however, to limit the number of patients in his care to those he can know personally.

Although much emphasis was placed on the relationship between physician and patient, moral treatment embraced a much larger psychological approach than individual psychotherapy. Indeed, perhaps the greatest asset of moral treatment was the attention it gave to the value of physical setting and social influences of hospital life as curative agents. In his book "Curability of Insanity" (1887) (7) the fore mentioned Dr. Butler repeatedly pointed out the importance of scrutinizing the hospital environment to find and remove whatever is depressing or disturbing. He insisted that a cheerful, sympathetic atmosphere and esthetic appeal are essential for the cure of many patients. His goal was to make hospital wards as homelike as possible, for he placed great faith in the value of family-like gatherings in which patients could discuss their problems among themselves and with the physician. He also believed that confidential interviews with patients were essential, but he was convinced that the turning point in many a patient's illness took place in group discussions. He also insisted that appropriate social influences could not be maintained if hospitals were allowed to care for more than 200 patients at one time. He considered monotony to be the greatest obstacle to be overcome in mental hospitals and believed heartily in promoting a wide variety of activities for patients.

The theoretical foundation of early American psychiatry and the success of its therapeutic approach to insane individuals as persons were a source of inspiration to those who believed in the dignity of man and sought to improve his condition. Horace Mann and Charles Dickens were particularly impressed by the experience of seeing moral treatment in action. In his 1833 report (16), as chairman of the board of trustees of the Worcester State Hospital, Horace Mann told a moving story of 32 fellow beings who had been restored to their reason under the influences of the hospital whose loss to their families would otherwise have been mourned without hope. He told further of the unbelievable changes which had taken place in those patients who had not recovered. When the hospital was first opened, there were at least one hundred patients who would assail any human being who came near them. In less than a year only 12 of these patients were still assaultive. Similarly, of 40 patients who would tear off their clothing in the beginning, only eight still did so at the time of the report. He commented on the civility and kindness which had come to prevail among the patients. Wailing, raving, and desponding were dispelled, and the facial expression of patients reflected their improved state of mind. He credited these heartening results to the efforts "of all those engaged in administering the daily affairs of the institution to exclude, as far as in any manner possible, all causes of mental disquietude, by substituting persuasion by force, by practicing forbearance, mildness, and all the nameless offices of humanity, by imbuing in every practicable way, the minds of the patients with a new set of pleasing, cheerful, grateful and benevolent emotions." He summed up the idea of moral treatment in the following words: "In fine, the whole scheme of moral treatment is embraced in a single idea—humanity—the law of love—that sympathy which appropriates another's consciousness of pain and makes it a personal relief from suffering whenever another's sufferings are relieved."

Charles Dickens' account (9) of his visit to the Boston State Hospital in 1842 brings to light still more facets of hospital life in the moral treatment era. He commented on the wide variety of activities available to patients including carriage rides in the open air, fishing, and gardening and several kinds of indoor and outdoor games. Patients worked with sharp-edged tools and ate their meals with knives and forks. The patients organized themselves in a sewing circle which held meetings and passed resolutions. They also attended dances which were held weekly. Dickens was particularly surprised with the self-respect which was inculcated and encouraged in the patients by the superintendent's attitude toward them. He made special note that the superintendent and his family dined with the patients and mixed among them as a matter of course.

The psychological orientation of moral treatment and the recoveries from psychosis accompanying its application cannot be lightly dismissed. Modern psychiatry would do well to regard the mental hospitals of the early nineteenth century as pilot hospitals which demonstrated the value of social and psychological factors in treatment. The reason this finding was largely disregarded for nearly one hundred years is a story in itself. The least we can do is borrow a leaf from our psychiatric forefathers and give full attention to the possibilities of treating psychoses by social and psychological means in the many state and federal hospitals which have so long considered psychosis curable *only* by physical or chemical means.

Bibilography

1. Annual Reports of the Worcester State Hospital, 1881.
2. Annual Reports of the Worcester State Hospital, 1882.
3. Annual Reports of the Worcester State Hospital, 1883.
6. BUCKNILL, J. C., and Tuke, D. H.: *A Manual of Psychological Medicine*. London: John Churchill, 1858, page 9.
7. BUTLER, J. S.: *Curability of Insanity* and *The Individualized Treatment of the Insane*. New York: G. P. Putnam's Sons, 1887.
9. DICKENS, C.: *American Notes*. Leipzig: Bernard Tauchnitz, 1842.
16. Mann H, Taft B, Calhoun WB, Foster AD, Gray FC. First annual report of the turstees of State Lunatic Hospital. Boston: Dutton and Wentworth, 1833.

5

Szasz, T. S. (1961). *The myth of mental illness: Foundations of a theory of personal conduct.* New York: Hoeber-Harper

First-time readers of Szasz's book, expecting a manifesto or diatribe proclaiming that mental illness does not exist, may be surprised to find in the introduction a more sober critique of the "vague, capricious, and generally unacceptable character" (p. ix) of psychiatry as a branch of knowledge that claims to be a science. They might also be surprised to learn that Szasz thought psychiatry had the potential to be *become* a science. In order to achieve such a status, he argued, the discipline needed to move away from what he described as its circular logic—that mental illness in a person is demonstrated by the fact that psychiatrists have diagnosed mental illness in that person. Szasz proposed that psychiatry move away from its focus on mental illness as an entity, in imitation of biologically focused medicine, and toward seeing it a process, with emphasis on observation of behavior. Thomas Scheff, writing 5 years after *The Myth of Mental Illness* was published, praised Szasz's analysis of the social functions that the concept of mental illness served but thought Szasz went too far in suggesting, or appearing to suggest, that many identified patients are shamming mental illness. Others have criticized Szasz for paying too little attention to the anguish and suffering that serious mental illness visits upon people. Whatever one's assessment, *The Myth of Mental Illness* is one of the most influential, and likely the best known, works of the antipsychiatry movement. The excerpt included here is from the first edition of the book.

Introduction

Karl R. Popper (1957, p. 177)

Sooner or later every scientific enterprise comes to a fork in the road. Scientists must then decide which of two paths to follow. The dilemma that must be faced is: How shall we conceive of what we do? Should we think of what we do in terms of *substantives* and *entities*—for example, elements, compounds, living things, mental illnesses, and so forth? Or should we think of it in terms of *processes* and *activities*—for example, Brownian movement, oxidation, or communication? We need not consider the dilemma in the abstract, other than to note that these two modes of conceptualization represent a developmental sequence in the evolution of scientific thought. Entity-thinking has always preceded process-thinking. Physics, chemistry, and certain branches of biology have long ago supplemented substantive conceptualizations by process-theories. Psychiatry has not.

Scope and Methods of the Study

I submit that the traditional definition of psychiatry, which is still in vogue, places it alongside such things as alchemy and astrology, and commits it to the category of pseudo science. Psychiatry is said to be a medical specialty concerned with the study and treatment of mental illness. Similarly, astrology was the study of the influence of planetary movements and positions on human behavior and destiny. These are typical instances of defining a science by specifying the subject matter of study. These definitions completely disregard method and are based instead on false substantives (Szasz, 1958a, 1959b). The activities of alchemists and astrologers—in contrast to the activities of chemists and astronomers—were not bound by publicly disclosed methods of observation and inference. Psychiatrists, likewise, have persistently avoided disclosing fully and publicly what they do. Indeed, whether as therapists or theorists, they may do virtually anything and still be considered psychiatrists. Thus, the behavior of a particular psychiatrist—as a member of the species "psychiatrist"—may be that of a physician, clergyman, friend, counselor, teacher, psychoanalyst, or all manner of combinations of these. He is a psychiatrist so long as he claims that he is oriented toward the problem of mental illness and health. But suppose, for a moment, that there is no such thing as mental illness and health. Suppose, further, that these words refer to nothing more substantial or real than the astrological conception of planetary influences on human conduct. What then?

Methods of Observation and Action in Psychiatry

Psychiatry stands at the crossroads. Thus far, thinking in terms of substantives—for example, neurosis, disease, treatment—has been the rule. The question is: Shall we continue along the same road, or branch off in the direction of process-thinking? Viewed in this light, my efforts in this study are directed first *at demolishing some of the major false substantives of contemporary psychiatric thought,* and second *at laying the foundations for a process-theory of personal conduct.*

Discrepancies between what people say they do and what they actually do are encountered in all walks of life, science included. The principle of operationism, made into a systematic philosophy of science by Bridgman (1936), was succinctly formulated by Einstein (1933) in connection with exactly this discrepancy in physics:

> If you want to find out anything from the theoretical physicists about the methods they use, I advise you to stick closely to one principle: Don't listen to their words, fix your attention on their deeds (p. 30).

Surely there is no reason to assume that this principle is any less valid for understanding the methods—and hence the nature and subject—of psychiatry.

Briefly stated, an operational definition of a concept is one that relates if to actual "operations." A physical concept is defined by physical operations, such as measurements of time, temperature, distance, and so forth. In physics, operational definitions may be contrasted with idealistic definitions, the latter being exemplified by the classic, pre-Einsteinian notions of Time, Space, and Mass. Similarly, a psychological or sociological concept, defined operationally, relates to psychological or sociological observations or measurements. In contrast, many psychosocial concepts are defined on the basis of the investigator's self-proclaimed intentions or values. The majority of present-day psychiatric concepts belong in the latter category.

The answer to the question "What do psychiatrists do?" depends, therefore, on the kind of psychiatrist one has in mind. He might be any of the following (the list is not necessarily complete): one who physically examines patients, administers drugs and electric shock treatments, signs commitment papers, examines criminals and testifies concerning them in courts, or, most commonly, perhaps, listens and talks to patients. In this book, I shall be concerned mainly with psychiatry as a special discipline whose method is, rather derisively but nevertheless quite correctly, often spoken of as "only talking." If the word "only" is disregarded as gratuitous condemnation, and if the meaning of "talking" is enlarged to encompass communications of all kinds, we arrive at the formulation of a basic method of psychiatry to which surprisingly few psychiatrists really subscribe. In fact, there is a split, perhaps even an unbridgeable gap, between what most psychotherapists and psychoanalysts do in the course of their work and what they say concerning the nature of it. What they do, of course, is to communicate with patients by means of language, nonverbal signs, and rules. Further, they analyze, by means of verbal symbols, the communicative interactions which they observe and in which they themselves engage. This, I believe, correctly describes the actual operations of psychoanalysis and psychosocially oriented psychiatry. But what do these psychiatrists tell themselves and others concerning their work? They talk as though they were physicians, physiologists, biologists, or even physicists! We hear about sick patients, instincts, and endocrine functions and of course "libido" and "psychic energies," both "free" and "bound." While the need for clarity in regard to scientific method is no longer a new idea among scientists, it requires re-emphasis in our field.

Psychiatry, using the methods of communication analysis, has much in common with the sciences concerned with the study of languages and communicative behavior. In spite of this connection between psychiatry and such disciplines as symbolic logic, semiotic,[1] and sociology, problems of mental health continue to be cast in the traditional framework of medicine. The conceptual scaffolding of medicine, on the other hand, has rested on the principles of physics and chemistry. This is entirely reasonable, for it has been and continues to be the task of medicine to study—and if necessary to alter—the physicochemical structure and function of the human body. Man's sign-using behavior, however, does not seem to lend itself to exploration and understanding in these terms.

The distinction between psychology and physics is, of course, a familiar one. The differences, however, are not usually taken seriously enough. The lack of commitment to psychology as a legitimate science is revealed by some scientists' outspoken expectation that in the end all scientific observations and statements will be phrased in a mathematico-physical idiom. More specifically, in the language of psychiatry and psychoanalysis infidelity to subject and methods is expressed in the persistent imitation of medicine. Thus we continue to speak of and presumably believe in such notions as "psychopathology" and "psychotherapy." This, at least, is the manifest state of our science. At the same time, ideas concerning object relationships and communications have gained greater acceptance, especially in recent decades. But a science can be no better than its linguistic apparatus permits. Hence our continued reliance on such notions as "neurosis," "psychosis," "emotional illness," "psychoanalytic treatment," and so forth cannot be lightly dismissed. We remain shackled to a scientifically outmoded conceptual framework and its terminology. We cannot, however, forever hold fast to and profit from the morally judgmental and socially manipulative character of our traditional psychiatric and psychoanalytic language without paying a price. I believe that we are in danger of purchasing superiority and power over nonpsychiatrists and patients at the cost of scientific self-sterilization and hence ultimate professional self-destruction.

Causality and Historicism in Modern Psychiatry

The issues of historical constancy and predictability are of the utmost importance for all of psychiatry. Questions such as whether hysteria was "always the same disease" revolve around it, as does also the question of whether a psychotherapist can "predict" whether Mr. X will be happy in marriage with Miss Y. It is implicit in traditional psychoanalytic thought that prediction is a legitimate concern of this science. One often hears, nowadays, about how prediction ought to be used to "validate" psychoanalytic hypotheses. I believe we should have serious reservations concerning such preoccupations with controlling and predicting psychosocial occurrences. Caution and skepticism require that we pay attention to the epistemology of psychiatry, and especially to the implications of deterministic and historic explanations of human behavior.

The psychoanalytic theory of man was fashioned after the causal-deterministic model of classical physics. The errors of this transposition have been amply documented in recent years (for example, Gregory, 1953; Allport, 1955). I wish to call attention here to that application of the principle of physical determinism to human affairs which Popper (1944–1945) aptly termed "historicism." Examination of much of modern psychiatric thought discloses the fundamental role of antecedent historical events as alleged *determinants* of subsequent behavior. The psychoanalytic theory of behavior is, therefore, a species of historicism. As long as this type of explanation is considered satisfactory, there is no need for other types of explanations, such as will be presented in this book. It should be kept in mind, in this

[1] The term "semiotic" will be used to designate the *science of signs* (Morris, 1946, 1955).

connection, that historicist theories of behavior preclude explanations of valuation, choice, and responsibility in human affairs.

Briefly stated, historicism is a doctrine according to which historical prediction is essentially no different from physical prediction. Historical (e.g., psychological, social) events are viewed as fully determined by their antecedents, in the same manner as physical events are by theirs. The prediction of future events is, therefore, possible in principle. In practice, prediction is considered to be limited by the extent to which past and present conditions can be accurately determined. Insofar as these can be adequately ascertained, successful prediction is assured.

Popper's models of historicist social thinkers were men like Plato, Nietzsche, Marx, and the modern totalitarian dictators and their apologists. According to historicist doctrine the future is determined—in a sense, irrevocably—by the past: "Every version of historicism expresses the feeling of being swept into the future by irresistible forces" (Popper, 1944–1945, p. *160*). Compare this with Freud's thesis that human conduct is determined by "unconscious forces" which, in turn, are the results of instinctual drives and early experiences. The crucial similarity between Marxism and classical psychoanalysis lies in the selection of a single type of antecedent cause as sufficient explanation of virtually all subsequent human events. In Marxism, human nature and conduct are determined by economic conditions; in psychoanalysis they are determined by family-historical (genetic-psychological) factors. Paradoxically, therapy is based on the expectation that reason and understanding might help to mitigate the otherwise irresistible forces of historicism. But whether the past is, in fact, so powerful a determinant of future human actions as it is of future physical events is a moot question. It is by no means the established fact that Freud claimed it was. This unsupported—and, I submit, false—theory of personal conduct has become widely accepted in our present *day*. It even has received legal approval, so to speak, by the American criminal statutes that codify certain types of actions as potentially the results of "mental illnesses."

The principal basis for the failure of historicism is that, in the social sciences, we are faced with a full and complicated interaction between observer and observed. Specifically, the prediction of a social event itself, may cause it to occur or may lead to its prevention. The so-called self-fulfilling prophecy—in which the predictor helps bring about the predicted event—exemplifies the empirical and logical complexities with which prediction in the social sphere is fraught. All this is not intended to deny or minimize the effects and significance of past experiences—that is, of historical antecedents—on subsequent human performances. The past does mold the personality and the human organism, as it may also mold machines (Wiener, 1960). This process, however, must be conceptualized and understood not in terms of antecedent "causes" and subsequent "effects" but rather in terms of modifications in the entire organization and functioning of the object acted upon.

In view of the rather obvious empirical and logical inadequacies of historicist theories, one may ask: What is the value of subscribing to an historicist position? In addition to providing a painstaking refutation of historicism, Popper (1944–1945) suggested an explanation of why many people adhere to it. He stated:

> It really looks as if *historicists were trying to compensate themselves for the loss of an unchanging world* by clinging to the belief that *change can be foreseen* because it is ruled by an *unchanging law* ([italics added] p. 161)

Let us recall in this connection that Freud (1927) proposed a similar explanation for why men believe in religion. He attributed religious belief to man's inability to tolerate the loss of the familiar world of childhood, symbolized by the protective father. Thus, a "father-in-heaven" and a replica of the protective childhood game are created to replace the father and the family lost in the here-and-now. The difference between religion and political historicism, from this point of view, is only in the specific identities of the "protectors." They are God and the theologians in the first instance, while in the second they are the modern totalitarian leaders and their apologists.

It is especially important to emphasize, therefore, that although Freud criticized organized religion for the patent infantilism that it is, he failed to apprehend the social characteristics of the "closed society" and the psychological characteristics of its loyal supporters. The paradox that is psychoanalysis—consisting on the one hand of an historicist theory and on the other of an antihistoricist therapy—thus came into being. Whatever the reasons— and many have been suggested—Freud (1940) adopted and promoted a biopsychological world view embodying the principle of constancy and resting squarely on it. We may assume that historicism had the same function for him, and for those who joined with him in the precarious early psychoanalytic movement, as it had for others: it provided a hidden source of comfort against the threat of unforeseen and unpredictable change. This interpretation is consonant with the current use of psychoanalysis and "dynamic psychiatry" as means for obscuring and disguising moral and political conflicts as mere personal problems (Szasz, 1960c).

In this connection, Rieff (1959) suggested that: "The popularity of psychoanalysis, in an age suffering vertigo from the acceleration of historical events, may be partly ascribed to *Freud's rehabilitation of the constant nature underlying history*" ([italics added] p. 214).

I am in agreement with Popper, however, that there is no such "constant nature underlying history"! Both man and society change, and, as they do, 'human nature" changes with them.

In the light of these considerations, what could we say concerning the relationship between psychosocial and physical laws? The two are not similar. Psychosocial antecedents do not "cause" human sign-using behavior in the same manner as physical antecedents "cause" their effects (Ryle, 1949). Furthermore, physical laws are relativistic with respect to physical circumstances, in particular to the size of the mass. The laws governing the behavior of large bodies (Newtonian physics) differ from those that govern the behavior of very small ones (quantum physics). It seems to me that as physical laws are relativistic with respect to mass, so psychological laws are relativistic with respect to social conditions. In other words, *the laws of psychology cannot be formulated independently of the laws of sociology.*

Psychiatry and Ethics

From the point of view which will be presented here, *psychiatry, as a theoretical science, consists of the study of personal conduct*—of clarifying and "explaining" the kinds of games that people play with each other; how they learned these games; why they like to play them; and so forth.[2] Actual behavior is the raw data from which the rules of the game are inferred. From among the many different kinds of behavior, the verbal form—or communication by means of conventional language—constitutes one of the central areas of interests for psychiatry. Thus, it is in the structure of language games (Sellars, 1954) that the interests of linguistics, philosophy, psychiatry, and semiotic meet. Each of these disciplines has addressed itself to different aspects of the language game: linguistics to its structure, philosophy to its cognitive signification, and psychiatry to its social usage.

---

[2] A systematic analysis of personal conduct in terms of game-playing behavior will be presented in Part V. *The model of games*, however, is used throughout the book. Unless otherwise specified, by "games" I refer to ordinary card games, board games, or sports. Although it is difficult to give a concise definition of the concept of game, game situations are characterized by a system of set roles and rules considered more or less binding for all of the players.

It is hoped that this approach will effect a much-needed and long overdue *rapprochement* between psychiatry on the one hand and philosophy and ethics on the other. Questions such as: "How does man live?" and "How ought man to live?" traditionally have been in the domains of philosophy, ethics, and religion. Psychology—and psychiatry, as a branch of it—was closely allied to philosophy and ethics until the latter part of the nineteenth century. Since then, psychologists have considered themselves empirical scientists whose methods and theories are allegedly no different than those of the physicist or biologist. But insofar as psychologists address themselves to the two questions raised above, their methods and theories do differ, to some extent, from those of the natural scientists. If these considerations are valid, psychiatrists cannot expect to solve ethical problems by medical methods.

In sum, then, inasmuch as psychiatric theories seek to explain, and systems of psychotherapy to alter, human behavior, statements concerning goals and values ("ethics") will be considered indispensable parts of theories of personal conduct and psychotherapy.

Hysteria as a Paradigm of Mental Illness

Modern psychiatry, if dated from Charcot's work on hysteria and hypnosis, is approximately one hundred years old. How did the study of so-called mental illnesses begin and develop? What economic, moral, political, and social forces helped to mold it into its present form? And perhaps most important, what effect did medicine, and particularly the concept of bodily illness, have on the development of the concept of mental illness?

The strategy of this inquiry will be to answer these questions, using conversion hysteria as a paradigm of the sort of phenomena to which the term "mental illness" may refer. Hysteria was selected for the following reasons:

Historically, it is the problem that captured the attention of the pioneer neuropsychiatrists (e.g., Charcot, Janet, Freud) and led to the gradual differentiation of neurology and psychiatry.

Logically, hysteria brings into focus the need to distinguish bodily illness from imitations of such illness. It thus presented the physician with the task of distinguishing the "real" or genuine from the "unreal" or false. The distinction between fact and facsimile—often apprehended as the distinction between object and sign, or between physics and psychology—remains the core-problem of contemporary psychiatric epistemology.

Psychosocially, conversion hysteria provides an excellent example of how so-called mental illness can best be conceptualized in terms of sign-using, rule-following, and game-playing because: (1) Hysteria is a form of non-verbal communication, making use of a special set of signs. (2) It is a system of rule-following behavior, making special use of the rules of helplessness, illness, and coercion. (3) It is a game characterized, among other things, by the end-goals of domination and interpersonal control and by strategies of deceit.

Everything that will be said about hysteria pertains equally, in principle, to all other so-called mental illnesses and to personal conduct generally. The manifest diversity of mental illnesses—for example, the differences between hysteria, obsessions, paranoia, etc.—may be regarded as analogous to the manifest diversity characterizing different languages. Behind the phenomenological differences, we may discover certain similarities. Within a particular family of languages, as for instance the Indo-European, there are significant similarities of both structure and function. Thus, English and French have much in common, whereas both differ greatly from Hungarian. Similarly, hysterical picture language and dream language are closely allied, whereas both differ significantly from a paranoid systematization. To be specific, both hysteria and dreams make extensive use of iconic signs, whereas paranoia makes extensive use of conventional signs (that is, everyday speech). The characteristic impact of paranoid transactions derives not from the peculiarity of the signs used but from the function to which they are put—noncognitive, promotive, object-seeking. To the analysis of personal conduct as communication, similar analyses in terms of rule-following and game-playing will be added. Of the three models, the game is most comprehensive, since it encompasses the other two (i.e., sign-using and rule-following).

Sociohistorical and Epistemological Foundations of Modern Psychiatry

In Part I, our task will be to examine how the modern concepts of hysteria and mental illness arose, developed, and now flourish. The sociohistorical contexts in which medicine, neurology, and later psychiatry were practiced, as well as the logical foundation of basic medical and psychiatric concepts, will be the main targets of interest and critical scrutiny. In the terminology of Gestalt psychology, this means that, at least at the beginning, we shall be more interested in the "ground" than in the "figure." The ground is the historical and sociopsychological context in which hysteria appears as the figure, or problem, to be studied and comprehended. As varying the background in an experiment in visual perception may make an object appear, become intensified, or disappear—so it is with problems of so-called mental illness. When the social background of behavioral phenomena is treated as a variable, the phenomena of mental illness can be seen to appear, become intensified, diminish, or disappear. It has long been known that an hysterical paralysis, for example, may disappear when a person is threatened by an acute danger, say a fire. Similarly, the disappearance of all sorts of neurotic illnesses in people sent to concentration camps is an illustration of how changes in the "ground" affect the perception—or perhaps in this case we may say the very existence—of the "figure."

In as much as psychoanalysis has gradually become identified as the branch of psychology especially concerned with the *intrapersonal* dimensions of human problems, it fell to other branches of the science of man to take cognizance of the *sociohistorical* background in which the phenomena studied are imbedded—first, to so-called dissident schools of psychoanalysis, lately to so-called social psychiatry. I believe that the identification of psychoanalysis with the purely, or even principally, intrapersonal dimension is false. From its inception psychoanalysis has been concerned with man's relationship to his fellow man, and to the group in which he lives. Unfortunately, this concern has been obscured by an ostensibly medical orientation.

Scrutiny of the sociohistorical context in which the modern concept of hysteria arose will necessitate an examination of the problem of imitation. We will thus be led to the logic of the relation between "real" and "false," irrespective of whether this distinction is encountered in medicine, psychiatry, or elsewhere. Since the distinction between "real" and "false" requires human judgment, the criteria on which such judgments in medicine and psychiatry are based, and the persons institutionally authorized to render such judgments, will be of the greatest significance and will be discussed in detail. In medicine, the criteria for distinguishing the genuine from the facsimile—that is, real illness from malingering—were based first on the presence or absence of demonstrable changes in the *structure* of the human body. Such findings may be obtained by means of clinical examination, laboratory tests, or post-mortem studies of the cadaver.

The beginning of modern psychiatry coincided with a new criterion for distinguishing real from false disease, namely, *alteration in function.* Conversion hysteria was the prototype of so-called *functional illness.* As paresis, for example, was considered a structural disease of the brain, so hysteria and mental illnesses generally were considered to be functional diseases of the same organ. So-called functional illnesses were thus placed in the same category as structural illnesses and were distinguished from imitated illnesses by means of the criterion of *voluntary falsification*. Accordingly, hysteria, neurasthenia, obsessive-compulsive neurosis, depression, paranoia, and so forth were regarded as diseases that happened to people. Mentally sick persons did not "will" their pathological behavior and were considered not "responsible" for it. These "mental diseases" were henceforth contrasted with malingering, which was the voluntary imitation of illness. In recent decades psychiatrists have claimed that malingering, too, is a form of mental illness. This poses a logical dilemma—the dilemma of the existence of an alleged entity called "mental illness" which, even when deliberately counterfeited, is still "mental illness."

Beside the empirical criteria for judging illness as real or false, the sociology of the judge officially authorized to render such judgments is of decisive significance. Some of the questions that arise are: What sorts of persons have the social power to make their judgments heard and to implement them? How do social class standing and the political makeup of society affect the roles of the judge, and the potentially sick person?

To answer these questions, an inquiry into medical and psychiatric practices in late nineteenth-century Western Europe, contemporary America, and Soviet Russia will be presented.

The conceptual and sociohistorical roots of the notion of mental illness are intertwined. Each root must be clearly identified. This work of clarification will be continued in Part II by (1) re-examining Breuer and Freud's "Studies on Hysteria," (2) surveying contemporary psychiatric attitudes toward hysteria, and (3) critically analyzing the connections between conversion hysteria and modern concepts of psychosomatic medicine.

Foundations of a Theory of Personal Conduct

The Sign-Using Model of Behavior

Although the concept of psychiatry as an analysis of communication is not novel, the full implication of the idea that so-called mental illnesses may be like languages, and not at all like diseases of the body, has not been made sufficiently explicit. Suppose, for instance, that the problem of hysteria is more akin to the problem of a person speaking a foreign tongue than it is to that of a person having a bodily disease. We are accustomed to believe that diseases have "causes," "treatments," and "cures." If, however, a person speaks a language other than our own, we do not usually look for the "cause" of his peculiar linguistic behavior. It would be foolish—and, of course, fruitless—to concern ourselves with the "etiology" of speaking French. To understand such behavior, we must think in terms of *learning* (Hilgard, 1956) and *meaning* (Ogden and Richards, 1930; Ryle, 1957). Accordingly, we might conclude that speaking French is the result of living among people who speak French. The sociohistorical context of the learning experience must not be confused with the history of the subject. The former is the concern of genetic psychology, psychiatry, and psychoanalysis—the latter the concern of philology and the history of languages. It follows, then, that if hysteria is regarded as a special form of communicative behavior, it is meaningless to inquire into its "causes." As with languages, we shall only be able to ask how hysteria was *learned* and what it *means*. This is exactly what Freud (1900) did with dreams. He regarded the dream as a language and proceeded to elucidate its structure and meanings.

If a so-called psychopathological phenomenon is more akin to a language problem than to illness, it follows that we cannot meaningfully talk of "treatment" and "cure." Although it is obvious that under certain circumstances it may be desirable for a person to change from one language to another—for example, to discontinue speaking French and begin speaking English—this change is not usually formulated in terms of "treatment." Speaking about learning rather than about etiology permits one to acknowledge that among a diversity of communicative forms each has its own *raison d'être* and that, because of the particular circumstances of the communicants, each is as valid as any other.

It is my thesis that hysteria—meaning thereby communication by means of bodily signs and complaints—constitutes a special form of sign-using behavior. Let us call this type of communication *protolanguage*. This language has a twofold origin. Its first source is man's bodily make-up. The human body is subject to disease and disability, manifested by means of bodily signs (e.g., paralysis, convulsion, etc.) and bodily feelings (e.g., pain, fatigue, etc). Its second source resides in cultural factors, especially in the apparently world-wide custom of making life easier, at least temporarily, for those who are ill. These two basic factors account for the development and use of the language of hysteria. *I submit that hysteria is nothing other than the "language of illness," employed either become another language has not been learned well enough, or because this language happens to be especially useful.* There may be, of course, various combinations of these two reasons for using this language.

In sum, then, our task in Part III will be to undertake a semiotical rather than a psychiatric or psychoanalytic analysis of hysteria. First, a detailed examination of the structure and function of protolanguage will be presented. This will be followed by an exposition of the relation of protolanguage to the general class of nondiscursive languages. Considerations of the problem of indirect communication—that is, scrutiny of the structure and function of alluding, hinting, implying, etc.—will conclude the semiotic analysis of hysteria.

The Rule-Following Model of Behavior

The concepts of rule-following and role-taking both derive from the premise that personal conduct may be studied fruitfully by considering man's "mind" mainly as a product of his social environment. In other words, although there are certain biological invariants in behavior, the precise pattern of human actions is determined largely by roles and rules. Accordingly, anthropology, ethics, and sociology are the basic sciences of human action, since they are concerned with the values, goals, and rules of human behavior (Kroeber, 1954; Kluckhohn, 1949; Sellars and Hospers, 1952).

With the introduction of the rule-following model, as a frame of reference for hysteria and mental illness, two questions naturally arise: (1) What kinds of roles are there, and how do they influence behavior? (2) Among a diversity of rules, which are the most relevant for understanding the historical development of the concept of hysteria?

My thesis is that two general types of rules are especially significant in the genesis of behavior which has been variously labeled "witchcraft," "hysteria," and "mental illness." One pertains to the essential helplessness of children and, hence, to the more-or-less biologically required help-giving activity of the parent. This results, especially among human beings, in complicated patterns of paired activities *characterized by the helplessness of one member and the helpfulness of the other.* The second source of rules which will be examined in detail are the teachings and practices of the Judeo-Christian religions. The New Testament in particular will be surveyed to discern the specific rules of conduct it prescribes. It will be apparent that for centuries Western man has been immersed—or has immersed himself—in an ocean of unserviceable social rules in which he has wallowed and nearly drowned. What I mean by this is that social life—through the combined impact of ubiquitous childhood experiences of dependence and of religious teachings—is so structured that it contains endless exhortations commanding man to behave childishly, stupidly, and irresponsibly. These exhortations to helplessness, although perhaps most powerful in their impact during the Middle Ages, have continued to influence human behavior to the present day.

The thesis that we are surrounded by an unseen ocean of human commands to be incompetent, impoverished, and sick will be illustrated mainly by references to the New Testament. In each person's actual life experiences, however, such influences need not necessarily come from officially organized religious sources. On the contrary, they derive usually from social intercourse with father, mother, husband, wife, employer, employee, and so on. However, the roles of the priestly and medical professions are especially significant in this connection, since their succoring activities rest squarely on the premise that the sinful, the weak, the sick—in brief, the disabled—should be helped. By implication, those who exhibit effective, self-reliant behavior need not be helped. They may even be taxed, burdened, or coerced in various ways. The *rewarding of disability*—although necessary in certain instances—is a potentially dangerous social practice.

The Game-Playing Model of Behavior

The communicational frame of reference implies that the communicants are engaged in an activity that is meaningful to them. By "meaningful" I refer to purposeful, goal-directed activity, and to the pursuit of goals in certain predetermined ways. If it appears that human beings are not so engaged, it is useful nevertheless to assume that they are and that we have been unable to comprehend the goals and the rules of their game. This position in regard to human behavior is not novel. It is a reformulation of the classic Shakespearean assertion that there is "method in madness." Similarly, in everyday life when a person acts in an incomprehensible fashion, the observer may ask, in the idiom of American slang, "What is his game?" or "What is his racket?" The basic psychoanalytic attitude toward "neurotic behavior" reflects the same premise. The analyst seeks to uncover and understand conduct in terms of unconscious motives, goals, roles, and the like. In the terms proposed here, the analyst seeks to unravel the game of life that the patient plays. The disposition to regard personal conduct as an expression of game-playing will constitute the theoretical basis of the last portion of this study.

A systematic exposition of the game-playing model of human behavior, based largely on the works of Mead and Piaget, will form the introduction to this subject. This will be supplemented by the construction of a game-hierarchy, with first-level or *object games* distinguished from higher-level or *metagames.*

Hysteria may be regarded as a heterogeneous mixture of metagames. As such, it—and mental illness generally—may be contrasted with uncomplicated cases of bodily illness and its treatment. The latter, being concerned with bodily survival, may be regarded as an object game. The former, being concerned with the problem of how man should live, is an example of a metagame.

Attempts simultaneously to pursue object games and metagames may bring a person into irreconcilable conflicts. Patrick Henry's famous declaration, "Give me liberty or give me death!" illustrates the potential conflict between physical survival and the ethical ideal of liberty. In this example, the end-goal of the metagame—that is, to live as a free man—takes precedence over the end-goal of the object game—that is, to survive at any cost. Conversely, adherence to the object game in this dilemma implies scuttling the metagame.

Games on any logical level may be played well or poorly. This holds true for hysteria, too. However, inasmuch as hysteria is composed of a mixture of several games, and inasmuch as the person trying to play this complex game is unaware of the rules by which he plays and the goals which he has set for himself, the likelihood of serious conflict in pursuing the goals and obeying the rules of the constituent games is great. This type of analysis will help us to see that while so-called psychiatric problems have significant intrapersonal, interpersonal, and social dimensions, they invariably have ethical dimensions as well. Once man rises above the level of playing the simplest sort of object game—the survival game—he is inevitably confronted by ethical choices. The analysis and rational scrutiny of the historical antecedents of "neurotic symptoms" or "character" cannot alone resolve an ethical dilemma. It is obvious that this can be accomplished only by making a human choice and committing one's self to it. This does not negate—on the contrary, it reemphasizes—the fact that the ability and the wish to make choices are themselves influenced by personal experiences.

The game-analytic description of human behavior unites elements of the sign-using and rule-following models into a coherent pattern. This approach to psychiatry is considered to be especially fitting for an integration of ethical, sociopolitical, and economic considerations with the more traditional concerns of the psychiatrist. Thus, the beginnings of a science and technology of human living, free of the errors of organicism as well as historicism, seem to be within reach.

Bibliography

Allport, G. W. (1955). *Becoming. Basic Considerations for a Psychology of Personality.* New Haven: Yale University Press.
Bridgman, P. W. (1959). *The Way Things Are.* Cambridge, Mass.: Harvard University Press.
Einstein, A. (1933). "On the Methods of Theoretical Physics." In, A. Einstein. *The World as I See It,* pp. 30–40. New York: Covici, Friede, 1934.
Freud, S. (1900). "The Interpretation of Dreams" (I & II). In, *The Standard Edition of the Complete Psychological Works of Sigmund Freud.* Vols. IV and V, pp. 1–621. London: Hogarth Press, 1953.
Freud, S. (1927). *The Future of an Illusion.* New York: Liveright, 1949.
Freud, S. (1940). *An Outline of Psychoanalysis.* New York: W. W. Norton.
Gregory, R. L. (1953). On physical model explanations in psychology. *Brit. J. Phil. Sc., 4:*192.
Hilgard, E. R. (1956). *Theories of Learning.* Second Edition. New York: Apple-ton-Century-Crofts.
Kluckhohn, C. (1949). *Mirror For Man. A Survey of Human Behavior and Social Attitudes.* New York: Premier Books, 1959.
Kroeber, A. L. (1954). *Anthropology Today. An Encyclopedic Inventory.* Chicago: The University of Chicago Press.
Ogden, C. K., and Richards, I. A. (1930). *The Meaning of Meaning. A Study of the Influence of Language upon Thought and of the Science of Symbolism.* With Supplementary Essays by B. Malinowski and F. G. Crookshank. Third Revised Edition. New York: Harcourt, Brace.
Popper, K. R. (1944–45). *The Poverty of Historicism.* Boston: Beacon Press, 1957.
Rieff, P. (1959). *Freud, The Mind of the Moralist.* New York: Viking.
Ryle, G. (1949). *The Concept of Mind.* London: Hutchinson's University Library.
Ryle, G. (1957). "The Theory of Meaning." In, C. A. Mace (ed.). *British Philosophy in the Mid-Century,* pp. 237–264. New York: Macmillan.
Sellars, W., and Hospers, J. (eds.) (1952). *Readings in Ethical Theory.* New York: Appleton-Century-Crofts.
Szasz, T. S. (1958a). Psychoanalysis as method and as theory. *Psychoanalyt. Quart., 27:*89.
Szasz, T. S. (1959b). The classification of "mental illness." A situational analysis of psychiatric operations. *Psychiat. Quart., 33:*77.

6

Goffman, E. (1961). *Asylums: Essays on the social situation of mental patients and other inmates.* New York: Anchor Books

Under the guise of being the athletic director's assistant, Goffman studied the lives of inmates and staff of a large mental hospital. People who enter the hospital as patients, Goffman says, are immersed in a strange world where their lives become the business of other people. Through a series of degradation rites, they experience a gradual "disculturation" and loss of self-efficacy, and their very characters are transformed as they learn to live as supplicants in "total institutions." Their presence in the institution, Goffman writes, is prima facie evidence that they are mentally ill. Their history, as captured in the hospital record, is a psychiatric version of the past constructed to demonstrate their need for treatment and their failure as persons. They are encouraged to learn and subscribe to this official version of their pasts and are said to have poor insight if they do not. Over time, they internalize this external version of self, along with a myriad of rules and assumptions that presuppose and dictate a loss of choice, self-determination, and knowledge of how to live outside the institution. Goffman notes, however, that patients of total institutions often find creative ways, out of view from staff, to make life within the institution more comfortable and interesting. *Asylums*, often regarded as a key document of the "antipsychiatry" movement, influenced a rising tide of public and professional repugnance for psychiatric hospitals that helped to fuel deinstitutionalization. The excerpt here is from Goffman's discussion of "The Moral Career of the Mental Patient.

Tom Dinzeo

Asylums: Essays on the Social Situation of Mental Patients and Other Inmates

Traditionally the term *career* has been reserved for those who expect to enjoy the rises laid out within a respectable profession. The term is coming to be used, however, in a broadened sense to refer to any social strand of any person's course through life. The perspective of natural history is taken: unique outcomes are neglected in favor of such changes over time as are basic and common to the members of a social category, although occurring independently to each of them. Such a career is not a thing that can be brilliant or disappointing; it can no more be a success than a failure. In this light, I want to consider the mental patient.

One value of the concept of career is its two-sidedness. One side is it linked to internal matters held dearly and closely, such as image of self and felt identity; the other side concerns official position, jural relations, and style of life, and is part of a publicly accessible institutional complex. The concept of career, then, allows one to move back and forth between the personal and the public, between the self and its significant society, without having to rely overly for data upon what the person says he thinks he imagines himself to be.

This paper, then, is an exercise in the institutional approach to the study of self. The main concern will be with the *moral* aspects of career—that is, the regular sequence of changes that career entails in the person's self and in his framework of imagery for judging himself and others.[1]

The category "mental patient" itself will be understood in one strictly sociological sense. In this perspective, the psychiatric view of a person becomes significant only in so far as this view itself alters his social fate—an alteration which seems to become fundamental in our society when, and only when, the person is put through the process of hospitalization.[2] I therefore exclude certain neighboring categories: the undiscovered candidates who would

---

[1] Material on moral career can be found in early social anthropological work on ceremonies of status transition, and in classic social psychological descriptions of those spectacular changes in one's view of self that can accompany participation in social movements and sects. Recently new kinds of relevant data have been suggested by psychiatric interest in the problem of "identity" and sociological studies of work careers and "adult socialization."

[2] This point has recently been made by Elaine and John Cumming, *Closed ranks* (Cambridge: Commonwealth Fund, Harvard University Press, 1957), pp. 101–102: *"Clinical experience supports the impression that many people define mental illness as 'that condition for which a person is treated in a mental hospital.'...Mental illness, it seems, is a condition which afflicts people who must go to a mental institution, but until they go almost anything they do is normal."* Leila Deasy has pointed out to me the correspondence here with the situation in white-collar crime. Of those who are detected in this activity, only the ones who do not manage to avoid going to prison find themselves accorded the social role of the criminal.

be judged "sick" by psychiatric standards but who never come to be viewed as such by themselves or others, although they may cause everyone a great deal of trouble[3]; the office patient whom a psychiatrist feels he can handle with drugs or shock on the outside; the mental client who engages in psychotherapeutic relationships. And I include anyone, however robust in temperament, who somehow gets caught up in the heavy machinery of mental-hospital servicing. In this way the effects of being treated as a mental patient can be kept quite distinct from the effects upon a person's life of traits a clinician would view as psychopathological.[4] Persons who become mental-hospital patients vary widely in the kind and degree of illness that a psychiatrist would impute to them, and in the attributes by which laymen would describe them. But once started on the way, they are confronted by some importantly similar circumstances and respond to these in some importantly similar ways. Since these similarities do not come from mental illness, they would seem to occur in spite of it. It is thus a tribute to the power of social forces that the uniform status of mental patient cannot only assure an aggregate of persons a common fate and eventually, because of this, a common character, but that this social reworking can be done upon what is perhaps the most obstinate diversity of human materials that can be brought together by society. Here there lacks only the frequent forming of a protective group life by ex-patients to illustrate in full the classic cycle of response by which deviant subgroupings are psychodynamically formed in society. This general sociological perspective is heavily reinforced by one key finding of sociologically oriented students in mental-hospital research. As has been repeatedly shown in the study of non-literate societies, the awesomeness, distastefulness, and barbarity of a foreign culture can decrease to the degree that the student becomes familiar with the point of view to life that is taken by his subjects. Similarly, the student of mental hospitals can discover that the craziness or "sick behavior" claimed for the mental patient is by and large a product of the claimant's social distance from the situation that the patient is in, and is not primarily a product of mental illness. Whatever the refinements of the various patients' psychiatric diagnoses, and whatever the special ways in which social life on the "inside" is unique, the researcher can find that he is participating in a community not significantly different from any other he has studied. Of course, while restricting himself to the off-ward grounds community of paroled patients, he may feel, as some patients do, that life in the locked wards is bizarre; and while on a locked admissions or convalescent ward, he may feel that chronic "back" wards are socially crazy places. But he need only move his sphere of sympathetic participation to the "worst" ward in the hospital, and this, too, can come into social focus as a place with a livable and continuously meaningful social world. This in no way denies that he will find a minority in any ward or patient group that continues to seem quite beyond the capacity to follow rules of social organization, or that the orderly fulfillment of normative expectations in patient society is partly made possible by strategic measures that have somehow come to be institutionalized in mental hospitals.

The career of the mental patient falls popularly and naturalistically into three main phases: the period prior to entering the hospital, which I shall call the prepatient phase; the period in the hospital, the inpatient phase; the period after discharge from the hospital,

---

[3.] Case records in mental hospitals are just now coming to be exploited to show the incredible amount of trouble a person may cause for himself and others before anyone begins to think about him psychiatrically, let alone take psychiatric action against him. See John A. Clausen and Marian Radke Yarrow, "Paths to the mental hospital," *Journal of Social Issues,* XI (1955), pp. 25–32; and August B. Hollingshead and Fredrick C. Redlich, *Social class and mental illness* (New York: Wiley, 1958), pp. 173–174.

[4.] An illustration of now this perspective may be taken to all forms of deviancy may be found in Edwin Lemert, *Social pathology* (New York: McGraw-Hill, 1951), see especially pp. 74–76. A specific application to mental defectives may be found in Stewart E. Perry, "Some theoretic problems of mental deficiency and their action implications," *Psychiatry,* XVII (1954), pp. 45–73, see especially pp. 67–68.

should this occur, namely, the ex-patient phase.[5] This paper will deal only with the first two phases.

The Prepatient Phase

A relatively small group of prepatients come into the mental hospital willingly, because of their own idea of what will be good for them, or because of wholehearted agreement with the relevant members of their family. Presumably these recruits have found themselves acting in a way which is evidence to them that they are losing their minds or losing control of themselves. This view of oneself would seem to be one of the most pervasively threatening things that can happen to the self in our society, especially since it is likely to occur at a time when the person is in any case sufficiently troubled to exhibit the kind of symptom which he himself can see. As Sullivan described it,

> What we discover in the self-system of a person undergoing schizophrenic change or schizophrenic processes, is then, in its simplest form, an extremely fear-marked puzzlement, consisting of the use of rather generalized and anything but exquisitely refined referential processes in an attempt to cope with what is essentially a failure at being human— a failure at being anything that one could respect as worth being.[6]

Coupled with the person's disintegrative re-evaluation of himself will be the new, almost equally pervasive circumstance of attempting to conceal from others what he takes to be the new fundamental facts about himself, and attempting to discover whether others, too, have discovered them.[7] Here I want to stress that perception of losing one's mind is based on culturally derived and socially engrained stereotypes as to the significance of symptoms such as hearing voices, losing temporal and spatial orientation, and sensing that one is being followed, and that many of the most spectacular and convincing of these symptoms in some instances psychiatrically signify merely a temporary emotional upset in a stressful situation, however terrifying to the person at the time. Similarly, the anxiety consequent upon this perception of oneself, and the strategies devised to reduce this anxiety, are not a product of abnormal psychology, but would be exhibited by any person socialized into our culture who came to conceive of himself as someone losing his mind. Interestingly, subcultures in American society apparently differ in the amount of ready imagery and encouragement they supply for such self-views, leading to differential rates of *self-referral;* the capacity to take this disintegrative view of oneself without psychiatric prompting seems to be one of the questionable cultural privileges of the upper classes.[8]

For the person who has come to see himself—with whatever justification—as mentally unbalanced, entrance to the mental hospital can sometimes bring relief, perhaps in part because of the sudden transformation in the structure of his basic social situation; instead

---

[5.] This simple picture is complicated by the somewhat special experience of roughly a third of ex-patients— namely, readmission to the hospital, this being the recidivist or "repatient" phase.

[6.] Harry Stack Sullivan, *Clinical studies in psychiatry,* edited by Helen Swick Perry, Mary Ladd Gawel, and Martha Gibbon (New York: Norton, 1956), pp. 184–85.

[7.] This moral experience can be contrasted with that of a person learning to become a marihuana addict, whose discovery that he can be "high" and still "op" effectively without being detected apparently leads to a new level of use. See Howard S. Becker, "Marihuana Use and Social Control," *Social Problems* III (1955), pp. 35–44; see especially pp. 40–41.

[8.] See Hollingshead and Redlich, *op. cit.,* p. 187, Table 6, where relative frequency is given of self-referral by social-class grouping.

of being to himself a questionable person trying to maintain a role as a full one, he can become an officially questioned person known to himself to be not so questionable as that. In other cases, hospitalization can make matters worse for the willing patient, confirming by the objective situation what has theretofore been a matter of the private experience of self.

Once the willing prepatient enters the hospital, he may go through the same routine of experiences as do those who enter unwillingly. In any case, it is the latter that I mainly want to consider, since in America at present these are by far the more numerous kind.[9] Their approach to the institution takes one of three classic forms: they come because they have been implored by their family or threatened with the abrogation of family ties unless they go "willingly"; they come by force under police escort; they come under misapprehension purposely induced by others, this last restricted mainly to youthful prepatients.

The prepatient's career may be seen in terms of an extrusory model; he starts out with relationships and rights, and ends up, at the beginning of his hospital stay, with hardly any of either. The moral aspects of this career, then, typically begin with the experience of abandonment, disloyalty, and embitterment. This is the case even though to others it may be obvious that he was in need of treatment, and even though in the hospital he may soon come to agree.

The case histories of most mental patients document offenses against some arrangement for face-to-face living —a domestic establishment, a work place, a semi-public organization such as a church or store, a public region such as a street or park. Often there is also a record of some *complainant,* some figure who takes that action against the offender which eventually leads to his hospitalization. This may not be the person who makes the first move, but it is the person who makes what turns out to be the first effective move. Here is the *social* beginning of the patient's career, regardless of where one might locate the psychological beginning of his mental illness.

The kinds of offenses which lead to hospitalization are felt to differ in nature from those which lead to other extrusory consequences—to imprisonment, divorce, loss of job, disownment, regional exile, non-institutional psychiatric treatment, and so forth. But little seems known about these differentiating factors; and when one studies actual commitments, alternate outcomes frequently appear to have been possible. It seems true, moreover, that for every offense that leads to an effective complaint, there are many psychiatrically similar ones that never do. No action is taken; or action is taken which leads to other extrusory outcomes; or ineffective action is taken, leading to the mere pacifying or putting off of the person who complains. Thus, as Clausen and Yarrow have nicely shown, even offenders who are eventually hospitalized are likely to have had a long series of ineffective actions taken against them.[10]

Separating those offenses which could have been used as grounds for hospitalizing the offender from those that are so used, one finds a vast number of what students of occupation call career contingencies.[11] Some of these contingencies in the mental patient's career have been suggested, if not explored, such as socio-economic status, visibility of the offense, proximity to a mental hospital, amount of treatment facilities available, community regard

---

[9.] The distinction employed here between willing and unwilling patients cuts across the legal one of voluntary and committed, since some persons who are glad to come to the mental hospital may be legally committed, and of those who come only because of strong familial pressure, some may sign themselves in as voluntary patients.

[10.] Clausen and Yarrow, *op. cit.*

[11.] An explicit application of this notion to the field of mental health may be found in Edwin Lemert, "Legal commitment and social control," *Sociology and Social Research,* XXX (1946), pp. 370–78.

for the type of treatment given in available hospitals, and so on.[12] For information about other contingencies one must rely on atrocity tales: a psychotic man is tolerated by his wife until she finds herself a boy friend, or by his adult children until they move from a house to an apartment; an alcoholic is sent to a mental hospital because the jail is full, and a drug addict because he declines to avail himself of psychiatric treatment on the outside; a rebellious adolescent daughter can no longer be managed at home because she now threatens to have an open affair with an unsuitable companion; and so on. Correspondingly there is an equally important set of contingencies causing the person to by-pass this fate. And should the person enter the hospital, still another set of contingencies will help determine when he is to obtain a discharge—such as the desire of his family for his return, the availability of a "manageable" job, and so on. The society's official view is that inmates of mental hospitals are there primarily because they are suffering from mental illness. However, in the degree that the "mentally ill" outside hospitals numerically approach or surpass those inside hospitals, one could say that mental patients distinctively suffer not from mental illness, but from contingencies.

Career contingencies occur in conjunction with a second feature of the prepatient's career—the circuit of agents—and agencies—that participate fatefully in his passage from civilian to patient status.[13] Here is an instance of that increasingly important class of social system whose elements are agents and agencies which are brought into systemic connection through having to take up and send on the same persons. Some of these agent roles will be cited now, with the understanding that in any concrete circuit a role may be filled more than once, and that the same person may fill more than one of them.

First is the *next-of-relation*—the person whom the prepatient sees as the most available of those upon whom he should be able to depend most in times of trouble, in this instance the last to doubt his sanity and the first to have done everything to save him from the fate which, it transpires, he has been approaching. The patient's next-of-relation is usually his next of kin; the special term is introduced because he need not be. Second is the *complainant,* the person who retrospectively appears to have started the person on his way to the hospital. Third are the *mediators*—the sequence of agents and agencies to which the prepatient is referred and through which he is relayed and processed on his way to the hospital. Here are included police, clergy, general medical practitioners, office psychiatrists, personnel in public clinics, lawyers, social service workers, schoolteachers, and so on. One of these agents will have the legal mandate to sanction commitment and will exercise it, and so those agents who precede him in the process will be involved in something whose outcome is not yet settled. When the mediators retire from the scene, the prepatient has become an inpatient, and the significant agent has become the hospital administrator.

While the complainant usually takes action in a lay capacity as a citizen, an employer, a neighbor, or a kinsman, mediators tend to be specialists and differ from those they serve in significant ways. They have experience in handling trouble, and some professional distance from what they handle. Except in the case of policemen, and perhaps some clergy, they tend to be more psychiatrically oriented than the lay public, and will see the need for treatment at times when the public does not.[14]

[12.] For example, Jerome K. Meyers and Leslie Schaffer, "Social stratification and psychiatric practice: A study of an outpatient clinic," *American Sociological Review,* XIX (1954), pp, 307–310; Lemert, *op. cit.,* pp. 402–403; *Patients in mental institutions, 1941* (Washington, D.C.: Department of Commerce, Bureau of the Census, 1941), p. 2.

[13.] For one circuit of agents and its bearing on career contingencies; see Oswald Hall, "The stages of a medical career," *American Journal of Sociology,* LIII (1948), pp. 327–336.

[14.] See Cumming and Cumming, *op. cit.,* p. 92.

An interesting feature of these roles is the functional effects of their interdigitation. For example, the feelings of the patient will be influenced by whether or not the person who fills the role of complainant also has the role of next-of-relation—an embarrassing combination more prevalent, apparently, in the higher classes than in the lower.[15] Some of these emergent effects will be considered now.[16]

In the prepatient's progress from home to the hospital he may participate as a third person in what he may come to experience as a kind of alienative coalition. His next-of-relation presses him into coming to "talk things over" with a medical practitioner, an office psychiatrist, or some other counselor. Disinclination on his part may be met be threatening him with desertion, disownment, or other legal action, or by stressing the joint and exploratory nature of the interview. But typically the next-of-relation will have set the interview up, in the sense of selecting the professional, arranging for time, telling the professional something about the case, and so on. This move effectively tends to establish the next-of-relation as the responsible person to whom pertinent findings can be divulged, while effectively establishing the other as the patient. The prepatient often goes to the interview with the understanding that he is going as an equal of someone who is so bound together with him that a third person could not come between them in fundamental matters; this, after all, is one way in which close relationships are defined in our society. Upon arrival at the office the prepatient suddenly finds that he and his next-of-relation have not been accorded the same roles, and apparently that a prior understanding between the professional and the next-of-relation has been put in operation against him. In the extreme but common case, the professional first sees the prepatient alone, in the role of examiner and diagnostician, and then sees the next-of-relation alone, in the role of adviser, while carefully avoiding talking things over seriously with them both together.[17] And even in those non-consultative cases where public officials must forcibly extract a person from a family that wants to tolerate him, the next-of-relation is likely to be induced to "go along" with the official action, so that even here the prepatient may feel that an alienative coalition has been formed against him.

The moral experience of being third man in such a coalition is likely to embitter the prepatient, especially since his troubles have already probably led to some estrangement from his next-of-relation. After he enters the hospital, continued visits by his next-of-relation can give the patient the "insight" that his own best interests were being served. But the initial visits may temporarily strengthen his feeling of abandonment; he is likely to beg his visitor to get him out or at least to get him more privileges and to sympathize with the monstrousness of his plight—to which the visitor ordinarily can respond only by trying to maintain a hopeful note, by not "hearing" the requests, or by assuring the patient that the medical[17] authorities know about these things and are doing what is medically best. The visitor then nonchalantly goes back into a world that the patient has learned is incredibly thick with freedom and privileges, causing the patient to feel that his next-of-relation is merely adding a pious gloss to a clear case of traitorous desertion.

[15] Hollingshead and Redlich, *op. cit.*, p. 187.

[16] For an analysis of some of these circuit implications for the inpatient, see Leila Deasy and Olive W. Quinn, "The wife of the mental patient and the hospital psychiatrist," *Journal of Social Issues*, XI (1955), pp. 49–60. An interesting illustration of this kind of analysis may also be found in Alan G. Gowman, "Blindness and the role of the companion," *Social Problems*, IV (1956), pp. 68–75. A general statement may be found in Robert Merton, "The role set: Problems in sociological theory," *British Journal of Sociology*, VIII (1957), pp. 106–120.

[17] I have one case record of a man who claims he thought *he* was taking his wife to see the psychiatrist, not realizing until too late that his wife had made the arrangements.

The depth to which the patient may feel betrayed by his next-of-relation seems to be increased by the fact that another witnesses his betrayal—a factor which is apparently significant in many three-party situations. An offended person may well act forbearingly and accommodatively toward an offender when the two are alone, choosing peace ahead of justice. The presence of a witness, however, seems to add something to the implications of the offense. For then it is beyond the power of the offended and offender to forget about, erase, or suppress what has happened; the offense has become a public social fact.[18] When the witness is a mental health commission, as is sometimes the case, the witnessed betrayal can verge on a "degradation ceremony."[19] In such circumstances, the offended patient may feel that some kind of extensive reparative action is required before witnesses, if his honor and social weight are to be restored.

Two other aspects of sensed betrayal should be mentioned. First, those who suggest the possibility of another's entering a mental hospital are not likely to provide a realistic picture of how in fact it may strike him when he arrives. Often he is told that he will get required medical treatment and a rest, and may well be out in a few months or so. In some cases they may thus be concealing what they know, but I think, in general, they will be telling what they see as the truth. For here there is quite relevant difference between patients and mediating professionals; mediators, more so than the public at large, may conceive of mental hospitals as short-term medical establishments where required rest and attention can be voluntarily obtained, and not as places of coerced exile. When the prepatient finally arrives he is likely to learn quite quickly, quite differently. He then finds that the information given him about life in the hospital has had the effect of his having put up less resistance to entering than he now sees he would have put up had he known the facts. Whatever the intentions of those who participated in his transition from person to patient, he may sense they have in effect "conned" him into his present predicament.

I am suggesting that the prepatient starts out with at least a portion of the rights, liberties, and satisfactions of the civilian and ends up on a psychiatric ward stripped of almost everything. The question here is how this stripping is managed. This is the second aspect of betrayal I want to consider.

As the prepatient may see it, the circuit of significant figures can function as a kind of betrayal funnel. Passage from person to patient may be effected through a series of linked stages, each managed by a different agent. While each stage tends to bring a sharp decrease in adult free status, each agent may try to maintain the fiction that no further decrease will occur. He may even manage to turn the prepatient over to the next agent while sustaining this note. Further, through words, cues, and gestures, the prepatient is implicitly asked by the current agent to join with him in sustaining a running line of polite small talk that tactfully avoids the administrative facts of the situation, becoming, with each stage, progressively more at odds with these facts. The spouse would rather not have to cry to get the prepatient to visit a psychiatrist; psychiatrists would rather not have a scene when the prepatient learns that he and his spouse are being seen separately and in different ways; the police infrequently bring a prepatient to the hospital in a strait jacket, finding it much easier all around to give him a cigarette, some kindly words, and freedom to relax in the back seat of the patrol car; and finally, the admitting psychiatrist finds he can do his work better in the relative quiet and luxury of the "admission suite" where, as an incidental consequence, the notion can survive that a mental hospital is indeed a comforting place. If the prepatient

[18.] A paraphrase from Kurt Riezler, "Comment on the social psychology of shame," *American Journal of Sociology,* XLVIII (1943), p. 458.

[19.] See Harold Garfinkel, "Conditions of successful degradation ceremonies," *American Journal of Sociology,* LXI (1956), pp. 420–424.

heeds all of these implied requests and is reasonably decent about the whole thing, he can travel the whole circuit from home to hospital without forcing anyone to look directly at what is happening or to deal with the raw emotion that his situation might well cause him to express. His showing consideration for those who are moving him toward the hospital allows them to show consideration for him, with the joint result that these interactions can be sustained with some of the protective harmony characteristic of ordinary face-to-face dealings. But should the new patient cast his mind back over the sequence of steps leading to hospitalization, he may feel that everyone's current comfort was being busily sustained while his long-range welfare was being undermined. This realization may constitute a moral experience that further separates him for the time from the people on the outside.[20]

I would now like to look at the circuit of career agents from the point of view of the agents themselves. Mediators in the person's transition from civil to patient status —as well as his keepers, once he is in the hospital—have an interest in establishing a responsible next-of-relation as the patient's deputy or guardian; should there be no obvious candidate for the role, someone may be sought out and pressed into it. Thus while a person is gradually being transformed into a patient, a next-of-relation is gradually being transformed into a guardian. With a guardian on the scene, the whole transition process can be kept tidy. He is likely to be familiar with the prepatient's civil involvements and business, and can tie up loose ends that might otherwise be left to entangle the hospital. Some of the prepatient's abrogated civil rights can be transferred to him, thus helping to sustain the legal fiction that while the prepatient does not actually have his rights he somehow actually has not lost them.

Inpatients commonly sense, at least for a time, that hospitalization is a massive unjust deprivation, and sometimes succeed in convincing a few persons on the outside that this is the case. It often turns out to be useful, then, for those identified with inflicting these deprivations, however justifiably, to be able to point to the co-operation and agreement of someone whose relationship to the patient places him above suspicion, firmly defining him as the person most likely to have the patient's personal interest at heart. If the guardian is satisfied with what is happening to the new inpatient, the world ought to be.[21]

Now it would seem that the greater the legitimate personal stake one party has in another, the better he can take the role of guardian to the other. But the structural arrangements in society which lead to the acknowledged merging of two persons' interests lead to additional consequences. For the person to whom the patient turns for help—for protection against such threats as involuntary commitment—is just the person to whom the mediators and hospital administrators logically turn for authorization. *It* is understandable, then, that some patients will come to sense, at least for a time, that the closeness of a relationship tells nothing of its trustworthiness.

---

[20] Concentration-camp practices provide a good example of the function of the betrayal funnel in inducing co-operation and reducing struggle and fuss, although here the mediators could not be said to be acting in the best interests of the inmates. Police picking up persons from their homes would sometimes joke good-naturedly and offer to wait while coffee was being served. Gas chambers were fitted out like delousing rooms, and victims taking off their clothes were told to note where they were leaving them. The sick, aged, weak, or insane who were selected for extermination were sometimes driven away in Red Cross ambulances to camps referred to by terms such as "observation hospital." See David Boder, *I did not interview the dead* (Urbana: University of Illinois Press, 1949), p. 81; and Elie A. Cohen, *Human behavior in the concentration camp* (London; Jonathan Cape, 1954), pp. 32, 37, 107.

[21] Interviews collected by the Clausen group at NIMH suggest that when a wife comes to be a guardian, the responsibility may disrupt previous distance from in-laws, leading either to a new supportive coalition with them or to a marked withdrawal from them.

There are still other functional effects emerging from this complement of roles. If and when the next-of-relation appeals to mediators for help in the trouble he is having with the prepatient, hospitalization may not, in fact, be in his mind. He may not even perceive the pre-patient as mentally sick, or, if he does, he may not consistently hold to this view.[22] It is the circuit of mediators, with their greater psychiatric sophistication and their belief in the medical character of mental hospitals, that will often define the situation for the next-of-relation, assuring him that hospitalization is a possible solution and a good one, that it involves no betrayal, but is rather a medical action taken in the best interests of the prepatient.[1] Here the next-of-relation may learn that doing his duty to the prepatient may cause the prepatient to distrust and even hate him for the time. But the fact that this course of action may have had to be pointed out and prescribed by professionals, and be defined by them as a moral duty, relieves the next-of-relation of some of the guilt he may feel.[23] It is a poignant fact that an adult son or daughter may be pressed into the role of mediator, so that the hostility that might otherwise be directed against the spouse is passed on to the child.[24]

Once the prepatient is in the hospital, the same guilt-carrying function may become a significant part of the staff's job in regard to the next-of-relation.[25] These reasons for feeling that he himself has not betrayed the patient, even though the patient may then think so, can later provide the next-of-relation with a defensible line to take when visiting the patient in the hospital and a basis for hoping that the relationship can be re-established after its hospital moratorium. And of course this position, when sensed by the patient, can provide him with excuses for the next-of-relation, when and if he comes to look for them.[26]

Thus while the next-of-relation can perform important functions for the mediators and hospital administrators, they in turn can perform important functions for him. One finds, then, an emergent unintended exchange or reciprocation of functions, these functions themselves being often unintended.

The final point I want to consider about the prepatient's moral career is its peculiarly retroactive character. Until a person actually arrives at the hospital there usually seems no way of knowing for sure that he is destined to do so, given the determinative role of career contingencies. And until the point of hospitalization is reached, he or others may not conceive of him as a person who is becoming a mental patient. However, since he will be held against his will in the hospital, his next-of-relation and the hospital staff will be in great need of a rationale for the hardships they are sponsoring. The medical elements of the staff will also need evidence that they are still in the trade they were trained for.

[22.] For an analysis of these non-psychiatric kinds of perception, see Marian Radke Yarrow, Charlotte Green Schwartz, Harriet S. Murphy, and Leila Deasy, "The psychological meaning of mental illness in the family," *Journal of Social Issues, XI* (1955), pp. 12–24; Charlotte Green Schwartz, "Perspectives on deviance— Wives' definitions of their husbands' mental illness," *Psychiatry*, XX (1957), pp. 275–291.

[23.] This guilt-carrying function is found, of course, in other role complexes. Thus, when a middle-class couple engages in the process of legal separation or divorce, each of their lawyers usually takes the position that his job is to acquaint his client with all of the potential claims and rights, pressing his client into demanding these, in spite of any nicety of feelings about the rights and honorableness of the ex-partner. The client, in all good faith, can then say to self and to the ex-partner that the demands are being made only because the lawyer insists it is best to do so.

[24.] Recorded in the Clausen data.

[25.] This point is made by Cumming and Cumming, *op. cit.,* p. 129.

[26.] There is an interesting contrast here with the moral career of the tuberculosis patient. I am told by Julius Roth that tuberculous patients are likely to come to the hospital willingly, agreeing with their next-of-relation about treatment. Later in their hospital career, when they learn how long they yet have to stay and how depriving and irrational some of the hospital rulings are, they may seek to leave, be advised against this by the staff and by relatives, and only then begin to feel betrayed.

These problems are eased, no doubt unintentionally, by the case-history construction that is placed on the patient's past life, this having the effect of demonstrating that all along he had been becoming sick, that he finally became very sick, and that if he had not been hospitalized much worse things would have happened to him—all of which, of course, may be true. Incidentally, if the patient wants to make sense out of his stay in the hospital, and, as already suggested, keep alive the possibility of once again conceiving of his next-of-relation as a decent, well-meaning person, then he, too, will have reason to believe some of this psychiatric work-up of his past.

Here is a very ticklish point for the sociology of careers. An important aspect of every career is the view the person constructs when he looks backward over his progress; in a sense, however, the whole of the prepatient career derives from this reconstruction. The fact of having had a prepatient career, starting with an effective complaint, becomes an important part of the mental patient's orientation, but this part can begin to be played only after hospitalization proves that what he had been having, but no longer has, is a career as a prepatient.

7

Brenner, M. H. (1973). *Mental illness and the economy.* Cambridge, MA: Harvard University Press

Brenner's study of the relationship between mental illness and changes in the economy involves the use of data on economic and hospital admissions in New York State in sum and by gender, education, ethnic background, marital background, and other domains, from the nineteenth century to the early 1970s. Brenner's argument, built on the premise of hospital admissions as the best indicator, in the pre–"community psychiatry" era, of rates and intensity of mental illness in the population, is simple and elegant: "First," he writes, "it is clear that instabilities in the national economy have been the single most important source of fluctuation in mental-hospital admissions or admission rates. Second, this relation is so consistent for certain segments of the society that virtually no major factor other than economic instability appears to influence variation in their mental hospitalization rates" (p. ix). From this basis, Brenner argues that socioeconomic and social-structural changes are better predictors of individual mental disorder than are individual effort, characteristics, and vulnerabilities. The excerpts here come from the book's conclusion. In the first excerpt, Brenner summarizes his case for the link between psychiatry and the social system and against a view of mental illness as residing primarily in the individual diagnosed with the mental illness. In the second excerpt, he concludes with the larger implications of his findings for the ideology of individualism in American society.

Conclusion and Implications

In Chapter 9 we proposed and examined various mechanisms whereby mental hospitalization could be increased through economic change. These mechanisms included possible increases in (1) intolerance of mental illness, (2) development of psychiatric symptoms, and (3) the use of the mental hospital as an almshouse. At that point it was concluded that any or all of these mechanisms might in some way be responsible for mental hospitalization. It was found, however, that for many population groups probably neither intolerance of mental illness nor the need for the material necessities of life was the *primary* factor intervening between economic change and mental hospitalization. It was therefore suggested that fluctuations in pathological behavior in the population at risk might in many cases be a major, if not *the* major, intervening variable. In any case, it appears that both the presence of psychiatric symptoms and intolerance of these symptoms are necessary components in hospitalization, and both of these inferences are consistent with prevailing theory and research evidence bearing on mental illness and psychiatric hospitalization.

Social and Personality Disorganization During Economic Change

At this juncture, it might be useful to speculate on the implications of various interpretations of the findings. Two interpretations of the data that do not require great imagination are simply that economic change has a substantial impact on psychiatry as an institution and on the lives of persons who eventually become mentally hospitalized. The data of this study consistently indicate that, historically, the role of psychiatry as an institution has been intimately tied to dislocations in the economic system.

This is a very different perspective on psychiatry from the one that is frequently seen in popular and even in professional literature. A common image is that of a face-to-face relation between a clinician and a distraught individual whose emotional and intellectual personality development is largely responsible for his mental disorder. This study, by contrast, emphasizes the institutional aspect of psychiatry and offers the view that psychiatry is an arm of the social system which has been called upon largely to assist in patching up ruptures resulting from poor economic and social integration. In this sense, psychiatry is seen as having a large-scale structure analogous to that of the economy itself.

Such a structure is, of course, an abstraction, as is the concept of the national economy as a system. Much as the economy is highly organized in terms of industries and occupations, the mentally ill have historically been cared for (for the most part) in large-scale organizations and with the participation of psychiatrists and other clinicians loosely allied

95

to such organizations. Moreover, psychiatry is organized through professional associations and through the training of professionals in schools of medicine and allied clinical institutions and settings.

It is interesting, however, that the clinicians who are involved in psychiatric care, in the United States in particular, operate under a set of values and beliefs that are probably antithetical to the perspective of this study. The data shown here clearly portray psychiatry historically as an agent of social repair, whereas traditionally the strategies of psychiatric care have, theoretically, been largely irrelevant to large-scale societal disequilibria.

Moreover, psychiatric care has traditionally not been focused even on major *individual* problems other than the disorder itself. The underlying theory is that the source of mental disorder lies not within the network of an individual's relations, but within the individual himself. We thus find responsibility for the disorder placed on the irrational and largely unconscious activities of the individual in whom it is observed. This assumption, that it is reasonable as well as possible to treat the individual's disorder apart from becoming involved in the social context in which it is enmeshed, may be debated on the ground that the disorder itself may largely depend on *continuing* interactions in which the individual is involved.

However, there is now a substantial accumulation of research evidence which indicates that the development of psychotic patterns of behavior and schizophrenic patterns in particular may occur through familial patterns of interaction.[1] Presented with a dynamic model of this sort, it becomes difficult for the independent observer to ascertain which of several family members may be most "sick." In fact, it might require an unusually severe set of precipitating stresses to bring about the classical pattern of disturbed intellectual or emotional functioning in any one of these family members.

Given data such as those found in this study, questions may be raised as to the relative effectiveness and appropriateness of much of traditional psychiatric practice. It appears from this study that many of the major reasons for psychiatric hospitalization—the most prominent modality of psychiatric treatment of severe mental illness—have to do with disruption of the social ties of individuals; furthermore, these disruptions are not initially under the control of, or in any way due to, the behavior of the individuals in question. The probability is quite strong that the person who becomes psychiatrically hospitalized is reacting to social changes affecting not only his own immediate style of life, but those of many other people as well. The needs of such persons probably encompass far more than has been traditionally considered the province of psychiatric care.

It is even possible that, in a substantial fraction of cases, psychiatric care may not be necessary in order to alleviate what were initially problems related to large- or small-scale social change. This possibility may present itself in at least two ways. First, once the problems of social disruption are dealt with, it is possible either that the individual will cease to react symptomatically or that the family might be better able emotionally to cope with his disorder. Second, it is possible that once the major social stresses have been moderated the individual may be better able to tolerate his own disorder and therefore, in fact, *be* less sick, that is, feel less uncomfortable with his own feelings and thoughts.

This view of the social processes by which mental illness may become more or less of a severe problem points to the potential importance of the clinician's ability to affect the social situation in which he finds his patient. It also suggests that the clinician ideally ought to be able to exert some control over the flow of social stresses that continuously disrupt his patients' social relations. The traditional psychiatric approach, however, does not focus on problems of social interaction or on the implications of social or economic change.

The fact that the psychiatric professions have traditionally not been able to deal with the major stresses which lead to mental hospitalization may simply be one way of referring to mental hospitalization as a social problem. However, hospitalization is not only a psychiatrically inappropriate response to economic stress; it actually compounds the social impact of economic stress enormously. Under conditions of economic stress, mental hospitalization represents the culmination of a process of disruption and disintegration of family and other close relations. It closes off and isolates an individual from his normal social context, placing him in a situation in which the focus of his life consists of adaptation to the routine of a highly bureaucratic organization.

The needs of the hospital as an organization, in turn, frequently bear little relation to the needs of the hospitalized patient in terms of his adjustment to social life. The image of the mental hospital as a place of confinement, rather than of readjustment, of the patient is partly responsible for the development of the community mental-health-center model which includes forms of psychiatric treatment that are fundamentally integrated with community life.

Within the scheme of mental hospitalization, the patient's economic and social careers can be very seriously damaged. There is not only immediate disruption of his career itself, which removes the patient from his usual socioeconomic matrix, but, more important, there may be a lasting impression of the former patient as a relatively high risk for potentially severe mental disorder which may disqualify him from a position that has even a modest level of responsibility attached to it. In addition, there is evidence that removal of an individual from a specific social group, such as friends or family, changes the structure and functioning of the group so that it may be quite difficult to reintegrate him into such a group.[2] The overall economic and social disruption brought about by economic stress may thus be greatly compounded by the intervention of hospitalization or another isolating experience.

Aside from examining the implications of economic change for the operation of psychiatry as a therapeutic endeavor, or for hospitalization in particular, we are interested in exploring some of the rather diffuse, but more socially pervasive, implications of economic stress. Two somewhat related concepts that describe disruptive characteristics of mental hospitalization are "pathology" and "social disintegration." Pathology refers especially to individual personality disorganization, whereas social disintegration implies breakdown in the functioning of the structure of social groups. It is entirely possible that personality disorganization rarely occurs except under conditions of social disorganization. The reverse may also be true, that is, there may be social structural decay only under conditions of personality disorganization. The two phenomena can, however, be separately investigated, and they have somewhat different implications.

For example, in the intensive examination of violent crimes among specific individuals, we may discover patterns of individual psychopathology or a disturbance in personality integration. If, on the other hand, we compare *rates* of violent crimes among various populations, we would probably not say that the population showing the highest rates was necessarily the most pathological, although we might wish to describe it as the least well integrated. In common parlance, "pathological" is a term that is most closely identified with unusual and probably severe social disruption, especially behavior for which a person may be criminally liable. Social disintegration, on the other hand, ordinarily refers to the more commonplace, and less precipitous, breakdown in cultural, political, institutional, or family systems.

The findings of this study raise the possibility that, for a substantial portion of the mentally hospitalized population, a primary reaction to economic stress occurs in the form of psychiatric symptoms. If this inference is correct, then it is probably true that other indicators of psychopathology would increase in the population at large during periods of economic stress. The data of this study on hospitalization of the criminally insane appear to substantiate this speculation. Admissions to hospitals for the criminally insane are as closely related (inversely) to economic change as are admissions to state or private psychiatric hospitals. It is only recently, however, that we have routinely begun to define and treat as psychiatrically ill a considerable number of persons judged to have committed crimes.

Nevertheless, the implication is that criminal behavior generally, and crimes against persons in particular, may respond as sharply to economic change as does mental hospitalization. There does appear to be some evidence supporting this hypothesis among scattered reports published during the last century.[3] Realistically, then, both the mental hospital and the prison might be considered agents of social control that are brought into play particularly during periods of economic disruption. On an institutional level, in fact, we might expect to see that the administration of the prison behaves very much like that of the mental hospital during economic changes.

Again, there is considerable evidence of an inverse relation between mortality from suicide and economic change.[4] Suicide is another example of an act that is frequently thought to be fundamentally psychopathological or, at least, to be a symptom of an underlying pathological condition. Moreover, in the case of suicide there are some studies that show very similar relations with economic change (in terms of age and sex) to the ones found in the present study of mental-hospital admissions. In fact, one of the major hypotheses of the present study—that the pattern of hospital admissions of higher socioeconomic groups would be more directly related to economic changes than those of lower socioeconomic groups—is drawn from studies of suicide in the United States.

Although we may consider relatively high rates of criminal behavior or suicide as unusually strong evidence of the lack of social integration, the concept of social integration is perhaps more directly understood as the overall cohesiveness of social ties. Similarly, whereas mental hospitalization provides a strong inferential indication of disruption in social relations, we do not have first-hand evidence of dramatic changes in the structure of families or friendships that might be assumed to have preceded hospitalization. In fact, it may be true that economic change can bring about mental hospitalization only as the conclusion of a lengthy causal chain of breakdowns in social relations.

Yet for most of the population that experiences economic stress, mental hospitalization is not an outcome. The implication may be that large-scale social disintegration nearly always produces some mental hospitalization. And finally, in speaking of mental hospitalization as one indicator of social disintegration, we imply that there are probably a number of such indicators of breakdown in family and other social relations that are the consequences of economic stress.

References

1. Gregory Bateson, Don D. Jackson, Jay Hayley and John Weakland, "Toward a Theory of Schizophrenia," *Behavioral Science*, 1:251–264 (1956); Theodore H. Lidz, Steven Fleck, and Alice R. Cornelison, *Schizophrenia and the Family* (New York: International Universities Press, 1965); Howard E. Freeman and Ozzie G. Simmons, "Mental Patients in the Community: Family Settings and Performance Levels," *American Sociological Review*, 23:147–154 (1958).
2. H. E. Freeman and O. G. Simmons, *The Mental Patient Comes Home* (New York: Wiley, 1963); J. B. Myers and L. Bean, *A Decade Later: A Follow-up of Social Class and Mental Illness* (New York: Wiley, 1968).

3. Harold Phelps, "Cycles of Crime," *Journal of Criminal Law and Criminology,* 20:107–121 (May–June 1929); Ray Mars Simpson, "Unemployment and Prison Commitments," *Journal of Criminal Law and Criminology,* 23:404–414 (September–October 1932); Andrew F. Henry and James F. Short, *Suicide and Homicide* (Glencoe, Ill.: Free Press, 1954).

4. Henry and Short, *Suicide and Homicide.* B. McMahon, S. Johnson and T. F. Pugh, "Relation of Suicide Rates to Social Conditions, Evidence From U. S. Vital Statistics," *Public Health Reports*, 78:285–293 (1963).

The Theme of Individualism

Perhaps the most important factors responsible for the relation between economic change and mental hospitalization that have not been reported earlier are those surrounding the theme of individualism in Western, and particularly American, intellectual and political life. The general cultural theme of individualism has had a pervasive impact on our understanding of both mental hospitalization and economic success and failure. Traditionally, it has been taken for granted that, since the mentally hospitalized patient is psychiatrically ill, mental hospitalization could be explained in accordance with prevailing theories of mental illness. These theories assumed that mental illness could be described within two broad categories, functional and organic. Until very recently, moreover, one or another unicausal model of mental illness was assumed to be operative. Under such models, mental disorder was thought to result from one specific agent of either a biochemical or a psychological nature. In both of these models, the broad social environment was largely ignored. Among the mental disorders that were attributed to organic (that is, nervous-system) damage, the proposed remedies were surgical or chemical, whereas among the functional illnesses efforts to alter personality structure were also used.

Even where psychotherapeutic methods of treatment were utilized, they usually relied upon theories of human behavior that were based on a perspective of individual psychology. Under the theme of individual psychology, even the major Freudian psychoanalytic writings came to be regarded as involving individual behavior as distinguished from what was thought of as social behavior. We need not dwell on the frequently unjustified critiques of Freudian psychology that base themselves on Freud's alleged disregard of the interpersonal foundations of personality development. The essential point is that there is a substantial intellectual tradition which has treated Freudian psychology as though it regarded the influences of cultures and social systems as irrelevant to the development of personality.[19] We may go so far as to say that since nearly all of the traditional psychotherapeutic techniques have as their aim the adjustment of the patient to the requirements and norms of society, the theories are individual-centered. By individual-centered we mean largely uninvolved with those changes that are initiated in the individual's social environment, which may have caused his failure to adjust to that environment.

The approach of individual psychology to the understanding of abnormal behavior is not peculiar to clinicians, but is probably the most prevalent viewpoint among the lay public (particularly within the United States). Among the general public, the occurrence of mental disorder is almost by definition an individual phenomenon which is unintelligible in social terms and is usually interpreted as irrational. Simply because mental illness connotes bizarreness to the general public, it must be viewed as an individual aberration.

The themes of individual psychology in clinical theory and mental disorder as individual abnormality may be closely related, however, to the theme of individualism that has been developed in Western, and especially American, culture. It is probably no accident, for example, that individual psychology has not predominated in the psychiatric practice of socialist countries.[20] For the general American public, the theme of individualism underlies concepts not only of just government but of an equitable legal system as well. Both the democratic process and much of the legal system are, to a great degree, founded on the philosophical concepts that include "free will." The free-will concept philosophically negates empirically based theories which argue that the behavior of an individual is strongly influenced by forces originating outside of himself.

Politically, free will has been used to justify the right of each individual to participate in the choice of his government on the ground that he exercises real choice—in other words, that he is free to exercise his choice. This freedom of choice is then distinguished from the procedures of dictatorial governments, in which the individual citizen submits blindly to those in authority. Similarly, the legal concept of criminality is grounded on the theological presupposition that individuals actually choose between right and wrong, and that it is not the society that influences them to choose one or the other, because, if society did provide the influences which determined that the individual should choose to engage in criminal behavior, then the society in general, and not the individual, would justifiably be attacked. Thus, for any individual, the only alternative to the legal assumption of free will and implicit rationality is of course irrationality, and therefore insanity.

Elements of the same individualistic philosophy can early be seen in the thinking of many Americans about the economic success or failure of individuals. The assumption is that an individual succeeds or fails by his own talents, abilities, and efforts. Almost in the same conceptual terms of individual psychology, individual achievement is seen as the product of the personality. In other words, allegedly stable individual personality characteristics are deemed responsible for the individual's motivation and capability. But there is an equally important ideological element in the theme of individualism in economic life. The theme originates in the arguments that underlie the laissez-faire capitalism of such 19th-century political economists as John Stuart Mill.[21]

The theme was further developed under the influence of the social Darwinists who gave birth to notion of "ragged individualism."[22] This general philosophical theme of individualism in economic behavior has been somewhat attenuated by the introduction of social-welfare policies and governmental manipulation of the economy during the Great Depression and the post-Second World War periods. Despite the significant de-emphasis of individualism as a nationally proclaimed economic ideology, the theme of individual competence has not been replaced as the major perspective by which success or failure is judged.

The fact that ability to succeed in economic life is substantially determined by an individual's position in the social structure appears to contradict the American ideal of equality of opportunity. It is apparent that the clear and well-publicized fact that the social class (or socioeconomic position) of one's parents has an overwhelming influence on personality development and life chances in general has not been accepted. Instead, the ideology of the Protestant ethic continues to be perpetuated, even though the sense of urgency over achievement may have abated somewhat.[23]

Perhaps the heart of the problem is that, where large aggregations of individuals are not organized in common pursuit of an objective, the belief takes hold, buttressed by the individualistic perspective, that the behavior of these individuals is not subject to social influence. In other words, the conception of what is *social* tends to be defined as that which is *organized*. It is relatively easy to identify social movements, and frequently even riots, as social behavior, but the image of the individual working alone, or even within a small group, fails to take on a sociocultural appearance. What then remains is that there is little appreciation of the fact that human behavior is constantly influenced by the sociological characteristics of the individuals involved (such as their sex, age, occupation, education, ethnicity) and the social and cultural context in which the behavior takes place.

There may be certain gains for political democracy by a continuance of the ideology of individualism. However, it is difficult to imagine that there are long-range benefits to the political or legal systems of any modern nation in the illusion that individual personality and behavior are *not* intimately related to the culture and institutions of the overall society. In fact, as the present study has shown, it can be extremely harmful for the society not to recognize that instabilities in the economic system can have a substantially disruptive effect on many social institutions, including the family.

Finally, it is important that economic instability be understood not only in terms of major economic downturns such as depressions or recessions, but more generally as any departure from smooth economic development during which a significant number of people are excluded.

References

19. See the literature in Herbert Marcuse, *Eros and Civilization: A Philosophical Inquiry into Freud* (New York: Random House, 1955), pp. 217–251.
20. Ari Kiev, *Psychiatry in the Communist World* (New York: Science House, 1968).
21. J. S. Mill, *Principles of Political Economy* (Toronto: University of Toronto Press, 1965; first published in 1848).
22. Richard Hofstadter, *Social Darwinism in American Thought* (Philadelphia: University of Pennsylvania Press, 1944).
23. David Reismann, Nathan Glazer, and Reuel Denney, *The Lonely Crowd* (New Haven, Conn: Yale University Press, 1961); W. W. Rostow, *The Stages of Economic Growth: A Non-Communist Manifesto* (Cambridge, England: Cambridge University Press, 1957).

8

Scull, A. T. (1976). The decarceration of the mentally ill: A critical view. *Politics and Society, 6*: 173–212

Scull's critique of deinstitutionalization includes a debunking of the oft-cited importance of the new psychiatric drugs—the phenothiazines—in fueling the movement to close down hospital beds and discharge patients to treatment in their home communities. Deinstitutionalization, he argues, proceeded in response to increased costs of maintaining hospital beds and the administrative policies that followed. The phenothiazines were introduced on a large scale only after the policy of early discharge and limited admissions had been implemented. Asylums once provided a convenient means of relieving families of the burden of caring for a mentally ill or otherwise unproductive member. As Social Security laws changed and the expense of maintaining asylums increased, treatment of the mentally ill resulted in mounting losses to the state, thus fueling interest in community care and privatization. Community treatment agencies began to fill this need, providing cheaper, often unregulated, and community-located but, still, institutional care. Thus, Scull contends, states transferred much of the responsibility of care for persons with mental illness to local providers and the federal government and rid themselves of a fiscal millstone. There is much more in this dense but compelling article, which the author edited for this volume from its original, longer form.

Luis Bedregal

The Decarceration of the Mentally Ill: A Critical View

In a colossal refuge for the insane, a patient may be said to lose his individuality and to become a member of a machine so put together, as to move with precise regularity and invariable routine; a triumph of skill adapted to show how such unpromising materials as crazy men and women may be drilled into order and guided by rule, but not an apparatus calculated to restore their pristine condition and their independent self-governing existence. In all cases admitting of recovery, or of material amelioration, a gigantic asylum is a gigantic evil, and figuratively speaking, a manufactory of chronic insanity.

John Arlidge, 1859

It is not well to sneer at political economy in its relations to the insane poor. Whether we think it right or not, the question of cost has determined and will continue to determine their fate for weal or woe.

George Cook, 1866

In recent years, a state-sponsored effort to deinstitutionalize deviant populations had become a central element in the social control practices of a number of advanced capitalist societies. In varying degrees, control of such deviant groups as criminals, juvenile offenders, and the mentally ill has increasingly become "community based." Yet despite the enormous importance of this change in social policy, surprisingly little effort has been made to unravel the reasons for its appearance. Most of the time it is discussed simply in passing. Only rarely does one come across sustained discussions of the problem.

In this paper we shall consider in some detail one very important aspect of this change, the decline of the mental hospital and the shift toward community treatment as a means of handling the mentally disturbed. It is frequently suggested that this development can be attributed to the discovery in the mid-1950s of an effective antipsychotic medication, the phenothiazines, and to the demonstration by liberal social scientists that mental hospitals were fundamentally antitherapeutic institutions, having detrimental effects on their inmate populations. We shall contend here that explanation in these terms is radically implausible and unsatisfactory, that, even though the work of liberal critics of incarceration and the advent of psychoactive drugs may have been used to justify recent trends toward deinstitutionalization, the causes of the switch lie elsewhere. Briefly, and at the risk of oversimplification, we shall argue that the primary factor behind the adoption of a policy of deinstitutionalization has been a drive to control the soaring costs of incarceration, and that the need to retrench in this fashion, in turn, reflects important recent changes in the nature of advanced capitalist social formations. More specifically, it reflects the qualitative transformation that has taken place in the role of the state, and the expansion of social welfare programs that has formed an important part of that transformation. Their availability has rendered the social control functions of incarcerating the mentally ill much less salient;

indeed, it has meant that other forms of social control have become equally functional. So it is that the state has maneuvered to cut back expenditures on mental hospitals and the like, even as it continues to spend money on other social services in increasing amounts.

Most of the key features that distinguish deviance and its control in modern society from the shapes that these phenomena assume in other types of society emerged in England and America during the early part of the nineteenth century. Of particular importance for our concerns in this paper, this period witnessed the substantial and sustained involvement of the state in this area, and the concomitant emergence of a centrally administered and directed social control apparatus committed to the treatment of many types of deviance in institutions (Scull 1974; Rothman 1971; Grob 1966, 1973). With only relatively minor changes and additions (the most notable of which was the adoption of probation and parole as a secondary mechanism for dealing with the criminal), the dominant response to problem populations until quite recently continued to rest on a policy of segregative control, more often than not in large custodial warehouses remote from large population centers and insulated from public view.

Within the past quarter of a century, however, this policy has, for the first time since its adoption, been seriously challenged and modified, though by no means entirely abandoned. Perhaps the most striking manifestation of this change is to be found in that segment of the social control apparatus that is concerned with the management of the mad. From the establishment of the first publicly supported asylums in the early nineteenth century, a pattern of consistent year-by-year increases in the number of inmates confined in mental hospitals swiftly established itself, and persisted right through the nineteenth century and the first half of the twentieth century. There appeared to be a remarkably consistent tendency to underestimate the demand for asylum accommodation, no matter how careful the effort to estimate the local requirements. Moreover, as additional facilities were built to meet the apparent excess demand, they too swiftly became filled to capacity, prompting repetitions of the original cycle for as long as money was forthcoming for buildings. In England, where the asylum system developed more rapidly than in America, the number of insane people grew from 21,000 (a rate of 12.66 per 10,000 people) in 1845—when provision of asylums at public expense became compulsory—to 95,600 (a rate of 30.30 per 10,000 people) by the end of the century; by 1954, the year when the mental hospital population finally peaked, the number of patients resident in mental hospitals had grown to 148,000 (a rate of 33.45 per 10,000 people). Over the same period, the United States experienced an increase of similar magnitude, though the timing here was somewhat different. Prior to 1955, for example, the public mental hospital population had quadrupled during the previous half century, whereas the general population had only doubled.

Since the mid-1950s, however, both countries have witnessed an abrupt reversal of this trend. Dating from 1954 and 1955 respectively, the number of patients resident in mental hospitals in each country has decreased in each and every year (see Tables 8.1 and 8.2) and there has emerged in both countries an explicit commitment to a policy, which has gathered momentum over the past two decades, of decarcerating the mentally disordered. Initially, doubts were expressed in some quarters about the significance of the decline in numbers and the likelihood of its long-term persistence, but these seem to have disappeared as the fall has continued without interruption (and in some places even at an accelerated pace) for two decades now. In their place, we have seen an increasingly confident projection of existing trends to their logical limits, typified by the 1961 forecast by the British minister of health in which he expected "the acute population of mental hospitals to drop by half in the next fifteen years and the long-stay population ultimately to dwindle to zero" (quoted in Hoenig and Hamilton 1969: 2).

Table 8.1 Resident Population in State and County Mental Hospitals in the U.S., 1954–1972

1954	554,000	1961	527,500	1967	426.000
1955	558,900	1962	515,600	1968	400,700
1956	551,400	1963	504,600	1969	no data
1957	548,600	1964	490,400	1970	no data
1958	545,200	1965	475,200	1971	309,017
1959	541,900	1966	452,100	1972	275,995
1960	535,500				

SOURCES: NIMH Statistical Note # 1; and K. A. Pollack and C. A. Taube, "Trends and Projections in State Hospital Use" (paper presented at the symposium on the future role of the state hospital, SUNY, Buffalo, October 11, 1973), Table 7 (for 1971 and 1972).

Table 8.2 Resident Population of Mental Patients in England and Wales 1951–1970

1951	143,196	1958	142,815	1965	123,600
1952	144,583	1959	139,083	1966	121,600
1953	146,643	1960	136,162	1967	118,900
1954	148,080	1961	135,400	1968	116,400
1955	146,867	1962	133,800	1969	105,600
1956	145,593	1963	127,600	1970	103,300
1957	143,220	1964	126,500		

SOURCES: E. M. Brooke, "Factors Affecting the Demand for Psychiatric Beds," *The Lancet,* December 1962 (for 1951–60); and Department of Health and Social Security figures (for 1961–70).

II

Curiously enough, while the numbers resident in mental hospitals have fallen dramatically over the past two decades, this fall has been accompanied by a steep rise in the overall admission rates. Statistically, the decline reflects a policy of greatly accelerated discharge. There is a strange historical parallel here. The establishment of the asylum system, particularly in the United States, depended heavily on the institution's presumed ability to cure. During the era of the "cult of curability," superintendents of existing institutions engaged in a bizarre competitive struggle to achieve the highest cure rates—a contest that eventually led to claims to be able to cure 100 percent of one's patients. If the asylum system thus had its roots in one sort of statistical version of cutthroat competition, its imminent demise seems to have provoked another—only this time, the hospitals, racing to discharge 100 percent of their intake within three months, seem largely unconcerned with labeling their output as cured.

An explanation of the policy of early release and consequent decline in mental hospital populations that enjoys a considerable measure of popularity in some psychiatric and official circles attributes the transformation simply to the growing use and effectiveness of psychoactive drugs. In the words of the Joint Commission on Mental Illness and Health (1961: 39), "tranquillizing...drugs have revolutionized the management of psychotic patients in American mental hospitals, and probably deserve primary credit for reversal of the upward spiral of the state hospital inpatient load." This account possesses the twin virtues of simplicity and of reinforcing the medical model of insanity by suggesting that the advent of psychoactive drugs signals a medical breakthrough in this area paralleling earlier ones allowing the successful treatment of other hitherto intractable chronic diseases. Yet despite its evident appeal, as an explanation it is distinctly flawed.

Not only does such an account tend to exaggerate the therapeutic achievement that these drugs represent but, as Mechanic (1969: 61–62) indicates, it is empirically inaccurate and inadequate in other ways as well. For example, studies of a number of English mental hospitals "show that new patterns of release were observable prior to drug introduction, and they suggest that the tremendous change which took place is largely due to alterations in administrative policies." In the late 1940s and early 1950s, "well before the new drugs were introduced," certain hospitals had already adopted a policy of placing "an emphasis on early discharge, or the avoidance of admission altogether, in order to prevent the accumulation of long-stay institutionalized patients,' … the pioneers' use of social techniques began in certain hospitals well before the national swing was noticed in 1955, and the underlying statistical trends must have long antedated the change in overall bed occupancy" (Wing and Brown 1970: 174, 179).

Even if this contradictory evidence had not been uncovered, to rest content with an explanation couched in these terms would imply the acceptance of a naively deterministic relationship between technological advances and changes in social control styles and practices, to the neglect of the influence of the social context in determining the uses to which these advances are put. In other contexts, for example, might not the more subtle and less visible control of patient behavior that the new drugs supposedly offered have been used simply to ease internal management problems and decrease the incidence of overt, blatant physical constraint within the institution (as, indeed, has been done to some extent) while having little or no effect on discharge patterns? Nor is it easy to see how a simple technological determinism of this sort can account for such things as the sudden acceleration of the decline in American mental hospital populations from the mid-1960s on when no comparable change occurred in England; or the other important aspect of the policy of decarceration, the conditions of existence endured by the mentally disabled discharged into the community.

But there remains a still more damaging objection that proponents of the pharmacological explanation have been forced to finesse, namely, a growing volume of evidence that suggests that claims about the therapeutic effectiveness of so-called antipsychotic medication—mainly the phenothiazines—have been greatly exaggerated. It is becoming clear, for example, that for a substantial proportion of those labeled schizophrenic, psychoactive drugs are largely ineffective. For example, a recent double-blind study of young male acute schizophrenics by Rappaport et al. (n.d.) found that patients randomly assigned placebos while hospitalized and not taking phenothiazines at follow-up "showed significantly greater clinical improvement and less pathology at follow-up, significantly fewer rehospitalizations and significantly less overall functional disturbance in the community than any other group of patients…. Also, significantly fewer patients in the placebo group became worse from discharge to follow-up. …In the long run, most patients *not* given phenothiazine medication do better…." There can now be no question but that the extreme optimism that greeted the advent of psychoactive drugs, and that persisted for a number of years, reflected the weakness and poor design of many of the evaluations made at that time far more than the actual efficacy of the drugs themselves. Subsequent careful review of the relevant literature has shown that "uncontrolled studies" of a sort that remain surprisingly common in this area "gave a systematically more positive evaluation of drug effect than controlled studies" (Davis 1965; Glide 1962).

All of this should not be taken to imply that administration of such drugs has no behavioral effects. To the contrary, the preponderance (though by no means all) of well-designed,

well-conducted studies "show that these drugs are better than placebo" if given in sufficiently high dosage (Davis 1965: 553). There can be no question, for example, that "excessive doses of neuroleptics produce severe reductions of motor activity and a general loss
of spontaneity "—function, in effect, as "chemical straitjackets" (Crane 1973: 126; Davis
1965: 561). However, it has been well-established that the phenothiazines are ineffective
for substantial portions of the target population and that, in any event, the types of maintenance doses generally prescribed are largely ineffective. Given this, how can anyone
seriously contend that the advent of drug therapy is the primary reason for the decline in
mental hospital populations (the more so since the drugs are apparently least effective with
the groups whose release has been most crucial to the running down of mental hospital
populations—the old, chronic cases)?

Even if most studies of the effectiveness of psychoactive drugs were far more uniformly
favorable than we have seen that they are, serious difficulties would remain for proponents
of the idea that the introduction of such drugs is the primary factor in the fall of mental
hospital populations. For one thing, most of the studies we now possess consider short-term
effects only. Where long-term follow-up studies do demonstrate the existence of a drug
effect (and because of "generally faulty research designs" evidence on this point is muddled
and contradictory), this effect is generally quite small (Gittleman et al. 1965; Englehardt et
al. 1960, 1963, 1964, 1967). Moreover, "the difference between those patients treated with
drugs and those not treated with drugs decreases over time. …As for the quality of the
patient's adjustment after he leaves the hospital, the results of drug therapy are even less
encouraging: the majority of those who live in the community continue to be unproductive and are often a burden to their families" (Crane 1973: 125). At best, therefore, one is
left with the conclusion that the introduction of psychoactive drugs may have facilitated
the policy of early discharge by reducing the incidence of florid symptoms among at least
some of the disturbed, thus easing the problems of managing them in the community (and
perhaps also by persuading doctors with an exaggerated idea of the drugs' efficacy of the
feasibility of such a policy). But that their arrival can be held primarily responsible for the
change is clearly highly implausible.

III

Recognizing the force of the criticism that serious account must be taken of social factors, others have sought an explanation of the decline in mental hospital populations in the
growing disenchantment in this period with the adequacy of such institutions as a response
to mental illness. In this view, a decisive factor underlying the transformation was the
superior understanding achieved in this period of the effects of these institutions on their
inmates. As Hoenig and Hamilton (1969: 245) put it, "the policy of avoiding long-term
hospitalization derives its main justification from the belief that it will protect the patient
from institutionalization." A spate of social scientific research in the 1950s and 1960s (the
most famous example of which was Goffman's *Asylums*) was devoted to the elucidation
of the baneful effects on the patient of prolonged incarceration in a mental institution. All
this research had shown, purportedly for the first time, that the defects in existing mental
hospitals were hot simply the consequence of administrative lapses or the lack of adequate
funds, but rather reflected fundamental and irremediable flaws in the basic structure of
such places, flaws so serious as to call into question their therapeutic usefulness—or rather
to suggest that they were fundamentally antitherapeutic.

The consensus was clear. Presented most persuasively by Goffman (1961), it was that the
crucial factor in forming a mental hospital patient was not his "illness," but his institution;

that his reactions and adjustments, pathological as they might seem to an outsider, were the product of the ill-effects of his environment rather than of intrapsychic forces; and, indeed, that they closely resembled those of inmates in other types of "total institutions," a term that came to symbolize this whole line of argument. The mental hospital, it now appeared, far from sheltering and helping to restore the disturbed to sanity, performed "a disabling custodial function." The work of men like Duncan Macmillan and T. P. Rees, British pioneers of the concept of the open hospital, had demonstrated "beyond question that much of the aggressive, disturbed, suicidal, and regressive behaviour of the mentally ill is not necessarily or inherently a part of the illness as such but is very largely an artificial byproduct of the way of life imposed on them [by hospitalization]." Major American psychiatrists expressed fears that "the patients are infantile... because we infantilize them" (Hunt 1957: 13, 21). Studies of institutions as diverse as research hospitals closely associated with major medical schools, expensive, exclusive, and well-staffed private facilities, and undermanned and underfinanced state hospitals, all revealed a depressingly familiar picture. To the researchers, the very "similarity of these problems strongly suggests that many of the serious problems of the state hospital are inherent in the nature of mental institutionalization rather than simply in the financial difficulties of the state hospitals" (Belknap 1956: 232).

The conclusion was inescapable. Mental hospitals "are probably themselves obstacles in the development of an effective program of treatment for the mentally ill" (Belknap 1956: xi). Policy recommendations followed naturally: "The time has come when we should ask ourselves seriously whether the interests of the mentally ill are best served by providing more psychiatric beds, building bigger and better mental hospitals. Perhaps we should concentrate our efforts on treating the patients within the community of which they form a part, and teach that community to tolerate and accept their idiosyncrasies" (Rees 1957: 527). After all, considering what current research had shown, surely "the worst home is better than the best mental hospital..." (Cumming and Cumming 1957: 55), so that "in the long run the abandonment of the state hospitals might be one of the greatest humanitarian reforms and the greatest financial economy ever achieved... (Belknap 1956: 212).

In place of the traditional stress on the need for institutionalization, there developed an increasingly elaborate attempt to convince the public, and, more importantly, the policy makers, of "the value and safety of community care" (Hunt 1957: 21). In some circles, "community treatment" came to be elevated into a new therapeutic panacea, and, supported by ever larger injections of federal funds in the United States, "community psychiatrists" became an increasingly important segment of the psychiatric profession as a whole. Particularly during the 1960s, an influential group of community psychiatrists, clinical psychologists, and other professionals were being listened to increasingly at the state and federal levels. In combination, it is suggested such discoveries and propaganda both logically implied and naturally produced a change in social policy.

No one familiar with the climate of contemporary liberal intellectual opinion can avoid recognizing the depths of current pessimism there concerning the value of institutional responses to all forms of deviance, or the degree to which decarceration has been elevated, in such circles, to the status of a new humanitarian myth, comparable only with the similar myth that attended the birth of the asylum. But, in general, social policy proves only mildly susceptible to the shifting intellectual fads and fashions of the day. The question remains as to why this one at least appears to have had so profound an impact. Granted that the advocates of the community approach vigorously proselytized on behalf of their cause, why were they listened to—particularly when their proposals ran counter to the deeply entrenched interests of institutional psychiatry, long a powerful interest group in the political arena?

The conventional answer to these questions has three basic elements: the emergence of a renewed concern on the part of the state for the patient's social and therapeutic rights; the therapeutic promise of community care, an appeal bolstered by the favorable outcome of early efforts in this direction; and an alleged increasing tolerance on the part of the community toward the mentally disturbed. Each of these arguments, though, is seriously defective. It is all very well to assert that "the higher level of tolerance for deviance in the post-World War II period has raised the prospect that the mentally ill and retarded could be returned to families and retained in residential neighborhoods" (Wolpert and Wolpert 1974: 72). But where this increased tolerance comes from is not explained; nor is evidence offered to demonstrate its existence— unless, of course, it is a mere tautology (such people have been returned to the community, which shows that the community must be more tolerant than it once was; therefore increased tolerance must account for the return of the insane to the community). And the issue is still more complicated than is suggested by asking why or whether a changed tolerance for deviant behavior has developed: there is also the question of whether this change is an independent (as the Wolperts would have it) or a dependent variable; whether it helped to produce the change in policy, or was itself the product of the changed policy. What evidence we do have bearing on this issue suggests the latter is the more plausible causal sequence. It quite clearly became official policy in this period to discourage the admission or readmission of patients who in an earlier era would have been taken without question, and whom relatives or neighbors actively sought to have institutionalized (Brown et al. 1966). Neither are the vociferous community protests that usually accompany a policy of community treatment the reaction one would expect from those becoming more tolerant of the presence of deviance.

In view of what we know of the circumstances surrounding the return of the mentally ill to the community, the claim that this change was motivated by either concern for the patients' rights, or because of the therapeutic benefits likely to ensue, seems if anything still more disingenuous. Indeed, the Wolperts' own findings reveal this to be so. In the first place, "the massive release of patients to facilities in residential neighborhoods" *preceded* "substantial data collection and analysis" on the likely effects of decarceration (1974: 14). In fact, even now we lack "substantiation that community care is advantageous for clients." Put bluntly, "data have not been generated by the mental health sector nor by the evaluators of their programs nor by those who fund the care system ... for determining what kinds of facilities are most beneficial or where those facilities should be sited." Furthermore, "the hospital release trend is independent of community after-care facilities," and for at least one important class of ex-patients, discharge in such circumstances, far from proving therapeutic, has been positively fatal: "mortality rates for elderly patients increases [sic] dramatically upon release ..." (Wolpert and Wolpert 1974: 19, 25).

Overall, there has been no adequate licensing, supervision, or inspection of board and care facilities for released mental patients, and no effort to avoid their "ghettoization" in the poorest, least desirable of neighborhoods. And, "in the absence of adequate after-care and rehabilitation services, the term 'community care' ... [remained] merely an inflated catch phrase which concealed morbidity in the patients and distress in the relatives" (Brown et al. 1966). As a natural consequence, "one form of confinement has been replaced by another, and the former patients are just as insulated from community attention and care as they were in the state hospital" (Wolpert and Wolpert 1974: 61). As far back as 1961, the Joint Commission on Mental Illness and Health (1961: 184), itself engaged in promoting the notion of decarceration, was forced to concede that "generally little attention is given to the psychological and social needs of these patients." Over the past thirteen years, the situation has not changed, and, to judge from the continuing official inaction, this does not greatly concern the authorities. Recent research has shown that it remains true that "for the long-term hospitalized patient, the move is usually into a boarding home facility... where little, effort is directed toward social and vocational rehabilitation." In practice, "it is only an illusion that patients who are placed in boarding or family care homes are 'in the community.' .... These facilities are in most respects like small long-term state hospital wards isolated from the community. One is overcome by the depressing atmosphere, not because of the physical appearance of the boarding home, but because of the passivity, isolation and inactivity of the residents..." (Lamb and Goertzel 1971: 29, 31). The picture is a grim one, and scarcely what one would gather from reading the liberal rhetoric on decarceration.

IV

As we have seen, a crucial element in rendering plausible the standard accounts of the move toward a noninstitutional response to mental illness has been the purported discovery by social scientists in the 1950s and 1960s of the institutional syndrome—the notion that confinement in an asylum may amplify and even produce disturbance, that in the "moral career of the mental patient" the institution may be more important than the illness. Supposedly, what had formerly been held to be the natural products of an unfolding infraindividual pathology were finally, and for the first time, seen as in large part the reflection of a natural response to a grossly deforming environment. But such claims reflect the narrow and an historical vision of those making them. Despite the pretensions of those sociologists convinced that the understanding of society waits upon advances in their peculiar discipline, recognition of the baneful effects of incarceration emerged early in the history of the asylum and took sophisticated forms. A number of nineteenth-century critics, both English and American, developed criticisms of institutionalization that in their essentials, and with respect to either their intellectual cogency or empirical support, were in no way inferior to the modern critique elaborated by Goffman and others (Howe 1854; Maudsley 1867; Bucknill 1880).

As this suggests, what we need to explain are the reasons why advocates of deinstitutionalization finally found a receptive audience in the 1950s and 1960s. If the shift toward community treatment was not the automatic product of advances in social scientific understanding, or of some miraculous technological breakthrough, then how else can we account for this change? To answer this question requires that we grasp the intimate relationships that exist between the nature of the social control apparatus and the social system as a whole, and the ways in which changes in the one prompt changes in the other. This is what we shall now attempt to do.

During the second half of the nineteenth century, whatever criticisms some intellectuals and professionals might make of asylums, so far as most people were concerned, such places remained a convenient way of getting rid of inconvenient people. The community was used, by now, to disposing of the derelict and troublesome in this fashion, placing them where, as one physician put it, "they are for the most part harmless because they are kept out of harm's way" (Hanwell Annual Report 1856: 36). Asylums' earlier association with social reform gave a lingering humanitarian gloss to the huge, cheap, and avowedly custodial dumps where the refuse of the community was now gathered together. Meanwhile, medical control of these institutions, and the rhetoric about cure that went with that control, provided a further legitimation of the custodial warehousing of these, the most difficult and troublesome elements of the disreputable poor. The working people, lacking an alternative means of ridding themselves of what, in the context of nineteenth-century working-class existence, was undoubtedly an intolerable burden—caring for their sick, aged, decrepit, or otherwise incapacitated relatives—had little option but to make use of the asylum. From the upper classes' perspective, the existence of asylums to treat the insane at public expense could be invoked as a practical demonstration of their own humanitarian concern for the less fortunate.

Far from asylums having been altruistic institutions detached from the social structures that perpetuate poverty, they were clearly important elements in sustaining those structures. For in this period, the influential classes in both England and America were all but unanimous in their unwillingness to insulate the population as a whole from the twin spurs of poverty and unemployment. Under the conditions characteristic of early industrial capitalism, relief threatened to undermine radically the whole notion of a labor market. It interfered with labor mobility. It encouraged the retention of "a vast inert mass of redundant labor" in rural areas, where the demand for labor was subject to wide seasonal fluctuations. It distorted the operations of the labor market, most especially on account of its tendency, via the vagaries of local administration, "to create cost differentials as between the various parts of the country" (Polanyi 1957: 301). And by its removal of the threat of individual starvation, it had a pernicious effect on labor productivity and discipline. On the ideological level, this determination to restrict relief was at once reflected and strengthened by the hegemony of classical liberalism. The latter's insistence that every man was to be free to pursue his fortune and at the same time was to be held responsible for his own success or failure, coupled with its dogmatic certainty that interference with the dictates of the free market could only be counterproductive in the long run (a proposition that could even be theoretically "proved"), rendered the whole notion of social protectionism an anathema.

Hence came the stress on the principle of "less eligibility" (enforced in large part through the discipline of institutions like workhouses and asylums) and the abhorrence of payments to individuals in the community (so-called outdoor relief) as the two central elements in dealing with the problems of extreme incapacity of one sort or another. For despite the ferocity of their ideological proclamations, as a practical political matter, the upper classes were aware of the impossibility of adhering rigidly to the dictates of the market. But though "the residuum of paupers could not, admittedly, be left actually to starve" (Hobsbawm 1969: 88), the pressures of the marketplace must be interfered with as little as possible. Here, an institutionally based system allowed the maintenance of conditions of relief that ensured that no one with any conceivable alternatives would seek public aid. In such a context, the asylum played its part, removing from lower-class families the impossible burdens imposed by those incapable of providing for their own subsistence, and thus ensuring that a potent source of discontent could be neutralized without having to alter society's basic structural arrangements.

The rejection of anything resembling a modern system of social protection or welfare and the use of the asylum were intimately connected in yet another way, for an important implication of the highly restricted welfare policies characteristic of the United States and England until well into the twentieth century was that asylums represented one of the few costs of production that were socialized, i.e., taken over by the state rather than the private sector. Thus the fiscal pressures from this source on the state were relatively slight, and the expenses associated with a system of segregative control were more readily absorbed.

As capitalism developed further, however, so the demands on the poor-law system changed, from instilling discipline and industriousness in a period of abundant unskilled human labor, to maintaining the capacity and willingness to work of an increasingly valuable resource. By now, the "workers' physical strength and good will had become important assets. Social insurance became one of the means of investing in human capital" (Rimlinger 1971: 10). Though slowed in varying degrees by the persisting appeal of classical liberal ideology, both societies began to construct the basic elements of the modern welfare state. In the remainder of this paper, I shall advance and attempt to document the contention that this development, coupled with a virtually simultaneous and massive expansion of the role of the state in other sectors of English and American society, decisively transformed the social context within which the social control apparatus was embedded; and that the ramifications of these changes account in large part for the move toward community treatment for the deviant.

To summarize my thesis briefly at the outset, I shall argue that, with the coming of the welfare state, the asylum system became, in relative terms, far more costly and difficult to justify. Formerly, there had been little or no alternative to keeping the chronically disabled cases of insanity in the asylum, for although the overwhelming majority were harmless, they could not provide for their own subsistence and no alternative sources of support were available to sustain them in the outside world. However, with the advent of a wide range of welfare programs providing just such support, the opportunity cost of neglecting community care in favor of asylum treatment—inevitably far more costly than the most generous schemes for welfare payments—rose sharply. Simultaneously, the increasing socialization of production costs by the state, something that has been taking place at an increasing pace during and since the Second World War, and of which modern welfare measures are merely one very important example, produced a growing fiscal crisis, as expenditures continuously threatened to outrun available revenue. In combination, a focus on the interplay of these factors enables us to resolve what at first sight is a paradox—namely, the emergence and persistence of efforts at retrenchment at a time when general expenditures on welfare items were expanding rapidly. For it is precisely the expansion of the one that made both possible and desirable the contraction of the other.

Clearly, the advent of the welfare state reflected in some measure a lessened resistance to such legislation on the part of a capitalist class increasingly led to confront the implications of the fact that, in an advanced economy, "human faculties are as important a means of production as any other kind of capital" (Marshall 1920: 229). Equally, however, the historical genesis of the welfare state is also the product of political struggles on the part of increasingly organized labor movements. To this extent, welfare measures represent social concessions made under the threat of, or in anticipation of, popular discontent and struggle. More specifically, "the greater security enjoyed by many during wartime, despite the absolute fall in living standards,...[and] the political necessity for capitalist states to avoid a return to slumps of the inter-war scale, and their ability to implement this by means of Keynesian policies...made demands for extended state intervention in the field of welfare irresistible..." (Gough 1975: 69).

The postwar growth in the relative strength of the labor movement, substantially a reflection of the largely successful pursuit of full-employment policies during this period, has produced a consolidation and extension of these earlier gains. All this has formed part of a process whereby, in all advanced capitalist societies (and particularly since 1945), there has been a prolonged expansion of government expenditures as the state moves to take on "a qualitatively expanded role in capitalist social formations." Especially notable, apart from the rising outlays on social services, has been the growing expenditure on such things as aid to private industry and on items designed to improve the economic infrastructure (e.g., roads, education, and government-supported research and development) (Gough 1975: 53, 60). The budgetary impact of all this has been startling. Even if one leaves aside the other components of state spending, in the United Kingdom, the social services have swallowed a proportion of the G.N.P. that has risen from 10.9 percent in 1937 to 24.9 percent by 1973, and an essentially similar pattern has been observable in the United States, where such outlays have risen from 9 percent of the G.N.P. in 1955 to 15 percent in 1969.

A number of factors besides real improvements in the level of services have contributed to the upward pressure on state budgets in this period. The United States and England, like other developed economies in the capitalist world system, have found that the costs of state services (especially social services) rise faster than the average price level, everywhere forcing an ever higher level of expenditure merely to maintain services at the same level in real terms. Undoubtedly this reflects the fact that on the average the level of productivity rises less fast in the state than in the private sector of the economy, which, in turn, reflects the relative predominance of low-productivity labor-intensive services in the state sector. Then, too, in addition to the technical difficulties associated with any effort to raise productivity in service occupations, the situation is "undoubtedly exacerbated in the case of state services by the absence of competitive pressure to reduce costs" (Gough 1975; 76). Furthermore, it is clear that the size of income maintenance expenditures has been heavily influenced by the growing proportion of aged in Britain and America, and indeed, by the general tendency of the dependent population to expand as a proportion of the total.

The budgetary strains on state mental hospitals reflected the impact of these general factors making for severe cost inflation, as well as two more specific conjunctural factors. The widespread unionization of state employees and the associated "advent of the eight-hour day and forty-hour week in state institutions... virtually doubled unit costs..." (Dingman 1974: 48). On top of this, a number of class action suits on behalf of hospital inmates were brought during the 1960s and 1970s (in the United States at least). Decisions such as *Wyatt v. Stickney* (1972) attempted to lay down minimum standards of treatment, while others sought to eliminate "institutional peonage," the employment of unpaid patient labor to reduce institutional costs. To the extent that they are implemented, these decisions unquestionably "force upon the states huge expenditures..." (Greenblatt 1974: 3–17), but they will obviously have no force if institutions can be emptied and closed instead.

In such circumstances, the continuation of an increasingly costly social control policy that, in terms of effectiveness, possesses few advantages over an apparently much cheaper alternative becomes increasingly difficult to justify; and the attractiveness of that alternative to governments under ever greater budgetary pressures, whatever the political difficulties in the way of its realization, becomes steadily harder to resist. In the words of those who have served as bureaucratic managers of the system, "rising costs more than any other factor have made it obvious that support of state hospitals is politically unfeasible... this is the principal factor behind the present push to get rid of state hospitals" (Dingman 1974: 48). To put it bluntly, "in a sense our backs are to the wall; it's *phase out* before we go *bankrupt* (Greenblatt 1974: 8, emphasis in the original).

To the extent that psychoactive drugs have played a role in the adoption of a policy of decarceration, I would suggest that it is the existence of these structural pressures that in large measure accounts for their being used in this way, rather than simply to ease the problems of internal management in asylums. Similarly, the impact of these pressures explains the differential susceptibility of the relevant audiences to the substantially identical criticisms of the asylum put forward in the 1860s and 1870s, and again in the 1950s and 1960s. The arguments had not changed, but the structural context in which they were advanced clearly had. Their contemporary reappearance allowed governments to save money while simultaneously giving their policy a humanitarian gloss. And to take the argument a step further, it is the intensity and extent of such pressures that account for the persistence of this policy despite public resistance to it, and despite the accumulation of evidence showing that, in terms of its ostensible goals, community care is substantially a failure.

As states realized that decarceration was feasible, they began to maneuver to obtain the cost savings it offered. Some of the largest savings immediately realizable came from the cancellation of planned new construction, and decisions to do this were widespread (Brill and Patton 1959). In the United States, large cost savings for hard-pressed local governments were also available where patients could be discharged from state hospitals (where they were provided for at state expense) to private, profit-making convalescent homes—not just because provision in such places was less costly, but also because changes in the social security laws in the late 1950s made it possible for these people to collect social security (and thus be supported at federal expense) so long as they were not in psychiatric institutions. A number of states followed California's lead in providing financial inducements to counties to avoid sending patients to state hospitals for inpatient care. In England, ministerial calls for ruthless cutbacks in the number of psychiatric beds were coupled with plans that included virtually no provision for increased community care. The plans promised major cost savings, and as a consequence, drew extensive support from right wing political figures.

For reasons we have already discussed, the pace of expansion of state expenditures on social services in both countries increased markedly during the 1960s and 1970s. As it did so, so the incentives to accelerate the movement toward deinstitutionalization likewise intensified. And it is precisely in this period that the momentum of the drive to shut down institutions and minimize incarceration gathered its greatest force. The range of devices used to divert potential inmates away from institutions was further expanded, and those already in existence were applied with greater urgency and effect. Welfare regulations were changed to make aid to mental patients discharged into the community more readily available. Screening projects were set up to encourage placement of potential admissions, particularly geriatric cases, in nonhospital settings (Epstein and Simon 1968). Involuntary commitment was made far more difficult in some jurisdictions, also helping to reduce hospital intakes. Perhaps most elaborate and effective of all was the system devised by the state of California in the Lanterman-Petris-Short Act (1967). Under this approach, counties were, in effect, bribed not to use state hospitals—a scheme that led to a further acceleration in the decline of state hospital populations, allowed the closure of four state hospitals within a five-year period, and produced substantial cost savings for the state.

Once the drive for control of soaring costs is seen as the primary factor underlying the move toward decarceration, both these and a number of other aspects of this change, which formerly appeared either fortuitous or inexplicable, become readily comprehensible. Ever since segregative control became the dominant mode of managing deviance, the public has shown consistently little desire or inclination to have officially labeled serious deviants returned to their midst. Studies made in the earlier phases of the decarceration movement indicated a continuing attitude of hostility, fear, and intolerance toward the mentally ill (Cumming and Cumming 1957; Nunnally 1961), and the presence and strength of these feelings have been amply documented by subsequent reactions, as efforts have continued to return the mentally ill to the community. Residents have fought hard to ensure that if the mental patients are released, they are not released into *their* neighborhoods, a favorite tactic in this battle being the enactment of restrictive zoning ordinances. Similar measures have frequently been employed to exclude such undesirable elements as criminals and addicts; and a recent study of the diversion of juvenile delinquents likewise concluded that "the actual establishment of group homes in local communities is often vehemently resisted by residents" (Coates and Miller 1973: 67).

These resistance strategies have naturally been most successfully employed by middle and upper class communities. Even those who have devoted their well-paid expertise to developing public relations techniques for the "neutralization of community resistance to group homes" have been forced to concede that these community homes have the best chance of being established in transient neighborhoods, "or where the local residents are not particularly capable of organized opposition." And they confess there are but "few strategies with potential for gaining access to a community that has the ability to organize itself in opposition, or in support of, issues" (Coates and Miller 1973: 78–79). In any event, on cost grounds, there has been little pressure to place ex-patients or other types of deviants in such respectable settings. Instead decarceration has produced "the growing ghettoiza-tion of the returning ex-patients along with other dependent groups in the population: the growing succession of inner-city land-use to institutions providing services to the depen-dent and needy... [and] the forced immobility of the chronically disabled within deterio-rated urban neighborhoods..., areas where land-use deterioration has proceeded to such a point that the land market is substantially unaffected by the introduction of community services and their clients..." (Wolpert and Wolpert 1974: 33, 38).

In such areas there is also an absence of organized community opposition to the presence of these people. As if they are industrial wastes that can without risk be left to decompose in some well-contained dump, these problem populations have increasingly been dealt with by a resort to their ecological separation and isolation in areas where they are by and large no longer visible, and where they may be safely left to prey on one another.

But in many places, the sheer numbers involved have led to spillovers into residential, usually working- or lower-middle-class, communities. The opposition this has aroused has been further stimulated by complaints over the scope of after-care facilities provided (or rather not provided). If the decarceration program was to live up to rhetorical claims about its being undertaken for the ex-patients' welfare, these aftercare facilities would have had to be extensively present, but this would have been extremely costly, and if the program was to realize financial savings they had to be substantially absent. They are absent. Thus, "the actual transfer of patients has tended to favor the preferred reassignment according to economy goals. For patients who have been 'dumped' by hospitals prematurely, both therapeutic and civil rights have been violated, as well as the rights of the recipient com-munities" (Wolpert and Wolpert 1974: 22). Governments have consistently made the most of the opportunity to secure "a major retrenchment in the psychiatric services program, made possible by a rapidly declining hospital population. The professional administrators were unable to convince the... government of the necessity to greatly expand community services and to redeploy staff and resources from institutional to community services" (Stewart et al. 1968: 87). In a number of instances, the complaints provoked by this situa-tion have grown so vociferous as to force the slowdown or halting of the release program.

In the burgeoning field of community corrections, the situation is essentially no different. In 1972, for example, when Massachusetts abruptly and virtually overnight closed down all juvenile reform schools in the state, not even token efforts had been made to develop an infrastructure capable of providing community supervision or control over those released. As for adult criminals, the most authoritative national survey in recent years of the cor-rections field pointed out that "the United States spends only 20 percent of its corrections budget and allocated only 15 percent of its total staff to service the 67 percent of offenders in the corrections workload who are under community supervision...," with the result that 67 percent of felons and 76 percent of misdemeanants were dealt with in case leads of over one hundred per staff member (President's Commission on Law Enforcement 1967: 4–5). Six years later, following major efforts to accelerate the diversion of criminals away from prison, the situation was essentially unchanged, perhaps worse, with the average probation officer's workload "far too great to permit adequate investigation for assessment or control purposes, let alone for appreciable assistance" (Glaser 1973: 99).

It is quite clear, of course, that from the point of view of state expenditures, incarcerating problem populations of all descriptions in state institutions is extraordinarily costly, usu-ally (though perhaps not universally) far more so than a deliberate policy of coping with them in the community. This is particularly obvious when, as has unquestionably been the case with the contemporary decarceration movement, the rhetoric of promoting rehabilita-tion through community treatment is taken no more seriously than similarly hyberbolic

Table 8.3 Cost Savings in California through Transfer to Community
Facilities in 1970

Age	Minimum to Moderate Care
18–64 State hospital ($16.25/day)	$5,691.25
Boarding home ($7.13/day)	$1,391.06
Net savings per patient year	$4,300.19
0–17 State hospital ($16.25/day)	$5,691.25
Family care ($5.33/day)	$2,151.32
Net savings per patient year	$3,539.93
Intermediate Care	
0–17 State hospital ($16.25/day)	$5,691.25
Private institution ($9.00/day)	$3,578.00
Net savings per patient year	$2,113.25
Nursing Care	
65+ State hospital ($19.25/day)	$7,026.25
Nursing home ($12.04/day)	$4,394.60
Net savings per patient year	$2,361.60

SOURCE: California Department of Mental Hygiene Data, 1971.

talk about treatment in the institution. Under such conditions, there emerge quite startling discrepancies in comparative costs on a per capita basis. This holds true whether one looks at the case of dependent and neglected children, criminals, juvenile delinquents, or mental patients.

A breakdown of some of the cost savings produced by community care, based on California data, is presented in Table 8.3. As these figures show (and as one would expect), the amount saved varies with the degree of disability (and hence care), but is always substantial. Moreover, the figures given tend to understate the actual savings realized, since the Community Services Division's calculations include administrative, placement, service, and Medi-Cal costs, while the Department of Mental Hygiene figures for state hospital costs fail to include all administrative costs.

One must grant, however, that reality is more complicated than these simple comparisons might suggest. Thus, in the short run at least, many of the costs of a mental hospital (or prison) system are fixed and unchangeable, regardless of the number of inmates occupying the institutions. As a consequence, a sizeable fraction of the savings potentially available from decarceration may not be immediately realizable, being postponed until the number of those incarcerated falls far enough to allow the state to close institutions and thereby eliminate fixed costs. But, on the other hand, to the extent that the adoption of diversionary policies obviates the need for massive expansion of the physical capacity of the existing institutional system (as has indubitably been the case with both asylums and prisons), decarceration provides a direct and immediate source of relief to the state's fiscal crisis whose importance is obvious, even while its dimensions are extraordinarily difficult to estimate with any precision.

For example, on the capital budget side, by the mid-1950s much of the existing physical plant of the mental hospital systems in both England and America, largely an inheritance from the nineteenth century, was rapidly approaching a degree of decay and decrepitude that would have made replacement mandatory. Moreover, annual admissions were already displaying a persistent tendency to rise markedly from one year to the next, a trend that, as Table 8.4 shows, grew still more prominent over the next decade and a half. If the

Table 8.4 First Admissions to U.S. State and County Mental Hospitals, 1950–1968

1950	114,054	1957	128,124	1963	131,997
1951	112,979	1958	137,280	1964	138,932
1952	118,213	1959	137,795	1965	144,090
1953	123,854	1960	140,015	1966	162,486
1954	121,430	1961	146,393	1967	164,219
1955	122,284	1962	129,698	1968	175,637
1956	123,539				

SOURCES: U.S. Department of Health, Education and Welfare: Public Health Service: Patients in Mental Institutions, Part H State and County Mental Hospitals 1950–1965, NIMH statistical note # 14.

NOTE: Figures for 1962 and all subsequent years were artificially deflated by changes in recording practices introduced at the end of 1961.

proportion of admissions becoming chronic long-stay cases had remained at or close to its historic levels, substantial new construction would obviously have been called for. Instead, as retention rates fell sharply, mental hospitals were pictured as dying institutions on which it was naturally foolish to spend any more by way of renovation—and capital expenditure on them was reduced to a minimum.

There can be no question but that the most careful efforts to derive estimates of the cost savings deinstitutionalization can produce have been with respect to the policy's impact on the handling of criminals rather than the mentally ill. In all probability, this reflects political demand for more precise data on cost differentials with respect to this problem population. Humanitarianism (otherwise known as being lenient or "soft" on criminals) has a distinct lack of political appeal in this context, so that in general the decarceration of criminals has been much more universally sold on cost grounds. As a result, estimates do exist of how much particular decarceration programs have saved the state. Best documented of all are those for the California Probation Subsidy Program: "Between 1966 and 1972 (using projections based on limited information for the 1971–72 fiscal year only) California can demonstrate that it has saved $185,978,820 through cancelled construction, closed institutions, and new institutions constructed but not opened. Total expenditure for probation subsidy ... for the same period of time, will be $59,925,705" (Smith 1971: 69).

By contrast, for the mentally ill, adequate data on the savings thus produced unfortunately do not exist. Such data as we do possess are highly fragmentary and incomplete. One useful indicator, however, is provided by the information presented in Table 8.5. As these figures show, state expenditure on mental hospitals, excluding capital items, as a proportion of state expenditures had consistently fallen since the mid-1950s, paralleling the fall in patient numbers. In many states the decline has been steep and dramatic: between 1955 and 1974, from 5.26 to only 1.7 percent in Illinois, from 5.86 to 2.40 percent in Massachusetts, and from 7.04 to 3.20 percent in New York. And overall, the proportion of state expenditures absorbed by the mental hospital sector has almost halved over the same period. These drastic reductions are all the more remarkable since they have been achieved in the face of a series of developments that appeared to threaten equally drastic increases in the proportion of state revenues absorbed by mental hospitals. We have already discussed a number of these: the general tendency of productivity to rise less fast in the state sector; the unionization of hospital workers and the advent of the forty-hour work week; the "right to treatment decisions" by the courts; and rising admissions rates. Given these circumstances, merely to have held state hospital costs down to a constant proportion of state budgets would clearly have been out of the question without vigorous attempts to divert

Table 8.5 Expenditures on Mental Hospitals as a Percentage of General State Expenditures, 1955–1974 (Selected States and Nationally)

	California	Illinois	Indiana	Massachusetts	Michigan	New York	Washington	All States
1955	2.57	5.26	3.53	5.86	2.73	7.04	1.79	3.38
1956	2.56	5.03	2.98	5.28	2.67	7.60	1.88	3.32
1957	2.60	4.48	3.29	4.93	2.63	7.41	2.00	3.25
1958	2.60	4.02	3.58	5.60	2.72	6.88	1.92	3.25
1959	2.43	4.00	3.38	5.36	2.61	6.66	1.91	3.09
1960	2.42	3.88	3.24	5.18	2.50	5.92	1.98	2.98
1961	2.36	4.01	3.06	5.67	2.34	5.73	2.15	2.99
1962	2.29	3.82	3.09	5.69	2.34	3.85	1.85	2.91
1963	2.23	3.79	3.02	5.13	2.34	5.37	1.64	2.79
1964	2.11	3.56	2.72	4.88	2.36	5.14	1.62	2.70
1965	1.97	4.08	2.65	4.65	2.37	5.45	1.61	2.68
1966	1.83	3.92	2.65	4.49	2.14	4.85	1.50	2.53
1967	1.72	4.12	2.51	4.18	2.08	4.69	1.50	2.46
1968	1.49	3.40	2.56	3.92	2.07	4.41	1.40	2.37
1969	1.34	3.10	2.51	3.49	1.99	4.12	1.49	2.29
1970	1.24	2.63	2.43	3.43	1.91	4.07	1.28	2.20
1971	1.10	2.45	2.23	3.16	1.92	3.74	1.18	2.03
1972	1.00	2.26	2.12	2.93	1.79	3.06	1.07	1.90
1973	0.93	2.07	2.08	2.51	1.69	3.04	1.04	1.90
1974	0.86	1.79	2.05	2.40	1.61	3.20	0.90	1.87
Change	67%	66%	42%	59%	41%	55%	50%	45%

1955–74

SOURCE: U.S. Bureau of the Census: State Finances.

NOTE: The above figures are calculated on the basis of current expenditures. Capital expenditures are excluded.

Table 8.6 Average Duration of Hospitalization at State Mental Hospitals in California, in Days, by Fiscal Year

Hospital	1966–67	1967–68	1968–69	1969–70
Agnews	135.9	111.0	96.5	18.0
Mendocino	108.7	88.0	72.2	8.0
Napa	150.6	135.1	108.3	61.0
Dewitt	104.1	96.9	80.3	24.0
Camarillo	145.2	123.5	128.1	18.0
Metropolitan	122.6	108.9	81.7	14.0

SOURCE: ENKI 1972, p. 195.

potential patients away from the hospital, so as to at least slow the rate at which admissions were rising, and continuing efforts to shorten the stay of those who did end up as hospital inmates. Table 8.6 provides evidence of just how far the latter approach has gone in certain jurisdictions.

An important caveat should be added here: obviously, one needs to know whether decreases in expenditures on mental hospitals have been partially offset by associated rises in state expenditures elsewhere (for example, on welfare, or community treatment programs). Regrettably for the United States (as for England), "on a nationwide basis only speculation is possible about this question" (Wolpert and Wolpert 1974: 22–23). However,

Table 8.7 California Mental Health Budget, Including Local (Short-Doyle) Programs, as a Percentage of the Total State Budget, by Fiscal Year

1959–60	2.58	1963–64	2.15	1967–68	1.80
1960–61	2.53	1964–65	2.26	1968–69	1.63
1961–62	2.46	1965–66	2.12	1969–70	1.71
1962–63	2.39	1966–67	2.00		

SOURCE: Calculated from figures in ENKI Research Institute, *A Study of California's New Mental Health Law*, p. 6.

where data do exist, as in the case of California, they demonstrate that the financial advantages do persist even when these other factors are taken into account. Table 8.7 shows that incorporating expenditures on local (noninstitutional) mental health programs still leaves a substantial downward trend of state outlays in this area.

The promise of such cost savings largely explains the curious political alliance that has fostered and supported decarceration. Social policies that allegedly benefit the poorest and most desperate segments of the community do not ordinarily arouse particular enthusiasm among the so-called fiscal conservatives. The goal of returning mental patients to the community is clearly an exception, for from the outset, in addition to the liberal adherents one might expect, it has attracted prominent, sometimes decisive, support from conservative ranks. This congruence of opinion between what are the two poles of "legitimate" political discourse has helped to render decarceration politically irresistible, since it has reduced the possibility of the movement's central premises being subjected to political scrutiny, and has lent the whole enterprise the character of being self-evident. This broad political base also helps to account for the consistency with which the policy has been pursued over time, and in places as disparate politically as New York or Massachusetts and Reagan's California.

The drive for financial savings has been evident in all phases of the program. One consequence has been ineffectual complaints from individuals who take seriously the rhetorical concern with the welfare of those who formerly ended up as "long stay," that is, life-long, inmates of mental institutions, that the actual implementation of the policy is producing "a relatively good service for the acutely ill...side by side with a second class service, or no service at all, for the chronic patient" (Wing 1971: 190). But this is clearly the most desirable approach on cost effectiveness grounds—to concentrate one's efforts on those one has some prospect of restoring to the work force and to self-sufficiency, and to abandon the rest to the cheapest alternative one can find.

One group for whom restoration in those terms is by definition a hopeless goal is the aged, particularly those past the official retirement age. And despite the growing proportion of elderly people in the populations of both England and America, largely successful efforts have been made to prevent this being reflected in a parallel accumulation of the aged in mental hospitals. Restrictive admissions policies have been adopted, whose effect has been substantially to exclude the hopeless aged. For example, "in New York State a selective admission policy was introduced in 1968," aimed at diverting as many of the aged as possible to general hospitals, or to "foster homes for the aged." Within a year, this policy had effected a 42 percent reduction in the number of aged persons admitted into mental hospitals (Pollack and Taube 1973:14). More generally, in the United States between 1955 and 1968, while the number of admissions (all ages less those over 65) rose more than 55 percent, from 89,144 to 138,474, admissions of those over 65 fell by almost 20 percent, from 33,140 to 26,594 (NIMH Statistical Note # 114).

Moving from admissions to length of stay, a similar policy has been pursued to clear elderly long-stay patients out of the mental hospitals into less expensive alternative situations. In the United States, the overall size of the resident mental hospital population fell by a relatively constant amount each year from 1955 to 1964 (1.2 percent per annum), but since 1964, there has been "an accelerated rate of discharge from year to year" (NIMH Statistical Note #1: 1). By 1970, for example, the rate was 9 percent a year. During this period, "discharge of the elderly patients has involved considerable transfer from the state hospital facilities to community nursing and convalescent homes" (Wolpert and Wolpert 1974: 27). A substantial proportion "of the acceleration of the population decreases in the State and county mental hospitals in the 1960's was undoubtedly due to the placement of long-term chronic patients into nursing homes," and it now "seems fairly certain that the entire range of purely *psychiatric* facilities cares for less than half of the aged mentally ill" (Pollack and Taube 1973: 32–33).

Most significantly, given our present concerns, NIMH (Statistical Note # 107) data reveal that:

> the reductions in the numbers of elderly patients resident in and admitted to inpatient psychiatric services, particularly State mental hospitals, in recent years appear not to have shifted the locus of care to community-based psychiatric facilities (community mental health centers and other out-patient psychiatric services) to any great degree. Instead, they have been accompanied by substantial increases in the number of mentally ill and mentally disturbed residents in nursing and personal care homes.

As Table 8.8 shows, between 1963 and 1969, there was a near doubling of the number of mentally ill patients resident in these homes, from about 222,000 in 1963 to almost 427,000 in 1969, and by 1972, the number had grown again, to 640,000. More detailed data from the same source provide powerful support for the contention that the driving force behind this transfer has been the cost savings that result. In the first place, "the state mental hospitals which have released large numbers of elderly over the past ten or more years, have failed to play a significant role in the follow-up support of these released patients." More seriously, "there appears to be a disproportionate utilization of homes offering personal (i.e., custodial-type) care only, by those elderly being transferred from mental hospitals," so that what we seem to be seeing is the emergence of a new pattern in custodial care for the mentally ill elderly. Even within the larger category of old-age homes, "as the level of provided service [and cost!] declines—from nursing-care homes to personal care homes— the admissions coming from mental hospitals as a percent of total admissions to these homes increases" (NIMH Statistical Note # 107: 6).

Table 8.8 Number of Patients with Mental Disorders Resident in Mental Hospitals and Nursing Homes in the U.S. in 1963 and 1969, Classified by Age

| | 1963 | | 1969 | |
	State and County Mental Hospitals	*Nursing Homes*	*State and County Mental Hospitals*	*Nursing Homes*
Total	504,604	221,721	369,969	426,712
Under 65	355.762	34,046	258,549	59,126
65 and over	148,842	187,675	111,420	367,586

SOURCE: Adapted from NIMH Statistical Note # 107, Table 2.

As this suggests, one indirect consequence of decarceration has been a much greater involvement of the private sector in coping with problem populations that were formerly the exclusive province of the state. The pattern of "the socialization of loss and the privatization of profit" (Birnbaum 1971: 283), already well-established in the military-industrial complex, is now imprinting itself on new areas of social existence. Particularly in America, an effort is under way to transform "social junk" into a commodity from which various "professionals" and entrepreneurs can extract a profit. Medicare and the nursing home racket are merely the largest and most blatant examples of this practice. At the other end of the age spectrum, for the very young who become dependent and neglected, the system of foster care involves increasingly "heavy reliance upon the purchase by the public social welfare sector of child care services from private agencies" (Fanshell and Shinn 1972: 3). In between, there have appeared whole chains of enterprises seeking to capitalize on this emerging market, ranging from privately run drug treatment franchises to fair-sized corporations sprawled across several states dealing with derelicts and discharged mental patients. Largely free of state regulation or even inspection, and lacking the bureaucratic encrustations of state-run enterprises, such places have found ways to pare down on the miserable subsistence existence characteristically provided in state institutions. For our present purposes, what is important about these places is that while, in an obvious sense, they are the creatures of change in state policy, yet on another, admittedly secondary, level they came to provide one of that policy's political supports and a source of pressure for its further extension.

In this context, the reality that community care frequently involves no more than a transfer from one institution to another institution or quasi-institutional setting is by no means confined to the case of the aged. Table 8.8 shows that in 1969 over 59,000 of those under the age of 65 and officially designated mentally ill were confined in nursing homes of various types. Many others are in so-called halfway houses, or ex-welfare hotels. In the words of a recent report on the situation in Michigan, many such patients have been dumped "in facilities having fifty or more residents..., large quasi-institutional settings [that] cannot be expected to provide the anticipated [therapeutic] benefits of community placement" (New York Times, March 22, 1974). But, of course, they do provide the benefit of substantial cost savings to the state.

The discharge pattern for the elderly closely corresponds to the expanding provision of subsistence level support for them by federal and local governments, with the most rapid decrease coming in the late 1960s and 1970s, following the passage of Medicare. Similarly, the decarceration of other inmates has coincided with administrative reorganizations and changes in bureaucratic regulations that have facilitated granting of the minimal outside support that permits the return of patients to the community. One should notice here the effects produced by the more fragmented nature of the United States' political structure and the differential impact within that structure of the fiscal crisis, felt more acutely at the state and local levels. Welfare has increasingly become a federal responsibility (or at least is federally funded) whereas institutional programs like mental hospitals have remained a state (occasionally a county) responsibility. This situation has greatly magnified the attractions of decarceration for states hard pressed for money, for with some administrative juggling with "conditions of eligibility," it permits the transfer of costs to a different level of government and thus relieves, temporarily at any rate, some of the local fiscal crisis. Almost certainly, this has had much to do with the more rapid decline in institutional populations in the United States, as compared with England.

Summary

Placing the decarceration movement in its structural context, this paper has argued that this shift in social control styles and practices must be viewed as a response to the changing exigencies of domestic pacification and control under welfare capitalism. In particular, it reflects structural pressures to sharply curtail the costly system of segregative control, once welfare payments, providing a subsistence existence for elements of the surplus population, make available a viable alternative to management in an institution. Such structural pressures are greatly intensified by the fiscal crisis encountered in varying degrees at the different levels of the state apparatus, a crisis engendered by advanced capitalism's need to socialize more and more of the costs of production—the welfare system itself being one aspect of this process of socialization.

It is the pervasiveness and intensity of these pressures, and their mutually reinforcing character, that account for most of the characteristic features of the new system of community care, and that enable us to comprehend the continued adherence to this policy even where it provokes considerable opposition. The significance of the introduction of psychoactive drugs has been shown to be much less than is commonly supposed, and I have suggested that in any event their use to lessen the difficulties of managing some patients in the community, rather than as merely an additional, less visible means of control to be used in the mental hospital, has been largely shaped by this same set of pressures. Finally, the critics of the asylum and advocates of community care on therapeutic grounds are shown to have had little influence on the actual course of policy, decarceration in practice displaying little resemblance to liberal rhetoric on the subject. Neither the arguments nor the evidence presented in their support by such people are in the least part novel, having been substantially anticipated at least a century ago. Thus their primary significance (though far from their authors' intent) would seem to be their value as ideological camouflage.

References

Belknap, I. (1956) *Human Problems of a State Mental Hospital* New York: McGraw-Hill.
Birnbaum, N. (1971) *Toward a Critical Sociology* New York: Oxford University Press.
Brill, H., and Patton, R. (1961) "Clinical Statistical Analysis of Population Changes in the New York State Hospitals Since the Introduction of Psychotropic Drugs," *American Journal of Psychiatry* 109:20–35.
Brown, G., Bone, M., Dalison, B., and Wing, J. (1966) *Schizophrenia and Social Care* London: Oxford University Press.
Bucknill, J. C. (1880) *The Care of the Insane and Their Legal Control* London: Macmillan.
Coates, R., and Miller, A. (1973) "Neutralization of Community Resistance to Group Homes," in Y. Bakal (ed.) *Closing Correctional Institutions* Lexington, MA: Lexington Books.
Crane, G. (1973) "Clinical Psychopharmacology in its Twentieth Year," *Science* 181:124–128.
Cumming, E., and Cumming, J. (1957) *Closed Ranks* Cambridge MA: Harvard University Press.
Davis, J. M. (1965) "Efficacy of Tranquilizing and Anti-Depressant Drugs," *Archives of General Psychiatry* 13:552–572.
Dingman, P. (1974) "The Case for the State Mental Hospital," in *Where Is My Home?* Scottsdale, AZ.
Engelhardt, D., Freedman, N., Glick, L., Hankoff, L., Mann, D., and Margolis, R. (1960) "Prevention of Psychiatric Hospitalization with the Use of Psychopharmacological Agents," *Journal of the American Medical Association* 173:147–149.
— (1963) "Phenothiazines in Prevention of Psychiatric Hospitalization II Duration of Treatment Exposure," *Journal of the American Medical Association* 186:981–983.

— (1964) "Phenothiazines in Prevention of Psychiatric Hospitalization III Delay or Prevention of Hospitalization," *Archives of General Psychiatry* 11:162–169.

— (1967) "Phenothiazines in Prevention of Psychiatric Hospitalization, IV. Delay or Prevention of Hospitalization: A Re-evaluation," *Archives of General Psychiatry* 16:98–101.

Epstein, L. J., and Simon, A. (1968) "Alternatives to State Hospitalization for the Geriatric Mentally Ill," *American Journal of Psychiatry* 124:955–961.

Fanshell, D., and Shinn, E. (1972) *Dollars and Sense in the Foster Care of Children* New York: Child Welfare League of America.

Gittelman, R. K., Klein, D. F., and Pollack, M. (1965) "Effectiveness of Psychotropic Drugs on Long Term Adjustment," *Psychopharmacology* 5:317–338.

Glaser, D. (1973) "Correction of Adult Offenders in the Community," in L. Ohlin (ed.), *Prisoners in America* Englewood Cliffs, N.J.: Prentice Hall

Glick, L., and Margolis, R. (1962) "A Study of the Influence of Experimental Design on Clinical Outcome in Drug Research," *American Journal of Psychiatry* 118:1087–1096.

Goffman, E. (1961) *Asylums* Garden City, New York: Doubleday.

Gough, I. (1975) "State Expenditure in Advanced Capitalism," *New Left Review* 92:53–92.

Greenblatt, M. (1974) "Historical Forces Affecting the Closing of State Mental Hospitals," in *Where Is My Home?* Scottsdale, AZ: NTIS.

Grob, G. (1966) *The State and the Mentally Ill: A History of Worcester State Hospital* Chapel Hill: University of North Carolina Press.

— (1973) *Mental Institutions in America: Social Policy to 1875* New York: Free Press.

Hanwell Lunatic Asylum (1856) *Annual Report*

Hobsbawm, E. (1969) *Industry and Empire* Harmondsworth: Penguin Books.

Hoenig, J., and Hamilton, M. (1969) "Extramural Care of Psychiatric Patients," *Lancet* i: 1322–1325.

Howe, S. G. (1854) *A Letter to [the] Commissioners of the State Reform School for Girls* Boston.

Hunt, R. C. (1957) "Ingredients of a Rehabilitation Program," Proceedings of the 34th Annual Conference of the Milbank Memorial Fund.

Joint Commission on Mental Illness and Health (1961) *Action for Mental Health* New York: Basic Books.

Marshall, A. (1920) *Principles of Economics* 8th ed. New York: Macmillan.

Maudsley, H. (1867) *The Physiology and Pathology of Mind* London: Macmillan.

Mechanic, D. (1969) *Mental Health and Social Policy* Englewood Cliffs, N.J.: Prentice Hall.

Nunally, J. C. (1961) *Popular Conceptions of Mental Health* New York: Holt.

Polanyi, K. (1957) *The Great Transformation* Boston: Beacon.

Pollack, E. S., and Taube, C. A. (1973) "Trends and Projections in State Hospital Use," unpublished paper presented at the Symposium on the Future Role of the State Mental Hospital, SUNY Buffalo, October 11,1973.

President's Commission on Law Enforcement and the Administration of Justice (1967) Washington, D.C.

Rothman, D. (1971) *The Discovery of the Asylum* Boston: Little, Brown,

Rappaport, M., Hopkins, H., Hall, K., Belleza, T., and Silverstein, J. (n.d.) "Schizophrenics for Whom Phenothiazines May Be Contraindicated or Unnecessary," unpublished paper, Langley Porter Neuropsychiatric Institute, San Francisco.

Scull, A. (1974) "Museums of Madness," unpublished Ph.D. dissertation, Princeton University.

Smith, R. (1971) *A Quiet Revolution—Probation Subsidy* Washington D.C: Department of Health, Education, and Welfare,

Stewart, A., Lafave, H., Grunberg, F., and Herjanic, M. (1968) "Problems in Phasing Out a Large Psychiatric Hospital," *American Journal of Pvschiatrv* 125:82–88.

Wing, J. (1971) "How Many Psychiatric Beds?" *Psychological Medicine* 1: 188–190.

Wing, J., and Brown, G. (1970) *Institutionalism and Schizophrenia* Cambridge: Cambridge University Press.

Wolpert, E., and Wolpert, J. (1974) "The Relocation of Released Mental Hospital Patients into Residential Communities," unpublished paper, Princeton University.

Practice and Research Texts

9

Hollingshead, A. B., & Redlich, F. C. (1958). *Social class and mental illness: A community study.* New York: John Wiley & Sons Inc.: New York

Hollingshead and Redlich's study of mental illness in New Haven, Connecticut, involved a census of persons receiving both public and private psychiatric treatment in that city. The study drew on extensive data from interviews with service providers and chart reviews and compared these to data from a general population sample of New Haven. The authors emphasize the importance of locating people in their life contexts, including the impact of factors such as income, religion, area of residence, culture and education, and relationships within the community. Study results indicated that low class was associated with higher rates of treated mental illness, controlling for religion, age, gender, and race. Diagnostic labels differed by class, with lower class status correlated with higher incidences of psychotic diagnoses. Differences in treatment setting and modality were associated with class status as well, with those in higher classes treated more often by private practitioners and hospitals and those in lower classes treated in public clinics and state hospitals. *Social Class and Mental Illness* was a landmark study that led to greater attention to the epidemiology of psychiatric disorders in the emerging field of community psychiatry. The excerpt here is from Chapter 6, "Paths to the Psychiatrist."

Rebecca Miller

Paths to the Psychiatrist

Introduction

Every person who follows a path that leads him eventually to a psychiatrist must pass four milestones. The first marks the *occurrence of "abnormal" behavior;* the second involves the *appraisal* of his behavior as "disturbed" in a psychiatric sense; the third is when the decision is made that psychiatric treatment is indicated; and the fourth is reached when the *decision is implemented* and the "disturbed" person actually enters the care of a psychiatrist. Due to the limitations of the data available to us because of the nature of our research design, the paths between the first two milestones will be sketched only in outline and illustrated by typical cases. The paths between the third and fourth milestones will be traced in detail with statistical materials accumulated on all cases in the study. In our discussion of the events that link each milestone, we will focus attention upon the question: Is class status a salient factor in the determination of what path a person follows on his way to a psychiatrist?

"Abnormal" Behavior

"Abnormal" behavior is used here to indicate actions that are different from what is expected in a defined social situation. Thus abnormal acts can be evaluated only in terms of their cultural and psychosocial contexts. Homicide, for example, is abnormal in a peaceful community; it is normal when inflicted on the enemy during war.

Viewed psychiatrically, the range of abnormal behavior is very great, covering in intensity mild neuroses to severe psychoses, and in duration from acute, transient "disturbances" to chronic reactions. It encompasses such well-defined phenomena as various types of schizophrenia, and many psychosocial maladjustments that never bring most persons to the attention of psychiatrists.[2] "Abnormality" depends upon appraisal.

"Appraisal"

The perception and "appraisal," by other person, of an individual's abnormal behavior as psychiatrically disturbed is crucial to the determination of whether a given individual is to become a psychiatric patient or be handled some other way. By appraisal we mean the evaluations of family members and proximate groups of abnormal behavior of person. The appraisal of behavior as psychiatrically abnormal precedes decisions concerning therapeutic intervention. Appraisal is carried on by individuals and groups through the interpretation of interacting responses. It may be conscious, preconscious, or unconscious; usually, it is a combination of all three. It is both interpersonal and intrapersonal. As a lay response, appraisal corresponds to the professional diagnosis. As an intrapsychic process, it designates how the prospective patient perceives his actions, particularly his disturbed actions. Appraisal, as an interpersonal process, entails how a disturbed person and his actions are perceived and evaluated by the individual and by other persons in the community. Appraisal will determine what is judged to be delinquency, bad behavior, or psychiatric troubles.

Class Status and Appraisal

Inferences drawn from clinical practice, the tape-recorded interviews with persons in the 5 percent sample, and patients and members of their families in the Controlled Case Study and the Psychiatric Census indicate that class I and II persons are more aware of psychological problems than class IV and V persons. Class I and II persons are also more perceptive of personal frustration, failure, and critical intrapsychic conflicts than class IV and V persons. Perception of the psychological nature of personal problems is a rare trait in any person and in any class, but it is found more frequently in the refined atmosphere of classes I and II than in the raw setting of class V. As a consequence, we believe that far more abnormal behavior is tolerated by the two lower classes, particularly class V, without any awareness that the motivations behind the behavior are pathological, even though the behavior may be disapproved by the class norms. We will illustrate these points by drawing upon the clinical histories of several patients in our study.

The first patient is an example of a higher status who is able and willing to utilize the help of a psychiatrist to overcome self-perceived disturbances. This patient is a 25-year-old graduate student, the son of a salaried, minor professional man in an established class II family. The patient's chief complaint is a feeling that he is not able to work to his full capacity. He first noted this difficulty as an undergraduate in a state university near his home. He discussed this problem with a college friend who was being treated by psychotherapy and, upon his friend's advice, consulted the psychiatrist in charge of the college mental hygiene clinic. However, he did not enter treatment at that time. He knew little about psychiatry when he went to the clinic, but he began to read Freud, Horney, and others; after a period of conscious aversion, he found the materials interesting. The information gathered from them led him, after he had entered graduate school, to discuss his feeling with his friend. Upon this occasion he entered treatment. He was skeptical about psychiatric help in the first weeks of therapy, but he convinced himself that obtaining psychotherapy does not mark a person as "crazy." From this point on he was able to profit from psychiatric treatment. In the course of several months of psychotherapy, he was able to discuss with the therapist his relationships with a stern, driving father and a brother who had disgraced the family on many occasions. The discussions made him realize he was far too critical of himself and inordinately ambitious; unconsciously he was identifying with his stern father while competing with and outdoing the "bad" brother. Gradually, he realized that his unconscious motivations were related to his depression, anxiety, and inability to do graduate work the way he desired.

The patient we shall use to illustrate the lack of sensitivity to psychopathological behavior in the lower segments of the status structure is an elderly class IV man. This man's clinical history indicates that he had exhibited psychopathological behavior throughout his life, but it was not interpreted as such by his family or his associates. A few incidents will clarify the lack of appraisal by the family. In 1940, he took his thermos bottle to a chemist for examination to see if his wife was trying to poison him. Every night before his wife went to bed she secreted butcher knives and other sharp instruments to keep them away from him. He did not trust his daughter to measure medicine "prescribed" for him by a corner druggist, and he accused her of trying to poison him to get his money. He entered his daughters' bedrooms while they were dressing or undressing unless they locked their doors. He kept a razor-sharp hunting knife in the cellar. A daughter and son-in-law knew about the weapon and his constant preoccupation with sharpening it, but no action was taken. The man became violent whenever anyone told him to stop cursing or stop anything he might be doing. When this occurred, he would shout and pound on the walls; on numerous occasions he broke the plaster with the force of his blows. The family avoided bringing any liquor into the home because the father became unmanageable when drunk.

The day before Christmas, however, he requested a bottle for the holidays, and the eldest daughter and son-in-law, in order to humor him, bought a fifth of whiskey. On Christmas Eve, he drank too much, became angry, and used his full vocabulary of obscenity and profanity on the family. The daughter and son-in-law put him to bed and removed his weapons from the room. The next morning he demanded to know what had happened the previous evening, and when he was told he began to yell and curse until the entire building of flats where the family lived was aroused. His daughter in desperation called the police who took the man to the city jail. He was held until after New Year's Day before he was tried, found guilty of breach of the peace, and was sentenced to sixty days in the county jail. After transfer to the jail, he became violent, and a psychiatrist was called to the jail by the sheriff. The psychiatrist recommended commitment to the state hospital.

This man had been in the state hospital two years at the time of the Psychiatric Census. His family did not want him in the home but they did not feel it was right for him to remain in the state hospital. His eldest daughter, who took charge of the situation, did not think he was "crazy." However, she made no active plans to care for him or to have him discharged. While the study was in progress the man died in the state hospital.

Although the patient presents a lifelong history of hostility, suspicion, and extreme lack of consideration of others, so far as we are able to determine neither his family nor others in his environment—even when his behavior became violent—considered him a "psychiatric problem." Such an appraisal of behavior is more typical of class V than of class IV, although people in all strata have blind spots regarding psychopathological implications of unusual behavior or even deliberately avoid thinking about them. The lower status patient will attribute his troubles to unhappiness, tough luck, laziness, meanness, or physical illness rather than to factors of psychogenic origin. The worst thing that can happen to a class V person is to be labeled "bugs," "crazy," or "nuts." Such judgment is often equal to being sentenced for life to the "bughouse." Unfortunately, this sentiment is realistic.

The case histories of two compulsively promiscuous adolescent females will be drawn upon to illustrate the differential impact of class status on the way in which lay persons and psychiatrists perceive and appraise similar behavior. Both girls came to the attention of the police at about the same time but under very different circumstances. One came from a core group class I family, the other from a class V family broken by the desertion of the father. The class I girl, after one of her frequent drinking and sexual escapades on a weekend away from an exclusive boarding school, became involved in an automobile accident while drunk. Her family immediately arranged for bail through the influence of a member of an outstanding law firm; a powerful friend telephoned a newspaper contact, and the report of the accident was not published. Within twenty-four hours, the girl was returned to school. In a few weeks the school authorities realized that the girl was pregnant and notified her parents. A psychiatrist was called in for consultation by the parents with the expectation, expressed frankly, that he was to recommend a therapeutic interruption of the pregnancy. He did not see fit to do this and, instead, recommended hospitalization in a psychiatric institution to initiate psychotherapy. The parents, though disappointed that the girl would not have a "therapeutic" abortion, finally consented to hospitalization. In due course, the girl delivered a healthy baby who was placed for adoption. Throughout her stay in the hospital she received intensive psychotherapy and after being discharged continued in treatment with a highly regarded psychoanalyst.

The class V girl was arrested by the police after she was observed having intercourse with four or five sailors from a nearby naval base. At the end of a brief and perfunctory trial, the girl was sentenced to a reform school. After two years there she was paroled as an unpaid domestic. While on parole, she became involved in promiscuous activity, was caught by the police, and sent to the state reformatory for women. She accepted her sentence as deserved "punishment" but created enough disturbance in the reformatory to attract the attention of a guidance officer. This official recommended that a psychiatrist be consulted. The psychiatrist who saw her was impressed by her crudeness and inability to communicate with him on most subjects. He was alienated by the fact that she thought masturbation was "bad," whereas intercourse with many men whom she hardly knew was "O.K." The psychiatrist's recommendation was to return the girl to her regular routine because she was not "able to profit from psychotherapy."

This type of professional judgment is not atypical, as we will demonstrate in Chapter 11, because, on the one hand, many psychiatrists do not understand the cultural values of class V, and on the other, class V patients and their families rarely understand common terms in the psychiatrists' vocabulary, such as "neuroses," "conflict," and "psychotherapy." The lack of communication between psychiatrist and patient merely adds to the hostility felt toward the psychiatrist and fear of what will happen to a member of the family if he is "taken away." A lack of understanding of the psychiatrist's goals occurs, in part, because lower class persons are not sufficiently educated, but also their appraisal of what is disturbed behavior differs greatly from that of the psychiatrist.

In class V, where the demands of everyday life are greatest, awareness of suffering is perceived less clearly than in the higher levels. The denial, or partial denial, of the existence of psychic pain appears to be a defense mechanism that is linked to low status. Also, class V persons appear to accept physical suffering to a greater extent than do persons in higher status positions. This may be realistic and in keeping with the often hopeless situations these people face in day-to-day living. In classes I and II, by way of contrast, there is less willingness to accept life as unalterable. Consequently, there is a marked tendency to utilize a psychiatrist to help ease subjective malaise or disease. Nevertheless, the individual usually tries to hide his "shame" until it is no longer concealable. Even members of the immediate family may not be told that the patient is in psychiatric treatment. For example, in an extreme case, a middle-aged class III Jewish woman takes great pains to let nobody except her favorite sister know that she is a patient. The sister, who usually brings the patient to the psychiatrist's office, insists that the patient be administered anesthesia before she receives electro-convulsive therapy. She does not think the patient should know about her "shameful" treatment.

Social Factors and Appraisal

The social factors influencing appraisal fall into two major categories: (1) access to existing technical knowledge and (2) sociocultural values. There is little doubt about the first point; without any knowledge of psychiatric therapy there can be no therapy, but prescription and application of therapy depend, upon a group's access to knowledge, particularly in a popular form. The consequences of this, however, have not been understood. Only recently has health education in mental illness begun to be developed by mass communication media. We mentioned in Chapter 5 that 300 years ago psychotics were considered to be witches and sorcerers. Even today, symptoms of neurosis and psychosis are thought to be caused by the "evil eye" by many class V Italians in this community. Naturally, such appraisal determined by culture is not compatible with modern psychiatric treatment.

We have begun barely to understand the appraisal process and the effects it has on who is treated by a psychiatrist and by what therapeutic techniques. A number of different things enter into it. The process of appraisal depends on individual factors of specific personality development and experience; it depends also on the values of our culture and the specific class subcultures as well as the knowledge and techniques which are available to the expert and to others who perceive and evaluate behavior in a given social situation.

Where people take their "troubles" depends on the value orientation of the individual which, in turn, depends upon group appraisal. Both interpersonal and intrapersonal appraisals are influenced by psychosocial and sociocultural factors. For example, a class I or II person who informs himself about diagnosis and treatment and who has access to the best medical opinion will appraise himself differently from the way in which a poorly informed class IV or V person will. The reasons for such differences in self-appraisal may be "deep" or "superficial." At this point, we are less concerned with individual differences than with responses to abnormality which are an integral part of a group's way of life.

Speaking broadly, a community can function adequately only by controlling members who create troubles of one kind or another for themselves and for other members of society. Through the years, special institutions have been developed to deal with particular types of chronically recurring troubles or dysfunctions, such as delinquency, poverty, and disease. Delinquency is handled by police, lawyers, judges, probation officers, and other legal functionaries. Poverty is alleviated by public and private welfare agencies. Medical institutions have been assigned the function of caring for personal crises that society defines as illness.

This neat tripartite separation of common dysfunctions works well so long as society makes clear judgments as to what agency is to care for what dysfunction. When lines of responsibility and function are unclear, as at present, problems arise. The objectives and responsibilities of psychiatric institutions often overlap with those of older welfare, legal, and medical institutions. Psychiatrists and psychiatric institutions are often asked to solve problems that involve several areas of social dysfunctions. Because of their characteristics which are as yet unclear, psychiatric institutions may be viewed as bridges between older institutions that have evolved to cope with social dysfunctions, When legal, economic, organic, and emotional factors play concomitant roles in an individual's troubles, that person may be referred to a psychiatrist mainly because traditional welfare, legal, and medical institutions have failed to handle the individual's multiple problems, possibly because no one institution is so equipped. In this sense, the psychiatrist is a community trouble shooter without a clearly defined role in relation to traditional institutions whose functions are more clearly defined and commonly accepted.

A person whose behavior is acceptable to his family, the community, and to himself is not likely to come to the attention of responsible institutional officers—parents, teachers, police, social workers, physicians, or such medical specialists as psychiatrists. However, when behavior is viewed as abnormal and a threat to the community, an individual may be brought to the attention of some official. For example, an adult male who exposes himself in public will not be tolerated by the community; at present, however, it is a moot point whether he will become a psychiatric patient or a legal case, inasmuch as our values assign the control of this kind of behavior to both penal and mental institutions. For another kind of behavior, that of a mildly hysterical class I or II female, the physician may recommend psychiatric care, but resistance to psychiatrists is so strong in our community that the chances are high she will not follow his advice. However, should she attempt suicide, she is likely to be brought forcibly into psychiatric treatment, for the class I and II subcultures attribute motivations toward self-destruction to psychopathology in the individual. In short: *Abnormal behavior that is appraised as being motivated by psychopathological disturbance in the individual is the province of the psychiatrist.*

Whether abnormal behavior is judged to be disturbed, delinquent, or merely idiosyncratic depends upon who sees it and how he appraises what he sees. To be sure, normal behavior is occasionally appraised as disturbed. Persons who perceive and appraise behavior may be classified into a number of categories: (1) the prospective patient, (2) members of the prospective patient's family, (3) friends, co-workers, neighbors, persons supplying and selling commodities, as well as leaders in community associations such as lodges and clubs, (4) professionals in the field of health (physicians, nurses, medical and psychiatric social workers, clinical psychologists), (5) professionals outside the field of health (ministers, lawyers, teachers, family case workers), and (6) officers of the community (police, attorneys, judges, and various other functionaries). Although there is some overlapping in these groups, they represent the major types of persons who perceive and evaluate behavior as normal or abnormal. Above all, these are the persons who decide whether abnormal behavior is delinquent or disturbed and who make referrals to psychiatric agencies.

Appraisals and Decisions to Act on Them

What is done about abnormal behavior that is appraised to be of psychogenic origin depends upon a number of factors. These include the assumed danger the behavior has for the disturbed individual as well as for other members of society, the attitudes, conscious and unconscious, of the individual and his family toward psychiatric treatment, and the availability of treatment. The implementation of appraisal is social, in large part, because the behavior of the persons involved, patients, therapists, or second parties, is defined in terms of cultural norms.

Among professional persons there are sharp differences in the ways behavior is perceived and appraised. Professionals—lawyers, ministers, teachers, physicians—also differ in their judgments from the perceptions and appraisals of lay persons. For example, conflicts are apt to occur when psychiatrists are asked to evaluate delinquent behavior among children and adolescents who are brought before juvenile courts. The judge may think that a child should be punished for his acts, whereas the psychiatrist may take the position that the child is disturbed and in need of treatment, not punishment. Such professional disagreements lead to fundamentally different ways of dealing with abnormal behavior which may block or delay a decision that a person is in need of psychiatric help. This is especially true when the evaluation of the expert does not coincide with "common-sense" opinion.[4] Even minor professional disagreements block the implementation of a decision by a competent person that an individual ought to be treated by a psychiatrist.

These disagreements are accentuated by the ambiguous role the psychiatrist plays in our society. Law, custom, and tradition have assigned the care of the obviously psychotic person to the medical profession, but the much broader area of deviant and maladjusted behavior, although viewed as abnormal by some members of society, is not accepted fully by the public as an appropriate area for psychiatric treatment. Psychiatrists, particularly those with a dynamic orientation, consider this not only a legitimate but a most important area of professional activity.

When a psychiatrist enters the area of maladjusted behavior, he works with problems not clearly defined as being within the traditional province of medicine. As a "social" practitioner, the psychiatrist shares the appraisal of abnormal behavior with the lawyer, the clergyman, the teacher, the social worker, and the psychologist on the professional level and with parents and volunteer advisors on the lay level. The psychiatrist's role as a therapist is complicated further by the vague definitions of what facets of abnormal behavior should be handled by what agencies in the society. To be specific, delinquency as a legal problem is in the province of the courts and the penal system. Dependency is assigned to public and private welfare agencies. Yet both delinquency and dependency may be symptomatic of emotional disturbance and therefore amenable to psychiatric treatment. This is one of the areas in the society where the role and function of the psychiatrist are least clear.

Closely related to this issue is the question: Should a sex deviant be prosecuted via the courts and prison system, or should he be regarded as ill and treated in a psychiatric setting? Historically, the sexually deviant individual has been viewed as a legal case and punished by the judicial system. In more recent years some lawyers, social workers, and parole officers have held that deviant sex behavior is a psychiatric problem, but this is a minority viewpoint. What actually happens to a sexual deviant may be determined more by his class status than by what is defined by the law or by the most enlightened theory of social scientists or "progressive" dynamically oriented psychiatrists.

The differential impact of class status on what is done about disturbed behavior after psychiatrists are consulted is clear-cut when an individual's abnormal behavior has come to the attention of the police and the courts. In such cases, offenders in classes I and II are far more likely to retain a psychiatrist to protect them from the legal consequences of their acts than are offenders in classes IV and V. While this research was in progress, a class I married man, whose wife was pregnant, was arrested for exposing himself to a little girl. He was referred to a psychiatrist to avoid a possible prison sentence. This accused man retained a shrewd lawyer, well acquainted with persons in high political circles and also with the judge, a political appointee, who tried the case. The lawyer's primary expectation of the psychiatrist was to make a statement in court that would, in his words, "get his client off the hook." The accused was found guilty of breach of the peace and "sentenced" to two years of psychotherapy. From a psychiatric viewpoint, this is not a miscarriage of justice, but an enlightened sentence. The point is that such "sentences" are given rarely to the class IV and V sexual deviates, alcoholics, and drug addicts who face higher and lower courts but usually land in prison, not on a psychoanalyst's couch. Class IV and V sex delinquents, if found by psychiatric consultants to be disturbed, are committed, at best, to public mental institutions rather than sent to jail.

The generally negative attitudes toward psychiatrists and psychiatric agencies in all social strata result in persons turning in many directions for help before they go to a psychiatrist. Often this is a last resort, "a cry for help."[5] To see a psychiatrist is a rather desperate step for most persons; it is taken reluctantly after other resources, mechanisms, and compensations have failed and when the suffering person feels at "the end of his rope." Even then the patient and his associates must overcome various resistances, individual and familial, these are often linked with class status. A physician may advise a patient to see a psychiatrist, and the patient may be willing to follow the physician's advice; however, the patient's family may object strongly because they fear the social criticism that will result, or because they do not believe in it or are unfamiliar with the practice of psychiatry. On the other hand, they may want the patient committed to a mental hospital to get him out of the family, even though they fear the resulting stigma. In most cases, the motivation to obtain psychiatric help involves ambivalent feelings and conflicting evaluations among the several persons involved.

The decision to turn to the psychiatrist is made generally only after there has been a serious breakdown in social relationships. Even when a person seeks help for a very circumscribed problem, there usually is more personality disintegration than surface manifestations may indicate. To be sure, there are differences between individuals as to the amount and kind of stress that lead to despair. There are also class-linked differences in perception of what one may do to relieve conscious and unconscious feelings of displeasure, disease, or malaise. Accordingly, in all classes there are many instances of outright refusal to cooperate to the point of physical violence among both neurotic and psychotic patients.

Awareness of disease or malaise, psychosocial sensitivity to it, and the ability to express one's feelings regarding disease are the antecedents of the action to cope with the causes of distress. In trying to understand subsequent actions, it is also important to know how psychological suffering is viewed in the several strata. It will make a difference whether suffering is considered a result of ill fate, as it tends to be in class V, or something amenable to remedial action as in the higher classes. Only when the suffering is viewed as remediable is it compatible with therapeutic intervention. Actual knowledge of the causal factors by the suffering person may be small—and need not be large—so long as the psychiatrist is accepted as a person who can help him.

A physician may form an opinion about a person with psychiatric difficulties; he may advise him to see a psychiatrist, or he may force him to enter a mental hospital by the use of an emergency certificate. The patient, though not consciously, may want the physician to do this in order to extract him from a difficult, threatening, and frustrating situation. Underlying motivations may include escape from an unbearable situation, a vague wish for love and support, and, probably, less frequently, a constructive desire to work through a problem with the aid of a competent doctor.

Implementation of Decisions to Seek Psychiatric Help

A decision to obtain psychiatric help is not identical with the implementation of that decision. Implementation may not be possible because the help which is sought is not always available. Many persons who want psychiatric help or who are referred to psychiatrists are seriously frustrated when they learn that, for geographic, social, and economic reasons, psychiatry is not available to them. We want to note here, however, that the data we will present in this chapter are limited to cases where the decision to refer an individual to a psychiatrist or psychiatric agency *was* implemented by the person's entry into treatment; instances where the decision was not implemented are not included in our figures.

Sources of Referral

The decision that a person's behavior is disturbed and is amenable to psychiatric treatment may result in a recommendation for action. For our purposes, a decision made by any person that an individual, who later became a patient and was counted in the Psychiatric Census, needed psychiatric care is called a *referral*. The name of the person responsible for the referral, ascertained from the clinical record of each patient, was entered on the Psychiatric Census schedule. We pointed out in a previous paragraph that one or more of six types of responsible persons ordinarily makes the decision that a person exhibiting disturbed behavior be treated by a psychiatrist. Each type of referral will be characterized briefly before we investigate class status as a significant factor in the question of *who* makes the decision to refer disturbed persons to psychiatrists.

1. SELF-REFERRALS. An individual who has enough knowledge of psychiatry and insight into himself to realize he is emotionally disturbed may decide to consult a psychiatrist about his problems. Such an individual is motivated by self-perception to seek relief through psychiatric treatment. Self-referrals are associated primarily with individuals who later are diagnosed as psychoneurotics.

2. FAMILY REFERRALS. Family perceptions of disturbance mean that some member of the immediate family recognizes the nature of an individual's symptoms and recommends psychiatric treatment. The individual may or may not accept the family's decision. When the sick individual refuses to accept the family's view of his difficulty, a psychiatrist may be called to the home or the patient may be brought forcibly to a psychiatrist's office. On the other hand, if his behavior is not considered too severe by his family and associates, nothing may be done until the patient's behavior becomes intolerable. The realization that a person is emotionally disturbed may be made by friends and close private associates; for present purposes, such referrals will be included with the family referrals.

3. MEDICAL REFERRALS. Medical perception of psychiatric illness usually occurs when an individual or some member of his family realizes that the person is ill but is not aware of the nature of his illness. The patient and his family may assume that the difficulty is organic and should be treated by a general practitioner or a medical specialist other than a psychiatrist. In this case, a general practitioner or a specialist concludes that the individual's difficulties are not within his domain and recommends psychiatric help. The general practitioner or specialist usually acts as an intermediary between the patient and the psychiatrist. Medical and psychiatric social workers and visiting nurses are the persons who frequently refer patients of the lower classes to psychiatric agencies.

4. NONMEDICAL PROFESSIONAL REFERRALS. Nonmedical professional personnel may observe an individual's behavior and, on the basis of their knowledge of emotional involvements, decide he needs psychiatric help. Guidance teachers in the school system and family case workers are the most common nonmedical professional persons making referrals. Ministers and lawyers may observe the behavior of disturbed persons, but lawyers make singularly few referrals.

5. OFFICIAL REFERRALS. Policemen, of all community officials, are the most likely to perceive that a psychotic individual is disturbed or in need of psychiatric care. This may occur when an officer is called to a home to calm or take charge of a violent individual or where a disturbed individual is being disorderly in a public place. When police officers come in contact with a disturbed individual in classes IV and V, they usually arrest him and hold him in jail until a psychiatrist examines him; if the individual is particularly disturbed he may be taken to the Emergency Room of the community hospital.

Usually when the police arrest a disturbed individual, they perceive the nature of his difficulty before his family does. The family may know the individual is "difficult," "quarrelsome," "ornery," "abusive," "vulgar," or "profane," but seldom realizes that the individual is mentally ill. The police officer's perception and evaluation of an individual's behavior is crucial in deciding whether the individual is to be sent to jail or to the state hospital. If the police in their investigation decide that the patient is responsible for his behavior, he will be held for trial and, in all probability, sentenced to a term in a local jail or the state penitentiary. On the other hand, if the police conclude that the individual does not understand the nature of his behavior, and therefore is not psychologically responsible for what he has done, the chances are high that he will be turned over to psychiatric authorities. Policemen are Very Important Persons in the process of "diagnosing" severely disturbed and antisocial behavior. We believe that police officers, especially in their training schools, should be given systematic training in the nature and recognition of mental illness. They should be taught also something of the reactions of frightened relatives and what is to be done with a disturbed person.

Let us examine the question of interrelationships between class status and who refers whom to psychiatric agencies. Our discussion is limited to patients in their *first course of treatment* because it is impossible in most cases to determine who made the original referral for patients who have experienced a previous course of psychiatric treatment. Also we are interested in who made the decision that first brought the disturbed person into psychiatric treatment. The data on referrals of patients in their first course of treatment are presented according to the two major groups, neurotics and psychotics. Among the psychotic patients, the schizophrenics are treated separately because of the size of the group and their referral patterns.

Sources of Referrals for Neurotics—by Class

The sources of first referrals among neurotic patients are divided, for purposes of presentation, into medical and nonmedical. Medical referrals are subdivided, in turn, into those made by private physicians and those made by clinic physicians. The nonmedical referrals are tabulated according to the typology described in the preceding section. All first referrals for neurotic patients are summarized in Table 9.1. Examination of the data presented in Table 9.1 shows a direct relationship between class status and the percentage of referrals to psychiatrists by private physicians. On the other hand, referrals from clinic physicians show an inverse relationship to class status. Although referrals from private and clinic physicians form class-linked gradients that run in opposite directions, there is no appreciable difference in the percentages of referrals to psychiatrists by clinic physicians between classes I–II and III, but there is a sharp increase in clinic physician referrals at the class IV level of the social hierarchy. Here the increase is from 9.2 percent in class III to 29.1 percent in class IV. Class V referrals from clinic physicians are essentially in the same proportion as in class IV. The percentage of referrals to psychiatrists from private physicians traces a distinctly different gradient, as a glance at Table 9.1 will show. However, the reader should keep in mind that clinics are associated with people in the two lower classes, whereas private practice is correlated with persons in the higher classes.

Referrals by nonmedical persons reveal an interesting series of variations from class to class. There is a definite class-linked gradient in police and court referrals, the higher the class, the lower the percentage of referrals, with a heavy concentration of referrals in class V. A few referrals are made by family and welfare agency social workers and teachers from classes I–II through IV. In class V, there are more referrals from social agencies and public health nurses than from all other nonmedical persons combined. Only clinic physicians approach officials in social agencies in the frequencies of referrals of class V persons to psychiatrists. If we view the clinic physician as a "community professional" along with teachers, social workers, and nurses, then we see that almost two out of three referrals in class V are made by professional workers in the community agencies. When official referrals that are made by the police and courts are added, the proportion becomes approximately four out of five. Few referrals in any class are made by lawyers and clergymen. Referrals by family members and friends are important in the four higher classes but not in class V. Self-referrals are almost as important as referrals by family members

Table 9.1. Percentage of Referrals from Specified Sources for Neurotics
Entering Treatment for the First Time—by Class

	Class			
Source of Referral	*I–II*	*III*	*IV*	*V*
Medical				
Private physicians	52.2	47.4	30.8	13.9
Clinic physicians	7.2	9.2	29.1	27.8
Nonmedical				
Police and courts*	0.0	1.3	5.1	13.9
Social agencies	1.4	5.3	4.3	36.1
Other professional persons	2.9	5.3	6.8	2.8
Family and friends	20.3	13.2	17.1	0.0
Self	15.9	18.4	6.8	5.5
n =	69	79	117	36

χ^2 = 74.26, 9 *df, p* < .001.
* χ^2 computed with *courts, social agencies,* and *other professional persons* combined; also with *family* and *self* combined.

and friends in classes I–II and III, but in class IV there are distinctly fewer self- than family referrals; there are as many self-referrals in class V as in class IV. The chi square in Table 9.1 reveals that who decides to refer disturbed persons later diagnosed as neurotic to psychiatric agencies is linked definitely to class status.

Sources of Referral for Psychotic Patients—by Class

The sources of referral for disturbed persons who are diagnosed as psychotic are more strongly associated with class status than for those who are diagnosed as neurotic. Moreover, the percentage of referrals by particular types of persons is sharply different. Both private physicians and clinic physicians make relatively fewer referrals of patients who are diagnosed later as psychotic in comparison with those who are neurotic. In classes III and IV, private physicians make the highest proportion of referrals. In class I–II, some four out of five referrals are made by the patient, his family, or his friends. There are few self-referrals in class III. The family makes about one in six, but family physicians make some three referrals out of five. Other professionals and the police make a few referrals. In class V, clinic physicians, the police, and the courts make more referrals; social agencies play a minor role. Class V psychotics, unlike the higher classes, are referred in the same general ways as the class V neurotics, except that the percentage of referrals by clinic physicians and social agencies is lower, whereas the proportion of police and court referrals is over three times higher. A close study of Table 9.2 will show that in each class there is a concentration of referrals from one or two types of persons. The patient and the family are the major sources of referral in classes I–II. In class III, private physicians and the family are the two principal sources of referral. In class IV, the family and clinic physicians share the decision with the police. In class V, the police and the courts, social agencies, and clinic physicians make practically all referrals.

The class-linked gradients on self-referrals and referrals by family members and friends in Tables 9.1 and 9.2 corroborate the generalization stated earlier that persons in the higher classes are more perceptive of disturbed behavior and of the potential help psychiatry offers than persons in the lower classes. For example, in class IV, only 24 percent of the neurotic

Table 9.2. Percentage of Referrals from Specified Sources for Psychotics
Entering Treatment for the First Time—by Class

	Class			
Source of Referral	*I–II**	*III*	*IV*	*V*
Medical				
Private physicians	21.4	59.4	44.1	9.0
Clinic physicians	...	6.2	16.3	13.0
Nonmedical				
Social agencies	...	...	7.4	19.6
Police and courts	...	4.8	18.9	52.2
Family and friends	42.9	17.2	8.1	2.0
Self	35.7	6.2	2.6	...
Other professionals	...	6.2	2.6	4.2
n =	14	64	270	378

$\chi^2 = 243.16$, 12 *df, p* < .001.
*Classes I–II and III were combined for the computation of χ^2 because of the small frequencies in classes I and II.

patients and 11 percent of the psychotic patients entered treatment through appraisal of the patient or other persons in the primary group that the patient was disturbed. In class III, by way of comparison, the comparable figures are 32 percent for the neurotics and 23 percent for the psychotics. When we compare class V referrals by various members of the primary group with class IV referrals, we see even a greater difference than when we compare the class III's with the class IV's. In class V there are no family referrals among neurotics, and only 2 percent of the psychotics are brought into treatment by members of their families. In class V, persons outside the family and friendship groups make practically all referrals. In this class, responsible community agents make almost all appraisals of disturbed behavior. Consequently, they are the sources of effective referrals.

Sources of Referrals for Schizophrenics—by Class

The sources of referral for schizophrenics were studied separately to determine if they are different from all psychotics. We found that schizophrenic persons in each class are referred to psychiatric agencies in almost the same ways as the total psychotic patient population. This might have been expected because the schizophrenics compose some 53 percent of all psychotics in treatment for the first time. The sources of referrals for the schizophrenic patients are recorded in Table 9.3. Perhaps the most striking thing about these data is that there are no self-referrals from classes I–II. In these strata we might expect to find enough insight to impel a disturbed person who is diagnosed later as schizophrenic to seek out a psychiatrist, but this is not what happens. In classes I and II, most referrals are made by the family after some member realizes that the patient is ill and in need of psychiatric care. When an appraisal is made that a member's behavior is disturbed the family brings the patient to the psychiatrist or calls the psychiatrist directly. Usually class I and II persons are brought to psychiatric treatment by their families after heated discussions at home. In one instance, a patient became so violent that a psychiatrist had to be called, and male members of the family held the patient while he was subdued by sedatives. The patient was then taken to a private psychiatric hospital under sedative. Ordinarily, however, the patient is aware that he is being taken to a psychiatrist or mental hospital, and violent disturbance is the exception.

Table 9.3. Percentage of Sources of Referral for Schizophrenics Entering Treatment for the First Time—by Class

Source of Referral *	Class			
	I–II	III†	IV	V
Medical				
Private physicians	45.5	66.7	35.3	10.6
Clinic physicians	...	3.7	23.3	12.5
Nonmedical				
Police and courts	...	7.4	24.8	52.3
Social agencies	...	...	3.8	17.6
Other professionals	...	3.7	1.5	3.7
Family and friends	54.4	11.1	9.8	3.2
Self	...	7.4	1.5	...
n =	11	27	133	216

$\chi^2 = 129.68$, 8 *df*, $p < .001$.
* The χ^2 was computed with social agency and other professional referrals combined, and self-referrals combined with family and friend referrals.
† In this analysis, cases in class I–II and III were combined.

Five schizophrenic patients in classes I–II were referred to psychiatrists by private practitioners. Three of these referrals came from general practitioners and two from specialists. In one case, a woman went to her family physician for difficulties described as nervousness and visceral aches and pains. The physician treated her for three weeks before he came to the conclusion she was psychiatrically disturbed; then he referred her to a private psychiatrist. This woman resisted referral but after discussing the situation with her husband, her sister, and a friend in the medical profession, she went to the recommended psychiatrist. The other two persons attempted suicide. The family physicians were called by their families, and the physicians referred them to private psychiatrists. Suicidal attempts in the higher classes provoke rather drastic, often dramatic, action. The two specialists who made referrals were internists; their referrals were made after preliminary treatment for the patient's real or imagined symptoms.

Class III schizophrenics were referred by all types of persons except social agencies. Two persons, both students, went to psychiatrists as a result of their own feelings. One, in the premedical course, came to the conclusion that his difficulties were psychiatric in nature and, as he said, "turned himself in" when he realized he was "out of contact" with reality. He was hospitalized immediately. Three patients were perceived to be ill by their families and friends. One was taken to a psychiatrist after a friend had convinced her husband that she was mentally ill. The husband and friend took this woman to a psychiatrist who previously had treated the friend. The woman accepted the situation and began ambulatory treatment. Most referrals in class III involved situations where the sick member's behavior became so disturbed that the family could no longer cope with it and called a physician. The police brought two class III persons to the attention of a psychiatrist. In one case, a young man was wandering along the street at 3 a.m. when he was stopped by a police car. The police realized that he did not know what he was doing and took him home. The father called a physician who examined the young man and referred him to a private psychiatrist. This case is interesting in that the man was not arrested but was taken home by the police who realized that he was ill. We infer that this action was related to the policeman's perception of the man's middle class status.

Class IV individuals are referred to psychiatrists by all types of decision-making persons, but the greatest number are seen first by private practitioners. Clinic physicians and public officers see about an equal number. Outside the family there are few referrals from any one source.

In class V, the police and courts, social agencies, and clinic physicians make over four out of five referrals. The police and courts alone make over half the referrals. The general sequence of events in these cases is as follows: The disturbed individual attracts the attention of the police, often by breach of the peace or by molesting other persons. After a complaint has been made, the police arrest the disturbed person and take him to jail, where he usually remains until a psychiatrist is brought into the case. If the prisoner is obviously psychotic, the police may take him directly to the emergency room of the community hospital where he is seen by a psychiatrist who is on call at all times. Social workers and public health nurses make referrals when they perceive a person who is in need of psychiatric attention. This recommendation is often resisted by the patient. Schizophrenic individuals in class V often come to the attention of physicians when they come to the dispensary of the community hospital for some physical ailment. Upon examination, the physician may decide that they are in need of psychiatric care and personally take the patient to the psychiatric clinic; experience has shown that otherwise the patient may simply walk out. Systematic observance of practices in the emergency room of the community hospital shows that when lower status persons attempt suicide, little attention is given to the possibility that they may be disturbed. If the patient can be treated medically or surgically without being admitted to the hospital, this is done. Such a patient is discharged without a referral having been made to the psychiatric service. If the patient has to be admitted to the hospital, because of the near success of the suicidal act, a referral may be made to the psychiatric service. However, before the referral is made, the suicidal act must be appraised as the act of a disturbed individual by some responsible person in the hospital. One of our class V patients came to the attention of a clinic physician when he reported for work as an orderly. The physician realized that the man was psychotic and took him to the psychiatric dispensary. Within a matter of hours, he was in the state hospital.

References

1   We are indebted to Dr. John Clausen, Chief, Socio-Environmental Laboratory, National Institute of Mental Health, for this pharase.
2   For an extensive discussion of this question, see F. C. Redlich, "The Concecpt of Normality," *American Journal of Psychotherapy*, Vol. 3 (July 1952), pp. 551-576.
3   This class V lay judgment will be supported with statistical data in Chapter Nine when we discuss duration of treatment by class status.
4   In a paper, "The Concept of Health in Psychiatry" [Leighton, Clausen, and Wilson (editors), *Explorations in Social Psychiatry*, Basic Books, Inc., 1957], Redlich cites a striking example from the court-martial scene in Herman Wouk's *The Caine Mutiny*.
5   Verbal communication by J. Rakusin.

10

Leighton, A. H., Lambo, T. A., Hughes, C. C., Leighton, D. C., Murphy, J. M., & Macklin, D. B. (1963). Psychiatric disorder in West Africa. *American Journal of Psychiatry, 120*, 521–527

This study was one of the first to examine the prevalence of psychiatric disorders in a non-European culture, that of the Yoruba tribe of Nigeria. The researchers, using a combination of qualitative and quantitative methods, aimed to gain a richer understanding of the socio-cultural causes of psychiatric disorders among the Yoruba and compare findings to epidemiological studies in North America, particularly Leighton's seminal study of psychiatric disorders in Stirling County, Nova Scotia. In this article, Leighton and colleagues, noting the caveats of a brief study period and a small sample, report a lower incidence of psychiatric disorders but higher rates of psychosomatic, depressive, and anxiety disorders, among the Yoruba compared to the Stirling County group. This study not only broke new ground in terms of cross-cultural mental health research, but came at a time of disruptions in traditional cultures across the globe that were "taking place with thundering rapidity" (p. 525). These disruptions might well lead to widespread mental disintegration among individuals in traditional culture cultures, the authors warned. Such dire outcomes might be prevented, however, if steps can be taken to counteract social disintegration in those cultures. Much of that avoidable damage may already have occurred in native cultures across the globe, but the authors' sounding of the alarm remains relevant in today's global village.

Psychiatric Disorder in West Africa

In undertaking this study of the prevalence of psychiatric disorder in a West African tribe, one of our interests was to see if the task could be done. Could we draw an adequate sample? Could we use the same kind of interviewing technique employed in similar studies in North America? What meaning might the very interview situation have for tribal respondents? Would problems of cultural relativity prove insurmountable?

Another inducement was the hope of determining the range of psychiatric symptoms in a non-European culture group. Several writers have emphasized the lack of depression and the prevalence of excitement in Africa while the clinical experience of one of us (Lambo) has pointed to existence of pathoplastic symptoms among patients not touched by European culture. All of these observations, however, were based on hospital cases, most of whom were psychotic. The picture presented by a probability sample of community people was unknown.

These two goals bear on the fundamental preoccupation of the Cornell Program in Social Psychiatry with sociocultural causes of psychiatric disorder. To study these qualitatively and quantitatively in a West African group and to compare the findings with what has been learned in epidemiological investigations in North America would, we thought, advance ideas of cause. These considerations required that we attend not only to evidences of disorder but also to sociocultural characteristics of the group. Consequently, we investigated the Yoruba culture as a whole, as well as certain specific facets such as age and sex roles, the effects of modernization, and various levels of sociocultural integration.

Methods. The research area consisted of about 100 square miles around the Aro Hospital for Nervous Diseases, which is located near the city of Abeokuta (population approximately 80,000), in the Western Region of Nigeria. The people in this area are almost exclusively of the Yoruba tribe, whose membership numbers about 80,000. Abeokuta is the headquarters for the Egba subtribe.

Within the area a preliminary selection of 25 villages, and from these a final selection of 15, was made to provide a range in size, in modernization, and in state of sociocultural integration. Eight segments of Abeokuta were also chosen for study.

Psychiatric interviewing was done on a male and a female adult in each selected household in the villages and town and also on a non-random group of mental patients of the Aro Hospital. Anthropological data were gathered concomitantly, again using samples, and were concerned particularly with detecting cultural change and with determining various levels of integration. A team of 4 full-time and 2 part-time psychiatrists and 3 social scientists made up the behavioral research group together with numbers of interpreters and assistants, and a medical team that provided treatment for all comers in the villages while the interviewing was going on. Two of the psychiatrists, Lambo and Asuni, are themselves members of the Yoruba tribe.

Working intensively for three months, psychiatric data were collected on 262 villagers, 64 residents of Abeokuta, 59 mental hospital patients, 12 patients of native healers and a few miscellaneous others, making altogether 416. Interviews lasted 1½ to 2 hours each. During the same period 152 social science questionnaires were obtained in the villages and Abeokuta, as well as unstructured interviews with headmen and elders.

Findings. In brief we can say that the methods proved workable, although certain problems arose which we discuss in another publication (1). Likewise the patterning and types of psychiatric disorder among the Yoruba turned out to be qualitatively much like the disorders with which we in North America and Europe are familiar. In making these generalizations, however, we would like to caution that our study was a pilot venture, done in a short period of time and on a limited, even if representative, sample. Thus while we are confident that our village sample adequately represents the 15 villages, we cannot say how well it represents all the other hundreds of villages and the other subtribes of the Yoruba.

After the interviews a judgment about each respondent was made by at least two psychiatrists as to: 1) the confidence felt that the person had any condition of psychiatric significance; 2) the amount of impairment in functioning due to the psychiatric condition; and 3) the types of symptom patterns present. The first of these is a four-point scale where A means that the person shows clear psychiatric symptoms, B that he probably has psychiatric symptoms, C that the evaluator is not sure, and D that the respondent is entirely free of any evidence of psychiatric symptoms. Impairment was rated according to the scale in the *Diagnostic and Statistical Manual* of the American Psychiatric Association. For the symptom patterns we used the terminology of the Manual, but did so descriptively, not diagnostically.

Since the frame of reference for most of the research team is based on experience in North America, we shall present our North American Stirling County findings for comparison with the Yoruba findings (2–4). Table 10.1 shows the ABCD ratings, the significant impairment, and the main categories of symptom patterns.

Here we see that there are fewer people who probably have psychiatric disorder (A or B) among the Yoruba than in the Stirling County group, and more people without symptoms (D). Likewise, only about half as many Yoruba show significant impairment from this cause. At the same time the Yoruba greatly exceed the other group in psychophysiologic and psychoneurotic symptoms. It seems most likely that the high percentage with psychophysiologic patterns includes some who had symptoms on the basis of physical diseases since such are exceedingly prevalent and disabling in this area. The survey method used does not permit distinguishing the etiologies of the symptoms reported. When we break down the psychoneurotic category into sub-categories, the Yoruba sample shows many more people with anxiety and depressive symptoms than does the Stirling County sample. Thus it seems that, whatever the situation with hospitalized patients, there is no shortage of depressive symptoms among the population at large.

Two brief summaries may be useful for illustration:

1. A 30-year-old man. His wife had left him some 4 years previously because she had not become pregnant. His depressive symptoms included marked appearance of sadness and slowness in response during the interview. He said he sometimes felt tired in the morning and could not get going, and even occasionally lay in bed for as long as three days at a time. He often felt hopeless and in despair and was subject to mood swings. Food seemed tasteless and hard to swallow and he thought he lost weight from worry.

Table 10.1. Psychiatric Findings, Yoruba Sample and Stirling County

Number of Respondents	Yoruba† Sample 326	Stirling County 1010
Ratings		
A (clear psychiatric)	23%	31%
B (probable)	17	26
C (doubtful)	35	26
D (asymptomatic)	25	17
Significant impairment	16%	33%
Symptom patterns*(current only)		
Psychophysiologic	84%	59%
Psychoneurotic	72	52
Personality disorder	6	6
Sociopathic	2	6
Psychotic	1	1
Brain syndrome	6	3
Mental deficiency	2	5

* Since these are not mutually exclusive, the total exceeds 100%. It should be noted furthermore that in terms of our criteria many people have a few symptoms without being rated either A or B. This accounts for the relatively high percentages under the psychophysiological and psychoneurotic headings.

† Respondents from the villages and Abeokuta.

2. A 48-year-old woman, whose depressive symptoms were in a setting of having to care for a sick child. The symptoms included not only hopelessness and despair, but also the wish to die. She had difficulty making decisions, did not like to be among people (though formerly she used to) and worried to such an extent that she felt this of itself added to her troubles and caused her to lose weight. Her appetite was poor and she felt tired in the mornings.

These direct comparisons between the findings from an African sample and a North American sample are of course open to numbers of serious questions. It is here that problems of difference in culture and situation are apt to have their strongest effect. Hence, although we think these comparisons are worth making in order to see at least what they are like, it remains uncertain to what extent the similarities and differences in percentages lie in the phenomena or are due to variations in information, criteria and procedures brought about by the cultural and situational differences.

We shall turn now to the somewhat safer ground of comparisons within the Yoruba group and of trends rather than percentages between the Yoruba and Stirling County. We shall also switch from the use of percentages to the use of a score called the "ridit" (5). This provides a measure of mental health status, or of the risk that any member of a given group has psychiatric disorder as compared to the whole sample. The score is so adjusted that the mean for the whole sample is 0.5. Scores higher than this indicate greater risk of disorder, while lower scores signify less risk, or better mental health.

If we compare the mental health status of men and women, among the Yoruba the two sexes turn out to be about the same, both having a ridit of approximately .50. In Stirling County, by contrast, men had a ridit of .44 and women of .56, a difference that is statistically significant and considerable.

This sex difference in mental health is of some interest. In Cornell studies made of Eskimo and Mexican Indian groups, women have in general shown a greater prevalence of psychiatric disorder than men. While this obtains in Stirling County as a whole, we found that in some of the individual communities women have a prevalence rate equal to or lower than that of the men. These comparisons suggest that different kinds of sociocultural environment have a differential effect on men and women. The further elucidation of this is, obviously, a target of prime importance, both from the point of view of practical consequences and of basic research into the nature of personality, male-female relationships, and the functioning of families.

It is appropriate to note here that a major hypothesis in previous studies of the Cornell Program has been that mental health is related to the degree of integration of the sociocultural environment; more specifically, that a disintegrated environment will foster the development of mental disorder. The several ways in which this influence will be manifested throughout the life course have been set forth more fully in other project publications (2–4).

In the Stirling County study the characterization of an environment as disintegrated or integrated was based upon investigation of the small community, its patterns of institutional functioning and interrelationship, and the form and content of its salient sentiment systems. It was not possible to establish absolute standards of integration or disintegration, but contrasting communities from the same general cultural setting were chosen to exemplify different points on a range of integration-disintegration. The type of sociocultural concept employed, then, was a diffuse environmental one, as contrasted to a segmental and "unit-centered" one, such as status or expected role behavior. Given the level of first approximation of the research field at the time, a concept of this order was considered by the researchers to be more appropriate than one which would more narrowly focus the research effort.

An integrated community was characterized by the presence of factors such as an adequate economic base, homogeneous ethnic composition, active religious institutions, family stability, effective leadership-followership patterns, diversified voluntary associational life, and several other items which made up a pattern of functional social features. Conversely a disintegrated community tended to be lacking in these characteristics. In moving into a markedly different sociocultural environment (Yoruba) with the intention of studying sociocultural integration, one of our problems was to devise ways to index the abstract concept in terms appropriate to the new setting. The process is similar to the familiar one of attempting to infer a genotype from its phenotypic expressions.

The first step was to evaluate analytically the criteria originally developed in the Stirling County study in order to determine whether, and to what extent, they could be adapted for research in Yoruba communities. This required analysis of Yoruba culture as portrayed in the literature and as given us by Yoruba key informants, with the attempt to locate segments of the social structure, the breakdown of which would lead to disintegration in the same manner as in the Stirling County communities. In what things—and thoughts—did "poverty" consist, for example? What were the empirical dimensions of "family" and how did this relate to leadership? While with some of the Stirling County indicators the process was the relatively simple one of asking "how do the Yoruba do it?", with other indicators the answer turned on the question of whether such a feature was found at all in the Yoruba social system, and if so, in what particular functional social context? On the whole, however, the majority of the Stirling County study indicators were adaptable, at least in modified form, and there were some additions to the list. In the end, most useful indicators of disintegration among the Yoruba turned out to be poverty, secularization, family instability, weak leadership, and poorly developed associations and recreational institutions.

Table 10.2. Mental Health (ridits) and Level of Sociocultural
Integration in Yoruba Villages and in Stirling County

	Integration		
	High	*Medium*	*Low*
Yoruba villages	.40	.53	.53
Stirling County	.48	.50	.66

Table 10.3. Mental Health, Culture Change and Integration in
the Yoruba Villages

	Changing (Ridit)	*Traditional (Ridit)*
Integrated	.41	.39
Disintegrated	.46	.69

Several research approaches were used to gather information bearing on the prevalence or absence of these proposed indicators in the villages so that we could classify the 15 study villages as either "integrated," "disintegrated," or somewhere in the middle. These consisted of observations of village life and setting, interviews with key informants, and questionnaire interviews incorporating items designed to gather information from a sub-sample of the same people who had been interviewed with the psychiatric questionnaire. Effort was made during the field period to keep the psychiatrists in ignorance of the estimated level of integration of the villages where they were interviewing so that their evaluation of records would not be influenced by the social scientists' conclusions.

When the psychiatric interviews from the study villages were evaluated and the ridit calculated, the results indicated that among this Yoruba group, as in Stirling County, mental health appears to decline as the degree of sociocultural disintegration increases. Table 10.2 gives the trend. Analysis of variance shows, in each cultural area, a significant "level of integration" effect.

Since rapid cultural change, so apparent in West Africa and other areas of the world these days, is often alleged to be the principal cause behind the increasing prevalence of psychiatric disorder in Euro-American societies, it was important to examine the data from this study for the relationships shown between mental health levels and the degree to which cultural change had taken place. We also wanted to determine how the effects of integration and culture change could be compared. By considering as indicators of change such factors as relative amount of wage employment, development of modern political activities, level of education, overall orientation to the new urban culture, and the like, we were able to place all 15 study villages in one or the other of 4 cross-cutting categories: 1) Changing and integrated; 2) Changing and disintegrated; 3) Traditional and integrated; and 4) Traditional and disintegrated.

In Table 10.3, although the number of cases is relatively small and the statistics not very dependable, the face value of the figures for this comparison suggest that the greatest contrast in mental health risk is associated with sociocultural disintegration in traditional villages. In villages undergoing change, the state of integration seems to make much less difference. In villages that appear disintegrated, mental health risk is greater where traditional ways of life persist. Obviously the matter is not settled by this pilot study, but it does appear reasonably clear that culture change and disintegation are not synonymous, either theoretically or empirically.

Conclusion

We would like to suggest that these findings have bearing on work in community development of all kinds, and especially for work in those areas of the world where profound changes are taking place with thundering rapidity. It seems that it is possible to have change without deterioration of mental health provided disintegration of the social system is avoided. Once the sociocultural system becomes fragmented, people lose their bearings, symptoms of anxiety, depression, apathy and non-rational hostility set in, the deleterious effects of disintegration are compounded and downward spirals are set in motion in which social pathology and psychopathology reinforce each other.

It further seems that men and women are affected differently, both with respect to frequency and with respect to symptom types. Table 10.3 suggests that where disintegration is present, culture change may have a positive effect on mental health. There is hope that attention to the functional requirements of both the social system and personality may put in our hands the power to reverse such spirals, or prevent their occurrence.

Bibliography

1. Leighton, A. H., *et al.*: Psychiatric Disorder Among the Yoruba. Ithaca, N.Y.: Cornell Univ. Press, 1963.
2. Leighton, A. H.: My Name Is Legion. New York: Basic Books, 1959.
3. Hughes, C. C, *et al.*: People of Cove and Woodlot. New York: Basic Books, 1960.
4. Leighton, D. C, *et al.*: The Character of Danger. New York: Basic Books. In press.
5. Bross, I. D. J.: Biometrics, 14: 18, 1958.

11

Caplan, G. (1964). *Principles of preventive psychiatry.* New York: Basic Books

Caplan, writing at the beginning of the community mental health center movement, argued that a community-based psychiatry must move away from a mainly individualistic focus on identification and treatment of isolated individuals toward seeing mental illness as a community-wide problem with solutions that emphasize prevention of mental illness. We include here excerpts from the introduction to his book for its well-crafted political rationale as well as for its argument for a prevention-based approach to community mental health. Here, Caplan frames the ways in which the views of possibly competing interests support his argument for a paradigm shift in public policy from hospital- to community-based psychiatry. He begins with the late President Kennedy's message to Congress on mental illness and retardation, then contrasts Congress's support, in the Mental Health Study Act of 1955, for a focus on prevention with that of the Joint Commission on Mental Illness and Health, which the Mental Health Study Act established, favoring treatment of major mental illnesses. Caplan then cites the views of Harry Solomon, former President of the American Psychiatric Association, public health professionals, social scientists, and the U.S. Army's preventative approaches with soldiers as a lead-up to the new era of community mental health, before giving a definition of preventive psychiatry that guides his book.

■ Introduction

When the late President Kennedy issued his Message on Mental Illness and Mental Retardation to the Congress of the United States on February 5, 1963, he heralded the beginning of a revolution in American psychiatry. He said: "I propose a national mental health program to assist in the inauguration of a wholly new emphasis and approach to care for the mentally ill. ... Governments at every level—Federal, state, and local—private foundations and individual citizens must all face up to their responsibilities in this area" (Kennedy, 1963, p. 2).

The fact of the message itself—the first official pronouncement on this topic by the head of a government in this or any other country—as well as its content emphasize that henceforward the prevention, treatment, and rehabilitation of the mentally ill and the mentally retarded are to be considered a *community* responsibility and not a private problem to be dealt with by individuals and their families in consultation with their medical advisers. True, the problem has for many years not been entirely a private matter. State and, to a lesser degree, local governments have played major roles in providing facilities for the care of the mentally ill and the mentally retarded, but planned and comprehensive programs to reduce the dimensions of the community problem have been rare, and organized efforts have largely focused on the provision of custodial institutions. The president said of these: "Many such hospitals and homes have been shamefully understaffed, overcrowded, unpleasant institutions from which death too often provided the only firm hope of release."

In such a national setting, American psychiatry has been in the main obliged to focus on individual efforts to improve the lot of patients, and its proudest claim has been that both in private practice and in certain public institutions many patients have received as competent a diagnostic and therapeutic service in this country as anywhere in the civilized world. Moreover, the number of psychiatrists and other mental health specialists who have received high-level professional training to equip them to deal with patients has in recent years been proportionately larger in this country than anywhere else, and so has the amount of research into problems of both etiology and of treatment.

The promise contained in the president's message and in the legislation to secure its implementation is that for the first time an organized program is being prepared that will seek to reduce the problem radically at the community level and that this nation-wide program will be directed, controlled, and partially funded by the federal government and implemented by state and local governments and private organizations. This should provide a framework within which psychiatrists and their colleagues will have the possibility of meaningfully introducing a community and preventive focus into their work. They will in fact be called on to do so by the leaders of our nation.

This mandate will inevitably affect the goals of psychiatry, which will from now on include the reduction in frequency of mental retardation and mental illness in the community in addition to the diagnosis and treatment of individual patients. This demands not only a major increase in recruitment, but also substantial changes in professional training in order to prepare the psychiatrists of the future for community-oriented practice.

It is safe to predict that a substantial increase in the number of planned community programs and of the budgetary resources to energize them will mean not only that a new group of community psychiatrists will be added to the ranks of the profession, but also that a considerable portion of the time and energy of those psychiatrists who are currently treating patients along traditional lines in private offices and in clinics will in the future be diverted to community practice.

The time is therefore ripe for an examination of the problems of community psychiatry in order to begin to build a body of knowledge on which students and practitioners of psychiatry may draw in orienting themselves to their new opportunities and responsibilities. The present book is one contribution to this end. It is based largely on the experience and thinking of one man and his colleagues over the past twenty years, but there have luckily been many others exploring roughly similar problems in the same period, and their contributions provide valuable additional source material for the book.

The currents of opinion that have molded the views put forward in this book can also be seen to have laid the groundwork for the president's message and its associated legislation and governmental planning. It is to be hoped that a historian will one day make a systematic study of the unfolding of the significant ideas in this transitional period, assuming that events confirm our prediction that we are witnessing the beginning of a metamorphosis in the profession of psychiatry in the United States. Meanwhile, it may be useful to give a brief account of the background of current changes.

Mention must first be made of the increasing interest of state and federal legislators in the community problem presented by the need to care for mentally ill and mentally retarded persons in the light of their large number, the widespread suffering and social disorganization they cause, and the associated drain on community resources. An outstanding consequence of this interest was the Mental Health Study Act of 1955, whereby Congress directed the establishment of a Joint Commission on Mental Illness and Health in order to carry out a

> nationwide analysis and reevaluation of the human and economic problems of mental illness and of the resources, methods, and practices currently utilized in diagnosing, treating, caring for, and rehabilitating the mentally ill ... as may lead to the development of comprehensive and realistic recommendations ... as give promise of resulting in a marked reduction in the incidence or duration of mental illness, and in consequence, a lessening of the appalling emotional and financial drain on the families of those afflicted or on the economic resources of the States and of the Nation (Joint Commission, 1961, p. 303).

It is of interest to note that the legislators were primarily oriented to the development of preventive programs. This has been manifested also in the terms of a number of "community mental health services" bills which have been enacted during the past fifteen years in such states as New York, California, Minnesota, New Jersey, and Vermont and which have focused on the provision of programs in local communities for the prevention, early treatment, and rehabilitation of mental disorders by means of consultation, mental health education, outpatient clinics, psychiatric departments in general hospitals, and rehabilitation services.

In contrast to this approach, it is of interest to study the recommendations contained in the final report of the Joint Commission that appeared in 1961. This report was based on a series of excellent studies under the able leadership of Jack R. Ewalt, which explored a wide field—theories of positive mental health and methodological problems of epidemiological research, the economics of mental illness, mental health manpower trends, community and research resources in mental health, the role of schools and churches, and current developments in the inpatient and outpatient care of the mentally ill. The Joint Commission was supported by thirty-six national organizations in the medical, public health, mental health, welfare, education, and social science fields. Its individual members included leaders of American psychiatry, psychology, social work, education, and social science, and among its chief officers were Kenneth E. Appel and Leo H. Bartemeier, who are among the most respected of American psychiatrists.

With so impressive an array of members and supporters and with so careful a study of the mental health needs and resources of this country as a foundation, it is not surprising that the report of the Joint Commission provides a competent survey of the field. In contrast, however, to the comprehensive, preventive, community approach advocated by the national and state legislators, it is of interest to note that the recommendations of the mental health professionals were largely restricted to the adult mentally ill and did not deal with the mentally retarded or to any significant degree with children suffering from mental disorders. They also focused mainly on plans for improving the mental hospitals of the country through reducing their size, improving their resources, and extending their services into the community, in an effort to deal more effectively with the psychotic patients, both acute and chronic, whose care, they showed, is currently being so badly neglected. Their attitude to preventive psychiatry is well summarized in the following paragraph:

> Here, of course, we reveal the bias of this report—and give a little discomfort to some of our colleagues who have a strong commitment toward practices and programs aimed at the promotion of positive mental health in children and adults. Indeed, a few members of the Joint Commission have found themselves in the position of affirming this final report as it relates to the treatment of the mentally ill and to research, but of rejecting the view that achievement of maximum effort in behalf of the mentally ill would require the minimizing of emphasis on the mental health of persons who are not ill or in immediate danger of becoming so. We have assumed that the mental hygiene movement has diverted attention from the core problem of major mental illness. It is our purpose to redirect attention to the possibilities of improving the mental health of the mentally ill. It is not our purpose, however, to dismiss the many measures of public information, mental health education, and child and adult guidance that may enhance an understanding of one's own and others' behavior and so build self-confidence, reduce anxiety, and result in better social adjustment and greater personal satisfaction. But our main concern here, in recommendations for a program attacking mental illness, is with various levels of service beginning with secondary prevention—early treatment of beginning disturbances to ward off more serious illness, if possible—and continuing through intensive and protracted treatment of the acutely and chronically ill (Joint Commission, 1961, pp. 242–243).

The difference between this view and that of the legislators is one of emphasis, but this leads to the major difference between recommendations which see an enlarged and improved mental hospital system as the core of a program for the treatment and rehabilitation of the mentally ill and the legislators' support of a comprehensive community service to encompass the entire range of mental health and disorder, including improved mental hospitals in a wide variety of agencies and resources.

It is significant that the president, in his message, which followed the report of the Joint Commission, reaffirmed the second view. He said:

> Central to a new mental health program is comprehensive community care. Merely pouring Federal funds into a continuation of the outmoded type of institutional care which now prevails

would make little difference. We need a new type of health facility, one which will return mental health care to the main stream of American medicine, and at the same time upgrade mental health services (Kennedy, 1963, p. 4).

In the part of his message devoted to mental retardation, he said: "Prevention should be given the highest priority in this effort" (Kennedy, 1963, p. 9). He advocated developments in the general health, education, welfare, and urban renewal fields which made it clear that he was focusing on primary prevention.

The bill introduced into the House of Representatives following the president's message was called the "Community Mental Health Centers Act of 1963" and was designed to set up a country-wide system of community mental health centers, each of which would act as the fulcrum for a comprehensive community program, to provide "services for the prevention or diagnosis of mental illness, or care and treatment of mentally ill patients, or rehabilitation of such persons" (U.S. House of Representatives, 1963, p. 19).

It would be an oversimplification to give the impression that psychiatrists and their professional colleagues as a group were in favor of a treatment-institution program, in contrast to the community-oriented legislators. The previous quotation from the Joint Commission report attests to the dissenting voices among members of the commission itself, and, although its major recommendations have been approved by the psychiatric profession as a whole, many have expressed disappointment over the restriction of its focus to the adult mentally ill, its lack of enthusiasm for primary prevention, and its advocacy of a central role for the mental hospitals. These psychiatrists derived solid satisfaction from the terms of the president's message and the Community Mental Health Centers Act of 1963, although some felt that the pendulum swung a little too far and that the possible contribution of the mental hospitals was somewhat underplayed, particularly in relation to the many patients who need long-term care and treatment.

Outstanding among psychiatric leaders who have for several years advocated a comprehensive, community, preventive approach is Robert H. Felix, director of the National Institute of Mental Health, whose agency provided the staff work in the preparation of the president's message and will probably play a significant part in developing the regulations, and later administering the provisions, of the Community Mental Health Centers Act, if it should be passed by Congress. Dr. Felix has exerted a more important influence than any other American psychiatrist in providing legislative leaders with a body of professional data and concepts as a basis for their community, preventive approach to mental health and mental disorder.

Another psychiatrist who has had a major influence upon legislative opinion is Harry C. Solomon, former director of Boston Psychopathic Hospital. In his presidential address to the American Psychiatric Association in 1958, he said: "I do not see how any reasonably objective view of our mental hospitals today can fail to conclude that they are bankrupt beyond remedy. I believe therefore that our large mental hospitals should be liquidated as rapidly as can be done in an orderly and progressive fashion" (Solomon, 1958, p. 7). He advocated the replacement of the mental hospitals by a variety of community agencies closely linked to general hospitals. He viewed these new agencies as centers for community programs of treatment and rehabilitation of the mentally ill, and, although he did not place as much emphasis on primary prevention, his views were quite similar to those contained in the president's message. As commissioner of mental health of the Commonwealth of Massachusetts, he has already made considerable progress toward establishment of the first community mental health centers in line with his plans, and these may well serve as models for those to be constructed under the new federal legislation.

Another influential group which has been developing a positive approach to community programs for the prevention of mental illness and mental retardation over the past fifteen years are the leaders of the public health profession. Lemkau and associates reported in 1961 the results of a country-wide survey of the attitudes of leading public health officials toward their responsibility for the prevention and treatment of the mentally ill. They found general acknowledgment that mental health is an essential facet of public health programs (Lemkau et al., 1961).

An increasing number of state and local public health programs include the prevention and treatment of mental illness among their activities, and this has naturally stimulated the development of theories and practices in relation to these illnesses which are in line with the generally accepted public health approach of organized programs to lower the incidence and prevalence of illness in the community.

Systematic courses of instruction in mental health have been introduced into schools of public health during the past twenty years—first at Johns Hopkins by Paul V. Lemkau, then at Harvard by Erich Lindemann, at North Carolina by Roger Howell, at Columbia by Viola Bernard, and later at other schools, such as Pittsburgh and Michigan.

The American Public Health Association recognized the interest of its members in mental health matters by establishing a Mental Health Section in 1957; and in 1962 it published a "Guide to Control Methods for Mental Disorders," prepared by its Program Area Committee on Mental Health, under the chairmanship of Ernest M. Gruenberg. This guide presents a public health approach to mental disorder, and, in the words of its Introduction, it seeks to answer such questions as:

> What can be done through organized health programs by governments and voluntary agencies and through community action to reduce the size of the burden created by mental disorders? What can be done to reduce the number of people who acquire one or another type of mental disorder? What can be done to shorten the duration of mental disorders which have already occurred? What can be done to reduce the amount of disability and distress caused by unpreventable or nonterminable disorders? (A.P.H.A., p. viii).

The interest of public health authorities in problems of mental health was also given concrete expression by Surgeon General Leroy E. Burney, when, in August, 1959, he established an Ad Hoc Committee on Planning for Mental Health Facilities. This committee, under the chairmanship of Jack C. Halderman, chief of the Division of Hospital and Medical Facilities of the Public Health Service, issued its report in January, 1961, in which it recommended:

> That community-based mental health facilities be established as part of a coordinated system of statewide health services .... Construction and expansion of large mental institutions should be strongly discouraged, and state activities should be directed towards replacement of existing institutions of this type by smaller community or regional facilities offering a wide spectrum of services (U.S.P.H.S., 1961, p. v).

This report anticipated many of the provisions of the Community Mental Health Centers Act of 1963. For instance, it advocated that:

> Planning activity should encompass the entire complex of mental health facilities and services required by the State .... Facility planning should be coordinated with other planning programs in the field of public health and mental health.

It recommended the replacement of large mental institutions

> ... by smaller community or regional facilities offering a wide spectrum of services. These include activities such as out-patient and emergency services through hospital clinics or mental

health centers, increased use of general hospitals for the treatment of psychiatric patients, half-way houses, day and night hospitals, and nursing homes (U.S.P.H.S., 1961, p. 3).

This public health approach of organized community planning for comprehensive programs to include prevention, treatment, and rehabilitation of mental disorders and to be coordinated with other community programs in the health and welfare fields has found a ready ear among many psychiatrists and their specialist colleagues, who, over the past twenty years, and in some cases even longer, have been exploring possibilities of preventing mental disorders in particular settings.

Erich Lindemann's (1944) important contribution to this field is so well known that it requires only brief mention. In 1943, he studied bereavement reactions among the survivors of those killed in the Coconut Grove night club fire and developed the fundamentals of "crisis theory" as a conceptual framework for preventive psychiatry. He felt that the possible psychopathological sequelae of unhealthy coping with the crisis of bereavement could be prevented by clergymen and other community caretakers helping the bereaved to mourn adequately, and he began to develop techniques of preventive intervention in order to achieve this. In 1948, he established a community mental health program, the Wellesley Human Relations Service, in which he and his colleagues explored the implementation of his preventive ideas.

It is significant that this early experiment in preventive psychiatry was established with the financial support of the Grant Foundation. This foundation has consistently supported organized efforts to prevent mental disorder over the past twenty years and has had as marked an effect on this field as the Commonwealth Fund had in the 1920's in promoting the establishment and growth of the child guidance movement. This was in no small measure the result of the interest and initiative of W. T. Grant himself, and in any history of preventive psychiatry his name will certainly loom large. His foundation supported not only the Wellesley community studies, but also such work as that of Prescott (1957) and Ojemann (1955) in developing programs for the prevention of mental disorder among children by modifying the curriculums and teaching methods in schools; the epidemiological researches of Rennie and Woodward (1948) and Leighton (1959), which attempted to correlate the prevalence of mental disorder with sociocultural forces in the hope that those factors associated with a high prevalence might be identified and altered so as to reduce the risk of mental disorder on a community level; and that of the International Preparatory Commission of the International Association of Child Psychiatry and Allied Professions, which culminated in 1962 in the first international congress devoted entirely to the topic of preventing mental disorders in children.

A representative sample of studies on the primary prevention of mental disorder in children which were in progress in this country in 1961 is contained in a book (Caplan, 1961) produced as part of the activities of this International Preparatory Commission. Sixteen studies are described and discussed. They range from broad epidemiological research to family studies and researches on individual parent-child relationships, and they include studies which focus on biological factors, on psychosocial factors, and on sociocultural factors.

A significant impression conveyed by this collection of researches is that preventive psychiatry must continually take into account the *multifactorial* nature of the forces which may provoke or ameliorate mental disorders. A psychiatrist who focuses on individual patients may permit himself the luxury of specializing in one set of factors—physical, psychosocial, or sociocultural—whether in relation to his diagnostic or his therapeutic system. As long as he selects his patients appropriately or as long as others learn of his interest and refer only the appropriate cases to him, he will feel justified in his narrow definition of the field because his clinical results will be satisfactory. As soon, however, as the psychiatrist expands his focus to encompass the total problem of mental disorder and mental retardation in the community and as soon as he enlarges his goals to include the reduction of this community problem, he must broaden his interest to include the whole range of etiological factors and of the modalities of prevention, treatment, and rehabilitation. He can then no longer restrict his conceptual framework to a purely biological, psychosocial, or sociocultural theory.

It is important to realize that such a step, although conceptually and emotionally not without difficulty, need not lead to a "watering-down" of one's original set of individual-patient-oriented theories and methods. It is possible to retain these and in fact to enrich them by the addition of new theoretical and methodological dimensions to one's professional armamentarium. For instance, many of the pioneers of preventive psychiatry have been psychoanalysts. In extending their efforts into the preventive field, they have added nonpsychoanalytic theories and techniques to their practice, such as those which will be subsequently discussed in this book; but this has not impaired their psychoanalytic concepts and methodology. The latter continue to have their original relevance whenever the psychiatrists try to understand or treat an individual patient. Moreover, since *psychosocial* factors loom large in both the etiology and management of many mental disorders, the theories and practices of psychoanalysis have proved of fundamental importance in developing the body of knowledge that is basic to preventive psychiatry. Of the eighteen chapters in *Prevention of Mental Disorders in Children* (Caplan, 1961), nine were written by psychoanalysts.

Psychoanalytic writings, especially those on ego psychology, have exerted a profound influence on the development of the conceptual framework of preventive psychiatry. It would not be appropriate here to review this vast literature, but the following papers, chosen almost at random, from a bibliography on psychoanalytic principles relating to the prevention of mental illness currently being prepared by the Committee on Social Problems of the American Psychoanalytic Association under the chairmanship of Joseph J. Michaels, illustrate the richness of this material.

BENEDEK, THERESE. Psychoanalytic implications of the primary unit, mother-child. *Amer. J. Orthopsychiat.,* 1949, 19, 642-654.

ESCALONA, SIBYLLE K. An appraisal of some psychological factors in relation to rooming-in and self-demand schedules. In Milton J. E. Senn (Ed.), *Problems of early infancy.* Transactions of the First Conference on Problems of Infancy and Childhood, March 3-4, 1947. New York: Josiah Macy, Jr., Foundation. pp. 58-62.

JOSSELYN, I. *The happy child: A psychoanalytic guide to emotional and social growth.* New York: Random House, 1955.

KRIS, MARIANNE. A group educational approach to child development. *J. Soc. Casewk.,* 1948, 29, 163-170.

LINDEMANN, E., & DAWES, L. The use of psychoanalytic constructs in preventive psychiatry. *Psychoanalytic study of the child.* New York: International Universities Press, 1952. Vol. VII, pp. 429-448.

MURPHY G. Prevention of mental disorders: Some research suggestions. *J. Hillside Hosp.,* 1960, 9, 131-146.

MURPHY, LOIS B. Emotional first aid for the young child. *Menninger Q.,* 1956, 10, 19-22.

Psychic development and the prevention of mental illness. Panel discussion reported by M. Furer. *J. Am. Psychoanal. Assoc.,* 1962, 10, 606-615.

SPITZ, R. The smiling response: A contribution to the ontogenesis of social relations. *Genet. Psychol. Monogr.,* 1956, 46, 57-125.

In addition to such papers as these, the writings of Hartmann, Kris, and Lowenstein (1946) on healthy and unhealthy types of ego development, of Kubie (1954) on the relevance for prevention of flexibility or rigidity in ego structure, of Erikson (1950) on the influence of psychosocial and sociocultural factors in ego development, of Lois Murphy (1963) on the coping responses of children to the ordinary crises of growing up, and of Ackerman (1958) and Spiegel (1954) on interaction and transaction in the family have exerted an important influence by emphasizing the significance of psychoanalytic theory and research for preventive psychiatry.

Definition of "Preventive Psychiatry"

In this book, the term "preventive psychiatry" refers to the body of professional knowledge, both theoretical and practical, which may be utilized to plan and carry out programs for reducing (1) the incidence of mental disorders of all types in a community ("primary prevention"), (2) the duration of a significant number of those disorders which do occur ("secondary prevention"), and (3) the impairment which may result from those disorders ("tertiary prevention").

This body of knowledge is closely related to the rest of psychiatry and is based on an understanding of the nature and manifestations of mentally disordered behavior in individuals and on traditional theory and practice in the psychiatric treatment and rehabilitation of patients. The preventive psychiatrist must be first and foremost a competent psychiatrist. In addition, he must acquire knowledge of a wide range of issues—social, economic, political, administrative, and so on—which will enable him to plan and implement programs that focus not only on individual patients but beyond them on the community problems of which they are a part. He must also learn to coordinate his activities with those of many other professional and nonprofessional workers who are actively involved in dealing with the health, educational, legal, and social aspects of the community problems posed by the mentally ill and the mentally retarded and with community programs in allied fields. The close working relationships which psychiatrists in traditional clinical practice have developed with psychologists, psychiatric social workers, and nurses must therefore be extended in preventive psychiatry to include collaboration with social scientists, economists, legislators, citizen leaders, and professional workers in the public health, welfare, religious, and educational fields.

From this it follows that preventive psychiatry is a branch of psychiatry, but it is also part of a wider community endeavor in which psychiatrists make their own specialized contributions to a larger whole. Preventive psychiatry, in my view, must be comprehensive. It must deal with all types of mental disorder in persons of all ages and classes, because our focus is on the total problem confronting the community and not merely on the problems of particular individuals and groups. In this I differ sharply from the point of view of the report of the Joint Commission. I believe that preventive psychiatry must include primary prevention as an essential ingredient and must promote mental health among members of the community who are currently not disordered, with the hope of reducing the risk that they will become disordered. I admit that the inclusion of primary prevention will result in a reduced capacity to deploy our psychiatric efforts in the areas of secondary and tertiary prevention, as argued by the Joint Commission, but I believe that our collaboration with other community workers and a resulting improvement in community programs in the general health, welfare, education, and urban renewal fields may not only reduce the vulnerability of the population to mental disorder but also improve the care and rehabilitation of those who become mentally ill by inviting the efforts of others to augment our psychiatric programs.

My emphasis on a comprehensive approach is based on the belief that not only are mentally disordered behavior patterns part of a whole system of ecological responses of a population in its interaction with its environment, but that our own operations as preventive psychiatrists are also part of the total community security system whereby socially deviant responses and undue individual victimization are kept in check. To ensure professional effectiveness, we must define our functioning in a specialized manner in line with the understanding and skills we develop, but we should take care not to erect boundaries which artificially fragment the field itself and which result in reducing the free flow of information among the various disciplines and professions about the total problem which confronts all of us as an organized community group.

For this reason, I oppose not only the point of view expressed in the report of the Joint Commission, but also that of the protagonists of community mental health programs who restrict their focus to exclude the mental hospitals or to exclude the mentally retarded or the chronic psychotics. Such an approach may well result in an effective institution or agency to improve the lot of a certain number of individual patients, but it retards the development of a planned program to deal with the community problem. Such a program certainly needs specialized agencies, but the nature and distribution of these, as well as their patterns of exchange of resources, clients, and information, must be determined by the total community, and not merely by the predilections of their professional workers or their boards of directors. As will be seen later in this book, this does not imply commitment to a socialized form of centralized governmental control. On the contrary, the community problem of mental disorder is so huge and our ignorance so vast, that all contributions—governmental, voluntary, and private—are to be welcomed.

The fundamental prerequisite for comprehensive preventive psychiatry, however, is that workers and agencies look not only at what they want to do and what they have the skill to accomplish, but also beyond this to the total community problem and to how their contribution may best fit into the total community effort. To be sure, there will be some who will admit responsibility only for their individual patients and who will not accept the community approach. Insofar as they practice in the private sector and are not subsidized by community funds, they are perfectly entitled to operate in accordance with their point of view. As we will see in Chapter VI, such private practitioners are an important means of "taking up the slack" in community programs, which, however carefully planned, will inevitably be unable to cover the whole field. A comprehensive community program of preventive psychiatry must take all diagnostic and treatment resources into account, whether these are under governmental or private control.

References

ACKERMAN, N. W. *The psychodynamics of family life.* New York: Basic Books, 1958.

American Public Health Association. *Mental disorders: A guide to control methods.* New York: Author, 1962.

CAPLAN, G. *Prevention of mental disorders in children.* New York: Basic Books, 1961.

ERIXSON, E. H. *Childhood and society.* New York: Nortion, 1950.

HARTMANN, H., KRIS, E., & LOEWENSTEIN, R. M. Comments on the formation of psychic structure. *Psychoanalytic study of the child.* New York: International Universities Press, 1946. Vol. II, pp. 11–38.

Joint Commission on Mental Illness and Health. *Action for mental health.* New York: Basic Books, 1961.

KENNEDY, J. F. "Message from the President of the United States Relative to Mental Illness and Mental Retardation." February 5, 1963, 88th Congress, First Session, House of Representatives, Document No. 58.

KUBIE, L. S. The fundamental nature of the distinction between normality and neurosis. *Psychoanal. Quart.*, 1954, 23, 167–204.

LEIGHTON, A.H. *My name is legion.* New York: Basic Books, 1959.

LEMKAU, P. V. (Ed.) The mental health function of the public health worker. In *Mental Health Teaching in Schools of Public Health.* New York: Columbia University Press, 1961.

LINDEMANN, E. Symptomatology and management of acute grief. *Amer. J. Psychiat.*, 1944, 101, 141-148.

MURPHY, LORS B. *The widening world of childhood.* New York: Basic Books, 1963.

OJEMANN, R. H., LEVITT, E. E., LYLE, W. H., & WHITESIE, M. F. The effects of a "causal" teacher-training program and certain curricular changes on grade school children. *J. exp. Educ.*, 1955, 24, 97–114.

PRESCOTT, D. A. *The child in the educative process.* New York: McGraw-Hill, 1957.

RENNIE, T. A. C., & WOODWARD, L. E. *Mental health in modern society,* New York: Commonwealth, 1948.

SOLOMON, H. C. The American Psychiatric Association in relation to American psychiatry. *Amer. J. Psychiat.*, 1958, 115, 1–9.

SPIEGEL, J. New perspectives in the study of the family. *Marriage and Fam. Living*, 1954, 16, 4.

United States House of Representatives #3688, 88th Congress, First Session, 1963. *A bill to provide for assistance in the construction and initial operation of community mental health centers and for other purposes.*

United States Public Health Service. *Planning of facilities for mental health services.* Public Health Service Pub. No. 808. Washington, D.C.: U.S. Government Printing Office, 1961.

12

Fairweather, G. W., Sanders, D. J., Maynard, H., Cressler, D. L. with Bleck, D. S. (1969). *Community life for the mentally ill: An alternative to institutional care.* Chicago: Aldine Publishing Company

Many professionals who, in theory, endorse the notion of persons with mental illness taking charge of their own treatment and their own lives have experienced a quandary: How can they encourage movement toward autonomy among clients who have been disempowered in the past and appear not to be ready to run their own lives without substantial professional support or involvement? This understanding may leave those professionals feeling that they would be practicing a kind of reverse paternalism if they tell their clients, in effect, "Go ahead, you're empowered, run your own life," and then stand back to watch them fall apart on their own. Fairweather and colleagues' book provides a rich account of an experiment in communal living in a "lodge society" in Palo Alto during the 1960s for persons being discharged from state hospitals. It is difficult to choose an excerpt from a work that, by its nature, requires an immersion in the experience it describes, but it would be a shame to omit one for that reason. We include material from a section on "early adjustment problems" for clients in their movement from institutionalization toward interdependent living in the community. Along with other elements, the authors emphasize the importance of work, both as a meaningful personal activity that provides income for the person and for its importance in terms of the values we place on valued roles and employment, as a ticket to full membership in local communities and U.S. society at large. This theme resonates even more strongly today.

Overview of the Experiment

Persons who are hospitalized for mental illness nowadays are often destined to become long-term residents of mental hospitals or to return to the community after a relatively short stay. In either case, the results for those least capable of reassuming responsible community roles are often catastrophic. With the advent of more and more interest in the community treatment of mental illness, a nationwide emphasis upon the mental patient's return to the community has developed. Very often, even with excellent planning and the devoted efforts of mental health workers, finding meaningful and participative community roles for these individuals is not accomplished. For the majority of those who leave the hospital without a family to which to return and for many others who remain in the hospital a long time before leaving, the too frequent result is a lonesome and unrewarding life in the social status of ex-mental patient. Many of these persons feel, and perhaps rightfully, that they have been the unwitting victims of social forces aimed at segregating them from the larger society

Previous experimental work in the mental hospital (Fairweather, 1964) has shown, however, that many such individuals—at least when belonging to small groups—are capable of taking care of one another, can make realistic decisions about their lives and those of their group, and can adjust reasonably, adequately, and semiautonomously to the hospital setting. But such group living situations, where the strengths and weaknesses of various individuals can be balanced by their working as a team, are not typically available in the community setting. The goal of this research, therefore, was to discover if new and meaningful social statuses and roles for mental patients could be created in the society so these persons could participate more actively in the social processes accorded ordinary citizens in their everyday life. It was, in fact, an attempt to provide in mid-twentieth-century America an alternative to the large mental hospital. In order to achieve this goal, it was necessary for the researchers to create a new small society in the community where chronic mental patients could go to live and work in a supportive group situation.

But it is not alone sufficient to create a totally new treatment program that can be carried out in the community. It must be a demonstrated improvement over current practices before it can be realistically considered by society. It is, therefore, essential that such a program be directly compared with treatment programs currently available to mental patients in the community. So, in addition to creating and implanting an entirely new living and working situation in the community for mental patients, every phase of the new treatment program was carefully evaluated. A thorough presentation of both the background for the comparative research and its results are presented in the five parts of this book.

After planning the experiment, which included the creation of the assessment devices and the research design, all individuals on a selected open ward were questioned about volunteering to live in the lodge society. Those who volunteered were randomly assigned to either the lodge group or its control group. Those who refused to volunteer constituted the experimental group used later to discover the effects of the act of volunteering itself.

On a prearranged date, the action phase of the study began. Initial testing was completed for all individuals in the sample, and group meetings by the potential lodge members to plan the imminent move into the community were begun. The members decided who their leaders would be, what procedures for purchasing food were needed, and the type of work each member would do. At the end of 30 days, the lodge group moved into its community residence. The move to the lodge initially occurred with considerable confusion. As with most plans, changes needed to be instituted immediately. Difficulties soon arose concerning the taking of tranquilizing medication, and a system whereby a lodge member gave medication to those persons who would not take it was instituted. The planned janitorial and gardening work was not done well by the members. Work habits learned in the hospital seemed to have been more oriented toward avoiding than carrying out work. Accordingly, work-training programs were initiated. Problems arose in obtaining food and preparing it.

Finally, one member who demonstrated an interest in cooking emerged from the group and eventually became the lodge member continuously responsible for preparing and serving meals.

But management of the food problem was only the first step toward achieving full autonomy in the community. It was soon discovered that the members worked best in teams. Each work team had a leader who became responsible for its work. A business manager emerged with the responsibility for keeping the business records of the organization. To aid the members in establishing competence in the various areas of living and work, the services of a number of consultants also were obtained. Thus the medical problems of the lodge were handled by a house physician, an accountant consulted the business manager about the manner in which the books should be kept, and a janitorial consultant aided the lodge group in improving its work methods.

Initially, extensive supervision of the lodge society was required. This was provided by a coordinator, a psychologist with many years of professional experience in the mental health field. According to the research plan, he was replaced by a graduate student with much less experience, while at the same time a governing body, composed of lodge members, was given increased autonomy in the management of both the social and work life of the lodge members. After several months of leadership under the graduate student coincident with increasing autonomy of the governing body, the student was replaced by lay leaders responsible only for the work aspect of the lodge. The member governing body at this point became totally responsible for the development and operation of the lodge. This committee of lodge members established policy for governing the members and for allocating lodge resources. For example, they set salary levels, approved vacations, determined how the organization's money would be spent, and disciplined troublesome members. Under joint lay and member leadership, an extensive business was created, and lodge living conditions became more attractive to the members. Eventually, the lodge building was closed and the remaining members became a completely autonomous group residing on their own in a new location. Despite this physical change, they continued the work and living arrangements of the lodge organization without the aid of lay or professional persons. Occasionally lodge members did request help from these persons, who then functioned as their consultants.

What did this new society achieve? Did it fulfill the expectations of those who established it? Several questions like these asked at the outset of the study were answered once the full sequence of events leading to autonomy of the lodge society was completed. The first question concerned whether or not a small subsociety of ex-mental patients could be implanted in the community. The results of this study show definitely that such small societies can be established if appropriate attention is given to their location and the norms and values of the surrounding neighborhood, and can even thrive in the appropriate setting. A second question concerned the degree to which a small society providing living and working arrangements for its ex-patient members could increase their time in the community and their employment, as well as enhance their personal self-esteem. Again, this question can be answered in the affirmative. Compared with traditional aftercare programs, the lodge society significantly increased employment and time in the community. The self-esteem of the persons in all aftercare programs was enhanced, since merely living in the community by itself was such an overpowering positive influence.

But what happened to those who did not volunteer to live in the lodge, many of whom gave as reasons for not volunteering that they expected better future employment and improved living situations? The results show that the act of volunteering itself had no major influence upon a person's community adjustment. People who did not volunteer fared no better than people who volunteered but could not go to the lodge because they were in the control group. These results again show the overwhelming value of the posthospital social situation itself.

As expected, the new community society dramatically reduced costs. When all of the expenses were paid by outside sources, the cost was approximately half that of keeping an individual in the mental hospital. And it should be noted here that the members of the lodge society who remained in it eventually became a self-supporting group.

But what of the effects of previous long-term hospital residence (chronicity) which were shown to be exceedingly important in earlier studies (Fairweather et al., 1960; Fairweather and Simon, 1963; Fairweather, 1964)? In this study, longer-term patients continued to adapt poorly in traditional aftercare programs but these differences disappeared in the lodge society. Not only, therefore, did the lodge society enhance the community adjustment of all members, but it also had a comparatively greater effect on those members who had been hospitalized for the longest time.

It is also possible to compare the group processes in the hospital and community lodge societies. In the hospital situation, the group processes were found to involve three essential dimensions: task group leadership, performance of the group, and group cohesiveness. However, in the autonomous community society, the leadership dimension combined with performance to form one dimension and group cohesiveness became the second dimension. Thus, group processes in the community may be explained by two dimensions. The difference between group-process dimensionality in the hospital and in the community appears to be due to the fact that in the hospital the professional staff can never give true autonomy to patient groups so that actual patient leadership can develop. In the community lodge situation, by contrast, the members themselves ultimately had to provide the total leadership for the group. Under this latter condition, excellence in group leadership resulted in excellence in group performance. Under the former condition, because of the social situation in which the patients found themselves, it could not. The results also showed that group formation occurs rather rapidly; 180 days from the inception of a group, its processes are so well defined that an entire replacement of the patient population does not alter these basic group dimensions.

From this study, a series of principles for the operation of community treatment programs was derived. It became clear that as the members developed a greater stake in the social system, they become more responsible. The pride that came with personal independence and the ownership of a business, which is one symbol of successful achievement in this society, was obvious to all concerned. Community-treatment programs thus need to provide as much autonomy to their members as possible. Pride cannot develop with autonomy, however, unless meaningful work, as society defines it, is also available to members, so that the responsibilities implied by autonomy are themselves meaningful. This is extremely important when viewed from the perspective of professional mental health workers. The finding that mental health workers expect patients both in and out of the hospital to fail in their adjustment is often used to justify the continuance of the ex-mental patient in his subordinate social position. The results of this study show that such expectancies are not warranted, and that these negative attitudes urgently need to be changed. Clearly, the paramount implication of this study for both the mental patient, other marginal individuals, and those who manage this society is the urgent need to create new and more participative social statuses and roles for those members who only marginally belong to it.

Early Adjustment Problems

At this early stage of life in the community, a social atmosphere similar to that of freed prisoners prevailed. Lodge members were exuberant over merely being in the community. Several began spending time at a local cocktail bar and supper club. One of the more emotionally regressed members started nightly visits where he imbibed alcohol excessively. He became very sociable. He was "having fun." He discovered women for possibly the first time in his life. As he became more responsive to the outside world, he became more psychotic—throwing rocks at a neighboring service station and at cars traveling on the freeway and starting a fire against the freeway fence. These incidents were reported to the group and investigated by the staff coordinator. Upon exploring the matter, it become apparent that not only was the member's nightly drinking affecting his behavior, but he had not taken his tranquilizing medication for nine days. His psychotic behavior became so pronounced that he was finally returned to the hospital.

The stress of community living had begun to take its toll on the fledgling group. The group member who had disappeared while loading the trucks at the hospital (p. 46) began to disappear at the lodge. He criticized the group's work methods, their use of equipment, and many other procedures adopted by the group. He boasted of his adroitness in the use of janitorial and yard equipment, and, in answer to his boasting, the members promptly him leader of a work crew whose job was to keep the premises clean. After the appointment he failed to show up for work and was just as promptly demoted. It seemed obvious from the outset that this member was unwilling or unable to be a productive group member. In the general meetings held to discuss important issues, he frequently slept or failed to appear. Yet, he maintained a rather affable easygoing manner and frequently said, "I am just lazy." As a consequence of his attitude and inability to adjust to the community situation, this member was also returned to the hospital after only nine days at the lodge. Both members who returned to the hospital stated that they wanted to remain in the lodge despite their maladaptive behavior which ended their stay there. Another member stated soon after he arrived at the lodge that he wanted to return to the hospital. Four days after arriving at the lodge, he became isolated and depressed. He repeatedly asked to be returned to the hospital, and his wish was granted. Thus the original group of 15 members had dwindled to 12 in a little more than a week's time.

As a consequence, concern by members for their peers began to emerge. Members expressed the belief that the loss of three persons in such a short period of time was a "tragedy" that could have been avoided. As a result of these discussions, the members initiated an orienting program for new persons who entered the lodge from the hospital, in an attempt to lessen the shock that apparently occurs in the move from hospital to community. Toward this end, they assigned the orientation role to an interested member.

Because of the noticeable difference between the hospital and the community which culminated in the three failures just mentioned, the lodge members also became aware that not everyone could remain in the lodge. They also noticed that those who failed did so in the first few days. For this reason they adopted a rule specifically requiring that each new member be placed on a two-week trial period upon entrance into the lodge society. After this trial period, if he had demonstrated that he was unable or unwilling to work in some capacity, he was required to return to the hospital regardless of what his desire might be. The decision about his acceptance was made by the executive committee who interpreted the rule to mean that anyone coming to the lodge had to agree to work while there. People refusing to work or showing an incapacity for work would have to leave, according to the committee's interpretation.

Soon after the institution of this rule, three new members joined the lodge. Two of them satisfactorily completed their two-week trial period. The third newcomer lasted for two days and then was returned to the hospital. Mr. Taylor, the returnee, quickly discovered that work was an essential condition for living at the lodge. The first day, instead of working on the job, he sat down on the ground outside a customer's residence and threw lighted cigarette butts on the porch. He was immediately returned to the lodge where he was later publicly criticized by his crew chief for being a "goof-off." The new member was a rather convincing paranoid schizophrenic with ten years' previous hospitalization. He offered the opinion that the leaders of the lodge society were too well treated compared to the followers and that he should immediately be appointed to a crew chief's position despite the fact that he could not work the power equipment essential for his job. Even so, most members attempted to convince him that he should remain in the lodge and try to work. They failed in this attempt and he returned to the hospital. Later, when offered the chance to leave the hospital again and to return as a crew chief at the lodge, he initially accepted and then rejected the offer because of a condition attached by the lodge members. They required that he undergo a training program to achieve proficiency in the use of power equipment.

During this time, Mr. Mateo, who was one of the original members, left the lodge to live with his parents. Since coming from the hospital, he had worked about three hours every day washing dishes. Because of the increase in the lodge's business, he was told that in addition to his dishwashing job he would have to be assigned part-time to a janitorial crew. He immediately requested a two-day vacation to visit his parents and when he returned with them he left the lodge. He informed the general manager, Mr. Ring, at the time of his departure that he was going to return to barber college—an action that Mr. Ring perceived as an escape from the lodge, since Mr. Mateo had failed to complete the barber's course several times in the past. Willingness to work as a prerequisite for acceptance in the lodge was becoming a well-established norm. Both Mr. Taylor and Mr. Mateo were unwilling to work, while at the same time exhibiting few crippling psychiatric symptoms. On the other hand, severity of emotional problems and psychotic behavior were not considered barriers to membership as long as the person behaviorally displayed a willingness to work.

At the end of the sixth week, the coordinator (Dr. Moore), who had been responsible for the lodge from its inception, announced his resignation stating that he would depart in approximately two weeks. His resignation was announced in a general meeting where the group was also told that the staff member who had been responsible for the hospital side of the research project would now become the new lodge coordinator. The reaction of the group was ambivalent. Mr. Murray, the business manager, stated that he would miss the departing coordinator. An argument developed between Mr. Black and Mr. Rich about the relative merits of the old and the new coordinators. This was the beginning of a period of difficulty for the members that would only be resolved two weeks later when the new coordinator appeared. Flurries of business activity punctuated by periods of inactivity occurred during this time. The morale of the group again declined. Although obtaining jobs for pay was temporarily slowed, there was much work that needed to be done around the lodge. Even though various projects were approved by the men themselves, no one took the initiative in beginning work on them.

Then a prolonged period of inactivity occurred. It produced various kinds of agitation among the members of the group. On at least two separate occasions, the general manager, Mr. Ring, resigned his position, only to be reelected immediately to his office. The executive committee, which had been organized as the policy-making body with the hope that it would become the governing body of the organization, only rarely convened to make decisions. Almost all leadership was abandoned. Excessive alcoholic indulgence emerged as a serious problem. During this time, Mr. Ward, an alcoholic, became an acute problem. Although he occasionally drank in his room, he began a prolonged period of seclusive drinking. After numerous private attempts by the coordinator to convince Mr. Ward to stop drinking, the executive committee was convened to urge the members to solve the problem. Their solution was to adopt the rule that "drinking on the grounds" would not be tolerated. However, no action was taken with Mr. Ward, who continued his drinking as blatantly as before. At this, the executive committee decided that their "no drinking" rule could not be enforced and hence should be rescinded. Next they decided that if a member's drinking interfered with his work, he would be given a warning the first time, a second offense would result in loss of pay, and on the third infraction he would be asked to leave the lodge. Despite the new rule, no action was taken about Mr. Ward's behavior. The next day Mr. Ward was found by another member lying in a very shallow pool of water in an intoxicated condition. He was put to bed and then returned to the hospital where it was determined that he was suffering from the d.t.'s. Finally, the coordinator met with the group and imposed a rule against drinking on the grounds. The coordinator further informed the group that he would personally enforce the rule because the executive committee had not done so. Thus it was clear by the end of two months in the community that this embryonic society still required outside leadership to enforce its own social rules.

The First Shift in Supervision

When the new coordinator arrived on the scene, the remnants of leadership remained in the hands of the general manager, Mr. Ring. Upon occasion this member-manager assumed leadership which he then relinquished unpredictably. When challenged by other group members, he would resign his position but just as quickly reclaim it, saying that there was no one else who could occupy the role. Such disorganization required a new restructuring of the social situation. New work procedures were clearly needed. Methods for determining the implements needed on the job and procedures for loading equipment onto trucks were the first innovations developed. Written forms were used as memory aids wherever possible. The greatest change, however, was that the new staff coordinator assumed actual leadership of the lodge. He first broadened the powers of the executive committee so that this group could assume actual leadership of the lodge to replace the arbitrary decisions which continued to be made by the intermittent leader, Mr. Ring. As the first step in this new plan, an organizational chart was devised and posted on the bulletin board. Table 12.1 shows this new "chain of command" and the broadened responsibilities of the executive committee. The new coordinator also posted on the bulletin board, so that all members could be aware of them, the existing rules and regulations for living at the lodge. Even though most of these regulations had been created by the lodge

Table 12.1. Organizational Chart of the Lodge

Dr. Cochran				
Executive Committee				
Ring (Chairman)	Murray (Secty.)	Smith	Jones	Black
Crews and Crew Chiefs				
Business Admin.	Kitchen Food	Crew No. 1	Crew No. 2	Crew No. 3
Murray	Smith Hunt	Black	Jones	Ring
		Rich	Fish	Stacey
		Parker	Lee	Steele
		Strong	Gonzales	Walker

Executive Committee's Responsibilities	
1. Medication	Jones
2. Orientation and welcoming of new members	Jones
3. Lodge Reports (daily & weekly)	Ring
a. O.D. reports	
b. Visitors log	
c. Sign-out log	
4. Janitorial Reports (daily)	Ring (via janitorial crew chiefs)
a. Job sheets	
b. Job check list	
c. Job inspection list	
5. Executive committee actions	Ring
6. Coordination and dispatching of jobs	Murray
7. Kitchen and food	Smith
8. Grounds	Black
9. Living quarters	Ring
10. Inventory (janitorial)	Ring
11. Laundry	Murray
12. O.D. schedules	Jones

members themselves, the listing of them by the coordinator was intended to formalize these expectations of the members; they may be found in verbatim form in Table 12.2.

Approximately two weeks after the new coordinator arrived, a general meeting was held during which he announced that all decisions would thereafter be made by the executive committee. The group accepted this reaffirmation without dissent. After the general meeting, the coordinator presented the executive committee with its first problems to solve. Mr. Ring assumed the chairmanship of the executive committee and, accordingly, the committee delegated much of its authority to him since he was already the lodge's general manager. However, the new coordinator informed the committee that regardless of how it delegated its duties, *the committee itself* would be responsible for governing the lodge. While Mr. Ring often attempted to usurp the authority of the executive committee by discussing problems only with the coordinator, on each occasion the new coordinator referred the problem to the executive committee for solution. As the members of the executive committee assumed more responsibility for administering the lodge, Mr. Ring's influence diminished. After a disagreement with an aggressive and much admired new member who was rising in the lodge leadership hierarchy, the executive committee expelled Mr. Ring from membership by demoting him from crew chief status—a social position necessary for membership on the committee.

Table 12.2. Rules for Living at the Lodge

1. No drinking on grounds or in local area in public—only at recognized places for such purposes (bar, private home, etc.).
   a. No drinking anywhere during the regular work day is permitted.
   b. Any member found to have been drinking 3 times will be asked to leave the lodge.
   c. No form of alcohol is to be brought onto the grounds for any purpose.
2. No gambling on the grounds.
3. Everybody must work and be ready for work at the start of the regular work day no matter what activities they participated in during the previous evening.
4. There will be no women brought onto the grounds.
5. People (visitors) must be invited to the lodge before they can come onto the grounds.
6. Those fellows who are indigent will receive $10 per week. If $10 or more per week is earned, no money will be paid to him from the indigent fund. If he earns less than $10 per week, the difference between what he earns and $10 will be paid to him weekly from the indigent funds.
7. Those fellows receiving no pension or compensation as well as those receiving less than $10 per week are classified as indigent.
8. All lodge members must abide by the decisions of the Executive Committee.
9. Any group decision may be vetoed by Dr. Cochran, but this will be done only when, in his judgment, the group decision might jeopardize the functioning of the lodge or janitorial service.
10. Admission to and departures from the lodge are strictly voluntary. Any member may leave at any time. It is the function of the Executive Committee to merely recommend or advise in such matters. Where possible, a request to leave should come before the Executive Committee for recommendation.
11. All new members coming to the lodge are automatically placed on a two-week trial period (LOA from the hospital). At the end of that period, the man will be asked if he desires to remain or return to the hospital. The Executive Committee, at the same time, will decide if the man should remain or return to the hospital. If both the committee and the man agree on his remaining, he will remain and start receiving wages. If the committee feels he should remain but the man wants to return to the hospital, he will return to the hospital. If both the committee and the man agree on his leaving the lodge, he will return to the hospital and receive no wages. It is noted that at any time during the two-week trial period, the new man may return to the hospital for any reason he so desires.
12. All members receiving any type of medication must take their medication as presented by the physician with no deviations.
13. All members will serve as O.D.s unless otherwise excused by the Executive Committee for a definite reason.
14. Any member desiring to take work passes from the lodge to seek work in the community outside of the Janitorial Service, for the eventual purpose of leaving, must first receive permission from the Executive Committee. He must then abide by the Committee's decision. If work passes are approved, the member will receive no wages for the time off from work at the lodge.
15. All members (roommates) will be responsible for the cleanliness of their own rooms.
16. All new members are to be oriented by the Executive Committee member assigned and must complete the training program to the satisfaction of the coordinator and crew chiefs before he is assigned to a crew.
17. The Executive Committee, as the decision-making body of the lodge, is responsible for members' behavior and for taking necessary disciplinary measures.
18. Any member leaving the lodge may return at a future date, providing there is available space and it is approved by the Executive Committee. They will be on a two-week trial period upon their return and receive no wages.
19. Any crew member who is dissatisfied with his crew assignment or his assigned duties is to make this known to his crew chief. This will then be reported to the coordinator, who will decide whether or not it warrants Executive Committee discussion and/or action.

Table 12.2. Continued

20. If any money is to be borrowed, it is to be referred to Dr. Cochran providing it involves $5.00 or more. Money can only be borrowed for dire emergencies and is not to be used for drinking purposes or taxicab fares.
21. Members may change room assignments only upon the approval of the coordinator and the members involved in the change.
22. Night work and Saturday work will be accepted based upon the judgment of the coordinator. The members assigned to this work will be on a voluntary basis and they will receive future time off for the extra work done.
23. Money received for night work only will be distributed amongst only those members participating in this work.
24. The assigned O.D. may not leave his post unless he receives the approval of an Executive Committee member and a replacement is found.
25. Any O.D. who is relieved of his duty at his own request for personal reasons must make up this time in the reasonable future.
26. Anyone leaving the lodge during any day of the week other than for his work assignment must sign out and sign in upon his return, no matter where he may be going.
27. All members are to be well-shaven, in uniform, and reasonably neat and clean while working in the community.
28. All new members, prior to being placed on the O.D. list, will first become Junior O.D.s and be assigned to a Senior O.D., with whom he will serve and be instructed in the O.D. duties and responsibilities for at least a two-week period.
29. A regular Executive Committee meeting will be held every other Wednesday evening at approximately 6:00 p.m. Meetings, however, will be held more frequently if the situation warrants it.
30. All Executive Committee decisions are to be reported to the group-at-large as soon as possible after the decision is reached.
31. Members may own and operate automobiles or trucks only with the approval of Dr. Cochran. If a member owns an automobile or truck, he may not use it during the regular work day unless permission is received.
32. All cleaning and washing of personal clothing (other than uniforms) are the responsibility of the individual members, both financially and otherwise.
33. Members are to use their own rooms for sleeping purposes and not the O.D. office or recreation room.
34. Any member using the recreation room bathtub and/or shower is responsible for cleaning it up and removing the towels and wash cloths.
35. The telephone may be used for local personal calls only. Any long distance personal calls are to be made from a pay station.
36. No smoking in food or restricted areas. No smoking is permitted in bed.

Once the members of the executive committee knew that they could effectively discipline members for rule infractions, they began exploring different ways in which rewards and punishments could be used to shape individual behavior. Punishments took the form of warnings or reductions in wages. Rewards came from promotions, such as that from worker to crew chief, or from increases in pay, or both. For example, the committee suspended a member from his nightly duties as O.D. because of irresponsible behavior and later made him eligible for the O.D.'s work when his behavior improved.[1] In another case, a member was not given a salary for two weeks because of poor performance on the job

[1] Since no staff member was permitted on the grounds after the day's work, a member of the lodge was assigned responsibility for the grounds and the other members. This position was called Officer of the Day (O.D.) after a similar role held in the hospital by physicians.

and the committee further recommended that his job be changed. His performance on the new job improved and, consequently, his salary was increased. These new actions by the executive committee had such an immediate effect that no major infractions occurred for a period of several weeks. Their effective decision-making began to unify the group. This growing responsibility of the executive committee for the lodge's members is well indicated in the new coordinator's research journal notes:

> Shortly after Mr. Walker came to the lodge, I received a call on a Saturday morning from Mr. Sears, indicating that Mr. Walker was in the local county jail, ostensibly for drunkenness. I came down to the lodge and we called the police, who verified that he had been arrested on Friday evening and was, in fact, in jail for drunkenness only and no other charge. His bail was $29. I immediately called an executive committee meeting to decide what to do with Mr. Walker, i.e., allow him to remain in jail, pay his bail, send him back to the hospital, etc. The executive committee decided to grant him a loan of $29 to pay his bail from our operating expense fund which would be paid back via deductions from his salary. Secondly, during the time he was waiting to go before the court after release, he was to be restricted to the lodge and would not be able to sign out at all and would work only at the lodge itself. Thirdly, it was agreed that he was to serve whatever sentence that would be decreed by the judge and if it was a suspended sentence, he was to serve it at the lodge on a similar restricted basis.

As part of the plan to reorganize the lodge, the coordinator communicated all information concerning jobs, individual and group performance, role changes, finances, and the like, to the entire group. Thus executive committee decisions were reviewed by all members at the general weekly meeting. In this way, the entire group was made fully aware of changes in procedures and the rule infractions of the members as they occurred. This procedure not only kept the members informed, but some changes in the executive committee's decisions were made as a result. At the same time, a concentrated effort was made to create effective communications between the coordinator and the members. At first, most of the discussions were initiated by the coordinator, but eventually some members began to initiate conversations with him. Discussions were most often held between the coordinator and the lodge leaders—the business manager, cook, and janitorial leaders. Despite his attempts, the rest of the members communicated with the coordinator only when they needed something or when they had committed an infraction of a rule.

Morale improved rapidly during the initial tenure of the new coordinator. The improvement was due to several factors: an increase in the number of available jobs, the social reorganization itself, and increased customer satisfaction with the work of the janitorial services. Members had become more job-oriented. For example, one crew spontaneously volunteered to correct several poor jobs completed by another crew and did so. Joking among members became commonplace. All were concerned about doing a good job and promoting good will, even though some members did not do a good job and the group did not always promote good will. The high morale, developing pride, and job orientation all tended to create a social atmosphere for effective problem-solving. This is demonstrated by two events during this period of lodge development. The first involved the kitchen crew, when an assistant cook, whose performance had been on the decline, suddenly returned to the hospital. His departure left the kitchen crew short of necessary workers. Four members volunteered to take his place working on Saturday so that the kitchen crew chief could have his regular day off. The second incident involved Mr. Black, who persisted in referring to the lodge members as patients. The members asked Mr. Black to discontinue this practice. After a reprimand by a member in the presence of others, he stopped referring to members as patients.

The new coordinator also attempted to establish an eight-hour work day. This was the first attempt to import the work norms of the community into the lodge. When this was first tried, since few paying customer's jobs were available, the group was required to complete work on the lodge grounds. During this period, a fence and two storerooms for tools and equipment were built. Within two weeks, the work day became eight hours long. In addition, a second change in work-performance norms was developing: workers began to feel that quality work should be done even though the job might take longer than anticipated. To accomplish this, attempts were made by the crew chiefs themselves to reduce carelessness, sloppiness, and slowness on the job.

By the time the new coordinator had been on the job a month, rules that regulated drinking and job behavior were being strongly enforced by the executive committee. A verbatim account from the coordinator's journal suggests how these new work norms were developing at that time:

> The two janitorial crew chiefs, up to now, have been extremely critical of their deviant members. I have noted that the workers in the crews have been taking more pride in the group's work and they themselves have become as critical as the crew chiefs. ... I think the workers who are out on the jobs feel a little more at ease with the clients and certainly Mr. Black and Mr. Jones (crew chiefs) handle themselves well with the clients.

One of the key mechanisms that allowed the executive committee to act with good judgment was the feedback of information from the customers. The members found that poor behavior on the job could result in being fired and excellent job performance was often well rewarded. This immediate communication by the customer of his positive or negative evaluation of the job helped shape the work habits of the members so that they more readily conformed to those of the general community. Acceptable behavior on the job excluded any type of deviant behavior which might result in the loss of a job or that would offend a customer. At the same time there was tolerance for deviant behavior within the lodge environment itself. Thus the group readily accommodated an occasionally hallucinated or deluded person in the lodge setting, but they would not tolerate such behavior on the job.

The ideas of quality work, working hard, and pleasing the customer were being strongly advocated by the newly appointed crew chief, Mr. Sears, who had replaced the deposed general manager, Mr. Ring. Mr. Sears' rise to power started after only a few days at the lodge. He rapidly became popular because he impressed the members with his persuasiveness, suggestions, and leadership. Not only was his leadership demonstrated in his role of crew chief and in informal social situations, but also as a member of the executive committee, of which he eventually became chairman. His ability to lead the men effectively and to relate to them was so impressive that it seemed the time had finally arrived when a member could take over some of the duties of the staff coordinator.

The Trials of a Peer Coordinator

A plan was created to train Mr. Sears to assume supervision of the lodge. The staff coordinator would gradually relinquish his role as leader of the lodge group and become instead a consultant to Mr. Sears. The peer coordinator (Mr. Sears), however, would be directly responsible to the staff coordinator for the operation of the lodge. Mr. Sears was approached with this plan. He said he would try it. His training, however, was not initiated for approximately another month because the staff coordinator wanted to be certain that Mr. Sears' initial positive reaction was not a fleeting one. Such a change in leadership offered the opportunity to study the effects of this small society under the leadership of a layman who was himself an ex-mental patient.

The decision was announced to the lodge members at a general meeting that Mr. Sears would commence training as a coordinator. The members were told that his salary would remain the same until he completed training. Then it would probably be increased. Surprisingly, this announcement was received without comment from other members of the group. After the meeting, however, several spontaneous and facetious remarks were made. One member said, "Hi, Doc," to Mr. Sears; another referred to him as "Junior"; a third member called him "my driver" and asserted that he could drive the truck better than the staff coordinator. This duty became the first training task for the peer coordinator. During the subsequent two-week training period, he learned his way around town by driving the truck, took responsibility for its maintenance, and using it, obtained janitorial supplies from the supply warehouse. He was instructed in scheduling jobs, filling out work forms, making job estimates, and checking on medication. As part of his training he was required to perform competently in all these aspects of the coordinator's job, without the staff coordinator being present. Initially, he remained a somewhat dependent individual, preferring to be viewed as the staff coordinator's assistant rather than as the lodge coordinator.

After his training was completed, however, Mr. Sears performed satisfactorily and showed initiative in solving many vexing problems. For example, he created an improved training program for new members in which their job proficiency had to be approved by all three crew chiefs before the neophytes could be assigned to a work crew. Mr. Sears still had some question regarding how much responsibility the staff coordinator would allow him to take and how independent he could be. At first he asked the staff leader questions relating to his work, such as, "How does this job look to you?" and "Is this job okay?" Later, he wanted to know if he could "chew the men out" when it was appropriate. On one occasion, he went on to say that he had been drinking beer and asked the staff leader "What are you going to do about it?" The staff coordinator told him that even in his new position he was governed by the rules of the lodge, one of which pertained to drinking behavior. Accordingly, his beer drinking was reported to the executive committee for their action.

This testing of the limits by the new peer coordinator was merely a prelude to a major test which occurred about a week later. The situation is described in the following verbatim account from the staff coordinator's research journal.

> At 7:15 a.m., Monday, I received a call at home. Mr. Sears stated that he had been out all night and asked that I drive the truck to take the fellows on the San Agustin jobs and that he would appreciate this very much since he had not slept all evening. Not knowing what the situation was, I did not say yes or no, but merely told him to complete the local route and I would discuss this with him when I saw him. He returned to the office at about 8:30 a.m., at which time he was wearing a shirt and tie, plopped himself down in a seat, and asked if I was going to take the boys to San Agustin. I responded by saying no, I would not—that this was his job, his responsibility no matter how he felt, and that I myself had gone to bed at 3:00 a.m. the previous morning. I reiterated the rule indicating that he and the others could do whatever they pleased at night time but that they must be ready for work the following morning. He did not comment, but merely left the office indicating that he would change his clothes and be ready shortly. He returned approximately 10 minutes later and apparently his attitude had changed quite drastically. It was obvious that this was the big test... His role had now been established.

Afterwards, he performed duties without supervision and manifested a sensitivity to both organizational and individual needs. In addition, he showed a facility in handling customer complaints. He was keenly aware of the processes within the group and became chairman of both the general weekly meetings which all members attended and the executive committee meetings. The number of jobs increased under his leadership and the quality of the crews' work improved noticeably. The lodge became a businesslike organization. Individual specialization began occurring. Mr. Rich, for example, was officially designated as the "stove man" because he became an expert in cleaning stoves. Mr. Black became an expert in cleaning rugs and he was often sent to jobs where rug cleaning was necessary. And, of course, Mr. Sears, the member coordinator, had become the expert in administration.

New procedures were evolving rapidly. A plan for vacations was adopted. Each member was entitled to one week's leave for every six months of work. The executive committee initiated a training program for O.D.s (p. 62). The new members entering the lodge would start their O.D. duties by serving with an experienced O.D. while they were in training. The senior O.D.s wrote evaluative reports on these trainees. New members did not begin training until they had lived at the lodge one week so that they could become accustomed to the community situation.

Another development took place in regard to the operating expense fund (10 per cent of the gross income for a given pay period) which was set aside purportedly for the purchase of supplies. It had been used upon a few occasions for temporarily paying damages to customers' property until the insurance payment for the damage was received and for minor repairs at the lodge which were later reimbursed by the lessors. However, during the tenure of the peer coordinator, the executive committee approved a loan to one of the members in order that he could purchase a pair of work shoes. The loan, at no interest, was to be repaid in three installments which were to be deducted from his future earnings. Shortly thereafter, other members requested funds for the purchase of clothing and the use of the members' savings for personal loans became a tradition at the lodge.

As Mr. Sears' contacts increased with customers, suppliers, and others in the neighborhood and general community, he was treated by them as the manager of the janitorial service. He was almost never perceived by the customers and vendors as an ex-patient himself, even though they were fully aware that the work crews were ex-patients. Mr. Sears readily accepted this perceived status and he was pleased at being viewed by people in the community as a full citizen. The perception of the peer coordinator is exemplified in the following excerpt from the staff coordinator's research journal.

> Shortly after my return from leave, the owner of the service station jokingly said to me that he guessed I was out of a job as Mr. Sears was now "running things." ... When I told him that Mr. Sears was also an ex-patient who had come up through the ranks he was quite surprised. I am sure he felt that an ex-mental patient could not run an operation such as this. He then became very positive indicating that the fellows were doing extremely well and there had been no problem.

After two months of performing at an optimum level, the strain of ever-increasing responsibilities began to show in the peer coordinator's behavior. His fall from grace and eventual collapse started slowly when he did not arrive for work one day because of excessive drinking. Soon after this incident he was married and began living in an apartment in the neighborhood. He came to work as any citizen might who had steady employment. Although this situation could have been a step toward maturity, it created an almost insurmountable financial problem for him. He secured a loan from the lodge operating expense fund to pay for the rental of his apartment. Because of the increased expense of living in an apartment and supporting a wife, Mr. Sears was obliged to secure two additional large loans from the lodge fund, neither of which he was prepared to repay from his weekly salary.

Not too long after his first absence from work, he did not appear at the lodge for three days. Again, drinking was the reason. After this, the behavioral deterioration progressed rapidly. He began complaining about the paper work he had to do. He made sarcastic comments on official papers. His drinking continued to increase. He became intolerant of other members' behavior. He made unrealistic demands upon the men about the quality of their work. On several occasions he walked off the job and the staff coordinator had to be called to replace him. Although his demeanor was typically friendly and courteous when he was not drinking, his behavior could be so destructive at times that finally the coordinator felt Mr. Sears had to change his behavior or leave the lodge. He gave Mr. Sears that choice. Although he chose to remain, soon thereafter the staff coordinator reluctantly relieved him of his job when he learned that Mr. Sears had been driving the work truck while intoxicated. For this serious offense, Mr. Sears was demoted to worker status. After holding and enjoying the highest status in the lodge society, this demotion was especially humiliating. As a last blow to his self-esteem, the executive committee of which he had been chairman told him to "shape up or leave the lodge." He decided to leave.

When the peer coordinator departed, it appeared that the stability of the lodge might be shaken. However, three factors in the situation prevented the disintegration that might otherwise have occurred. First, the staff coordinator was well informed about the detailed developments of the lodge society as an integral part of his consulting role. Therefore, he immediately was able to resume the full responsibilities of the coordinator role. Second, the lodge's social structure had become by this time relatively stable. Finally, the demise of the peer coordinator was not a sudden and unforeseen occurrence for the members. The peer coordinator's maladaptive behavior and consequent decline had been perceived by all lodge members.

Although the changeover to the staff coordinator was not planned, it represented a step backward in the planned progression toward peer group autonomy from all staff supervision. Unfortunately, the reversion from peer coordinator to the previous staff coordinator occurred at an inopportune time as far as the research plan (pp. 40–41) was concerned. The plan required that this staff coordinator be replaced by a second coordinator with less professional experience. Since increased member autonomy was supposed to be introduced by the new coordinator—a graduate student—the last two months of the previous staff coordinator's tenure necessarily had to be spent in maintaining the status quo.

At the time of the transition to the new coordinator, some activities of the lodge members no longer required supervision and others required less supervision than in earlier stages of the lodge society's development. The operations of the kitchen and dining facilities were essentially free from supervision. Mr. Smith, the manager of the kitchen, ordered and prepared all the food. Although the tenure of the current business manager was of recent origin, he no longer required constant supervision. The janitorial and yard crews were far from performing independently, even though they had become more reliable as a consequence of their experience, training, and supervision. Thus, on an occasional job the men still damaged customers' property and most jobs required some supervision from the staff coordinator. This was the state of the organization when the new, less professionally experienced coordinator took over supervision of the lodge. The transition was accomplished over a two-week period during which the new coordinator learned the necessary procedures and finally assumed total responsibility for the lodge operation.

References

FAIRWEATHER, G. W., SIMON, R., GEBHARD, M. E., WEINGARTEN, E., HOLLAND, J. L., SANDERS, R., STONE, G. B., and REAHL., G. E. Relative effectiveness of psychotherapeutic programs: a multicriteria comparison of four programs for three different groups. *Psychol. Monogr.*, 1960, 74, No. 5 (whole no. 492).

FAIRWEATHER, G. W. and SIMON, R. A further follow-up comparison of phychotherapeutic programs. *J. Consult. Psycol.*, 1963, 27, 186.

FAIRWEATHER, G. W (Ed.), *Social psychology in treating mental illness: an experimental approach*. New York: John Wiley & Sons, Inc., 1964.

13

Lamb, H. R., & Goertzel, V. (1971). Discharged mental patients—Are they really in the community? *Archives of General Psychiatry, 24, 29–34*

"Community integration" is one present-day term for helping people with mental illness attain the status and sense of belonging that allows them to be and to feel they are part of the community rather than just being housed in it. (See Ware and colleagues' 2007 article, "Connectedness and citizenship: Redefining social integration," *Psychiatric Services* 58 (4), 469–474.) Exactly 40 years ago, Lamb and Goertzel addressed essentially the same question in their study of random assignment to high and low expectation community environments for discharged psychiatric hospital patients. High expectations in the former condition involved day treatment and workshop attendance and participant involvement in their own treatment and rehabilitation planning. Low expectations in the latter condition essentially meant no expectations. Participants were placed in boarding homes with no requirements or incentives for involvement in their own care. The positive findings for the high expectation group gave credibility to the ideal of productive lives in the community for persons with chronic mental illness and histories of long-term hospitalization. That there were few follow-ups to this successful experiment is true of other innovative and successful programs across our three eras of community psychiatry.

Discharged Mental Patients—Are They Really in the Community?

This study measures the effect of a high-expectation and a low-expectation environment on discharged long-term mental patients randomly assigned to one of two community settings. The high-expectation setting includes a halfway house, a day-treatment center, and a rehabilitation workshop. It demands much in the way of mobility, planning, and accepting responsibility. Low-expectation patients go to boarding homes where docility is valued and little initiative is expected. The boarding-home group is not really in the community. It is like a small ward moved to a community setting. The high-expectation group has a higher rehospitalization rate, but a longer time out of the hospital with a high level of instrumental performance. The high-expectation group is less segregated, is less likely to be labeled as deviate, and is less stigmatized.

In recent years there has been a mass exodus of long-term mental patients from state hospitals, an exodus generally assumed to further reintegration into the community. Is the widespread rejoicing about this movement really justified? For the long-term hospitalized patient, the move is usually to a boarding-home facility, which is described as "in the community." But are these persons really in the community? To what extent have they shed their mental patient role and identity? What are the implications for having been labeled "mentally ill"? Do they remain stigmatized? What is their potential for participation in terms of instrumental performance? This paper will examine these questions.

These issues emerged in the course of a research project concerned with the return of long-term hospitalized patients to the community. This controlled study measures the effects of two different environments on discharged mental patients, contrasting "high" and "low" expectation community environments.

Upon release from the state hospital, patients in the experimental group are placed in a high-expectation environment. The assumption is made that the discharged patient has a potential for some degree of functioning and integration into the community. By this we do not necessarily mean independent living and competitive employment; an attempt is made to meaningfully involve the patient in the community, at whatever level of functioning he is ultimately able to attain.

Patients in the comparison group are placed in a low-expectation environment in the community, usually in a boarding or family-care home, where little effort is directed toward social and vocational rehabilitation. Such ex-patient placement is typical in California (and elsewhere) for patients who do not return to parental or conjugal homes.

Social and vocational rehabilitation for the experimental group begins in a day-treatment center; hopefully most of the members can progress to a sheltered workshop, then into some type of work placement and eventually to paid competitive employment. The patients initially reside—after leaving the hospital—in a halfway house from which they can progress to a satellite housing program (apartments housing two to four ex-patients and with some supervision from halfway house staff), and then to independent living. Obviously, this is a theoretical model for progression from hospital dependency to independent living and competitive employment in the community. One of the major questions of this study is to determine to what extent the chronically hospitalized population in our project can, in fact, move through the program.

Method

A patient is referred to the project by the hospital staff if he has no family or if both staff and patient agree that he should not return to his family. Patients are then randomly assigned to the experimental or comparison group. Those patients who will return directly to their families are not included in this study. To be eligible for the project all patients prior to referral must have been hospitalized at least one half of the two preceding years; the average length of hospitalization was approximately eight years. The hospital experience for the two groups differs in only one respect. The experimental group members attend a weekly one-hour preleave group meeting conducted at the hospital by the project staff. Some of the comparison group attend a weekly preleave meeting for patients referred to boarding homes.

Results

What Happens in the First Six Months Following Referral to the Project?—There is considerably more movement in and out of the hospital for the experimental group than for the comparison group. At the end of six months 81% (25 out of 31) of the experimental group were separated from the hospital as compared to 45% (9 out of 20) of the comparison group. But one half of the experimental group who were rehospitalized at least once compared with one of the nine comparison-group patients. Four of the 12 in the experimental group who were rehospitalized were discharged for a second time into the community.

In the six-month period (180 days) following referral to the project, the total experimental group averaged 71 days in the community compared to only 43 days for the comparison group.

What Happens in the First 18 Months Following Referral to the Project?—Only 25 patients have been in the project long enough for an 18-month follow-up. In this smaller group are 15 from the experimental high-expectation group and 10 in the comparison group; all but one in each group were separated from the hospital within this 18-month period (540 days). The median time spent in the hospital before separation but after assignment to one of the two groups is 36 days for the experimental group and 114 days for the comparison group. Again, there is much more movement in and out of the hospital for the experimental-group members than for the comparison group.

In the 18-month period following referral to the project, the total experimental group averages 307 days in the community and the comparison group 266 days.

Where Do They Live?—During the first six months from referral to the project, when living outside of the hospital, the experimental-group member's live almost exclusively in the halfway house and the comparison group lives in boarding homes three quarters of the time.

In the smaller group for whom 18 months have passed since their referral, the experimental group spends only one-half its time out of the hospital in the halfway house; the other one-half is divided between satellite housing, living with family, living alone, and, only 2% of the time, in boarding homes. For the comparison group, 78% of the time out of the hospital during the 18-month period is still spent in boarding homes, with the remainder divided between family and living alone.

What Do They Do While Out of the Hospital?—During the first six months from referral to the project, when living outside of the hospital, the experimental group spent 76% of the time in the day-treatment center. The challenge of working with long-term psychiatric patients in the day-treatment center and a description of the treatment program has been published elsewhere.[1] Within the six-month period, 77% of the time of the experimental group patients in the community, after leaving the day-treatment center, is spent in some vocational activity as compared with 23% for the comparison group. Fully 77% of the comparison-group time is spent in no structured activity.

For the 18-month period, there is a greater variety of vocational activities in both groups. In the experimental group, two thirds of the time is spent in some vocational activity (sheltered workshop, work placement, volunteer job, paid employment with 11% functioning as housewives and mothers) as compared with only 40% of the comparison group.

Comment

Results reported here are based on small samples and thus are preliminary findings. We believe, however, that the following observations are justified: when a special effort at case finding and preleave preparation is undertaken by the staff of a coordinated community program—including a day-treatment center, halfway house, and rehabilitation workshop—more long-term patients can be moved out of a state mental hospital and in less time than are patients referred to a boarding-home facility. This is shown to be true even though this project is being conducted at a time when there is more than the usual effort being expended by hospital and local welfare workers to get patients out into boarding homes. Although a large proportion of patients the high-expectation setting will probably need to be rehospitalized, they will still have a longer total time living out of the hospital than will the patients from the low-expectation group. Despite the higher initial dollar cost of the high-expectation environment and the stormier course of these patients (reflected in many crises, only some of which result into rehospitalizations), we find that the level of functioning and integration in the community is higher after both 6 and 18 months than it is for those persons in the low-expectation environment.

The increased frequency of hospitalization for those persons who are in the high-expectations group is understandable. At the halfway house, the day center and the workshop, passivity, isolation, and inactivity are unacceptable modes of coping with an environment which stresses activity, movement, and responsibility. Halfway-house residents are expected to participate actively in the functioning of the house, to plan and prepare meals, to carry out most essential household tasks. They are also expected to examine their own behavior and the behavior of others when problems arise.[2] They are not permitted to sit passively in the halfway house during normal working hours; residents must have a regular structured daytime activity outside of the halfway house (i.e., job, sheltered workshop, day-treatment center, school). They are responsible for getting to their daytime activity by public transportation, on foot, or by arranging for a ride with someone who has the use of a car. Regularly scheduled group meetings are held at the day-treatment center, at the halfway house, and at vocational services to help patients assess their level of functioning. Active involvement is expected in regard to planning for both social and vocational aspects of their lives. Thus, patients feel pressured; life is turbulent but also stimulating. For some, their new life situation is invigorating and leads to achievement in terms of instrumental performance and achieving some measure of independence; others break under the strain and return to the hospital but usually for a relatively short time. The hospital to which they may have longed to retreat now seems dull and bleak and they usually want again to try the outside world.

Patients in Boarding Homes

We feel it is only an illusion that patients who are placed in boarding or family-care homes are "in the community." Indeed, the contrast between most boarding homes and a high-expectation halfway house is striking. Our observations of boarding homes are in close agreement with the extensive survey made by Silberstein.[3] These facilities are in most respects like small long-term state hospital wards isolated from the community. One is overcome by the depressing atmosphere, not because of the physical appearance of the boarding home, but because of the passivity, isolation, and inactivity of the residents. They lack spontaneity, spend much of their day watching television, and relate to boarding-home operators as children do to a parent. In many family-care and boarding homes, the residents are kept out of the kitchen and often no responsibility is given to them beyond some attempt at encouraging self-care.

Silberstein[3] describes the situation clearly:

All of the care homes (22) I visited were operated by women. Husbands, if any, were only peripherally involved in the operation of the homes. Most of the women, prior to becoming caretakers, had jobs in which they provided physical care to sick, aged, or disabled persons. The caretakers were quite maternal, met the physical needs of their guests, and related to them as they would to young children. They expected their residents to be docile recipients of services. Few caretakers delegated any responsibilities to their guests and did not feel these former patients were capable of handling them. However, in several homes, where the caretaker was suddenly hospitalized, the residents had immediately and competently taken over the management of the home until the caretaker returned whereupon they again became docile recipients of services. Patients feared the caretaker's displeasure. Disagreements between the caretaker and residents seldom occurred openly, and when they did, often resulted in the resident having to leave the home. Caretakers often viewed the expression of anger or annoyance by a resident as an indication of mental illness, and would then consult their doctor or social worker for medication for the patient. If the caretaker dealt with disagreement herself, she often did so by either ignoring them or reprimanding the patient as a mother would a young child.

Thus, boarding homes are for the most part so structured that they maximize the state-hospital-like atmosphere. The boarding-home operator usually needs or wants a group of quiet, docile, "good" patients. The monetary reward system of the boarding home encourages this, for the operator is being paid by the head, rather than being rewarded for rehabilitation efforts for her "guests."

The Long-term Hospitalized Patient

Scheff[4] believes that persons enter careers of long-term or recurring mental illness by coming to the attention of people in authority during a crisis situation, being offered the role of mental patient, and subsequently being rewarded for accepting this role and punished when they attempt to return to a nonpatient role. In time they acquire a concept of themselves based on the societal expectations of this role. We feel this formulation has some validity, but that other crucial factors are underemphasized in this approach.

As a group, these patients are characterized by an overwhelming dependency in a society where high value is placed upon independence. Independence is also part of one's prized self-image, as defined by Wilensky[5]; a sense of being excessively dependent can be a major contributor to a person's low self-esteem. Insufficient ego strength to deal with life stresses is an almost universal finding in this group. Some patients, because of their own lack of internal controls, seek the increased external social controls of the hospital. A host of other factors contribute to patients becoming long-term. Some patients alienate society by physical violence or by not meeting role expectations (either social or vocational) and are consequently relegated to the state hospital. They may also alienate the hospital subsociety which relegates them to a back ward, or in various ways puts them out of sight and mind, and little is done to encourage them to re-enter the outside community. In other cases a symbiotic relationship develops between patients and the hospital: the patients are dependent on the hospital and the hospital holds on to patients because they meet hospital needs for patients who are good workers or can serve as ward scapegoats.

Many patients, including those in this study, when they leave hospitals find themselves in what amounts to a sheltered subsociety. In some cases this is done deliberately. Fairweather et al[6] had concluded from their previous experience that most long-term hospitalized patients are not able to live independently in the community and engage in competitive employment. In our experience with long-term patients we also find a population characterized by overwhelming dependency and inadequacy in instrumental performance, social, vocational, or both. Even a "successful" rehabilitation effort with this hard-core group rarely results in the transformation into a highly productive person with a high-level job or the ability to live completely independently for a prolonged period of time, or both. Fairweather et al met these needs by carefully setting up a sheltered subsociety in the community for persons whom they felt could not meet the role expectations of the larger society. Here, ex-patients lived together and operated their own janitorial service. In this vocational enterprise each man was not expected to work at the normal pace of persons in the community but, as in the principle of the sheltered workshop, was expected to work up to his capacity and to be paid according to his performance. Our experimental-group ex-patients leaving the hospital also find themselves in a variety of sheltered rehabilitation facilities such as the halfway house, the day-treatment center, and the sheltered workshop.

The Deviant Label of Mental Illness

An important question in the discussion of different environments in the community for long-term patients who are no longer hospitalized are the implications for the delabeling process—to what extent have they lost their label as mental patients. Much has been written about the negative effects of labeling a person as "mentally ill"—and rightly so if we accept the definition of labeling as (1) acquiring a deviant label, (2) segregation, and (3) stigmatization.

Fully as important as a deviant label of mental illness are the role expectations that this label implies. Thus, recognition that a person needs tranquilizing medication and sheltered facilities to maintain him in the community involves making a diagnosis of mental illness. This need not imply, however, that such persons are disabled and should spend their lives in hospitals or in nonproductive passivity and dependency in the community. On the contrary, it can be stressed to both the patient and the public that just because one needs medication and sheltered facilities does not mean that one should not eventually be expected to take one's place in society to the full amount of his capabilities. It is crucial to separate the positive aspects of being a patient (i.e., a person recognizing that he needs medication) from the negative aspects (i.e., the careers of) mental patients as described by Scheff[4] and Goffman.[7]

It is eliminating the stigmatization that must concern us, not the deviant label per se or even the element of segregation. By accepting a position in an agency or in a sheltered subsociety, the patient may be segregated and acquire a deviant label; he need not, however, be stigmatized if he feels accepted by the staff and fellow clients in the agency, is treated with dignity, and feels he has options available to him, both socially and vocationally. The stigma is reduced if he is helped to reject seeing himself as inherently defective and inferior and if it is made clear to him that he has strengths which make him "not just a mental patient" but a person who has positive qualities, although he is handicapped by emotional problems which, hopefully, are transitory. If a person is seen and sees himself as having many positive qualities, in addition to whatever emotional difficulties he may have, then he is not self-stigmatized and is not so readily labeled by others.

Situational vs Characterological

In determining whether formerly hospitalized patients are in the community, we can also use Scheff's criterion "Is denial (normalization) occurring?" Are they accepted by those with whom they associate as persons who happen to have emotional problems, but more importantly also have other attributes, including the potential for a social role that is not stigmatized? Is the mental problem seen as characterological, as inherent in the person, or as situational, something that could have happened to anyone? This situational viewpoint can be encouraged by the staffs of community mental health facilities. It is not helpful to say "you need medications for life." It is better to say "It will be difficult for you to return to the community after being so long in the hospital. Take your medicines until you feel comfortable in the outside world. Take your medications to facilitate this transition." Such a strategy can be successfully continued for as long as necessary with the process always presented as temporary and situational (i.e., "Keep taking your medications for a while longer until you have adjusted to your new job. What's your hurry to stop?"). Further, a crucial aspect of the professional's role in this process is to stress the patient's strengths—both to the patient and to the agencies serving him.

It should be emphasized that the issue is not whether *in fact* the mental problem is characterological or situational—usually it is both, in varying degrees. What is important is that the person involved not see himself as inherently defective and inferior in a way that sets him apart from society and that he see himself as having strengths in addition to whatever problems he might have. He must feel that he has options available to him, aside from the role of mental patient, both socially and vocationally. His picture of himself must be reasonably congruent with his prized self-image, the way he would like to be and appear. Taking a situational point of view can often be a way of helping the patient maintain a positive self-image.

Inept Persons*

Status	Persons Labeled Mentally Ill		Persons Not Necessarily Labeled Mentally Ill	
	Segregated, Deviant Label, Stigmatized		*Segregated, Deviant Label, Not Stigmatized*	*Not Segregated, May or May Not Have Deviant Label, Not Stigmatized*
Type of Protection	State Hospital	Boarding and family-care homes	Sheltered subsocieties (that of Fairweather and our own, with "high" expectations)	Protection of the inept in industry, government, etc.
Vocational	Sheltered employment in some cases	Sheltered employment occasionally	Sheltered employment	Paid "competitive" employment (protected)
Living	Hospital	Boarding and family-care homes	Sheltered facility (halfway house, satellite housing program)	Family, alone, sometimes boarding house or residence club

*This scheme does not include persons who would be considered inept who are living with family or are alone and are dependent on welfare agencies or their families. These persons may or may not be mentally ill.

182

Protection of the Inept

Obviously not all long-term psychiatric patients, or marginal and inept persons in general, need a sheltered subsociety. Goode[8] has shown that most social institutions find ways to protect the inept. This is done without necessarily labeling these persons as inept or as mentally ill or as anything other than members of the institutions involved. Thus, industry, the military, governmental agencies, and so on, find ways to utilize and protect marginal persons who suffer from varying degrees of inadequacy and ineptness. Some industries, particularly some large public utilities, have formalized this arrangement of retaining persons who have become less productive by setting up sheltered workshops for the retraining of their employees who have become disabled.

Inept persons make other persons feel more secure by comparison; further, in the process of accommodating the inept, standards of performance for everyone are set at a reasonable level. Without the protection of the inept person, life would be a constant competitive jungle for everyone.

Generally speaking, the requirements for entering these competitive systems are higher than the requirements for remaining in them. A person must usually show some promise of productivity at the time of hiring and be able to maintain this for some time before the social institution feels an obligation to find a sheltered position for this person to keep him within their system. Consequently, many persons who might be considered by mental health professionals to be "psychiatrically disturbed" have found their niche in various institutions. Even though their productivity may be below par, they find support from a large organization and avoid being labeled.

We find it useful to regard the long-term mentally ill patient as one category of inept persons. Much of what has been said is summarized in the Table.

In the Community: Myth or Fact?

We recognize that we are presently setting up a small subsociety for our own experimental group. Fairweather et al[6] recognized the same phenomenon and consequently structured their program for discharged mental patients as a special subsociety for persons whom they felt could not ever meet the role expectations of the larger society.

Treatment personnel tend to judge being "in the community" by the amount of contact the patient has with nonpatients. Patients who are not able to progress beyond a type of subsociety, where patients associate only with other patients, although no longer in the hospital, are not really in the community, if we use as our criteria significant contacts with nonpatients and participation in nonpatient activities.[9,10] Certainly, however, he is much more in the community than is the patient who resides in boarding homes which are, essentially, small state hospital long-term wards set up in the community.

But segregation in a sheltered subsociety is not the only or even the most important criterion in determining whether a patient is in the community. Other sociological criteria would include such questions as, "Is denial (normalization) taking place? Are the role expectations those of acquiring a primary identity as citizens rather than as patients? Are the individual's potentials for social and vocational performance in the community being realized insofar as this is possible? Has stigmatization been reduced to a minimum?" Thus, the boarding home patients are not really in the community; they are referred to as "guests" but the stigmatization continues. The expectation is that the "guests" will remain regressed and dependent indefinitely. Denial and normalization are not employed. The labeling process remains relatively unchanged in the boarding homes.

In contrast, we feel that the high-expectation setting in the community as described in this paper facilitates the process of delabeling. Here ex-patients are less segregated, experience more normalization, are less likely to be labeled as deviate, experience less stigmatization, and see themselves as functioning members of the community.

References

1. Lamb HR: Chronic psychiatric patients in the day hospital. *Arch Gen Psychiatry* 17:615–621, 1967.
2. Richmond C: Transitional housing, in Lamb HR, et al (eds): *Handbook of Community Mental Health Practice.* San Francisco, Jossey-Bass, 1969, pp 145–174.
3. Silberstein SO: *A Survey of the Mental Health Functions of the Systems of Residential Home Care for the Mentally Ill and Retarded in the Sacramento Area.* Mimeographed, 1969.
4. Scheff TJ: *Being Mentally Ill. A Sociological Theory.* Chicago, Aldine Publishing Co, 1966.
5. Wilensky HL: Varieties of work experience, in Borow H (ed): *Man in a World of Work.* Boston, Houghton Mifflin Co, 1964, pp 125–149.
6. Fairweather GW, Sanders DH, Maynard H, et al: *Community Life for the Mentally Ill: An Alternative to Institutional Care.* Chicago, Aldine Publishing Co, 1969.
7. Goffman E: *Asylums—Essays on the Social Situation of Mental Patients and Other Inmates.* Garden City, NY, Doubleday & Co Inc, 1961.
8. Goode W: The protection of the inept. *Am Sociol Rev* 32:5–19, 1967.
9. Lampert JP: Action for community involvement. *Ment Hosp* 12:13–16, 1961.
10. Patterson CH: A suggested blueprint for psychiatric rehabilitation. *Commun Ment Health J* 1:61–68, 1965.

14

Feighner, J. P., Robins, E., Guze, S. B., Woodruff, R. A., Winokur, G., & Munoz, R. (1972). Diagnostic criteria for use in psychiatric research. *Archives of General Psychiatry, 26* (2), 57–63

DSM-III, or the third iteration of the American Psychiatric Association *Diagnostic and Statistical Manual of Mental Disorders*, was a response, as Nancy Andreasen, former president of the APA, would describe in a latter-day classic, to the lack of diagnostic precision of psychodynamically oriented psychiatry. This article was a response to what Feighner and his colleagues describe as the limitations of *DSM-III*'s predecessor, *DSM-II*, on best clinical judgment and experience. While noting that they do not consider their new diagnostic criteria to be definitive, the authors describe the process of culling elements for those criteria from a number of sources, including clinical descriptions, laboratory primary and follow-up studies of individual patients, exclusion criteria, and family studies. They present criteria for 14 psychiatric illnesses, including primary affective disorders, secondary affective disorders, schizophrenia, alcoholism, and drug dependence. The reform that *DSM-III* and source documents such as Feighner and colleagues' article represented would accumulate its own baggage, as we shall see in the two eras after this one.

Diagnostic Criteria for Use in Psychiatric Research

Diagnostic criteria for 14 psychiatric illnesses (and for secondary depression) along with the validating evidence for these diagnostic categories come from workers outside our group as well as from those within; it consists of studies of both outpatients and inpatients, of family studies, and of follow-up studies. These criteria are the most efficient currently available; however, it is expected that the criteria be tested and not be considered a final, closed system. It is expected that the criteria will change as various illnesses are studied by different groups. Such criteria provide a framework for comparison of data gathered in different centers, and serve to promote communication between investigators.

This communication presents specific diagnostic criteria for those adult psychiatric illnesses that have been sufficiently validated by precise clinical description, follow-up, and family studies to warrant their use in research as well as in clinical practice.

These criteria are not intended as final for any illness. The criteria represent a distillation of our clinical research experience, and of the experiences of others cited in the references. This communication is meant to provide common ground for different research groups so that diagnostic definitions can be emended constructively as further studies are completed. The use of formal diagnostic criteria by a number of groups, regardless of whether their interests are clinical, psychodynamic, pharmacologic, chemical, neuropsychological, or neurophysiological, will result in a solution of the problem of whether patients described by different groups are comparable. This first and crucial taxonomic step should expedite psychiatric investigation.

Diagnosis has functions as important in psychiatry as elsewhere in medicine. Psychiatric diagnoses based on studies of natural history permit prediction of course and outcome, allow planning for both immediate and long-term treatment, and make communication possible between psychiatrists and other physicians, as well as among psychiatrists themselves. Such functions are of obvious importance in research.[1-4]

In contrast to the American Psychiatric Association *Diagnostic and Statistical Manual of Mental Disorders (DSM-II)*, in which the diagnostic classification is based upon the "best clinical judgment and experience" of a committee and its consultants, this communication will present a diagnostic classification validated primarily by follow-up and family studies. The following criteria for establishing diagnostic validity in psychiatric illness have been described elsewhere and may be divided into five phases.[5]

The Five Phases

1. Clinical Description

In general, the first step is to describe the clinical picture of the disorder. This may be a single striking clinical feature or a combination of clinical features thought to be associated with one another. Race, sex, age at onset, precipitating factors, and other items may be used to define the clinical picture more precisely. The clinical picture thus does not include only symptoms.

2. Laboratory Studies

Included among laboratory studies are chemical, physiological, radiological, and anatomical (biopsy and autopsy) findings. Certain psychological tests, when shown to be reliable and reproducible, may also be considered laboratory studies in this context. Laboratory findings are generally more reliable, precise, and reproducible than are clinical descriptions. When consistent with a defined clinical picture they permit a more refined classification. Without such a defined clinical picture, their value may be considerably reduced. Unfortunately, consistent and reliable laboratory findings have not yet been demonstrated in the more common psychiatric disorders.

3. Delimitation From Other Disorders

Since similar clinical features and laboratory findings may be seen in patients suffering from different disorders (eg, cough and blood in the sputum in lobar pneumonia, bronchiectasis, and bronchogenic carcinoma), it is necessary to specify exclusion criteria so that patients with other illnesses are not included in the group to be studied. These criteria should also permit exclusion of borderline cases and doubtful cases (an undiagnosed group) so that the index group may be as homogeneous as possible.

4. Follow-up Study

The purpose of the follow-up study is to determine whether or not the original patients are suffering from some other defined disorder that could account for the original clinical picture. If they are suffering from another such illness, this finding suggests that the original patients did not comprise a homogeneous group and that it is necessary to modify the diagnostic criteria. In the absence of known etiology or pathogenesis, which is true of the more common psychiatric disorders, marked differences in outcome, such as between complete recovery and chronic illness, suggest that the group is not homogeneous. This latter point is not as compelling in suggesting diagnostic heterogeneity as is the finding of a change in diagnosis. The same illness may have a variable prognosis, but until we know more about the fundamental nature of the common psychiatric illnesses, marked differences in outcome should be regarded as a challenge to the validity of the original diagnosis.

5. Family Study

Most psychiatric illnesses have been shown to run in families, whether the investigations were designed to study hereditary or environmental causes. Independent of the question of etiology, therefore, the finding of an increased prevalence of the same disorder among close relatives of the original patients strongly indicates that one is dealing with a valid entity.

While no psychiatric syndrome has yet been fully validated by a complete series of steps, a great deal of work has been published indicating that substantial validation is possible. This communication is a summary of that work in the form of specific diagnostic criteria. The studies of validation for each illness are cited. In addition, we in this department have carried out a study of interrater reliability and validation of reliability with an 18-month follow-up study of 314 psychiatric emergency room patients (to be published) as well as a seven-year follow-up study of 87 psychiatric inpatients (to be published), each of whom was interviewed personally and systematically. There were four different raters in the emergency room study. Agreement ranged from 86% to 95% about diagnosis with diagnostic criteria similar to those outlined in this report. There were two different raters in the inpatient study; reliability between those raters was 92%. In the emergency room study and in the inpatient study, validity, as determined by correctly predicting diagnosis at follow-up by criteria such as those of this report, was 93% and 92%, respectively.

Not only are specific criteria necessary for each diagnosis, but criteria are also needed for scoring individual symptoms as positive. The following criteria have been used for this purpose. (1) The patient saw a physician (includes chiropractor, naturopath, healer, etc) for the symptom. (2) The symptom was disabling enough to interfere with the patient's usual routine. (3) The symptom led the patient to take medication on more than one occasion. (4) The examining physician believes that, because of its clinical importance, the symptom should be scored positive even though the aforementioned criteria were not present; eg, a spell of blindness lasting a few minutes that the patient minimizes, or hallucinations or delusions which the patient does not recognize as pathological, and which did not disrupt the patient's usual routine. (5) Symptoms are *not* scored positive if they can be explained by a known medical disease of the patient (this does not apply to organic brain syndrome and mental retardation).

It will be apparent below that certain diagnoses are mutually exclusive (primary affective disorders and schizophrenia), while others may be made in the same patient (antisocial personality disorder with alcoholism or drug dependency; hysteria or anxiety neurosis with secondary depression). More work will be necessary before the full significance of various diagnostic combinations becomes evident. It should also be clear that any of the diagnoses may be further subdivided according to various clinical, demographic, or other variables. For example, primary depression may be divided into psychotic and nonpsychotic, bipolar and unipolar, early onset and late onset. Similarly, schizophrenia may be subdivided into paranoid, hebephrenic, and catatonic subtypes.

Diagnostic Criteria

Primary Affective Disorders.[6-16]—*Depression.*—For a diagnosis of depression, *A* through *C* are required.

A. Dysphoric mood characterized by symptoms such as the following: depressed, sad, blue, despondent, hopeless, "down in the dumps," irritable, fearful, worried, or discouraged.

B. At least five of the following criteria are required for "definite" depression; four are required for "probable" depression. (1) Poor appetite or weight loss (positive if 2 lb a week or 10 lb or more a year when not dieting). (2) Sleep difficulty (include insomnia or hypersomnia). (3) Loss of energy, eg, fatigability, tiredness. (4) Agitation or retardation. (5) Loss of interest in usual activities, or decrease in sexual drive. (6) Feelings of self-reproach or guilt (either may be delusional). (7) Complaints of or actually diminished ability to think or concentrate, such as slow thinking or mixed-up thoughts. (8) Recurrent thoughts of death or suicide, including thoughts of wishing to be dead.

C. A psychiatric illness lasting at least one month with no preexisting psychiatric conditions such as schizophrenia, anxiety neurosis, phobic neurosis, obsessive compulsive neurosis, hysteria, alcoholism, drug dependency, antisocial personality, homosexuality and other sexual deviations, mental retardation, or organic brain syndrome. (Patients with life-threatening or incapacitating medical illness preceding and paralleling the depression do not receive the diagnosis of primary depression.)

Mania.—For a diagnosis of mania, *A* through *C* are required.

A. Euphoria or irritability.

B. At least three of the following symptom categories must also be present. (1) Hyperactivity (includes motor, social, and sexual activity). (2) Push of speech (pressure to keep talking). (3) Flight of ideas (racing thoughts). (4) Grandiosity (may be delusional). (5) Decreased sleep. (6) Distractibility.

C. A psychiatric illness lasting at least two weeks with no preexisting psychiatric conditions such as schizophrenia, anxiety neurosis, phobic neurosis, obsessive compulsive neurosis, hysteria, alcoholism, drug dependency, antisocial personality, homosexuality and other sexual deviations, mental retardation, or organic brain syndrome.

There are patients who fulfill the above criteria, but also have a massive or peculiar alteration of perception and thinking as a major manifestation of their illness. These patients are considered by some to have a "schizophreniform" or "atypical" psychosis, ie, an illness of acute onset (less than six months), in a patient with good premorbid psychosocial adjustment, with prominent delusions and hallucinations in addition to the affective symptoms. Clinical studies of this disorder indicate that from 60% to 90% of cases have a remitting illness and return to premorbid levels of psychosocial adjustment with a longitudinal course consistent with primary affective disorder.[17-22] The remaining 10% to 40% have a chronic illness consistent with schizophrenia. These patients are, therefore, classified as having an undiagnosed psychiatric disorder and are not included in either primary affective disorder or schizophrenia.

Secondary Affective Disorders.— Secondary depression, "definite" or "probable," is defined in the same way as primary depression, except that it occurs with one of the following: (1) A preexisting non-affective psychiatric illness which may or may not still be present. (2) A life-threatening or incapacitating medical illness which precedes and parallels the symptoms of depression.

Schizophrenia.[17-31]—For a diagnosis of schizophrenia, *A* through *C* are required.

A. Both of the following are necessary: (1) A chronic illness with at least six months of symptoms prior to the index evaluation without return to the premorbid level of psychosocial adjustment. (2) Absence of a period of depressive or manic symptoms sufficient to qualify for affective disorder or probable affective disorder.

B. The patient must have at least one of the following: (1) Delusions or hallucinations without significant perplexity or disorientation associated with them. (2) Verbal production that makes communication difficult because of a lack of logical or understandable organization. (In the presence of muteness the diagnostic decision must be deferred.)

(We recognize that many patients with schizophrenia have a characteristic blunted or inappropriate affect; however, when it occurs in mild form, interrater agreement is difficult to achieve. We believe that, on the basis of presently available information, blunted affect occurs rarely or not at all in the absence of *B*-1 or *B*-2.)

C. At least three of the following manifestations must be present for a diagnosis of "definite" schizophrenia, and two for a diagnosis of "probable" schizophrenia. (1) Single.

(2) Poor premorbid social adjustment or work history. (3) Family history of schizophrenia. (4) Absence of alcoholism or drug abuse within one year of onset of psychosis. (5) Onset of illness prior to age 40.

Anxiety Neurosis.[32]—For a diagnosis of anxiety neurosis, A through D are required.

A. The following manifestations must be present: (1) Age of onset prior to 40. (2) Chronic nervousness with recurrent anxiety attacks manifested by apprehension, fearfulness, or sense of impending doom, with at least four of the following symptoms present during the majority of attacks: (a) dyspnea, (b) palpitations, (c) chest pain or discomfort, (d) choking or smothering sensation, (e) dizziness, and (f) paresthesias.

B. The anxiety attacks are essential to the diagnosis and must occur at times other than marked physical exertion or life-threatening situations, and in the absence of medical illness that *could* account for symptoms of anxiety. There must have been at least six anxiety attacks, each separated by at least a week from the others.

C. In the presence of other psychiatric illness(es) this diagnosis is made *only* if the criteria described in A and B antedate the onset of the other psychiatric illness by at least two years.

D. The diagnosis of probable anxiety neurosis is made when at least two symptoms listed in A-2 are present, and the other criteria are fulfilled.

Obsessive Compulsive Neurosis[33,34]—For a diagnosis of obsessive compulsive neurosis, both A and B are required.

A. Manifestations 1 and 2 are required. (1) Obsessions or compulsions are the dominant symptoms. They are defined as recurrent or persistent ideas, thoughts, images, feelings, impulses, or movements, which must be accompanied by a sense of subjective compulsion and a desire to resist the event, the event being recognized by the individual as foreign to his personality or nature, ie, "ego-alien." (2) Age of onset prior to 40.

B. Patients with primary or probable primary affective disorder, or with schizophrenia or probable schizophrenia, who manifest obsessive-compulsive features, do not receive the additional diagnosis of obsessive compulsive neurosis.

Phobic Neurosis.[35,36]—For a diagnosis of phobic neurosis, both A and B are required.

A. Manifestations 1 and 2 are required. (1) Phobias are the dominant symptoms. They are defined as persistent and recurring fears which the patient tries to resist or avoid and at the same time considers unreasonable. (2) Age of onset prior to 40.

B. Symptoms of anxiety, tension, nervousness, and depression may accompany the phobias; however, patients with another definable psychiatric illness should not receive the additional diagnosis of phobic neurosis.

Hysteria.[37–39]—For a diagnosis of hysteria, both A and B are required.

A. A chronic or recurrent illness beginning before age 30, presenting with a dramatic, vague, or complicated medical history.

B. The patient must report at least 25 medically unexplained symptoms for a "definite" diagnosis and 20 to 24 symptoms for a "probable" diagnosis in at least nine of the following groups.

Group 1

Headaches
Sickly majority of life

Group 2

Blindness
Paralysis

Anesthesia
Aphonia
Fits or convulsions
Unconsciousness
Amnesia
Deafness
Hallucinations
Urinary retention
Trouble walking
Other unexplained "neurological" symptoms

Group 3

Fatigue
Lump in throat
Fainting spells
Visual blurring
Weakness
Dysuria

Group 4

Breathing difficulty
Palpitation
Anxiety attacks
Chest pain
Dizziness

Group 5

Anorexia
Weight loss
Marked fluctuations in weight
Nausea
Abdominal bloating
Food intolerances
Diarrhea
Constipation

Group 6

Abdominal pain
Vomiting

Group 7

Dysmenorrhea
Menstrual irregularity
Amenorrhea
Excessive bleeding

Group 8

Sexual indifference
Frigidity
Dyspareunia
Other sexual difficulties
Vomiting all nine months of pregnancy at least once, or hospitalization for hypermesis gravidarum

Group 9

Back pain
Joint pain
Extremity pain
Burning pains of the sexual organs, mouth, or rectum
Other bodily pains

Group 10

Nervousness
Fears
Depressed feelings
Need to quit working, or inability to carry on regular duties because of feeling sick
Crying easily
Feeling life was hopeless
Thinking a good deal about dying
Wanting to die
Thinking about suicide
Suicide attempts

Antisocial Personality Disorder.[40,41]—A chronic or recurrent disorder with the appearance of at least one of the following manifestations before age 15. A minimum of five manifestations are required for a "definite" diagnosis, and four are required for a "probable" diagnosis.

A. School problems as manifested by any of the following: truancy (positive if more than once per year except for the last year in school), suspension, expulsion, or fighting that leads to trouble with teachers or principals.

B. Running away from home overnight while living in parental home.

C. Troubles with the police as manifested by any of the following: two or more arrests for nontraffic offenses, four or more arrests (including tickets only) for moving traffic offences or at least one felony conviction.

D. Poor work history as manifested by being fired, quitting without another job to go to, or frequent job changes not accounted for by normal seasonal or economic fluctuations.

E. Marital difficulties manifested by any of the following: deserting family, two or more divorces, frequent separations due to marital discord, recurrent infidelity recurrent physical attacks upon spouse, or being suspected of battering a child.

F. Repeated outbursts of rage or fighting not on the school premises: if prior to age 18 this must occur at least twice and lead to difficulty with adults; after age 18 this must occur at least twice, or if a weapon (eg, club, knife, or gun) is used, only once is enough to score this category positive.

G. Sexual problems as manifested by any of the following: prostitution (includes both heterosexual and homosexual activity), pimping, more than one episode of venereal disease, or flagrant promiscuity.

H. Vagrancy or wanderlust, eg, at least several months of wandering from place to place with no prearranged plans.

I. Persistent and repeated lying, or using an alias.

Alcoholism.[42-45]—A "definite" diagnosis is made when symptoms occur in at least three of the four following groups. A "probable" diagnosis is made when symptoms occur in only two groups.

A. Group One: (1) Any manifestation of alcohol withdrawal such as tremulousness, convulsions, hallucinations, or delirium. (2) History of medical complications, eg, cirrhosis, gastritis, pancreatitis, myopathy, polyneuropathy, Wernicke-Korsakoff's syndrome. (3) Alcoholic black-outs, ie, amnesic episodes during heavy drinking not accounted for by head trauma. (4) Alcoholic binges or benders (48 hours or more of drinking associated with default of usual obligations: must have occurred more than once to be scored as positive).

B. Group Two: (1) Patient has not been able to stop drinking when he wanted to do so. (2) Patient has tried to control drinking by allowing himself to drink only under certain circumstances, such as only after 5:00 pm, only on weekends, or only with other people. (3) Drinking before breakfast. (4) Drinking nonbeverage forms of alcohol, eg, hair oil, mouthwash, Sterno, etc.

C. Group Three: (1) Arrests for drinking. (2) Traffic difficulties associated with drinking. (3) Trouble at work because of drinking. (4) Fighting associated with drinking.

D. Group Four: (1) Patient thinks he drinks too much. (2) family objects to his drinking. (3) Loss of friends because of drinking. (4) Other people object to his drinking. (5) Feels guilty about his drinking.

Drug Dependence (Excluding Alcoholism).[46]—This diagnosis is made when any one of the following is present. The drug type is specified according to *DSM-II*.

A. History of withdrawal symptoms.

B. Hospitalization for drug abuse or its complications.

C. Indiscriminate prolonged use of central nervous system active drugs.

Mental Retardation.—This disorder, which has different causes, is described both in terms of intellectual impairment as well as social maladaptation as described in *DSM-II*. In view of the fact that the social adaptation scales have not been standardized to the level of current intelligence tests, only the latter are used in making this diagnosis. The following criteria are used:

A. When the IQ is available from currently acceptable tests, the categories of *DSM-II* are used.

B. In the absence of IQ tests, the following will be accepted as evidence of suspected mental retardation: (1) Despite continued effort the individual fails the same grade two years in succession or (2) despite continued effort the individual fails to pass the sixth grade by the time he is16 years old.

(Caution should be used in making the diagnosis of mental retardation in the presence of another psychiatric illness, eg, schizophrenia, severe affective disorders, antisocial personality disorder.)

Organic Brain Syndrome.[47,48]—This diagnosis is made when either criterion *A* or criterion *B* is present.

A. Two of the following manifestations must be present. (In the presence of muteness the diagnosis must be deferred.) (1) Impairment of orientation. (2) Impairment of memory. (3) Deterioration of other intellectual functions.

B. This diagnosis is also made if the patient has at least one manifestation *(A)* in addition to a known probable cause for organic brain syndrome.

Homosexuality.[49-52]—For a diagnosis of homosexuality, *A* through *C* are required.

A. This diagnosis is made when there are persistent homosexual experiences beyond age 18 (equivalent to Kinsey rating 3 to 6).

B. Patients who fulfill the criteria for transsexualism are excluded.

C. Patients who perform homosexual activity only when incarcerated for a period of at least one year without access to members of the opposite sex are excluded.

Transsexualism.[53-55]—In order to receive a "definite" diagnosis of transsexualism, at least four of the five following manifestations must be present with at least one manifestation occurring prior to age 12. A diagnosis of "probable" transsexualism is made when three of the following manifestations are present, with at least one occurring prior to age 12.

A. A persistent desire to belong to the opposite sex, with a sense of having been born into the wrong sex.

B. A strong desire to resemble physically the opposite sex by any available means, eg, manner of dress, behavior, hormone therapy, and surgery.

C. A strong desire to be accepted by the community as a member of the opposite sex.

D. A negative feeling about the patient's external genitalia (breasts are included) including attempts at mutilation and a desire for surgery.

E. A negative feeling towards heterosexual activity and a persistent feeling that physical attraction to members of the same sex is not a homosexual orientation.

Anorexia Nervosa.[56-60]—For a diagnosis of anorexia nervosa, *A* through *E* are required.

A. Age of onset prior to 25.

B. Anorexia with accompanying weight loss of at least 25% of original body weight.

C. A distorted, implacable attitude towards eating, food, or weight that overrides hunger, admonitions, reassurance and threats; eg, (1) Denial of illness with a failure to recognize nutritional needs, (2) apparent enjoyment in losing weight with overt manifestation that food refusal is a pleasurable indulgence, (3) a desired body image of extreme thinness with overt evidence that it is rewarding to the patient to achieve and maintain this state, and (4) unusual hoarding or handling of food.

D. No known medical illness that could account for the anorexia and weight loss.

E. No other known psychiatric disorder with particular reference to primary affective disorders, schizophrenia, obsessive-compulsive and phobic neurosis. (The assumption is made that even though it may appear phobic or obsessional, food refusal alone is not sufficient to qualify for obsessive-compulsive or phobic disease.)

F. At least two of the following manifestations. (1) Amenorrhea. (2) Lanugo. (3) Bradycardia (persistent resting pulse of 60 or less). (4) Periods of overactivity. (5) Episodes of bulimia. (6) Vomiting (may be self-induced).

Undiagnosed Psychiatric Illness.—Some patients cannot receive a diagnosis for one or more reasons. Among the more common problems that cause a patient to be considered undiagnosed are the following: (1) cases in which only one illness is suspected but symptoms are minimal. (2) Cases in which more than one psychiatric illness is suspected but symptoms are not sufficient to meet the criteria of any of the possibilities. (3) Cases in which symptoms suggest two or more disorders but in an atypical or confusing manner. (4) Cases in which the chronology of important symptom clusters cannot be determined. (5) Cases in which it is impossible to obtain the necessary history to establish a definitive diagnosis.

Comment

There are many diagnoses listed in *DSM-II* not considered in this communication because sufficient clinical data for even limited diagnostic validation are not available. A recent attempt to delineate passive-aggressive personality disorder as a separate entity based on cross-sectional and longitudinal data brings to focus some of the problems in diagnostic validation. As the investigators of that study suggested, further studies are needed before the validity of that syndrome is established.[61]

Finally, the criteria presented in this report are "minimal" in two senses: First, all diagnostic criteria are tentative in the sense that they change and become more precise with new data. Second, we have made no effort to subclassify these illnesses. (For example, we have presented criteria to define primary affective disorders, unipolar type, without suggestions for further subdivision into forms of early and late onset, psychotic or nonpsychotic forms, agitated or retarded forms, and so forth. It is clear that primary affective disorder, unipolar type, is a reasonable major classification. The data to support its subclassifications are still tentative.) We and other investigators will continue to work toward modification and subclassification. What we now present is our synthesis of existing information, a synthesis based on data rather than opinion or tradition. We hope that such a presentation will help to promote useful communication among investigators

References

1. Kramer M: Cross-national study of diagnosis of the mental disorders: Origin of the problem. Amer J Psychiat 125(suppl):1–11, 1969.
2. Zubin J: Cross-national study of diagnosis of the mental disorders: Methodology and planning. Amer J Psychiat 125(suppl):12–20, 1969.
3. Cooper JE, Kendell RE, Gurland BJ, et al: Cross-national study of diagnosis of the mental disorders: Some results from the first comparative investigation. Amer J Psychiat 125(suppl):21–29, 1969.
4. Lehmann HE: A renaissance of psychiatric diagnosis, discussion, Amer J Psychiat 125(suppl):43–46, 1969.
5. Robins E, Guze SB: Establishment of diagnostic validity in psychiatric illness: Its application to schizophrenia. Amer J Psychiat 126:983–987, 1970.
6. Mendels J: Depression: The distinction between syndrome and symptom. Brit J Psychiat 114:1549–1554, 1968.
7. Lehmann HE: Psychiatric concepts of depression: Nomenclature and classification. Can Psychiat Assoc J 4:1–12, 1969.
8. Mendels J, Cochrane C: The nosology of depression: The endogenous-reactive concept. Amer J Psychiat 124(suppl):11, 1968.
9. Rosenthal SH: The involutional depressive syndrome. Amer J Psychiat 124(suppl):21–34, 1968.
10. Robins E, Guze SB: Classification of affective disorders, in Proceedings of the NIMH workshop, Psychobiology of Depression, to be published.
11. Cassidy WL, et al: Clinical observations in manic-depressive disease: A quantitative study of 100 manic-depressive patients and 50 medically sick controls. JAMA 164:1535–1546, 1957.
12. Gittleson NL: The effect of obsessions on depressive psychosis. Brit J Psychiat 112:253–259, 1966.
13. Clayton PJ, Pitts FN Jr, Winokur G: Affective disorder: IV. Mania. Compr Psychiat 6:313–322, 1965.

14. Lipkin KM, Dyrud J, Meyer GG: The many faces of mania. Arch Gen Psychiat 22:262–267, 1970.

15. Perris C: A study of bipolar (manic-depressive) and unipolar recurrent depressive psychoses. Acta Psychiat Scand 42(suppl 194):1–189, 1966.

16. Winokur G, Clayton PJ, Reich T: Manic Depressive Illness. St. Louis, CV Mosby Co, 1969.

17. Welner J, Strömgren E: Clinical and genetic studies on benign schizophreniform psychoses based on a follow-up. Acta Psychiat Neurol Scand 33:377–399, 1958.

18. Eitinger L, Laane CV, Language feldt G: The prognostic value of the clinical picture and the therapeutic value of physical treatment in schizophrenia and the schizophreniform states. Acta Psychiat Neurol Scand 33:33–53, 1958.

19. Stephens JH, Astrup C, Mangrum JC: Prognostic factors in recovered and deteriorated schizophrenics. Amer J Psychiat 122:1116–1121, 1966.

20. Vaillant GE: The prediction recovery in schizophrenia. J Nerv Ment Dis 135:534–543, 1962.

21. Vaillant GE: Prospective prediction of schizophrenic remission. Arc Gen Psychiat 11:509–518, 1964.

22. Clayton PJ, Rodin L, Winokur G: Family history studies: III. Schizoaffective disorder, clinical and genetic factors including a one to two-year follow-up. Compr Psychiat 9:31–49, 1968.

23. Bleuler E: Dementia praecox or the group of schizophrenics. J. Zinkin (trans), New York, International Universities Press, 1950.

24. Langfeldt G: The prognosis in schizophrenia. Acta Psychiat Neurol Scand 110(suppl):1-66, 1956.

25. Langfeldt G: Diagnosis and prognosis of schizophrenia. Proc R Soc Med 53:1047–1052, 1960.

26. Fish F: A guide to the Leonhard classification of chronic schizophrenia. Psychiat Q 38:438–450, 1964.

27. Wender PH: The role of genetics in the etiology of the schizophrenias. Amer J Orthopsychiat 39:447–458, 1969.

28. Wender PH, Rosenthal D, Kety S: A psychiatric assessment of the adoptive parents of schizophrenics, in Rosenthal D, Kety S (eds): The Transmission of Schizophrenia. Oxford, England, Pergamon Press, 1968.

29. Heston L: Psychiatric disorders in foster home reared children of schizophrenic mothers. Brit J Psychiat 112:819–825, 1966.

30. Heston L: The genetics of schizophrenic and schizoid disease. Science 167:249–256, 1970.

31. Fish F: Schizophrenia. Baltimore, Williams & Wilkins Co, 1962.

32. Wheeler EO, White PD, Reed EW, et al: Neurocirculatory asthenia (anxiety neurosis, effort syndrome, neurasthenia). JAMA 142:878–888, 1950.

33. Goodwin DW, Guze SB, Robins E: Follow-up studies in obsessional neurosis. Arch Gen Psychiat 20:182–187, 1969.

34. Pollitt J: Natural history of obsessional states: A study of 150 cases. Brit Med J 1:194–198, 1957.

35. Agras S, Sylvester D, et al: The epidemiology of common fears and phobia. Compr Psychiat 10:151–156, 1969.

36. Marks I: Fears and Phobias. New York, Academic Press, 1969.

37. Guze SB: The diagnosis of hysteria: What are we trying to do? Amer J Psychiat 124:491–498, 1967.

38. Perley MJ, Guze SB: Hysteria—the stability and usefulness of clinical criteria: A quantitative study based on a follow-up period of 6–8 years in 39 patients. N Engl J Med 421–426, 1962.

39. Purtell JJ, Robins E, Cohen ME: Observations on the clinical aspecs of hysteria: A quantitative study of 50 patients and 156 control subjects. JAMA 146:902–909, 1951.

40. Robins LN: Deviant Children Grown Up: A Sociological and Psychiatric Study of Sociopathic Personality. Baltimore, Williams & Wilkins Co, 1966.

41. Robins E: Antisocial and Dyssocial personality disorders, in Freedman M, Kaplan HI (eds): Comprehensive Textbook of Psychiatry. Baltimore, Williams & Wilkins Co, 1967.

42. Barchha R, Stewart MA, Guze B: The prevalence of alcoholism among general hospital ward patients. Amer J Psychiat 125:681–684, 1968.

43. Jellinek EM: The Disease Concept of Alcoholism. New Haven, Conn, Hillhouse Press, 1960.

44. Guze SB, Goodwin DW, Crane J: Criminality and psychiatric disorders. Arch Gen Psychiat 20:583–591, 1969.

45. Bailey MB, Haberman P, et al: The epidemiology of alcoholism in urban residential area. Q J Alcohol 26:19–40, 1965.

46. Isbell H, White WM: Clinical characteristics of addictions. Amer J Med 14:558–565, 1953.

47. Wolff HG, Curran D: Nature of delirium and allied states. Arch Neuropsychiat 33:1175–1215, 1935.

48. Guze SB, Cantwell DP: The prognosis in "organic brain" syndrome. Amer J Psychiat 120:878–881, 1964.

49. Kinsey AC, Pomeroy WR, Martin CE: Sexual Behavior in the Human Male. Philadelphia, WB Saunders Co.

50. Hemphill RE, Leitch A, et al: A factual study of male homosexuality. Brit Med J 1:1317–1323, 1958.

51. Saghir MT, Robins E: Homosexuality: I. Sexual behavior of the female homosexual. Arch Gen Psychiat 20:291–229, 1969.

52. Saghir MT, Robins E, et al: Homosexuality: II. Sexual behavior of the male homosexual. Arch Gen Psychiat 21:219–229, 1969.

53. Green R, Money J (eds): Trans-sexualism and Sex Reassignment. Baltimore, Johns Hopkins Press, 1969.

54. Pauly IB: The current status of the change of sex operation. J Nerv Ment Dis 147:460–471, 1968.

55. Green R: Childhood cross-gender identification. J Nerv Ment Dis 147:500–509, 1968.

56. Kay DWK, Leigh D: The natural history, treatment, and prognosis of anorexia nervosa, based on a study of 38 patients. J Ment Sci 100:411–431, 1954.

57. Warren W: A study of anorexia nervosa in young girls. J Child Psychol Psychiat 9:27–40, 1968.

58. Bruch H: Anorexia nervosa and its differential diagnosis. J Nerv Ment Dis 141:555–566, 1965.

59. King A: Primary and secondary anorexia nervosa syndromes. Br J Psychiat 109:470–479, 1963.

60. Dally P: Anorexia Nervosa. New York, Grune & Stratton Inc, 1969.

61. Small IF, Small JG, Alig VB, et al: Passive-aggressive personality disorder: A search for a syndrome. Amer J Psychiat 126:973–981, 1969.

15

Rosenhan, D. L. (1973). On being sane in insane places. *Science, 179, 250–258*

The study that Rosenhan reports on in this article involved an experiment in which he and seven friends, none of whom had a history of serious psychiatric problems, attempted to gain entrance to 12 different hospitals across five states, claiming only to hear voices that seemed to be saying things like "empty," "hollow," or "thud." All pseudopatients were admitted to the hospital and had lengths of stay ranging from 7 to 52 days. Once admitted, all ceased reporting any symptoms. All but one was diagnosed with schizophrenia and, when released, left with the diagnosis of "schizophrenia in remission." Along with misdiagnosis, Rosenhan describes the distressing experiences of the pseudopatients, particularly the phenomenon of depersonalization, and their observations of staff beatings, verbal abuse, and neglect of patients. Rosenhan and other pseudopatients also recorded their attempts to engage staff on the unit. The results were disturbing: The vast majority of psychiatrists, nurses, and attendants responded to questions such as, "When will I get grounds privileges?" by moving on with heads averted. Rosenhan's article sent shockwaves through the psychiatric community and had no small part in subsequent revamping of the diagnostic system and publication of the *DSM-III*. It is still cited today as an example of the inexactness of psychiatric diagnosis and the importance of social-institutional context in assessing an individual's mental health status.

Rebecca Miller

On Being Sane in Insane Places

If sanity and insanity exist, how shall we know them?

The question is neither capricious nor itself insane. However much we may be personally convinced that we can tell the normal from the abnormal, the evidence is simply not compelling. It is commonplace, for example, to read about murder trials wherein eminent psychiatrists for the defense are contradicted by equally eminent psychiatrists for the prosecution on the matter of the defendant's sanity. More generally, there are a great deal of conflicting data on the reliability, utility, and meaning of such terms as "sanity," "insanity," "mental illness," and "schizophrenia" (1) Finally, as early as 1934, Benedict suggested that normality and abnormality are not universal (2). What is viewed as normal in one culture may be seen as quite aberrant in another. Thus, notions of normality and abnormality may not be quite as accurate as people believe they are.

To raise questions regarding normality and abnormality is in no way to question the fact that some behaviors are deviant or odd. Murder is deviant. So, too, are hallucinations. Nor does raising such questions deny the existence of the personal anguish that is often associated with "mental illness." Anxiety and depression exist. Psychological suffering exists. But normality and abnormality, sanity and insanity, and the diagnoses that flow from them may be less substantive than many believe them to be.

At its heart, the question of whether the sane can be distinguished from the insane (and whether degrees of insanity can be distinguished from each other) is a simple matter: do the salient characteristics that lead to diagnoses reside in the patients themselves or in the environments and contexts in which observers find them? From Bleuler, through Kretchmer, through the formulators of the recently revised *Diagnostic and Statistical Manual* of the American Psychiatric Association, the belief has been strong that patients present symptoms, that those symptoms can be categorized, and, implicitly, that the sane are distinguishable from the insane. More recently, however, this belief has been questioned. Based in part on theoretical and anthropological considerations, but also on philosophical, legal, and therapeutic ones, the view has grown that psychological categorization of mental illness is useless at best and downright harmful, misleading, and pejorative at worst. Psychiatric diagnoses, in this view, are in the minds of the observers and are not valid summaries of characteristics displayed by the observed (3–5).

Gains can be made in deciding which of these is more nearly accurate by getting normal people (that is, people who do not have, and have never suffered, symptoms of serious psychiatric disorders) admitted to psychiatric hospitals and then determining whether they were discovered to be sane and, if so, how. If the sanity of such pseudopatients were always detected, there would be prima facie evidence that a sane individual can be distinguished from the insane context in which he is found. Normality (and presumably abnormality) is distinct enough that it can be recognized wherever it occurs, for it is carried within the person. If, on the other hand, the sanity of the pseudopatients were never discovered, serious difficulties would arise for those who support traditional modes of psychiatric diagnosis. Given that the hospital staff was not incompetent, that the pseudopatient had been behaving as sanely as he had been outside of the hospital, and that it had never been previously suggested that he belonged in a psychiatric hospital, such an unlikely outcome would support the view that psychiatric diagnosis betrays little about the patient but much about the environment in which an observer finds him.

This article describes such an experiment. Eight sane people gained secret admission to 12 different hospitals (6). Their diagnostic experiences constitute the data of the first part of this article; the remainder is devoted to a description of their experiences in psychiatric institutions. Too few psychiatrists and psychologists, even those who have worked in such hospitals, know what the experience is like. They rarely talk about it with former patients, perhaps because they distrust information coming from the previously insane. Those who have worked in psychiatric hospitals are likely to have adapted so thoroughly to the settings that they are insensitive to the impact of that experience. And while there have been occasional reports of researchers who submitted themselves to psychiatric hospitalization (7), these researchers have commonly remained in the hospitals for short periods of time, often with the knowledge of the hospital staff. It is difficult to know the extent to which they were treated like patients or like research colleagues. Nevertheless, their reports about the inside of the psychiatric hospital have been valuable. This article extends those efforts.

Pseudopatients and their Settings

The eight pseudopatients were a varied group. One was a psychology graduate student in his 20's. The remaining seven were older and "established." Among them were three psychologists, a pediatrician, a psychiatrist, a painter, and a housewife. Three pseudopatients were women, five were men. All of them employed pseudonyms, lest their alleged diagnoses embarrass them later. Those who were in mental health professions alleged another occupation in order to avoid the special attentions that might be accorded by staff, as a matter of courtesy or caution, to ailing colleagues (8). With the exception of myself (I was the first pseudopatient and my presence was known to the hospital administrator and chief psychologist and, so far as I can tell, to them alone), the presence of pseudopatients and the nature of the research program was not known to the hospital staffs (9).

The settings were similarly varied. In order to generalize the findings, admission into a variety of hospitals was sought. The 12 hospitals in the sample were located in five different states on the East and West coasts. Some were old and shabby, some were quite new. Some were research-oriented, others not. Some had good staff-patient ratios, others were quite understaffed. Only one was a strictly private hospital. All of the others were supported by state or federal funds or, in one instance, by university funds.

After calling the hospital for an appointment, the pseudopatient arrived at the admissions office complaining that he had been hearing voices. Asked what the voices said, he replied that they were often unclear, but as far as he could tell they said "empty," "hollow," and "thud." The voices were unfamiliar and were of the same sex as the pseudopatient.

The choice of these symptoms was occasioned by their apparent similarity to existential symptoms. Such symptoms are alleged to arise from painful concerns about the perceived meaninglessness of one's life. It is as if the hallucinating person were saying, "My life is empty and hollow." The choice of these symptoms was also determined by the *absence* of a single report of existential psychoses in the literature.

Beyond alleging the symptoms and falsifying name, vocation, and employment, no further alterations of person, history, or circumstances were made. The significant events of the pseudopatient's life history were presented as they had actually occurred. Relationships with parents and siblings, with spouse and children, with people at work and in school, consistent with the aforementioned exceptions, were described as they were or had been. Frustrations and upsets were described along with joys and satisfactions. These facts are important to remember. If anything, they strongly biased the subsequent results in favor of detecting sanity, since none of their histories or current behaviors were seriously pathological in any way.

Immediately upon admission to the psychiatric ward, the pseudopatient ceased simulating *any* symptoms of abnormality. In some cases, there was a brief period of mild nervousness and anxiety, since none of the pseudopatients really believed that they would be admitted so easily. Indeed, their shared fear was that they would be immediately exposed as frauds and greatly embarrassed. Moreover, many of them had never visited a psychiatric ward; even those who had, nevertheless had some genuine fears about what might happen to them. Their nervousness, then, was quite appropriate to the novelty of the hospital setting, and it abated rapidly.

Apart from that short-lived nervousness, the pseudopatient behaved on the ward as he "normally" behaved. The pseudopatient spoke to patients and staff as he might ordinarily. Because there is uncommonly little to do on a psychiatric ward, he attempted to engage others in conversation. When asked by staff how he was feeling, he indicated that he was fine, that he no longer experienced symptoms. He responded to instructions from attendants, to calls for medication (which was not swallowed), and to dining-hall instructions. Beyond such activities as were available to him on the admissions ward, he spent his time writing down his observations about the ward, its patients, and the staff. Initially these notes were written "secretly," but as it soon became clear that no one much cared, they were subsequently written on standard tablets of paper in such public places as the dayroom. No secret was made of these activities.

The pseudopatient, very much as a true psychiatric patient, entered a hospital with no foreknowledge of when he would be discharged. Each was told that he would have to get out by his own devices, essentially by convincing the staff that he was sane. The psychological stresses associated with hospitalization were considerable, and all but one of the pseudopatients desired to be discharged almost immediately after being admitted. They were, therefore, motivated not only to behave sanely, but to be paragons of cooperation. That their behavior was in no way disruptive is confirmed by nursing reports, which have been obtained on most of the patients. These reports uniformly indicate that the patients were "friendly," "cooperative," and "exhibited no abnormal indications."

The Normal are not Detectably Sane

Despite their public "show" of sanity, the pseudopatients were never detected. Admitted, except in one case, with a diagnosis of schizophrenia (10), each was discharged with a diagnosis of schizophrenia "in remission." The label "in remission" should in no way be dismissed as a formality, for at no time during any hospitalization had any question been raised about any pseudopatient's simulation. Nor are there any indications in the hospital records that the pseudopatient's status was suspect. Rather, the evidence is strong that, once labeled schizophrenic, the pseudopatient was stuck with that label. If the pseudopatient was to be discharged, he must naturally be "in remission"; but he was not sane, nor, in the institution's view, had he ever been sane.

The uniform failure to recognize sanity cannot be attributed to the quality of the hospitals, for, although there were considerable variations among them, several are considered excellent. Nor can it be alleged that there was simply not enough time to observe the pseudopatients. Length of hospitalization ranged from 7 to 52 days, with an average of 19 days. The pseudopatients were not, in fact, carefully observed, but this failure clearly speaks more to traditions within psychiatric hospitals than to lack of opportunity.

Finally, it cannot be said that the failure to recognize the pseudopatients' sanity was due to the fact that they were not behaving sanely. While there was clearly some tension present in all of them, their daily visitors could detect no serious behavioral consequences— nor, indeed, could other patients. It was quite common for the patients to "detect" the pseudopatients' sanity. During the first three hospitalizations, when accurate counts were kept, 35 of a total of 118 patients on the admissions ward voiced their suspicions, some vigorously, "You're not crazy. You're a journalist, or a professor [referring to the continual note-taking]. You're checking up on the hospital." While most of the patients were reassured by the pseudopatient's insistence that he had been sick before he came in but was fine now, some continued to believe that the pseudopatient was sane throughout his hospitalization (11). The fact that the patients often recognized normality when staff did not raises important questions.

Failure to detect sanity during the course of hospitalization may be due to the fact that physicians operate with a strong bias toward what statisticians call the type 2 error (5), This is to say that physicians are more inclined to call a healthy person sick (a false positive, type 2) than a sick person healthy (a false negative, type 1). The reasons for this are not hard to find: it is clearly more dangerous to misdiagnose illness than health. Better to err on the side of caution, to suspect illness even among the healthy.

But what holds for medicine does not hold equally well for psychiatry. Medical illnesses, while unfortunate, are not commonly pejorative. Psychiatric diagnoses, on the contrary, carry with them personal, legal, and social stigmas (12). It was therefore important to see whether the tendency toward diagnosing the sane insane could be reversed. The following experiment was arranged at a research and teaching hospital whose staff had heard these findings but doubted that such an error could occur in their hospital. The staff was informed that at some time during the following 3 months, one or more pseudopatients would attempt to be admitted into the psychiatric hospital. Each staff member was asked to rate each patient who presented himself at admissions or on the ward according to the likelihood that the patient was a pseudopatient. A 10-point scale was used, with a 1 and 2 reflecting high confidence that the patient was a pseudopatient.

Judgments were obtained on 193 patients who were admitted for psychiatric treatment. All staff who had had sustained contact with or primary responsibility for the patient— attendants, nurses, psychiatrists, physicians, and psychologists—were asked to make judgments. Forty-one patients were alleged, with high confidence, to be pseudopatients by at least one member of the staff. Twenty-three were considered suspect by at least one psychiatrist. Nineteen were suspected by one psychiatrist *and* one other staff member. Actually, no genuine pseudopatient (at least from my group) presented himself during this period.

The experiment is instructive. It indicates that the tendency to designate sane people as insane can be reversed when the stakes (in this case, prestige and diagnostic acumen) are high. But what can be said of the 19 people who were suspected of being "sane" by one psychiatrist and another staff member? Were these people truly "sane," or was it rather the case that in the course of avoiding the type 2 error the staff tended to make more errors of the first sort—calling the crazy "sane"? There is no way of knowing. But one thing is certain: any diagnostic process that tends itself so readily to massive errors of this sort cannot be a very reliable one.

The Stickiness of Psychodiagnostic Labels

Beyond the tendency to call the healthy sick—-a tendency that accounts better for diagnostic behavior on admission than it does for such behavior after a lengthy period of exposure— the data speak to the massive role of labeling in psychiatric assessment. Having once been labeled schizophrenic, there is nothing the pseudopatient can do to overcome the tag. The tag profoundly colors others' perceptions of him and his behavior.

From one viewpoint, these data are hardly surprising, for it has long been known that elements are given meaning by the context in which they occur. Gestalt psychology made this point vigorously, and Asch (13) demonstrated that there are "central" personality traits (such as "warm" versus "cold") which are so powerful that they markedly color the meaning of other information in forming an impression of a given personality (14). "Insane," "schizophrenic," "manic-depressive," and "crazy" are probably among the most powerful of such central traits. Once a person is designated abnormal, all of his other behaviors and characteristics are colored by that label. Indeed, that label is so powerful that many of the pseudopatients' normal behaviors were overlooked entirely or profoundly misinterpreted. Some examples may clarify this issue.

Earlier I indicated that there were no changes in the pseudopatient's personal history and current status beyond those of name, employment, and, where necessary, vocation. Otherwise, a veridical description of personal history and circumstances was offered. Those circumstances were not psychotic. How were they made consonant with the diagnosis of psychosis? Or were those diagnoses modified in such a way as to bring them into accord with the circumstances of the pseudopatient's life, as described by him?

As far as I can determine, diagnoses were in no way affected by the relative health of the circumstances of a pseudopatient's life. Rather, the reverse occurred: the perception of his circumstances was shaped entirely by the diagnosis. A clear example of such translation is found in the case of a pseudopatient who had had a close relationship with his mother but was rather remote from his father during his early childhood. During adolescence and beyond, however, his father became a close friend, while his relationship with his mother cooled. His present relationship with his wife was characteristically close and warm. Apart from occasional angry exchanges, friction was minimal. The children had rarely been spanked. Surely there is nothing especially pathological about such a history. Indeed, many readers may see a similar pattern in their own experiences, with no markedly deleterious consequences. Observe, however, how such a history was translated in the psychopathological context, this from the case summary prepared after the patient was discharged.

> This white 39-year-old male ... manifests a long history of considerable ambivalence in close relationships, which begins in early childhood. A warm relationship with his mother cools during his adolescence. A distant relationship to his father is described as becoming very intense. Affective stability is absent. His attempts to control emotionality with his wife and children are punctuated by angry outbursts and, in the case of the children, spankings. And while he

says that he has several good friends, one senses considerable ambivalence embedded in those relationships also ....

The facts of the case were unintentionally distorted by the staff to achieve consistency with a popular theory of the dynamics of a schizophrenic reaction (15). Nothing of an ambivalent nature had been described in relations with parents, spouse, or friends. To the extent that ambivalence could be inferred, it was probably not greater than is found in all human relationships. It is true the pseudopatient's relationships with his parents changed over time, but in the ordinary context that would hardly be remarkable—indeed, it might very well be expected. Clearly, the meaning ascribed to his verbalizations (that is, ambivalence, affective instability) was determined by the diagnosis: schizophrenia. An entirely different meaning would have been ascribed if it were known that the man was "normal."

All pseudopatients took extensive notes publicly. Under ordinary circumstances, such behavior would have raised questions in the minds of observers, as, in fact, it did among patients. Indeed, it seemed so certain that the notes would elicit suspicion that elaborate precautions were taken to remove them from the ward each day. But the precautions proved needless. The closest any staff member came to questioning these notes occurred when one pseudopatient asked his physician what kind of medication he was receiving and began to write down the response. "You needn't write it," he was told gently. "If you have trouble remembering, just ask me again."

If no questions were asked of the pseudopatients, how was their writing interpreted? Nursing records for three patients indicate that the writing was seen as an aspect of their pathological behavior. "Patient engages in writing behavior" was the daily nursing comment on one of the pseudopatients who was never questioned about his writing. Given that the patient is in the hospital, he must be psychologically disturbed. And given that he is disturbed, continuous writing must be a behavioral manifestation of that disturbance, perhaps a subset of the compulsive behaviors that are sometimes correlated with schizophrenia.

One tacit characteristic of psychiatric diagnosis is that it locates the sources of aberration within the individual and only rarely within the complex of stimuli that surrounds him. Consequently, behaviors that are stimulated by the environment are commonly misattributed to the patient's disorder. For example, one kindly nurse found a pseudopatient pacing the long hospital corridors. "Nervous, Mr. X?" she asked. "No, bored," he said.

The notes kept by pseudopatients are full of patient behaviors that were misinterpreted by well-intentioned staff. Often enough, a patient would go "berserk" because he had, wittingly or unwittingly, been mistreated by, say, an attendant. A nurse coming upon the scene would rarely inquire even cursorily into the environmental stimuli of the patient's behavior. Rather, she assumed that his upset derived from his pathology, not from his present interactions with other staff members. Occasionally, the staff might assume that the patient's family (especially when they had recently visited) or other patients had stimulated the outburst. But never were the staff found to assume that one of themselves or the structure of the hospital had anything to do with a patient's behavior. One psychiatrist pointed to a group of patients who were sitting outside the cafeteria entrance half an hour before lunchtime. To a group of young residents he indicated that such behavior was characteristic of the oral-acquisitive nature of the syndrome. It seemed not to occur to him that there were very few things to anticipate in a psychiatric hospital besides eating.

A psychiatric label has a life and an influence of its own. Once the impression has been formed that the patient is schizophrenic, the expectation is that he will continue to be schizophrenic. When a sufficient amount of time has passed, during which the patient has done nothing bizarre, he is considered to be in remission and available for discharge. But the label endures beyond discharge, with the unconfirmed expectation that he will behave as a schizophrenic again. Such labels, conferred by mental health professionals, are as influential on the patient as they are on his relatives and friends, and it should not surprise anyone that the diagnosis acts on all of them as a self-fulfilling prophecy. Eventually, the patient himself accepts the diagnosis, with all of its surplus meanings and expectations, and behaves accordingly (5).

The inferences to be made from these matters are quite simple. Much as Zigler and Phillips have demonstrated that there is enormous overlap in the symptoms presented by patients who have been variously diagnosed (16), so there is enormous overlap in the behaviors of the sane and the insane. The sane are not "sane" all of the time. We lose our tempers "for no good reason." We are occasionally depressed or anxious, again for no good reason. And we may find it difficult to get along with one or another person—again for no reason that we can specify. Similarly, the insane are not always insane. Indeed, it was the impression of the pseudopatients while living with them that they were sane for long periods of time—that the bizarre behaviors upon which their diagnoses were allegedly predicated constituted only a small fraction of their total behavior. If it makes no sense to label ourselves permanently depressed on the basis of an occasional depression, then it takes better evidence than is presently available to label all patients insane or schizophrenic on the basis of bizarre behaviors or cognitions. It seems more useful, as Mischel (17) has pointed out, to limit our discussions to *behaviors*, the stimuli that provoke them, and their correlates.

It is not known why powerful impressions of personality traits, such as "crazy" or "insane," arise. Conceivably, when the origins of and stimuli that give rise to a behavior are remote or unknown, or when the behavior strikes us as immutable, trait labels regarding the *behaver* arise. When, on the other hand, the origins and stimuli are known and available, discourse is limited to the behavior itself. Thus, I may hallucinate because I am sleeping, or I may hallucinate because I have ingested a peculiar drug. These are termed sleep-induced hallucinations, or dreams, and drug-induced hallucinations, respectively. But when the stimuli to my hallucinations are unknown, that is called craziness, or schizophrenia—as if that inference were somehow as illuminating as the others.

The Experience of Psychiatric Hospitalization

The term "mental illness" is of recent origin. It was coined by people who were humane in their inclinations and who wanted very much to raise the station of (and the public's sympathies toward) the psychologically disturbed from that of witches and "crazies" to one that was akin to the physically ill. And they were at least partially successful, for the treatment of the mentally ill *has* improved considerably over the years. But while treatment has improved, it is doubtful that people really regard the mentally ill in the same way that they view the physically ill. A broken leg is something one recovers from, but mental illness allegedly endures forever (18), A broken leg does not threaten the observer, but a crazy schizophrenic? There is by now a host of evidence that attitudes toward the mentally ill are characterized by fear, hostility, aloofness, suspicion, and dread (19). The mentally ill are society's lepers.

That such attitudes infect the general population is perhaps not surprising, only upsetting. But that they affect the professionals—attendants, nurses, physicians, psychologists, and social workers—who treat and deal with the mentally ill is more disconcerting, both because such attitudes are self-evidently pernicious and because they are unwitting. Most mental health professionals would insist that they are sympathetic toward the mentally ill, that they are neither avoidant nor hostile. But it is more likely that an exquisite ambivalence characterizes their relations with psychiatric patients, such that their avowed impulses are only part of their entire attitude. Negative attitudes are there too and can easily be detected. Such attitudes should not surprise us. They are the natural offspring of the labels patients wear and the places in which they are found.

Consider the structure of the typical psychiatric hospital. Staff and patients are strictly segregated. Staff have their own living space, including their dining facilities, bathrooms, and assembly places. The glassed quarters that contain the professional staff, which the pseudopatients came to call "the cage," sit out on every dayroom. The staff emerge primarily for caretaking purposes—-to give medication, to conduct a therapy or group meeting, to instruct or reprimand a patient. Otherwise, staff keep to themselves, almost as if the disorder that afflicts their charges is somehow catching.

So much is patient-staff segregation the rule that, for four public hospitals in which an attempt was made to measure the degree to which staff and patients mingle, it was necessary to use "time out of the staff cage" as the operational measure. While it was not the case that all time spent out of the cage was spent mingling with patients (attendants, for example, would occasionally emerge to watch television in the dayroom), it was the only way in which one could gather reliable data on time for measuring.

The average amount of time spent by attendants outside of the cage was 11.3 percent (range, 3 to 52 percent). This figure does not represent only time spent mingling with patients, but also includes time spent on such chores as folding laundry, supervising patients while they shave, directing ward cleanup, and sending patients to off-ward activities. It was the relatively rare attendant who spent time talking with patients or playing games with them. It proved impossible to obtain a "percent mingling time" for nurses, since the amount of time they spent out of the cage was too brief. Rather, we counted instances of emergence from the cage. On the average, daytime nurses emerged from the cage 11.5 times per shift, including instances when they left the ward entirely (range, 4 to 39 times). Late afternoon and night nurses were even less available, emerging on the average 9.4 times per shift (range, 4 to 41 times). Data on early morning nurses, who arrived usually after midnight and departed at 8 a.m., are not available because patients were asleep during most of this period.

Physicians, especially psychiatrists, were even less available. They were rarely seen on the wards. Quite commonly, they would be seen only when they arrived and departed, with the remaining time being spent in their offices or in the cage. On the average, physicians emerged on the ward 6.7 times per day (range, 1 to 17 times). It proved difficult to make an accurate estimate in this regard, since physicians often maintained hours that allowed them to come and go at different times.

The hierarchical organization of the psychiatric hospital has been commented on before (20), but the latent meaning of that kind of organization is worth noting again. Those with the most power have least to do with patients, and those with the least power are most involved with them. Recall, however, that the acquisition of role-appropriate behaviors occurs mainly through the observation of others, with the most powerful having the most influence. Consequently, it is understandable that attendants not only spend more time with patients than do any other members of the staff—that is required by their station in the hierarchy—but also, insofar as they learn from their superiors' behavior, spend as little time with patients as they can. Attendants are seen mainly in the cage, which is where the models, the action, and the power are.

I turn now to a different set of studies, these dealing with staff response to patient-initiated contact. It has long been known that the amount of time a person spends with you can be an index of your significance to him. If he initiates and maintains eye contact, there is reason to believe that he is considering your requests and needs. If he pauses to chat or actually stops and talks, there is added reason to infer that he is individuating you. In four hospitals, the pseudopatient approached the staff member with a request which took the following form:

Table 15.1. Self-Initiated Contact by Pseudopatients with Psychiatrists and Nurses and Attendants, Compared to Contact with Other Groups

Contact	Psychiatric hospitals		University campus (nonmedical)	University medical center		
				Physicians		
	(1) Psychiatrists	(2) Nurses and attendants	(3) Faculty	(4) "Looking for a psychiatrist"	(5) "Looking for a internist"	(6) No additional comment
Responses						
Moves on, head averted (%)	71	88	0	0	0	0
Makes eye contact (%)	23	10	0	11	0	0
Pauses and chats (%)	2	2	0	11	0	10
Stops and talks (%)	4	0.5	100	78	100	90
Mean number of questions answered (out of 6)	*	*	6	3.8	4.8	4.5
Respondents (No.)	13	47	14	18	15	10
Attempts (No.)	185	1283	14	18	15	10

*Not applicable.

"Pardon me, Mr. [or Dr. or Mrs.] X, could you tell me when I will be eligible for grounds privileges?" (or " ... when I will be presented at the staff meeting?" or "... when I am likely to be discharged?"). While the content of the question varied according to the appropriateness of the target and the pseudopatient's (apparent) current needs, the form was always a courteous and relevant request for information. Care was taken never to approach a particular member of the staff more than once a day, lest the staff member become suspicious or irritated. In examining these data, remember that the behavior of the pseudopatients was neither bizarre nor disruptive. One could indeed engage in good conversation with them.

The data for these experiments are shown in Table 15.1, separately for physicians (column 1) and for nurses and attendants (column 2). Minor differences between these four institutions were overwhelmed by the degree to which staff avoided continuing contacts that patients had initiated. By far, their most common response consisted of either a brief response to the question, offered while they were "on the move" and with head averted, or no response at all.

The encounter frequently took the following bizarre form: (pseudopatient) "Pardon me, Dr. X. Could you tell me when I am eligible for grounds privileges?" (physician) "Good morning, Dave. How are you today?" (Moves off without waiting for a response.)

It is instructive to compare these data with data recently obtained at Stanford University. It has been alleged that large and eminent universities are characterized by faculty who are so busy that they have no time for students. For this comparison, a young lady approached individual faculty members who seemed to be walking purposefully to some meeting or teaching engagement and asked them the following six questions.

1. "Pardon me, could you direct me to Encina Hall?" (at the medical school: "…to the Clinical Research Center?").
2. "Do you know where Fish Annex is?" (there is no Fish Annex at Stanford).
3. "Do you teach here?"
4. "How does one apply for admission to the college?" (at the medical school, "…to the medical school?").
5. "Is it difficult to get in?"
6. "Is there financial aid?"

> Without exception, as can be seen in Table 15.1 (column 3), all of the questions were answered. No matter how rushed they were, all respondents not only maintained eye contact, but stopped to talk. Indeed, many of the respondents went out of their way to direct or take the questioner to the office she was seeking, to try to locate "Fish Annex," or to discuss with her the possibilities of being admitted to the university.

Similar data, also shown in Table 15.1 (columns 4, 5, and 6), were obtained in the hospital. Here too, the young lady came prepared with six questions. After the first question, however, she remarked to 18 of her respondents (column 4), "I'm looking for a psychiatrist," and to 15 others (column 5), "I'm looking for an internist." Ten other respondents received no inserted comment (column 6). The general degree of cooperative responses is considerably higher for these university groups than it was for pseudopatients in psychiatric hospitals. Even so, differences are apparent within the medical school setting. Once having indicated that she was looking for a psychiatrist, the degree of cooperation elicited was less than when she sought an internist.

Powerlessness and Depersonalization

Eye contact and verbal contact reflect concern and individuation; their absence, avoidance and depersonalization. The data I have presented do not do justice to the rich daily encounters that grew up around matters of depersonalization and avoidance. I have records of patients who were beaten by staff for the sin of having initiated verbal contact. During my own experience, for example, one patient was beaten in the presence of other patients for having approached an attendant and told him, "I like you." Occasionally, punishment meted out to patients for misdemeanors seemed so excessive that it could not be justified by the most radical interpretations of psychiatric canon. Nevertheless, they appeared to go unquestioned. Tempers were often short. A patient who had not heard a call for medication would be roundly excoriated, and the morning attendants would often wake patients with, "Come on, you m-----f-----s, out of bed!"

Neither anecdotal nor "hard" data can convey the overwhelming sense of powerlessness which invades the individual as he is continually exposed to the depersonalization of the psychiatric hospital. It hardly matters which psychiatric hospital—the excellent public ones and the very plush private hospital were better than the rural and shabby ones in this regard, but, again, the features that psychiatric hospitals had in common overwhelmed by far their apparent differences.

Powerlessness was evident everywhere. The patient is deprived of many of his legal rights by dint of his psychiatric commitment (21). He is shorn of credibility by virtue of his psychiatric label. His freedom of movement is restricted. He cannot initiate contact with the staff, but may only respond to such overtures as they make. Personal privacy is minimal. Patient quarters and possessions can be entered and examined by any staff member, for whatever reason. His personal history and anguish is available to any staff member (often including the "grey lady" and "candy striper" volunteer) who chooses to read his folder, regardless of their therapeutic relationship to him. His personal hygiene and waste evacuation are often monitored. The water closets may have no doors.

At times, depersonalization reached such proportions that pseudopatients had the sense that they were invisible, or at least unworthy of account. Upon being admitted, I and other pseudopatients took the initial physical examinations in a semipublic room, where staff members went about their own business as if we were not there.

On the ward, attendants delivered verbal and occasionally serious physical abuse to patients in the presence of other observing patients, some of whom (the pseudopatients) were writing it all down. Abusive behavior, on the other hand, terminated quite abruptly when other staff members were known to be coming. Staff are credible witnesses. Patients are not.

A nurse unbuttoned her uniform to adjust her brassiere in the presence of an entire ward of viewing men. One did not have the sense that she was being seductive. Rather, she did not notice us. A group of staff persons might point to a patient in the dayroom and discuss him animatedly, as if he were not there.

One illuminating instance of depersonalization and invisibility occurred with regard to medications. All told, the pseudopatients were administered nearly 2100 pills, including Elavil, Stelazine, Compazine, and Thorazine, to name but a few. (That such a variety of medications should have been administered to patients presenting identical symptoms is itself worthy of note.) Only two were swallowed. The rest were either pocketed or deposited in the toilet. The pseudopatients were not alone in this. Although I have no precise records on how many patients rejected their medications, the pseudopatients frequently found the medications of other patients in the toilet before they deposited their own. As long as they were cooperative, their behavior and the pseudopatients' own in this matter, as in other important matters, went unnoticed throughout.

Reactions to such depersonalization among pseudopatients were intense. Although they had come to the hospital as participant observers and were fully aware that they did not "belong," they nevertheless found themselves caught up in and fighting the process of depersonalization. Some examples: a graduate student in psychology asked his wife to bring his textbooks to the hospital so he could "catch up on his homework"—this despite the elaborate precautions taken to conceal his professional association. The same student, who had trained for quite some time to get into the hospital, and who had looked forward to the experience, "remembered" some drag races that he had wanted to see on the weekend and insisted that he be discharged by that time. Another pseudopatient attempted a romance with a nurse. Subsequently, he informed the staff that he was applying for admission to graduate school in psychology and was very likely to be admitted, since a graduate professor was one of his regular hospital visitors. The same person began to engage in psychotherapy with other patients—all of this as a way of becoming a person in an impersonal environment.

The Sources of Depersonalization

What are the origins of depersonalization? I have already mentioned two. First are attitudes held by all of us toward the mentally ill—including those who treat them—attitudes characterized by fear, distrust, and horrible expectations on the one hand, and benevolent intentions on the other. Our ambivalence leads, in this instance as in others, to avoidance.

Second, and not entirely separate, the hierarchical structure of the psychiatric hospital facilitates depersonalization. Those who are at the top have least to do with patients, and their behavior inspires the rest of the staff. Average daily contact with psychiatrists, psychologists, residents, and physicians combined ranged from 3.9 to 25.1 minutes, with an overall mean of 6.8 (six pseudopatients over a total of 129 days of hospitalization). Included in this average are time spent in the admissions interview, ward meetings in the presence of a senior staff member, group and individual psychotherapy contacts, case presentation conferences, and discharge meetings. Clearly, patients do not spend much time in interpersonal contact with doctoral staff. And doctoral staffs serve as models for nurses and attendants.

There are probably other sources. Psychiatric installations are presently in serious financial straits. Staff shortages are pervasive, staff time at a premium. Something has to give, and that something is patient contact. Yet, while financial stresses are realities, too much can be made of them. I have the impression that the psychological forces that result in depersonalization are much stronger than the fiscal ones and that the addition of more staff would not correspondingly improve patient care in this regard. The incidence of staff meetings and the enormous amount of record-keeping on patients, for example, have not been as substantially reduced as has patient contact. Priorities exist, even during hard times. Patient contact is not a significant priority in the traditional psychiatric hospital, and fiscal pressures do not account for this. Avoidance and depersonalization may.

Heavy reliance upon psychotropic medication tacitly contributes to depersonalization by convincing staff that treatment is indeed being conducted and that further patient contact may not be necessary. Even here, however, caution needs to be exercised in understanding the role of psychotropic drugs. If patients were powerful rather than powerless, if they were viewed as interesting individuals rather than diagnostic entities, if they were socially significant rather than social lepers, if their anguish truly and wholly compelled our sympathies and concerns, would we not *seek* contact with them, despite the availability of medications? Perhaps for the pleasure of it all?

The Consequences of Labeling and Depersonalization

Whenever the ratio of what is known to what needs to be known approaches zero, we tend to invent "knowledge" and assume that we understand more than we actually do. We seem unable to acknowledge that we simply don't know. The needs for diagnosis and remediation of behavioral and emotional problems are enormous. But rather than acknowledge that we are just embarking on understanding, we continue to label patients "schizophrenic," "manic-depressive," and "insane," as if in those words we had captured the essence of understanding. The facts of the matter are that we have known for a long time that diagnoses are often not useful or reliable, but we have nevertheless continued to use them. We now know that we cannot distinguish insanity from sanity. It is depressing to consider how that information will be used.

Not merely depressing, but frightening. How many people, one wonders, are sane but not recognized as such in our psychiatric institutions? How many have been needlessly stripped of their privileges of citizenship, from the right to vote and drive to that of handling their own accounts? How many have feigned insanity in order to avoid the criminal consequences of their behavior, and, conversely, how many would rather stand trial than live interminably in a psychiatric hospital—but are wrongly thought to be mentally ill? How many have been stigmatized by well-intentioned, but nevertheless erroneous, diagnoses? On the last point, recall again that a "type 2 error" in psychiatric diagnosis does not have the same consequences it does in medical diagnosis. A diagnosis of cancer that has been found to be in error is cause for celebration. But psychiatric diagnoses are rarely found to be in error. The label sticks, a mark of inadequacy forever.

Finally, how many patients might be "sane" outside the psychiatric hospital but seem insane in it—not because craziness resides in them, as it were, but because they are responding to a bizarre setting, one that may be unique to institutions which harbor neither people? Goffman (4) calls the process of socialization to such institutions "mortification"—an apt metaphor that includes the processes of depersonalization that have been described here. And while it is impossible to know whether the pseudopatients' responses to these processes are characteristic of all inmates—they were, after all, not real patients—it is difficult to believe that these processes of socialization to a psychiatric hospital provide useful attitudes or habits of response for living in the "real world,"

Summary and Conclusions

It is clear that we cannot distinguish the sane from the insane in psychiatric hospitals. The hospital itself imposes a special environment in which the meanings of behavior can easily be misunderstood. The consequences to patients hospitalized in such an environment—the powerlessness, depersonalization, segregation, mortification, and self-labeling—seem undoubtedly countertherapeutic.

I do not, even now, understand this problem well enough to perceive solutions. But two matters seem to have some promise. The first concerns the proliferation of community mental health facilities, of crisis intervention centers, of the human potential movement, and of behavior therapies that, for all of their own problems, tend to avoid psychiatric labels, to focus on specific problems and behaviors, and to retain the individual in a relatively non-pejorative environment. Clearly, to the extent that we refrain from sending the distressed to insane places, our impressions of them are less likely to be distorted. (The risk of distorted perceptions, it seems to me, is always present, since we are much more sensitive to an individual's behaviors and verbalizations than we are to the subtle contextual stimuli that often promote them. At issue here is a matter of magnitude. And, as I have shown, the magnitude of distortion is exceedingly high in the extreme context that is a psychiatric hospital.)

The second matter that might prove promising speaks to the need to increase the sensitivity of mental health workers and researchers to the *Catch 22* position of psychiatric patients. Simply reading materials in this area will be of help to some such workers and researchers. For others, directly experiencing the impact of psychiatric hospitalization will be of enormous use. Clearly, further research into the social psychology of such total institutions will both facilitate treatment and deepen understanding.

I and the other pseudopatients in the psychiatric setting had distinctly negative reactions. We do not pretend to describe the subjective experiences of true patients. Theirs may be different from ours, particularly with the passage of time and the necessary process of adaptation to one's environment. But we can and do speak to the relatively more objective indices of treatment within the hospital. It could be a mistake, and a very unfortunate one, to consider that what happened to us derived from malice or stupidity on the part of the staff. Quite the contrary, our overwhelming impression of them was of people who really cared, who were committed and who were uncommonly intelligent. Where they failed, as they sometimes did painfully, it would be more accurate to attribute those failures to the environment in which they, too, found themselves than to personal callousness. Their perceptions and behavior were controlled by the situation, rather than being motivated by a malicious disposition. In a more benign environment, one that was less attached to global diagnosis, their behaviors and judgments might have been more benign and effective.

References and Notes

1. P. Ash, *J. Abnorm. Soc. Psychol.* 44, 272 (1949); A. T. Beck, *Amer. J. Psychiat.* 119, 210 (1962); A. T. Boisen, *Psychiatry* 2, 233 (1938); N. Kreitman, *J. Ment. Sci.* 107, 876 (1961); N. Kreitman, P. Sainsbury, J. Morrisey, J. Towers, J. Scrivener, *ibid.,* p. 887; H. O. Schmitt and C. P. Fonda, *J. Abnorm. Soc. Psychol.* 52, 262 (1956); W. Seeman, *J. Nerv. Ment. Dis.* 118, 541 (1953). For an analysis of these artifacts and summaries of the disputes, see J. Zubin, *Annu. Rev. Psychol. 18,* 373 (1967); L. Phillips and J. G. Draguns, *ibid.* 22, 447 (1971).
2. R. Benedict, *J. Gen. Psychol.* 10, 59 (1934).
3. See in this regard H. Becker, *Outsiders: Studies in the Sociology of Deviance* (Free Press, New York, 1963); B. M. Braginsky, D. D. Braginsky, K. Ring, *Methods of Madness: The Mental Hospital as a Lost Resort* (Holt, Rinehart & Winston, New York, 1969); C. M. Crocetti and P. V. Lemkau. *Am. Soc. Rev.* 30, 577 (1965); E. Goffman, *Behavior in Public Places* (Free Press, New York, 1954); R. D. Laing. *The Divided Self: A Study of Sanity and Madness* (Quadrangle, Chicago, 1960); D. L. Phillips, *Am. Soc. Rev.* 28, 963 (1963); T. R. Sarbin, *Psychol. Today* 6, 18 (1972); E. Schut, *Am. J. Soc.* 75, 309 (1969); T. Szasz, *Law, Liberty and Psychiatry* (Macmillan, New York, 1963); *The Myth of Mental Illness: Foundations of a Theory of Mental Illness* (Hoeber Harper, New York, 1963). For a critique of some of these views, see W. R. Gove, *Am. Soc. Rev.* 35, 873 (1970).
4. E. Goffman, *Asylums* (Doubleday, Garden City, NY, 1961).
5. T. J. Scheff, *Being Mentally Ill: A Sociological Theory* (Aldine, Chicago, 1966).
6. Data from a ninth pseudopatient are not incorporated in this report because, although his sanity went undetected, he falsified aspects of his personal history, including his marital status and parental relationships. His experimental behaviors therefore were not identical to those of the other pseudopatients.
7. A. Barry, *Bellevue Is a State of Mind* (Harcourt Brace Jovanovich, New York, 1971); I. Belknap, *Human Problems at a State Mental Hospital* (McGraw-Hill, New York, 1956); W. Caudill, F. C. Redlich, H. R. Gilmore, E. B. Brody, *Am. J. Orthopsychiat.* 22, 314 (1952); A. R. Goldman, R. H. Bohr, T. A. Steinberg, *Prof. Psychol.* 1, 427 (1970); unauthored, *Roche Rep.* 1 (No. 13), 8 (1971).
8. Beyond the personal difficulties that the pseudopatient is likely to experience in the hospital, there are legal and social ones that, combined, require considerable attention before entry. For example, once admitted to a psychiatric institution, it is difficult, if not impossible, to be discharged on short notice, state law to the contrary notwithstanding. I was not sensitive to these difficulties at the outset of the project, nor to the personal and situational emergencies that can arise, but later a writ of habeas corpus was prepared for each of the entering pseudopatients and an attorney was kept "on call" during every hospitalization. I am grateful to John Kaplan and Robert Bartels for legal advice and assistance in these matters.
9. However distasteful such concealment is, it was a necessary first step to examining these questions. Without concealment, there would have been no way to know how valid these experiences were; nor was there any way of knowing whether whatever detections occurred were a tribute to the diagnostic acumen of the staff or to the hospital's rumor network. Obviously, since my concerns are general ones that cut across individual hospitals and staffs, I have respected their anonymity and have eliminated clues that might lead to their identification.
10. Interestingly, of the 12 admissions, 11 were diagnosed as schizophrenic and one, with the identical symptomatology, as manic-depressive psychosis. This diagnosis has a more favorable prognosis, and it was given by the only private hospital in our sample. On the relations

between social class and psychiatric diagnosis, see A. deB. Hollingshead and F. C. Redlich, *Social Class and Mental Illness: A Community Study* (Wiley, New York, 1958).

11. It is possible, of course, that patients have quite broad latitudes in diagnosis and therefore are inclined to call many people sane, even those whose behavior is patently aberrant. However, although we have no hard data on this matter, it was our distinct impression that this was not the case. In many instances, patients not only singled us out for attention, but came to imitate our behaviors and styles.

12. J. Cumming and E. Cumming, *Commun. Ment. Health* 1, 135 (1965); A. Farina and K. Ring. *J. Abnorm. Psychol.* 70. 47 (1965); H. E. Freeman and O. G. Simmons, *The Mental Patient Comes Home* (Wiley, New York, 1963); W J. Johannsen, *Ment. Hygiene* 53, 218 (1969); A. S. Linsky, *Soc. Psychiat.* 5, 166 (1970).

13. S. E. Asch, *J. Abnorm. Soc. Psychol.* 41, 258 (1946); *Social Psychology* (Prentice-Hall, New York, 1952),

14. See also I. N. Mensh and J. Wishner, *J. Person.* 16, 188 (1947); *J.* Wishner, *Psychol. Rev.* 67, 96 (1960); J. S. Bruner and R. Tagiuri, *in Handbook of Social Psychology,* G. Lindsey, Ed. (Addison-Wesley, Cambridge, Mass., 1954), vol. 2, pp. 634–654; J. S. Bruner, D. Shapiro, R. Tagiuri, in *Person Perception and Interpersonal Behavior,* R. Tagiuri and L. Petrullo, Eds. (Stanford University Press, Stanford, Calif., 1958), pp. 277–288.

15. For an example of a similar self-fulfilling prophecy, in this instance dealing with the "central" trait of intelligence, see R. Rosenthal and L. Jacobson, *Pygmalion in the Classroom* (Holt, Rinehart & Winston, New York, 1968),

16. E. Zigler and L. Phillips, *J. Abnorm. Soc. Psychol. 63,* 69 (1961). See also R. K. Freudenberg and J. P. Robertson, *A.M.A, Arch. Neurol. Psychiatr.* 76, 14 (1956).

17. W. Mischel, *Personality and Assessment* (Wiley, New York, 1968).

18. The most recent and unfortunate instance of this tenet is that of Senator Thomas Eagleton.

19. T. R. Sarbin and J. C. Mancuso, *J. Clin. Consult. Psychol.* 35, 159 (1970); T. R. Sarbin, *ibid.* 31, 447 (1967); J. C. Nunnally, Jr., *Popular Conceptions of Mental Health* (Holt, Rinehart & Winston, New York, 1961).

20. A. H. Stanton and M. S. Schwartz, *The Mental Hospital: A Study of Institutional Participation in Psychiatric Illness and Treatment* (Basic, New York, 1954).

21. D. B. Wexler and S. E. Scoville, *Ariz. Law Rev.* 13, 1 (1971).

16

Stein, L. I., Test, M. A., and Marx, A. J. (1975). Alternative to the hospital: A controlled study. *American Journal of Psychiatry*, 132, 517–522

This article is one of several published by Stein, Test, and Marx, in different authorial combinations and orders, on the potential for persons with serious mental illness to live in the community after discharge from psychiatric hospitalization. It reports on the results of an intervention involving intensive training in daily living activities delivered by staff who were also discharged from their hospital positions to work in the community. (This intervention evolved into the current Assertive Community Treatment/ACT approach.) The goal of the research was to give people previously deemed too symptomatic to live outside the hospital support for accomplishing the tasks of everyday living and developing leisure activities that they would need in order to live stably in their home communities. One of the study's primary objectives was to give participants the opportunity to develop skills in coping with community life. As a means of decreasing dependency, which the authors hypothesized to be the key reason for rehospitalization, participants were exposed to social contingencies such as eviction for repeated disruptive behavior rather than being shielded from them by hospitalization. Using randomized assignment to experimental and control groups, they found that experimental intervention participants achieved higher rates of supported employment and had lower rates of unemployment and rehospitalization than control group participants, who received standard treatment. The Stein, Test, and Marx articles, among the most frequently nominated of all our classics, demonstrated that people with serious mental illness could lead stable lives outside hospitals, given the proper combination of treatment and supports.

Elizabeth Flanagan

Alternative to the Hospital:
A Controlled Study

The authors describe the evaluation of a treatment model that makes use of the community to help mentally ill patients acquire necessary coping skills. This approach is based on the assumption that deficiency in coping skills and aggressive dependency are primarily responsible for high readmission rates to mental hospitals and that coping skills and autonomy are best learned in the community, where the patient will be needing and using them. The treatment model is evaluated by comparing it with progressive in-hospital treatment and follow-up care. The results suggest that the model described can successfully treat patients with a high level of symptomatology in the community rather than in the mental hospital.

It is evident that psychiatry is not successfully meeting the treatment needs of a substantial number of patients who come to public mental hospitals. In spite of recent innovative and intensive approaches, such as novel in-hospital programs (1–3), dramatic shortening of patients' hospital stay (4–6), and attempts to make use of community agencies for treatment (7), a sizable percentage of patients continue to spend considerable time in mental institutions, function poorly between admissions, and experience high readmission rates.

It is our contention that this persisting high rate of "treatment failures" is caused by the fact that existing models of treatment do not effectively ameliorate certain disabilities shared by many of these patients. These disabilities, which have been mentioned frequently in the literature (8–11), can be described in two ways: as a limited repertoire of instrumental and problem-solving behaviors to meet the goals and demands of life, leading to persisting difficulties with work habits, socialization, leisure-time activities, etc., and as powerful dependency needs, frequently expressed as an aggressive dependency on family or institutions.

These problems lead to a tenuous community adjustment, keeping patients on the brink of rehospitalization. Patients thus disabled carry various diagnoses, ranging from schizophrenia to dependent personality. However, these disabling characteristics cut across diagnostic categories and can, in fact, represent the rock upon which treatment often founders. For example, the manifestations of an acute schizophrenic episode are managed relatively easily by means of phenothiazine drugs; however, if either a deficiency in coping skills or an aggressive dependency is also present, the problems of discharging and maintaining the patient in the community can be enormous.

In this paper we describe the evaluation of a clinical research program that is a radical departure from the present system of short-term hospitalization plus aftercare. The program, titled "Training in Community Living," was designed to help patients acquire the coping skills and autonomy necessary for a reasonable community adjustment. The model uses the community as a treatment arena; hospitalization is virtually eliminated. The rationale for this approach is based on theoretical and empirical work suggesting that the hospital itself frequently has a debilitating influence on patients (12–14) and, more importantly, that the community has much to offer as an arena for treatment of this population (15–17). The community, in contrast to the hospital, has stronger demand characteristics for appropriate behavior, has more healthy role models for the patients to emulate, and requires much less generalization to implement what is learned in treatment.

This new model for treating severely disturbed patients is being rigorously evaluated by comparing patients treated in the community with a control group receiving the presently available model of progressive in-hospital treatment of short duration plus aftercare services in the community. The relative success of the two models is being considered in terms of a number of patient outcome variables and in terms of social and economic costs. This paper outlines the clinical and research procedures and reports the results of the study to date.

Method

Subjects

The subjects for this ongoing study include all patients seeking admission for inpatient care at Mendota Mental Health Institute who meet the following criteria: 1) residence in Dane County, Wis., which consists of the city of Madison and the surrounding area; 2) age of 18 to 62; and 3) any diagnosis other than severe organic brain syndrome or primary alcoholism.

Experimental Design

Patients meeting the above criteria are randomly assigned to either the community treatment group or the control group by the admission office staff. Control patients are treated in the hospital for as long as deemed necessary and then linked with appropriate community agencies. Experimental patients do not enter the hospital. They are treated according to the training in community living approach for 14 months, after which the staff are no longer available to them. Assessment data on all patients are gathered at baseline (time of admission) and every 4 months for a period of 36 months by means of personal interviews by a research staff. This staff operates independently of both clinical teams.

Control Treatment

Patients assigned to the control group are screened upon admission by a member of the hospital's acute treatment unit serving Dane County. The patients are usually, although not necessarily, admitted to the hospital, where they receive progressive treatment aimed at preparation for return to the community. The Dane County unit serves as a stringent control for the experimental program because it has a high staff-to-patient ratio and offers a wide variety of services, including inpatient treatment, partial hospitalization, and out-patient follow-up. It is by no means a custodial unit; its median length of stay is only 17 days. This unit also makes liberal use of the aftercare services available in Madison for discharged patients.

Experimental Treatment

Work with patients. Patients assigned to the community program are interviewed upon admission by a member of the experimental staff. They are then taken from the admission office to the community to begin their treatment program. Every effort is made to avoid hospitalization, which is used only for patients who are imminently suicidal or homicidal or who are so severely psychotic that they require high doses of medication that can be given only in the hospital's structured environment. In the rare instances when hospitalization is used, it is of short duration so that community treatment can begin with minimal delay.

The community treatment approach focuses directly on an in vivo teaching of coping skills as well as on treating the acute problem that precipitated the patient's coming to the hospital. The patient's treatment consists of participation in a full schedule of daily living activities in the community. Pharmacotherapy is used when appropriate.

The therapeutic input from the staff consists of motivating, supporting, and often being with the patients day and evening. More specifically, staff members, who are "on the spot" in patients' homes and neighborhoods, teach and assist them in such daily living activities as laundry upkeep, shopping, cooking, going to restaurants, grooming, budgeting, and use of transportation. Patients are also given sustained and intensive assistance in finding a job or placement in a sheltered workshop. Staff then continue daily contact with patients and their supervisors or employers to help with on-the-job problem solving.

Patients are aided in the constructive use of leisure time and the development of effective social skills by staff prodding and supporting their involvement in relevant community recreation and social activities. This frequently involves staff members accompanying patients to such functions on a regular basis. In all of these activities, a "can do" philosophy is transmitted from staff to patient, the assets of the patients are stressed, and their symptomatology is played down. Daily, even hourly contact of staff with patients is emphasized initially and then gradually diminished according to each patient's progress in the treatment program.

The staff. To carry out the program, we retrained a mental hospital ward staff, which consisted of a psychiatrist, a psychologist, a social worker, an occupational therapist, nurses, and aides. These staff members spend their time dispersed throughout the community working with patients in such settings as their homes, their places of work, supermarkets, and recreational facilities. They help the patients learn the requisite skills to sustain a satisfactory community adjustment. Twice a day the staff members gather at the project's headquarters, a rented house in downtown Madison, to share information, revise treatment programs as necessary, and plan the next shift's work schedule. There are two shifts, so that the program is well staffed from 7 a.m. until 11 p.m., seven days a week. A member of the professional staff remains on call at night to give 24-hour-a-day coverage for patients as well as for community agencies.

Making use of mental hospital personnel in this kind of extrohospital program has advantages as well as disadvantages. The advantages include the experience of mental hospital personnel in and commitment to working with severely ill patients and their orientation toward working with patient behaviors as well as feelings and cognitions. These workers are also experienced with a team approach; they are willing to rotate shifts so that the program can be operational at all times. The major disadvantage lies in the transition from work in a highly structured hospital setting, where little is required in the way of individual decision making, to work in the inevitably unstructured setting of the community, where a great deal of initiative and willingness to make decisions on the spot is vital. Fortunately, with training and support this transition was possible and the staff members increasingly welcome greater responsibility.

Community agencies. A program of this nature cannot survive unless the community is carefully prepared for its implementation. Before we conducted the pilot study (18) upon which this program is largely based, we held conferences with every relevant community agency to establish the closest of working relationships. Our major goal was to influence them to respond to the patients in a manner that would promote responsible behavior rather than reinforce maladaptive modes of coping with stress. For example, if a patient's behavior was disruptive to other tenants in his apartment building, we would encourage the landlord to talk to the patient directly about his behavior and tell him he would be evicted if it continued. This is in contrast to the community's usual response, which is to see to it that the patient's disruptive behavior leads to rehospitalization. That action implicitly gives the patient the message that he is not responsible for his behavior, teaches the patient a maladaptive mode of coping with stress, and reinforces the chronic patient role.

The manner in which we gained and maintained the cooperation of the supporting agencies in the community in relating to patients as described above is most clearly communicated by the following illustration:

The local sheltered workshop is an agency that we use frequently; we regard its cooperation as essential. Early in our work in community treatment, therefore, we met with the administrative staff of the workshop to discuss our philosophy of treating patients as responsible individuals and to obtain their sanction for our sending highly symptomatic patients to the workshop. After this was accomplished we enrolled several patients in the workshop and gradually developed effective techniques for maintaining the cooperation of this agency. We soon learned that even though we had gained support from the workshop administration, daily contact with floor supervisors was a necessary and useful endeavor because these individuals were relating directly to our patients. Throughout these contacts we urged workshop personnel to operate only in the area of their own expertise, rather than to relate to the patients as if they were therapists.

Our contacts with personnel at the workshop took the following forms: 1) structured meetings were held to review patient progress and to solve problems collaboratively, 2) a member of our staff frequently worked alongside our patients in the workshop as a model for the workshop staff and to discuss with them techniques useful in relating effectively with our patients, and 3) our staff was available on a round-the-clock basis to aid in the handling of crises and to provide assistance in any matter relevant to our patients. While such crisis contacts were usually initiated by a telephone call from workshop personnel, we often found it helpful to go immediately to the site of the problem to demonstrate our willingness to help.

Our assistance most often took the form of consulting with workshop personnel on how they might handle a patient rather than our directly intervening with the patient. Repeated supportive contacts such as these gradually assured the workshop staff that we were not dumping our work on them and provided valuable opportunities for training and problem solving. The result was that many workshop personnel became highly skilled in our training in community living techniques, and the number of crisis calls from this agency greatly diminished.

Modifications of these techniques of constant availability, modeling, support, and collaborative problem solving were successfully used to gain the active cooperation of a wide variety of individuals and agencies in the community. These included landlords, employers, social and recreational leaders, restaurant owners, vocational counselors, mental health workers, the staffs of local emergency rooms, the police, and the district attorney's office.

Summary of guidelines. The community treatment approach focuses directly on the patient disabilities discussed and thus adheres to the following guidelines:

- In-hospital treatment, even with extremely symptomatic patients, is virtually eliminated so as not to reinforce dependency and to prevent institutionalization.
- Treatment concentrates primarily on teaching coping skills necessary to live in the community and enjoy a reasonable quality of life. The learning of these skills takes place solely in the community.
- Work with families and significant others is primarily directed toward the breaking of pathologically dependent relationships.
- Staff members relate to patients as responsible individuals and make maximal efforts to expose them to the natural contingencies of living in society.
- A close relationship is maintained with an exceptional variety of community facilities, from agencies to individuals, to ensure the consistency and continuity of our approach.
- Staff members are assertive in their approach, not only to minimize the possibility of patients dropping out of treatment, but to maximize their engagement in responsible, independent community living.

Measuring Instruments

At the time of their admission to the study, we administer the following measuring instruments to the patients in each group:

Demographic Data Form. We devised this form to collect standard demographic data on the patients' life situation and economic status.

Short Clinical Rating Scale (19). This scale measures symptomatology. We used a summary scale of this measure, the global symptomatology rating, which is a 9-point scale in which $0 =$ none and $8 =$ severe.

Community Adjustment Form. We devised this form to assess the patient's living situation, how much time he had spent in institutions, his employment record, his social relationships, the quality of his environment, his subjective satisfaction with life, and what leisure-time activities he participated in.

Family Burden Scale. At one month, the Family Burden Scale is administered to the most significant other in the patient's family if that person lives in Dane County. We devised this 3-point scale to assess whether or not the experimental approach of treating the patient in the community places more of an emotional and economic burden on family members than does the control approach. A score of 1 on this scale indicates that the family feels no extra burden; a score of 3 indicates severe burden.

Every four months, the global symptomatology rating, the community adjustment form, and the Family Burden Scale are readministered.

Results

The results presented here represent data collected on the first 60 patients in each group during their first four months in the study. These results are important primarily as a measure of the feasibility of implementing our model as an alternative to treatment in a mental hospital.

Characteristics of the Sample

Relevant characteristics of patients in the two treatment groups at the time of admission to the study are presented in Table 16.1. From this table it can be seen that the sample was

Table 16.1. Demographic Characteristics of Experimental Group (N = 60) and Control Group (N = 60) at Time of Admission to the Study

Characteristic	Experimental Group	Control Group	Significance
Sex			n.s.*
Male	33	34	
Female	27	26	
Marital status			n.s.*
Single	30	28	
Married	14	16	
Divorced or separated	16	16	
Mean age	31.3, SD = 10.4	30.6, SD = 11.5	n.s.**
Mean number of months spent in psychiatric institutions before admission to study	15.3, SD = 26.6	11.3, SD = 26.3	n.s.**
Mean global symptomatology rating	4.7, SD = 1.6	3.9, SD = 1.6	p < .01**

*By chi-square test.
**By two-tailed t test.

relatively young, that most patients (approximately 75 percent) were either single, separated, or divorced, and that the patients had accumulated a substantial amount of time in psychiatric institutions before admission to this study.

The only variable on which patients in the experimental group differed significantly from the patients in the control group was global symptomatology: the experimental patients were somewhat more symptomatic than the control patients. This difference is viewed as conservative bias.

Decision To Hospitalize

Only 6 of the 60 experimental patients were hospitalized in comparison with 54 of the 60 control patients (p < .001 by chi-square test). The 6 experimental patients spent a mean of 13.83 days in the hospital (SD = 15.60), and the 54 control patients spent a mean of 22.87 days in the hospital (SD = 20.35). Of the 54 control patients who were hospitalized, 14 were readmitted after being discharged within the first four months of the study, representing a readmission rate of 33 percent in four months.

Living Situation

Table 16.2 summarizes where patients lived during their first four months in the study. The amount of time spent in psychiatric hospitals was, of course, strikingly different in the two groups. There was no significant difference between the groups in the amount of time spent in medical or penal institutions. There was also no significant difference between the two groups in the amount of time spent in sheltered living situations. There was, however, a significant difference in the amount of time spent in independent settings: the experimental patients spent more time in independent settings than the control patients.

Employment Situation

The employment situation of patients in both groups during the first four months of study is shown in Table 16.3. It can be seen that experimental patients spent significantly less

Table 16.2. Living Situations of Experimental Group (N = 52) and Control Group (N = 53) During First Four Months of Study*

| Living Situation | Experimental Group | | Control Group | | |
	Mean	SD	Mean	SD	Significance
Psychiatric institution	1.77	5.77	22.09	21.10	p<.001**
Medical institution	1.15	5.33	0.96	2.93	n.s.**
Penal institution	5.25	16.70	3.52	10.87	n.s.**
Supervised setting***	7.17	18.03	12.34	22.36	n.s.**
Independent setting	84.65	25.40	61.09	32.75	p<.001**

*Expressed as mean percent of four-month period ±SD; the Ns represent the number of patients in each group on whom interviews were completed.
**By two-tailed t test.
***Refers to such places as semisheltered boarding homes, halfway houses, and family care homes.

Table 16.3. Employment Situations of Experimental Group (N = 52) and Control Group (N = 53) During First Four Months of Study*

| Employment Situation | Experimental Group | | Control Group | | |
	Mean	SD	Mean	SD	Significance
Unemployed	36.81	34.42	65.74	32.39	p<.001**
Sheltered employment	30.99	39.96	4.13	10.98	p<.001**
Competitive employment	32.32	38.19	30.04	32.05	n.s.**

*Expressed as mean percent of four-month period ±SD; the Ns represent the number of patients in each group on whom interviews wore completed.
**By two-tailed t test.

time unemployed and significantly more time in sheltered employment than did control patients. There was no significant difference between groups in the amount of time spent in competitive employment. Follow-up data will show whether or not time spent in sheltered employment leads to competitive employment.

Other Measures

As was shown in Table 16.1, both groups scored high (between "moderately" and "markedly" ill) upon entry into the study on the global symptomatology rating. By the end of four months patients in both groups revealed a significant decrease in symptomatology, with no significant difference between groups on amount of improvement. Preliminary measures of social relationships, leisure-time activities, quality of environment, and subjective satisfaction with life also revealed no significant differences between groups at the end of four months.

Family Burden Scale

One month after entry into the study the burden felt by the families of both groups was almost identical. The 18 relatives of patients in the experimental group had a mean rating of 1.89 (SD=.76), and the 16 relatives of patients in the control group had a mean rating of 1.81 (SD=.75). At four months there was a significant decrease in the burden felt by families of experimental patients; their mean rating was 1.44 (SD = .70) (p < .01 by two-tailed t test). However, there was no such decrease in the burden felt by control families; their mean rating remained 1.81 (SD = .75). These results indicate that our community treatment approach did not place excessive stress on the families of experimental patients in comparison with the traditional approach (p < .05 by two-tailed t test).

The relatively small numbers of 18 and 16 for the families of experimental and control groups, respectively, reflect the fact that a high percentage of our patients do not have family living near them.

Discussion

The above results clearly indicate that our extrohospital model is a feasible alternative to mental hospital treatment. While other studies have demonstrated successful alternatives to the mental hospital for selected populations such as patients with families close by (20–22), we used a randomly selected group of patients presenting for admission to a public hospital. Patients were included in the study regardless of symptomatology and regardless of the presence or absence of social resources.

While the longer range data currently being collected are certainly needed to assess the overall effectiveness of the model, the four-month data demonstrate that, in the new model, hospital stays were virtually eliminated, thereby reducing the disruption to life, the social stigma, and the reinforcement of dependency that result from hospitalization. The psychiatric hospital was used less, but there was no increase in the amount of time spent in penal institutions by our experimental patients, and no "mini-hospital" was created in the community. Rather, experimental patients spent most of their time in independent living situations, and the amount of time spent in overall productive functioning was increased. This was accomplished without reducing the individual patient's quality of life or his personal satisfaction with life. It is also important to note that this was accomplished without increasing the burden felt by the patient's family.

These results may be viewed as tautological: i.e., reduction of time in the hospital "creates" increased time in productive community living. To some extent this is true; however, the existence of third-rate boarding houses and hotels crowded with discharged mental patients makes it clear that simply being out of the hospital does not necessarily ensure satisfactory community functioning (23).

A cost-benefit analysis comparing the new model with traditional treatment is in progress to determine the economic feasibility of the program. Data from the economic study as well as data regarding the future clinical outcome of patients will be reported at a later time. Although the primary significance of the current data is in demonstrating that the training in community living model is a feasible alternative for patients who would otherwise be treated in public mental hospitals, it is our hope that the follow-up data will show that this model also enhances the long-range community adjustment of these patients.

References

1. Paul GL: Chronic mental patient: current status: future directions. Psychol Bull 71:81–94, 1969.
2. Sanders R, Smith RS, Weinman BS: Chronic Psychoses and Recovery. San Francisco, Jossey-Bass, 1967.

3. Fairweather GW: Social Psychology in Treating Mental Illness. New York, John Wiley & Sons, 1964.
4. Caffey EM Jr, Jones RD, Diamond LS, et al: Brief hospital treatment of schizophrenia—early results of a multiple-hospital study. Hosp Community Psychiatry 19:282–287, 1968.
5. Grad J, Lubach JE: An intensive treatment program for psychiatric inpatients: a description and evaluation. J Health Soc Behav 10:225–236, 1969.
6. Mendel WM: Effect of length of hospitalization on rate and quality of remission from acute psychotic episodes. J Nerv Ment Dis 143:226–233, 1966.
7. Glasscote RM, Kraft AM, Glassman SM, et al: Partial Hospitalization for the Mentally Ill: A Study of Programs and Problems. Washington, DC, Joint Information Service of the American Psychiatric Association and the National Association for Mental Health, 1969.
8. Mechanic D: Therapeutic intervention: issues in the care of the mentally ill. Am J Orthopsychiatry 37:703–718, 1967.
9. Ludwig AM, Farrelly F: The code of chronicity. Arch Gen Psychiatry 15:562–568, 1966.
10. Ludwig AM, Farrelly F: The weapons of insanity. Am J Psychother 21:737–749, 1967.
11. Braginsky BM, Braginsky DB, Ring K: Methods of Madness: The Mental Hospital as a Last Resort. New York, Holt, Rinehart & Winston, 1969.
12. Barton R: Institutional Neurosis. Bristol, England, John Wright & Sons, 1966.
13. Goffman E: Asylums. Garden City, NY, Doubleday & Co, 1961.
14. Gruenberg EM: The social breakdown syndrome—some origins. Am J Psychiatry 123:1481–1489, 1967.
15. Glasscote RM, Cumming E, Rutman ID, et al: Rehabilitating the Mentally Ill in the Community: A Study of Psychosocial Rehabilitation Centers. Washington, DC, Joint Information Service of the American Psychiatric Association and the National Association for Mental Health, 1971.
16. Fairweather GW, Sanders DH, Maynard H, et al: Community Life for the Mentally Ill: An Alternative to Institutional Care. Chicago, Aldine Publishing Co, 1969.
17. Weinman B, Sanders R, Kleiner R, et al: Community based treatment of the chronic psychotic. Community Ment Health J 6:13–21, 1970.
18. Marx AJ, Test MA, Stein LI: Extro-hospital management of severe mental illness—feasibility and effects on social functioning. Arch Gen Psychiatry 29:505–511, 1973.
19. French NH, Heninger GR: A Short Clinical Rating Scale for use by nursing personnel: I. Development and design. Arch Gen Psychiatry 23:233–240, 1970.
20. Pasamanick B, Scarpitti F, Dinitz S: Schizophrenics in the Community: An Experimental Study in the Prevention of Hospitalization. New York, Appleton-Century-Crofts, 1967.
21. Langsley DG, Kaplan DM: The Treatment of Families in Crisis. New York, Grune & Stratton, 1968.
22. Rittenhouse DJ: Endurance of effect: family treatment compared to identified patient treatment (abstract), in Proceedings of the 78th Annual Convention of the American Psychological Association, Vol 2. Washington, DC, APA, 1970, pp 535–536.
23. Murphy HBM, Pennee B, Luchins D: Foster homes: the new back wards? Canada's Mental Health, Sept-Oct 1972, pp 1–17.

III

The Community Support Movement and Its Demise (1977–1997)

Larry Davidson and Priscilla Ridgway

The 1977–1997 era was one of high promise and dashed hopes followed by increasing promise in the care and treatment of people with psychiatric disorders. By the time Jimmy Carter was inaugurated in January 1976, articles were beginning to appear in academic journals with titles such as, "Community mental health: A noble failure?" "Psychiatry under siege: The chronically mentally ill shuffle off to oblivion," and "Dying with their rights on."[1-3] These articles reflected a dawning awareness across the United States that the first 20 years of deinstitutionalization had depopulated institutions but changed little in the quality of life of many people with serious mental illnesses.

Regarding the process of deinstitutionalization, passage of the Social Security Act creating Supplemental Security Income (SSI), the income support program for people with permanent disabilities, and Medicare and Medicaid, which pay for community-based care and treatment for people living in poverty, had made possible the large-scale discharge of patients to their home communities. Previous to creation of these programs, few public resources had existed to serve those leaving long-term hospitalization to other settings or to replace other functions of the mental institution. By one report, only nine halfway houses, fewer than two dozen partial hospitals, and eight rehabilitation centers had been developed throughout the United States by the end of the 1950s.[4]

The Social Security Act of 1965 provided funding for psychiatric care and income support outside of state hospitals and thus made possible decreases in state hospital census on an average of 1.5% per year successively from 1955 to 1965 and 6% per year between 1965 and 1980.[4] A landmark class action suit removed one of the remaining incentives for keeping patients in state hospitals when, in 1973, the U.S. Supreme Court, in *Souder v. Brennan*, made it illegal for hospitals to continue to have inpatients perform work without pay. Having to adhere to the minimum wage and overtime provisions of the Fair Labor Standards Act deprived the hospitals of a source of free labor, thus undercutting state hospitals' ability to function as low-cost custodial institutions. By the time President Carter took office, the state hospital census had already been reduced by about half from its mid 1950s' peak of 559,000 patients.

Resources to adequately house and care for all those leaving institutions had to be found or generated somewhere. The local Community Mental Health Centers simply did not respond adequately to their needs, instead gearing most services to those with less complex needs and milder mental health concerns. If people were to be deinstitutionalized, their disposition would in large part be driven by the parameters under which providers could capture state or federal reimbursement. In fact, the 1970s became a time of "transinstitu-tionalization." Patients were discharged from state hospitals in the tens of thousands but were not discharged back to their communities of origin to live lives in the normal manner. Instead, they were transferred to nursing homes, board and care homes, and other equally institutional settings.[5] Between 1960 and 1970 alone the census of nursing homes doubled, from 470,000 to 925,000. While the census at state hospitals decreased from 500,000 to 370,000 between 1963 and 1969, the same period saw the total number of patients in institutions, including both state hospitals and nursing homes, increase from 725,000 to almost 800,000.

Deinstitutionalization was being judged as a failure not only because it had, in large part, become transinstitutionalization but also because many people who were not simply moved from state hospital to nursing home did not fare much better. With the introduction of Social Security Income in the early 1970s, the federal government began to provide a source of income for those determined to be permanently disabled, thereby allowing state hospitals to consider dispositions other than nursing homes or other institutions. Many patients were discharged to unprepared and unsupported families of origin or to low-income, primarily single-room occupancy, housing. Discharged to such residences based on the assumption that they would manage with their SSI checks, people faced life in the community with few supports beyond limited entitlement programs and the fledgling community mental health centers, which were reluctant to serve individuals who had severe mental disorders (and/or did not have private insurance).

While many former inpatients persevered and cobbled together services and supports as they could, many others were left to their own devices with few places to turn for assistance or support. It should be no surprise, therefore, that increasing numbers of individuals with serious mental illness who had been discharged began to appear on the streets, and in the jails, of cities across the country. As Morrissey and Goldman wrote:

> Deinstitutionalized patients encountered the hostility and rejection of the general public and the reluctance of community mental health and welfare agencies to assume responsibility for their care. Tens of thousands ended up in rooming houses, foster homes, nursing homes, run-down hotels, and on the streets. The transfer of patients from "the back wards to the back alleys" led to widespread concerns that deinstitutionalization was a disaster.[5,pp.21–22]

President Carter, responding to increasing awareness of the early failures of deinstitutionalization and acting on his stated commitment to human welfare issues, convened a new mental health commission and appointed First Lady Rosalynn Carter, a longtime advocate for improvements in mental health care, as honorary chairperson. At the same time, the Government Accounting Office undertook a year-long review of deinstitutionalization, and academic and policy experts expressed increasing concern over the need for a national plan to address the needs of persons with serious mental illnesses. The next several years saw a flurry of activity, energy, and optimism that has not been paralleled in community mental health since.

The Carter Administration also initiated in 1977 the Community Support Movement, with funding from the Community Support Program branch of the NIMH. The Community Support System (CSP) was predicated on the need for comprehensive, life-long, and broad-based systems of community support services for people with serious and prolonged psychiatric disabilities. The purpose of this new initiative was to consolidate the constructive ideas and successes of the previous two decades and bring mental health practitioners and researchers together with family members, individuals with serious mental illnesses, and legal advocates around an agenda that, in the event, was to shape the next three decades of community mental health policy and practice.

The CSP program branch supported the development of stakeholder knowledge building through Learning Community Conferences that brought together mental health consumers, family members, innovative providers, policy makers, and researchers to define the principles and components of a comprehensive service system and the values that would promote adequate care. Among the principles adopted were those of consumer self-determination and empowerment, natural supports, mutual self-help, and a wide range of flexible but coordinated services and supports. A comprehensive community support system was defined to include client identification and outreach, housing and residential services, vocational training and employment assistance, psychosocial rehabilitation services, protection and advocacy, treatment, crisis response services, healthcare, leisure and recreation, family and peer support, and income supports and benefits assistance.

The CSP initiative funded many pilot projects and systems development activities across the country, provided intensive technical assistance to programs and states, and led interagency efforts of the federal government on behalf of the target population. The growth of psychosocial rehabilitation and the consumer and family movements and of recovery-oriented knowledge were encouraged and flourished in many areas of the United States, through CSP initiatives and other technical assistance funded by the federal government. Much of the optimism and energy stimulated by the Community Support Movement, however, abruptly declined with the election of Ronald Reagan in 1980. With the Omnibus Reconciliation Act, passed at the outset of his first term, President Reagan not only eliminated the new $800 million that the Carters had requested from Congress to fund community support services and build community support systems but also reduced funding for Community Mental Health Centers (CMHCs) and the NIMH. Guidelines for essential services of CMHCs were abolished and budgets were reduced by 25%, while at the NIMH 400 central office positions were eliminated and funding for services was reduced by one-third. In addition, all NIMH regional offices were closed. To this day there are fewer federal resources for local systems to access for consultation, technical assistance, or training in order to introduce new interventions or improve delivery of care. The responsibility to fund systems change has largely fallen back to the states, which have taken up these responsibilities to widely varying degrees.

Under the Reagan Administration, the Social Security Administration also began to review most SSI cases for eligibility, resulting in tens of thousands of individuals with mental illnesses being discontinued. (On appeal several years later, many people were reinstated. In the interim, the federal government had saved millions of dollars.) With less money for community services and supports, fewer people receiving federal entitlements, and diminished infrastructure support for system development, prospects for individuals with serious mental illnesses were poor. Other economic factors associated with Reagan's new federalism compounded the problems of reduced funding and resources. The combination of urban renewal and gentrification, deep cuts in federal housing programs and low-income housing development, and additional cuts in federal entitlement programs led to the widespread advent of homelessness in the United States.[6] People with psychiatric disabilities were more likely than other Americans to experience homelessness because of their poverty, loss of benefits, fragmentation of helping systems, housing discrimination, lack of support systems, and the cyclical nature of their disorders.

In addition to cutting dollars for mental health services and leaving tens of thousands of people homeless, the policies of the Reagan Administration also led to consolidation of federal mental health grant dollars into state block grants. While reducing the amount of federal money allocated for mental health services, block grants gave states much more autonomy in how the remaining dollars were spent. As described by one observer, "Block grants broadly define supported activities, give substantial discretion to recipients in the use of funds, and attempt to limit federally imposed requirements to the minimum necessary to insure compliance with national goals."[7,p.236] The resulting autonomy introduced a tremendous amount of variability between states in terms of who is served, by what means, and with what expected outcomes.

The end of categorical funding and the increase in state autonomy allowed states to begin to look at ways of integrating what had become "unmanaged" systems or "nonsystems" of community-based care. The disparate array of outpatient, residential, and rehabilitative services that had emerged over the preceding 20 years to serve deinstitutionalized patients had been created in a gradual, piecemeal, and largely uncoordinated fashion. With no new money on the horizon, states were left to make the most of the funding they had. This translated into being pushed to reduce what duplication or redundancy in services might exist, limit the amount of resources allocated to the most expensive services, such as inpatient care, and find ways to derive the maximum benefit from those services which remained or could be funded through reallocating existing funds. Mechanic summed up this challenge in 1986:

> Developing integrated systems of community care for chronic patients is limited less by inadequate knowledge than by organizational, political, economic, and professional barriers. Providing the necessary spectrum of services and appropriate individualized care requires an organizational entity with sufficient authority to oversee expenditures from varying funding sources and to plan tradeoffs between alternative types of expenditures. These sources are diverse and complex, involve multiple funding agencies and eligibility criteria, and cut across sectors as varied as state and local mental health agencies, Medicaid, SSDI and SSI, and housing programs ... [Despite these complexities] developing such systems is a course preferable to institutional care [8, p. 894].

Mechanic made his case for developing integrated systems of community care at a time of renewed calls for a return to institutionalization, as more individuals fell through the cracks of what was to have been the societal safety net of the mental health system. While academic researchers focused on predictors of community tenure and quality of life among discharged patients[8] and social factors that affect social inclusion,[9] administrators were left with the daunting task of trying to bring some order into this chaos. The only realistic alternative to emerge at the time was to find ways to bring all of the different funding streams together to develop and "manage" systems of care that would integrate housing with Medicaid, federal Block grant dollars, and disability entitlements. As Geller wrote, "In community care, the 1980s was a decade of consolidating practices, evaluating efforts, and facing new problems. It was more of a decade of tinkering than it was of innovating."[10,p.49] In fact, with perhaps with the single exception of the demonstration project launched by the Robert Wood Johnson Foundation (RWJ) and the U.S. Department of Housing and Urban Development to evaluate the utility of an integrated local mental health authority, little progress was made in addressing these complexities and challenges until the next decade, with the introduction of managed care.

Creation of local mental health authorities was one attempt among several to consolidate and manage the loose array of services that had emerged over the preceding 30 years. While launched in 1989, the RWJ's Program on Chronic Mental Illness actually unfolded over the first half of the 1990s. The same was also true of the other primary strategies used to try to "manage" the fragmented array of community based services and supports. These attempts included case management and assertive community treatment, and the use of various financing strategies that could be traced back to the pre-1950s days of the state hospital. We focus on these strategies as representing the major advances of the 1990s, however, as all of these lines of development converged at this time under the general rubric of managed care. The need for managing care had been brought gradually to the policy forefront in the 1980s, as the situations of persons with serious mental illnesses further declined, but awareness did not lead to concerted action until the 1990s. During this decade, the RWJ invested $29 million in its Program on Chronic Mental Illness, the Clinton Administration tried to tackle broad health care reform, and the states began to experiment with ways to improve services for seriously mentally ill persons.

Case management had been introduced in the 1970s as an initial means of responding to the difficulties people had in gaining access to mental health and other health and social services. Initially, case management was conceptualized as providing a "brokering" function in which a single case manager would assess the needs of each client, make telephone calls, and fill out paperwork for services the client would receive from other programs and agencies. In the 1990s, however, it became clear that the brokerage model of case management was not adequate to meet the needs of individuals with serious mental illnesses, for two main reasons. First, due in part to their disability (such as their cognitive impairments), in part to their lack of resources (such as transportation), and in part to their previous negative experiences with health and social services (such as their involuntary hospitalization and the unresponsiveness of social welfare agencies), brokering services for these persons did not translate into their engagement in those services. Second, and equally important, was the fact that lone case managers could do little to fill the gaps, overcome the fragmentation, or override the seemingly arbitrary bureaucratic policies and procedures of community agencies in nonsystems of care.

In response to these facts, new models—the clinical case manager, therapist-case manager, and rehabilitation case manager—were developed. In these models, case managers provided the bulk of services and only referred their clients out to other programs or agencies for specific services that they could not provide directly.[11,12] These case managers also coordinated care among multiple providers, ensured continuity of care over time, and assisted clients with activities of daily living, including transporting and accompanying them to appointments with other service providers. Since the amount of work involved in supporting a single client in this manner could be extensive, case loads for such practitioners had to be limited. Eventually, different levels of need were distinguished so that case loads could be adjusted accordingly: Some clients required only traditional case management, others required the services of a clinical case manager but only for a few hours a week, and others still required intensive clinical case management. Still, advances in case management care fell short of making up for the deficiencies in overall systems of care.

The next step was progression from intensive clinical case management to Assertive Community Treatment (ACT). By the 1990s, ACT was being introduced and conceptualized primarily as a team-based form of intensive clinical case management, based on the reasoning that some clients were so disabled and had such complex needs that a single clinical case manager would not be sufficient to maintaining these clients in the community. If such persons were to remain outside of hospitals, a more intensive and team-based modality would be required. This became the function of ACT teams. No longer used to bring institutionalized patients out of the state hospital as with the original PACT model in Madison, Wisconsin, these teams were charged with keeping their clients in the community, eliminating or greatly reducing hospitalizations that were costly for the mental health system and disruptive for clients. In addition to being available 24 hours a day and 7 days a week, ACT teams attempted to overcome the gaps, fragmentation, and limitations of existing systems of care by providing all mental health services to its clients on their own. In theory, then ACT would replace the system of care by becoming its own system, with the exception of referral to acute inpatient care when needed.

As it evolved in the 1990s, however, ACT came to be seen more and more as only one component of an overarching system of care. Due to its service intensity and cost, ACT was introduced into systems as a solution to meeting the needs of only the most costly and resource intensive of its clients. When combined with the outreach and engagement strategies first learned through homeless outreach teams in the 1980s, the focus of ACT also shifted from the social learning theory approach of in vivo skills training to serving a continuous treatment function for "difficult-to-engage" clients. As a result, consumer advocates and social scientists criticized ACT for focusing too narrowly on training clients in the skills of being compliant psychiatric patients rather than for taking on valued social roles in their communities. Providing mobile crisis intervention, distributing medications to ensure adherence, and managing clients' entitlement income, ACT was charged, in Floersch's terms, with limit its scope to "meds, money, and manners."[13]

Local mental health authorities (LMHAs), as introduced through the RWJ initiative, were a system solution to a system problem rather than a service innovation. LMHAs were to bring together all of the various funding and factors influencing mental health services under one administrative umbrella, which could then allocate the combined resources equitably according to the needs and priorities of their local communities. By combining administrative, fiscal, clinical, and rehabilitative responsibilities under one entity, it was hoped that LMHAs would eliminate the fragmentation of a number of loosely affiliated services with separate missions, funding priorities, and parameters that had come to characterize community mental health services. By granting authority over funding to a central manager, fiscal incentives could be aligned with system goals, providers could be brought together into collaborative or coordinated relationships to offer integrated care, and a clear locus of decision making and accountability could be established. What remained to be determined was from whom LMHAs would derive their authority, over what funds and functions, and with what aims.

For example, while one priority of federal funding and state service provision into the 1980s was the population of persons who were determined to be "seriously and persistently mentally ill," this population was not necessarily given the same high priority at the level of local communities, which sometimes were more concerned about school dropout rates among youth or a loss of work due to untreated depression among adults. In addition to whatever political influence they could bring to bear on the systems they were to coordinate, then, LMHAs would only be able to blend, pool, or combine funding streams with the sanction of their funders, who had their own agendas apart from that of community mental health. Given the importance of consolidating funding to the potential for success of the LMHA model, we turn to financing strategies as the last cluster of attempts to find ways to manage community services.

As Mechanic noted, a primary concern of system managers had to be the fact that their funding streams were diverse and were subject to different eligibility criteria imposed by multiple funding agencies at state, local, and federal levles.[14] Different approaches to bringing these diverse streams together were tried out during the 1990s at the same time as various approaches to reforming general medical care were being implemented and evaluated. Among these approaches, the strategies that were thought to show the most promise in mental health care were capitation and mainstreaming.

In capitated systems, providers receive fixed payments for taking on the entirety of a person's or population's care and are then accorded the flexibility to determine how best to spend this fixed amount of money to meet the needs of that person or population of interest. Such an approach places a premium on increasing the cost-efficiency of care and encourages preventive and early intervention in order to avoid acute and costly care down the road. This approach also establishes a clear point of accountability, as all services are provided or purchased by a central entity. With its emphasis on reducing costs, however, people with serious and complex needs will typically be excluded by capitation plans or by providers negotiating capitation arrangements. Within mental health, therefore, a concerted effort has been required to evaluate the potential of capitation for people with serious and complex needs, as these are the same people who otherwise would bankrupt conventional capitation plans. Given the incentives built in to capitation to deny or minimize care in order to stay within budget or generate profits, such arrangements would still require independent monitoring of client outcomes and appropriateness and quality of care.[15]

Attempts to "mainstream" the care of persons with serious mental illnesses included provider arrangements, such as health maintenance organizations (HMOs), used for the general population or for populations with less serious and complex needs. In addition to having the same financial incentives to deny or minimize care as capitation plans, however, HMOs had little or no experience providing treatment to seriously mentally ill persons, or, often, no experience providing mental health care at all. Most HMOs "carved out" or sub-contracted responsibility for "behavioral health" (mental health and addiction treatment). The challenges faced by these subcontractors were the same as those faced by capitation plans and nonmanaged systems. It would seem that regardless of the funding strategy or arrangement, serving individuals with serious and persistent mental illnesses remains a costly, labor intensive, and complicated endeavor. The various experiments of the 1990s appear to have done little to change this fact or to offer long-term solutions to the challenges involved in doing so.

The essential failure of mental health managed care to make life better for persons with prolonged disorders was counterbalanced somewhat by the rise in interest, toward the end of this era, in the potential for recovery for this population. The recovery movement began with the emergence of a vibrant ex-patient movement and the stories of persons who had recovered, often despite poor care. During the 1980s and 1990s, a number of long-term outcomes studies showed that people with even very long careers as mental patients could rebound and reclaim a life, and successful outcomes were found in many psychosocial rehabilitation programs that helped people achieve stable housing, mainstream employment, and advanced education. Hope for systems change was again on the horizon.

References

1. Smith, W. G., Hart, D. W. (1975). Community mental health: A noble failure? *Hospital and Community Psychiatry, 26,* 581–583.
2. Reich, R., Siegel, L. (1975). Psychiatry under siege: The chronically mentally ill shuffle off to oblivion. *Psychiatric Annals, 3*(11), 35–55.
3. Treffert, D. A. (1973). Dying with their rights on. *American Journal of Psychiatry, 130*(9), 1041.
4. Johnson, A. B. (1990). *Out of bedlam: The truth about deinstitutionalization.* New York: Basic Books.
5. Morrissey, J. P., Goldman, H. H. (1986). Care and treatment of the mentally ill in the United States: Historical developments and reforms. *Annals of the American Academy of Political and Social Science, 484,* 12–27.
6. Mechanic, D., Rochefort, D. A. (1992). A policy of inclusion for the mentally ill. *Health Affairs, 11*(1), 128–150.
7. Buck, J. A. (1984). Block grants and federal promotion of community mental health services, 1946–1965. *Community Mental Health Journal, 20,* 236–247.

8. Solomon, P., Davis, J., Gordon, B. (1984). Discharged state hospital patients' characteristics and use of aftercare: Effect on community tenure. *American Journal of Psychiatry, 141*(12): 1566–1570.

9. Link, B. G., Cullen, F. T., Frank, J., Wozniak, J. F. (1987). The social rejection of former mental patients: Understanding why labels matter. *American Journal of Sociology, 92*(6), 1461–1500.

10. Geller, J. L. (2000). The last half-century of psychiatric services as reflected in *Psychiatric Services. Psychiatric Services, 51,* 41–67.

11. Anthony, W. A., Cohen, M., Farkas, M. D., Cohen, B. F. (1988). Case management: More than a response to a dysfunctional system. *Community Mental Health Journal, 24,* 219–228.

12. Harris, M., Bergman, H.C. (1988). Clinical case management for the chronically mentally ill: A conceptual analysis. In Harris, M., Bachrach, L. L. (eds.), *Clinical case management. New Directions for Mental Health Services, 40,* 5–13.

13. Floersch, J. (2002). *Meds, money, and manners: The case management of severe mental illness.* New York: Columbia University Press.

14. Mechanic, D. (1986). The challenge of chronic mental illness: A retrospective and prospective view. *Hospital and Community Psychiatry, 37*(9), 891–896.

15. Hoge, M. A., Davidson, L., Griffith, E. E. H., Jacobs, S. (1988). The crisis of managed care in the public sector. *International Journal of Mental Health, 27,* 52–71.

Government, Legislative, and Policy Classics

17

U.S. Government Accountability Office. (1977). *Returning the mentally disabled to the community: Government needs to do more.* Washington, D.C.: Author. GAO Publication No. HRD-76-152

This 1977 report, requested by Congress, describes the progress made since President Kennedy's 1963 speech proclaiming a national goal of deinstitutionalization of persons with mental illness and mental retardation. Five major cities and five states were directly sampled for the report. Local agencies, public institutions, private agencies, and service providers were contacted and surveyed; federal and state legislation and policy papers, administrative documents, and court decisions were reviewed; and fieldwork was used to document the lives of a number of persons with mental illness and mentally retardation who had been released from institutions to community services. The report details the experiences of many persons living in dirty, overcrowded residences that provided only medication treatment. Many people, it notes, were discharged from one form of institution separated, for the most part, from the communities in which they were located—state mental hospitals—and placed, without adequate services plans, in community institutions—nursing homes, shelters, and halfway houses. The report recommended increased funding for development of better community services, a review of Medicaid and SSI supplements, increased vocational services and help in finding work, and more and better low-income housing. Gerald Grob and Howard Goldman note the impetus the report gave to the emerging Community Support Movement in their 2006 book, *The Dilemma of Federal Mental Health Policy*. We include the summary of the government report here.

Dietra Hawkins

Returning the Mentally Disabled to the Community: Government Needs to Do More; Department of Health, Education, and Welfare and Other Federal Agencies

Digest

Care and treatment for the mentally disabled in communities rather than in institutions has been a national goal since 1963. Some federal courts have held that the mentally disabled have a constitutional right to be treated in communities when community care serves their needs more and restricts their freedom less. (See Ch. 1.)

Nevertheless, many mentally disabled needlessly enter, remain in, or reenter institutions. Others have been released from institutions before enough community facilities and services were available and without adequate planning for, and later review of, their needs. This review did not include the criminally insane and did not consider the quality of care in institutions. (See Ch. 2.)

Because federal programs provide the financing, states are encouraged to transfer the mentally disabled from institutions to nursing homes and other facilities that often are inappropriate. Federal programs can, do, or should affect "deinstitutionalization"—that is, serving only those needing institutional care in institutions and serving others in the community.

These programs need to be better managed, responsibilities and accountability of federal agencies need to be clearly defined, and federal agencies need to work harder together to help achieve deinstitutionalization. (See Ch. 3.)

There is no overall plan and management system to

—set forth specific steps needed to accomplish deinstitutionalization,
—define specific objectives and schedules,
—define acceptable community-based care, or
—provide central direction and evaluation.

Three organizations are responsible for directing and coordinating efforts of federal agencies: the Office of Management and Budget, federal regional councils, and the President's Committee on Mental Retardation.

The first two have not taken action on deinstitutionalization; the President's Committee has been only partly effective in coordinating the work of federal agencies.

Department of Health, Education, and Welfare

The Department of Health, Education, and Welfare's (HEW's) approach to deinstitutionalization was disorganized.

—Plans to make community placement work had not been made.
—Instructions to constituent agencies had not been issued.
—No one organization had been assigned responsibility for overseeing deinstitutionalization.

Although they are helpful, developmental disabilities programs and the community mental health centers program have not done as much as expected and have not provided the resources or services needed to place mentally disabled people in the community.

Developmental Disabilities Program

The developmental disabilities programs in the five states reviewed provided funds to develop and expand community resources and worked productively with other agencies. But success was not commensurate with need.

The Developmentally Disabled Assistance and Bill of Rights Act of 1975, if properly implemented, should resolve many problems. HEW and other federal agencies must support state developmental disabilities programs by identifying specific actions that other federally supported agencies need to take. Greater commitment and cooperation from other federally supported state and local programs also are needed. (See Ch. 4.)

Community Mental Health Centers and Clinics

Increased services available from community mental health centers and clinics have not always reduced unnecessary admissions to mental hospitals or provided services to people released from mental hospitals. Medication was the only service provided to many patients.

The mental health centers program has developed separately from the public mental hospital system, making integration of the two difficult. Funding for community-based mental health services has not grown in proportion to the need.

Allocations for mental hospitals still dominate most state mental health budgets, and restrictions and other problems have prevented the use of other funds to improve community-based care for the mentally ill. Declining federal funding for centers has caused several communities to avoid the program. (See Ch. 5.)

Medicaid

Lacking alternatives, local programs use money provided by the Medicaid program to place the mentally disabled in nursing homes. Many homes are not staffed or prepared to meet the special needs of the mentally disabled or are not the best setting for persons so placed.

People were also placed in nursing homes or elsewhere without any release plans, with plans that did not identify all services needed, or without adequate provisions for follow-up services.

HEW has started to improve the quality of care nursing homes provide but has not dealt specifically with the special needs of the mentally disabled in these homes. HEW can help by systematically evaluating and enforcing Medicaid requirements for deinstitutionalization and by integrating related requirements in Medicaid and other agency programs.

How do HEW standards for institutions for the retarded that participate in the Medicaid program affect a state's ability to help those inappropriately placed in such facilities or who risk being admitted to them?

HEW must answer this question, because states must improve facilities to comply with the standards by March 18, 1977, and must also expand community programs for the retarded. Sufficient funds often are not available to do both. (See Ch. 6.)

Under the Social Security Act, states must find and correct situations in which Medicaid recipients are wrongly placed in mental hospitals, institutions for the retarded, or nursing homes or do not receive appropriate services there. HEW must also survey these programs to validate their effectiveness.

State and HEW efforts in this area should be improved because they were inadequate to meet the needs of the mentally disabled. (See Ch. 7.)

Medicare

Medicare provides insurance for only limited outpatient care for the mentally ill. Because of this, many people may be placed unnecessarily in mental hospitals.

HEW monitors state surveys of mental hospitals for compliance with Medicare standards, including those on discharge planning, but this has been limited. HEW has recognized these problems and was trying to solve them. (See Ch. 8.)

Supplemental Security Income

Although Supplemental Security Income has helped mentally disabled people return to communities, some of these people have been placed in substandard facilities, placed without provision for support services, or placed inappropriately. Standards on group housing for Supplemental Security Income recipients were not required; this aggravated the problem.

Supplemental Security Income payments were reduced or not authorized when public agencies helped maintain or operated community residential facilities for the mentally disabled. Legislation enacted in August and October 1976 eliminated many of these reductions in Supplemental Security Income and authorized such payments to persons in certain publicly operated community residences. (See Ch. 9.)

Social Services

Although many mentally disabled have been released from public institutions without provision for needed services, many states have not used all federal funds available under social services programs. This is partly because of the controversy and confusion about the program and the inability or unwillingness of states to provide necessary matching funds.

HEW had not monitored or enforced its requirements that social service plans respond to individual needs or that foster placements be appropriate.

A new social services program started in 1975 does not include these requirements. Although deinstitutionalization is one goal of the new program, HEW does not require states to coordinate their program plans on this goal with those of mental health agencies, community mental health centers, or other agencies. (See Ch. 10.)

Vocational Rehabilitation

State vocational rehabilitation agencies have helped mentally disabled persons remain in and return to communities. Since the enactment of the Rehabilitation Act of 1973, these agencies have reported some increased efforts to rehabilitate persons with mental handicaps classified as severe disabilities. This act required emphasis on service to the more severely disabled.

Vocational rehabilitation for the mentally retarded has been provided primarily for the mildly retarded or persons with nearly normal intelligence quotients in the community (rather than in institutions). Vocational rehabilitation for the mentally ill often was focused on drug addicts, alcoholics, and persons with mental disabilities not considered severe by HEW.

HEW needs to improve its management of the vocational rehabilitation program so that appropriate emphasis is given to the more severely mentally disabled. (See Ch. 11.)

Department of Housing and Urban Development

Only one of eight local housing authorities contacted considered the needs of the lower income, mentally disabled people in its housing assistance plan. This consideration is required by the Housing and Community Development Act of 1974.

In 1971, the president directed the Department of Housing and Urban Development to help develop special housing for the retarded. However, the department had not

—made plans for this,
—told local housing authorities and managers or sponsors of HEW-assisted housing to consider the needs of the mentally disabled, or
—informed its headquarters and field staffs of their responsibilities under the president's directive. (See Ch. 12.)

Department of Labor

Labor job training and placement programs often have helped mentally disabled persons, but they have not been available to many mentally disabled persons in or released from institutions.

The Secretary of Labor had not informed the department staff of their responsibilities in helping accomplish deinstitutionalization, and program administrators had not considered their programs' effects on this objective.

Many people served by sheltered workshops were not placed into competitive, productive employment; others needed job training and placement to help them lead normal or nearly normal lives in the community. (See Ch. 13.)

Recommendations to the Congress

The Congress should consider:

—Designating a committee in each House with the responsibility for monitoring all federal efforts to help place the mentally disabled in the community so that Federal agencies work together and support state efforts to serve the mentally disabled. (See p. 182.)

—Requiring state developmental disabilities programs to concentrate on coordinating activities at the local level. (See p. 182.)

—Amending the Social Security Act to increase the outpatient mental health services available under Medicare. (See p. 183.)

—Consolidating the funds earmarked for mental health under the special health revenue sharing and the community mental health center programs into a formula grant to state mental health agencies. (See p. 183.)

The Congress should also consider whether additional legislation is needed to help federal, state, and local agencies provide more job training and placement services to the severely mentally disabled, who have particular disadvantages in the job market. (See p. 184.)

Recommendations to the Director, Office of Management and Budget

At least 135 federal programs—administered by 11 major departments and agencies of the government—affect the mentally ill or mentally retarded. Therefore, the Director should

—instruct federal agencies to develop and help implement deinstitutionalization,

—see that the responsibilities and specific actions to be taken by federal agencies are clearly defined, and

—direct Federal regional councils to mobilize, coordinate, and evaluate federal work affecting this goal throughout the country. (See p. 184.)

Recommendations to the Secretary of Hew

The Secretary should:

—Define responsibilities of and actions to be taken by HEW agencies.

—Designate an agency or official responsible for coordinating this work.

—Determine how to make sure that state and local agencies administering HEW-supported programs develop and implement effective case management systems for people being released from public institutions.

—Evaluate the need and desirability of providing incentives for care for the mentally disabled other than in intermediate care facilities.

—Determine a clear and consistent federal role in mental health and retardation programs and make recommendations to the Congress. (See p. 184.)

—Improve individual department programs. (See pp. 186 to 190.)

Recommendations to the Secretaries of Labor and Housing and Urban Development

The Secretaries should each make community care for the mentally disabled a departmental objective and improve existing programs. (See pp. 190 and 191.)

Agency Comments

The Office of Management and Budget; HEW; the Departments of Housing and Urban Development, Labor, and Justice; and the National Association of State Mental Health Program Directors generally agreed with GAO's findings.

The Departments of Labor and Housing and Urban Development generally agreed with the recommendations and outlined several actions they have taken, were taking, or planned to take to help return the mentally disabled to the community.

HEW did not specifically comment on the recommendations, but said that it would study them and develop a plan for implementing those it concurred in.

The Office of Management and Budget outlined actions it would take, but disagreed with the recommendations to it, arguing that they were unwarranted and would unjustifiably interfere with state and local responsibilities. GAO continues to believe that the actions recommended are needed and, if implemented, would not interfere with state and local responsibilities.

State agencies commented on findings related to them that were contained in separate reports GAO issued on each state reviewed.

18

Sharfstein, S. S. (1982). Medicaid cutbacks and block grants: Crisis or opportunity for community mental health? *American Journal of Psychiatry, 139* (4), 466–470

The Community Support Program initiative, begun under the Carter Administration with more fanfare than funding, never emerged as a robust federal program, although its concepts and approach continued to influence planners' and policy makers' thinking long after it faded as a program. During the Reagan Administration, funding cuts and changes in funding mechanisms further complicated planning for comprehensive community mental health care. Sharfstein discusses the growth of the mental health service industry as a whole and the shrinking of state hospital inpatient services from 1955 to 1977. This growth, he notes, was made possible by federal funding, including Medicaid, and private insurance. Possible upcoming changes in funding in the early 1980s included the use of block grants to the state, for which mental health would have to compete with other social programs, and caps on Medicaid spending resulting from a cutback in federal contributions. At a time when there was much concern about the future of public mental health services, Sharfstein argued that there were opportunities that mental health providers and planners might act on to sustain and even improve services. He proposes a form of "mental health HMO" (health maintenance organization) to provide continuity of care and comprehensive services organized and administered under the umbrella of community mental health centers and systems. HMO became a dirty word for health care patients in general during the 1990s and up to the present. In the 1970s and early 1980s, however, many consumers liked them because of the range of services they provided and the relative ease of gaining access to most of these services, mainly through a primary physician who coordinated the person's care, at one clinic.

Medicaid Cutbacks and Block Grants: Crisis or Opportunity for Community Mental Health?

The fourfold growth in the mental health service system since 1955 has been largely financed by federal monies and by federal and state funding through Medicaid. This growth represents expansion of both institutional and outpatient settings, even though there has been a total reversal of the proportion of inpatient to outpatient care over the last 22 years. Current proposals to cap Medicaid costs and to issue block grants challenge the delivery system to attempt alternatives, such as financing similar to what is done in a health maintenance organization (HMO). The author describes a model of a "mental health HMO" that would be appropriate from professional, consumer, and economic perspectives.

In his February 8, 1981, economic message, President Ronald Reagan declared to the Congress, "The taxing power of government must be used to provide revenues for legitimate government purposes. It must not be used to regulate the economy or bring about social change. We've tried that and surely must be able to see that it doesn't work." As part of an overall economic recovery program, President Reagan proposed a major change in the federal financing of community mental health services. These changes include limits on direct federal involvement with localities by "block granting" programs to the states and a cutback in third-party financing through a cap on the Medicaid program. In this paper I will review the potential impact of these policies on the community mental health movement, a major health initiative over the past 25 years supported in large part by the federal government. These efforts have led to substantial change in the practice and setting of psychiatric care. A major reassessment of the accomplishments and problems of this initiative took place in the last administration, and the challenge of the 1980s will be to sustain the gains as well as solve the problems of community approaches for individuals with mental illness.

Growth of the Mental Health Industry, 1955–1977

The decades of the 1960s and 1970s witnessed dramatic changes in psychiatric treatments and a massive shift in the proportion of inpatient to outpatient psychiatric care. These were decades of tremendous growth and diversification for mental health services, treatment opportunities, and the psychiatric and psychological professions. This growth was fueled by a substantial amount of federal financing through categorical support, especially community mental health center and training grants, and through third-party programs—most importantly Medicaid (Title 19). The number of patients seen in the general health and specialty mental health systems has expanded dramatically, and individuals of all socioeconomic backgrounds have the opportunity for a wide array of new treatment and rehabilitation programs (1).

From 1955 to 1977 the number of inpatient and outpatient care episodes in specialty mental health facilities almost quadrupled, from 1.7 million episodes in 1955 to 6.4 million in 1977. (Patient care episodes are defined as the number of residents in inpatient facilities [or the number of people on the rolls of non-inpatient facilities] at the beginning of the year plus the total additions to these facilities during the year. Total additions during the year include new admissions, readmissions, and returns from long-term leave. It is, therefore, a duplicated count of individuals, and it includes only episodes in organized psychiatric specialty settings. Episodes of psychiatric care in private office practice of mental health professionals, general medical practice and clinics, and other non-mental-health settings such as neighborhood health centers, general hospital medical services, and nursing homes are not included.)

When population growth was controlled for, the patient care episode rate per 100,000 population tripled in 1955–1977. During the same time span there was a substantial shift in the settings in which these episodes occurred. Three-quarters of all patient care episodes in 1955 took place in inpatient settings. By 1977, a little more than one-quarter of all episodes were in inpatient settings. Even though the overall number of patient care episodes increased by 40%, there was a proportional decline in inpatient episodes in state and county mental hospitals, where such episodes decreased from about half of all episodes in 1955 to only 9% in 1977. The tenfold increase in outpatient care episodes during these two decades is of major importance; the federal funding of 788 community mental health centers since 1963 and the growth of outpatient clinics are the leading reasons for this expansion (2) (see Table 18.1).

Although the number of state and county mental hospitals decreased only 2% from 1975 to 1977, the number of beds in these hospitals since 1955 decreased about 70%, far out of proportion to the actual number of hospitals that closed. The difficulty in closing state mental hospitals and the concomitant problem in shifting resources from the fixed costs of large public institutions to the variable costs of community care have been major obstacles to the funding of community care (4). Closing a mental hospital requires major economic dislocation for communities and has led to strong union protest and state legislative opposition. Psychiatric units in general hospitals and community mental health centers have accounted for the greatest growth in the facility sector of the mental health system (see Table 18.1).

The number of mental health professionals has grown along with the number of facilities, especially the number of psychologists and social workers. Many of these individuals are employed in the new facilities and many others are in private practice. The number of both psychologists and social workers has increased over 300% since 1955, and the number of psychiatrists has increased 183% (see Table 18.2). National Institute of Mental Health (NIMH) training grants have provided a subsidy for this growth in mental health professionals—especially psychiatrists, psychologists, psychiatric social workers, and psychiatric nurses.

This ferment and growth in service delivery and number of professionals would not have happened except for ever-expanding public and private third-party financial support sources, including federal "seed money" for community mental health centers and alcohol and drug treatment programs. Other major sources of funds include Medicaid, increased private health insurance, and federally subsidized insurance such as the Federal Employees Health Benefits Program. Coverage under private insurance today usually includes full care of short-term inpatient stays in general hospital settings. Short-term psychiatric units in general hospitals have expanded due to this increase in insurance

TABLE 18.1. Trends in the Specialty Mental Health System, 1955–1977

Item	1955	1977	Change
Patient care episodes[a]			
Inpatient			
State mental hospital	818,000	574,000	30% less
Other	478,000	1,243,000	160% more
Total	1,296,000	1,817,000	40% more
Outpatient			
Federally funded community mental health centers		1,741,000	
Other	379,000	2,835,000	648% more
Total	379,000	4,576,000	1,107% more
Total	1,675,000	6,393,000	282% more
Psychiatric beds			
Psychiatric hospitals			
State	623,000	184,000	70% less
VA[b]	56,000	34,000	40% less
Proprietary	16,000	17,000	6% more
Psychiatric units in nonfederal general hospitals	7,000	29,000	314% more
Community mental health centers		15,000	
Direct expenditures for mental illness	$1.2 billion[c]	$19.6 billion[d]	1,533% more

[a] Source of data, unless otherwise noted, is NIMH Division of Biometry and Epidemiology published and unpublished data.

[b] Includes VA psychiatric hospital beds and beds in psychiatric units of VA general hospitals.

[c] See Fein (3).

[d] Report of the Research Triangle Institute: "The Cost to Society of Alcohol, Drug Abuse, and Mental Illness." contract 283-79-001. Alcohol, Drug Abuse, and Mental Health Administration, Nov. 1980.

TABLE 18.2. Growth in Number and Rate of Mental Health Professionals, 1955–1980

Group of Professionals	1955	1980	Change
Psychiatrists[a]			
Number	10,600	30,023	183% more
Rate per 100,000 population[b]	6.4	13.7	114% more
Psychologists[c]			
Number	13,500	56,933	322% more
Rate per 100,000 population[b]	8.1	25.9	220% more
Social workers[d]			
Number	20,000	83,000	315% more
Rate per 100,000 population[b]	12.1	37.8	212% more

[a] Data until 1960 included American Psychiatric Association membership plus filled psychiatric residency positions. 1960–1980 data also included nonmembers of APA who reported their specialty as psychiatry to the American Medical Association. Approximately 10% of all psychiatrists in 1980 were child psychiatrists.

[b] Source for civilian population of the United States: U.S. Bureau of the Census: *Current Population Reports*, Series P-25, numbers 802 and 888.

[c] Data based on membership in the American Psychological Association. Until 1980, 37% of all psychologists were in clinical counseling or guidance psychology. In 1980 between 26,000 and 28.000 (52%) were licensed or certified health science provider psychologists.

[d] Data based on membership in the National Association of Social Workers. Approximately 20% to 25% of all social workers were in mental health practice. In 1980, 11,000 were on the register of "certified clinical social workers."

financing. Longer-term beds in state and county public mental hospitals have been phased out as deinstitutionalization policies have been implemented (5). Expenditure trends (see Table 18.1) indicate that there has been a major growth in the cost of care during this time period due to the combined effects of inflation and growth of the system.

Overgrowth or Appropriate Response to Need?

Trends of the last two decades have led to criticism of ever-expanding expectations of and disappointment with some of the original goals articulated for community mental health (6). Many questions are being raised by third-party payers as to what services for which conditions are medically necessary and appropriate (7). Further criticism has been leveled at community mental health centers for abandoning the clinical/medical model (8). A related issue and problem concerns the deinstitutionalization of chronic mental patients from state and county mental hospitals without adequate resource planning in communities and community support (9). The great neglect and the abandonment of these patients remain major public health problems for the 1980s.

The Medicaid program, which is the largest source of federal funds supporting the care of the mentally ill, emphasizes institutional care. It is mostly biased toward acute care in nonprofit general hospitals and chronic care in nursing homes. Increasing state resources are required for Medicaid as well. This is beginning to challenge the categorical state mental health programs for financial supremacy in the treatment of the chronic population. Over 90% of the costs are accounted for by inpatient or intermediate care facilities; there is very little support for outpatient or community mental health services. To date, Medicaid has been mostly a subsidy for the increasing costs of long-term care institutions and an opportunity for states to shift the costs from state to federal funds. A government report dated December 1980 (10) emphasized the possible opportunities for Medicaid as a funder of community-based care for the chronically ill by expanding the range of services through new intermediate care, day treatment, and psychosocial rehabilitation opportunities. This potentially represents a cost-effective approach that could consolidate some of the gains of the 1960s and 1970s in community care and provide a financial base for fledgling community programs which attempt to address the needs of the long-term patient. Currently, Medicaid is spread quite thin across outpatient alternatives, and in some states current reimbursement rates are so low as to discourage community providers from giving service to Medicaid recipients.

Proposals for Block Grants and Medicaid Caps

Two proposals have surfaced recently that create uncertainty and worry among providers and planners of community mental health services. The first proposal would put a "cap" on Medicaid spending through a limit on federal support. The second is the idea of block grants, which would give states money for a range of federal service programs in one lump, the money to be spent at the state's discretion. This would end federal categorical "seed money" as a mechanism to develop community services. The focus for planning of service delivery would shift to states and local communities. Priorities would be set locally, and funding decisions would be made within a context of overall state priorities.

Despite the obvious cost-containment aspects of these proposals, there are opportunities for a more rational service delivery system inherent in this kind of fiscal constraint. The cap on Medicaid might provide an impetus to review and reassess the heavy institutional biases of that program. Block grants, which would free local and state programs from federal regulations, could be critical in filling in the gaps and provide funding to develop a service and financial strategy that would shift resources from state institutions into the community.

One approach that would have a number of advantages would emphasize a planned system of prepaid per capita contracts with local providers to take care of the array of needs of the mentally ill. This would allow the system to develop cost-effective alternatives based on such prospective budgets. A "mental health maintenance organization" could initially be put into operation through the federal block grant as part of a proposal from the local community program such as a community mental health center (CMHC) within the state. Underfunded alternatives such as day treatment and psychosocial rehabilitation would be financed more adequately within fixed budgets as programs consolidated and focused on cost-effective approaches in the community.

The experience with health maintenance organizations (HMOs), which emphasize prepayment, enrolled populations, and comprehensive services, has been shown to be less costly than fees for service financed by insurance. The savings have been achieved primarily through lower hospital admission rates (11). This is true for savings in mental health services in HMOs as well (12). One study (13) found that costs for a comparable population were $500 less for patients in prepaid programs than for patients treated in a fee-for-service program.

A similar suggestion was made in the 1978 report of the Commission on Public General Hospitals (14). This report recommended strongly the development of organized ambulatory primary care programs based on preenrolled populations funded on a prepaid per capita basis. For the mental health system to develop such alternatives it is essential to consider the advantages to state agencies, general hospitals—especially in the voluntary nonprofit sector—and providers such as psychiatrists in private practice. The advantages and disadvantages of such an approach to each of these groups is beyond the scope of this paper. What follows is a description of what is required for any program, public or private, to put together such a mental health HMO.

Approaches to Capitation Contracting

HMOs have had four years of experience with capitation contracting with states for people eligible for Medicaid as one way of attempting to tie together the health care needs of the Medicaid population and the cost-containment goals of government. Although this experience is limited (15–17), the essential ideas of this approach could be a major innovation in the delivery of community mental health services in the 1980s.

Organizations of community mental health centers and systems would negotiate on a prepaid capitation approach a contract with states for all needed services for a defined enrolled population. The essence of the system would include an enrolled population and would offer comprehensive services for fixed periodic per capita payment. The actual nature of the system or center could vary, taking on many forms and shapes depending on local circumstances, history, and the ideas of planners and community leaders. The key concept is the capacity to plan and organize a rational delivery system that will contain costs yet assure accessibility and availability of appropriate services.

For a "mental health HMO" to work, it should contain the following five basic elements:

1. Hospital care must be limited. Expensive acute as well as longer-term hospital care can be avoided for the majority of the mentally ill. Alternatives or substitutes are available but have remained underfinanced by public funding and therefore have

been underutilized. These include outpatient alternatives, day treatment, 24-hour crisis intervention, and home care. An organized mental health HMO could develop this array of services with the proper prospective financing, organizing, and management.

2. Continuity of care must be promoted. The clinical, rehabilitation, and social services needed for an enrolled population with a wide variety of mental conditions should be available within one system or setting so that patients do not have to go shopping among a myriad of agencies and programs for needed care. The concept of "case managers" as a part of community support systems is an important aspect of this approach.

3. Access to needed care must be assured. Through a prepaid citation approach there should be no financial barrier to care. There also must be enough professionals and professional services for the enrolled population in order for services to be available without excessive waiting periods.

4. Preventive interventions should be encouraged. This is particularly relevant in the areas of secondary and tertiary prevention. Again, the key needs of the chronically mentally ill are for continuous community support and psychosocial rehabilitation opportunities.

5. There should be consumer options. Within a geographic area consumers should be able to select on a competitive basis the program in which they would like to enroll. Once the program has been selected, access would be restricted to services in that particular program, but, just as in the Federal Employees Health Benefits Program, there should be an "open season" when enrollees have the option of moving among the various plans if they are dissatisfied. Competition would encourage quality and accountability.

It is clear from this description that economic incentives are critical. The mental health HMO is "at risk" if patients do badly and need more expensive care. The positive incentives include the ability to plan cost-effective services and have a secure financial basis for planning and service delivery. Obviously, there are dangers associated with these incentives. First, it would be impossible for the current delivery system to continue in the same inefficient expensive way, and a number of programs within a geographic area would have to close down or cut back. It is also clear that within the mental health HMO system itself the substitution of alternatives for expensive care requires development and expansion. The second danger, which is a chronic issue for all HMOs, is the tendency to underserve and neglect patients. It is within this kind of system that management abuses can take place. These include abandonment of or underservice for the patient, contrasted to the overservice problem of so-called Medicaid "mills," which are based on fee-for-service arrangements. Accountability includes assurances to the public payers that patients are getting needed services, that they are not being abandoned in welfare hotels or jails, and that services are of decent quality. Peer review becomes an important factor in relation to the issue of quality.

The principal problem in negotiations with state agencies for both Medicaid funding and block grants is the need for good actuarial assumptions or estimates for the basis of the capitation rate. These include good data on the characteristics of the enrolled population, such as age, sex, cultural background, number of deinstitutionalized patients in the community, and people eligible for Medicaid, as well as the number and kind of services needed so that expected utilization can be predicted. Further, there is a need for decent cost measures of both units of service and episodes of care. In the first phase of this approach estimates will need to be validated over time and changed because this is a poorly known area at present.

This approach could provide many benefits to patients, providers, and the goals of community mental health. It could reduce the costly duplication and fragmentation of services that currently exist. The alternative in relation to cutbacks is mindless cost cutting, leading to further imbalances or limits on coverage that already skew service delivery inappropriately toward institutional alternatives. The 1980s could then be an era of "reinstitutionalization," and the economic focus could be economies of scale in the large asylums for the many and fee-for-service practice for the few.

References

1. Regier DA, Goldberg ID, Taube CA: The de facto US mental health services system: a public health perspective. Arch Gen Psychiatry 35:685–693, 1978.
2. Witkin MJ: Trends in Patient Care Episodes in Mental Health Facilities, 1955–1977: Statistical Note 154. Bethesda, Md, NIMH Division of Biometry and Epidemiology, 1980.
3. Fein R: Economics of Mental Illness. New York, Basic Books, 1959.
4. Sharfstein SS, Turner JE, Clark HW: Financing issues in the delivery of services to the chronically mentally ill and disabled, in The Chronic Mental Patient: Problems, Solutions, and Recommendations for a Public Policy. Edited by Talbott JA. Washington, DC, American Psychiatric Association, 1978.
5. Witkin M: State and Regional Distribution of Psychiatric Beds in 1978: Statistical Note 155. Bethesda, Md, NIMH Division of Biometry and Epidemiology, Jan 1981.
6. Sharfstein SS, Wolfe JC: The community mental health centers program: expectations and realities. Hosp Community Psychiatry 29:46–49, 1978.
7. Sharfstein SS: Third-party payers: to pay or not to pay. Am J Psychiatry 135:1185–1188, 1978.
8. Sharfstein SS: Will community mental health survive in the 1980s? Am J Psychiatry 135:1363–1365, 1978.
9. Ozarin LD, Sharfstein SS: The aftermaths of deinstitutionalization: problems and solutions: Psychiatr Q 50:128–132, 1978.
10. Toward a National Plan for the Chronically Mentally Ill. Washington, DC, US Department of Health and Human Services, Dec 1980.
11. Luft HS: How do health maintenance organizations achieve their "savings"? N Engl J Med 298:1336–1343, 1978.
12. Meier G: HMO experiences with mental health services to the long-term emotionally disabled. Inquiry, Summer 1981, pp 125–138.
13. Spiro HR, Siassi I, Crocetti G: Cost-financed mental health facility, II: utilization profile of a labor union program. J Nerv Ment Dis 160:241–248, 1975.
14. The Future of the Public General Hospital: Report of the Commission on Public General Hospitals. Chicago. Hospital Research and Educational Trust, 1978.
15. Martin E Segal Co: HMOs and Medicaid: Approaches to Capitation Contracting. Washington, DC, Health Services Administration Bureau of Medical Services, 1977 .
16. Report of the Joint Health Care Financing Administration Public Health Service Task Force on HMO-Medicaid Contracting. Washington, DC, US DHEW, Jan 1981.
17. Wilson D: Evaluating the Potential for Medicaid/HMO Contracting: Strategy for Selection of Target States. Bethesda, Md, Office of Health Maintenance Organizations, Public Health Service Jan 15, 1981.

First Person and Literary Classics

First Person and Literary
Classics

19

Chamberlin, J. (1978). *On our own: Patient-controlled alternatives to the mental health system.* New York: Hawthorn Books

Judi Chamberlin's first-person account of mental health in America was published at a time of soul searching about deinstitutionalization and the community mental health movement, as policy makers, practitioners, and researchers looked back in frustration and tried to determine where and how things had gone wrong. Chamberlin added a patient voice, one of the first with a distinctly collective and political message to go with that of personal experience. Her chapter titles—"A patient's view of the mental health system," "The making and unmaking of a mental patient," "Consciousness raising," "Inside the mental patient's association," "People not patients," and others—reflect this movement from the personal to the political and from an individual experience of oppression to a collective resistance and voice. Chamberlin's story ranges from a chilling and moving account of her own history as a mental patient to her discovery of consumer-run alternatives. Here is an excerpt from the chapter on consciousness raising, including Chamberlin's discovery of the Mental Patient's Liberation Project in New York, which marked a transition point in her passage from patient to advocate. Chamberlin was Director of Education and Training for the National Empowerment Center in Massachusetts at the time of her death in 2010.

Consciousness Raising

The barriers to instituting change in the mental health system are enormous. The "mental health industry" is an entrenched bureaucracy, resistant to change from within and almost totally unresponsive to outside pressures. Mental health is big business; in fiscal year 1974–1975, fourteen million dollars was spent on mental health services in the United States.[1] Psychiatrists, the most prestigious mental health professionals, like other doctors, are reluctant to allow nonphysicians to have very much input into what they see as purely medical matters. Other mental health specialties, such as psychology, occupational therapy, and social work, have their own power bases within the mental health system, positions they have won after struggling with the psychiatric establishment. The nonpsychiatric mental health disciplines have promoted their own alternative facilities, such as halfway houses and ex-patient social clubs. Although these alternatives are not (usually) run by psychiatrists, they are still firmly under professional control.

The alternative programs that form the subject of this book are different, because their underlying philosophy is different. Nonprofessional, client-controlled services don't divide people into "sick" and "well," "helper" and "helped." They see every person as having a combination of strengths and weaknesses, and the need for help in one area does not negate the ability to help others also. But in order to achieve these ends, people have to recognize their own strengths and abilities. They have to discover that sometimes there are no "experts" to turn to. People who seek out these alternatives, have experienced the harm that the "experts" and their methods can cause.

These alternatives have been begun in a spirit of anger and frustration, by people who have had firsthand experience with unresponsive, unhelpful mental health "care." But more than anger and frustration is necessary to enable people to set up functioning alternatives. People also need confidence in their own abilities—confidence that has often been damaged by contact with the mental health system. So, side by side with the work of setting up the alternative has gone another essential activity—building up the confidence and self-esteem of all the people involved in the work. This consciousness-raising process seems to have been independently arrived at by groups in many places as an important part of creating meaningful alternatives for people.

Many of the people involved in these alternatives are ex-mental patients, who face a special set of barriers. The crippling stereotypes about mental illness have often been internalized by ex-patients, many of whom believe (at least some of the time) that they are weak, incapable, untrustworthy, "sick," "crazy," or whatever. It is difficult or impossible to go through the experience of mental institutionalization without beginning, to some extent, to hate oneself. Part of the process of institutional "treatment" is convincing the patient that his or her former ideas, beliefs, and behaviors were wrong. One stands little chance of discharge without agreeing—or seeming to agree—with the staff's assessment of what constitutes mental health. Even a person who struggles successfully to maintain his or her own way of thinking can be damaged by this form of psychological assault. Also, there are many people who go looking for help with their problems, who are quite willing to acknowledge that they need new and more effective ways of coping, but who have not found that help from psychiatry. These people are now joining to set up alternatives in order to get help with their own problems, as well as to help others. They don't see themselves as inherently better than any other potential users of the service.

Mutual-support networks of some sort seem to be an essential part of getting alternatives started. They are directly analogous to the consciousness-raising groups that have served to get women involved in feminism. These leaderless women's groups had no "experts"; they developed their theory out of the examination of the lives of their members. Self-defeating behavior was not viewed as illness but rather as a response to a society that imposed a special set of pressures on women. The work of women's consciousness raising and that of ex-patients has enormous overlap. In both kinds of groups participants have often experienced the liberating realization that they were not "crazy" after all.

Consciousness raising is not "therapy." Therapy has as its goal adjusting the individual to the "reality" of his or her own life. Therapists (particularly in mental institutions) seldom question the assumption that the underlying social system is a benign influence on people's behavior. In a consciousness-raising group, on the other hand, people begin to see that much of what they had viewed as their own individual problems are responses to real frustrations. In mental patient consciousness-raising groups, people have discovered that their dissatisfactions with their own lives (and with the "treatment" they got in the hospital) were not "symptoms of mental illness" but were valid perceptions of what was wrong with their lives.

People do not "go crazy" for no reason. Often they are afraid to recognize that their "happy marriage" is making them miserable, that their "good job" is drudgery, that their "loving family" is a mass of unspoken, simmering tensions. These are pressures that can, indeed, drive one crazy. Psychiatry—especially in the mental hospital—seldom helps people to make these frightening, but potentially liberating, discoveries. The function of the mental hospital is to cool out the anger and rebellion, conveniently labeled "symptoms," so that the person can return to "normal" life.

Consciousness raising, on the other hand, helps people to see that their so-called symptoms are indications of real problems. The anger, which has been destructively turned inward, is freed by this recognition. Instead of believing that they have a defect in their psychic makeup (or their neurochemical system), participants learn to recognize the oppressive conditions in their daily lives.

The realization that a person has suffered at the hands of a system that is supposed to have helped him or her is an important first step. Often it takes a long time for an ex-patient to realize fully the extent of the damage that has been done. The belief that one has been harmed may coexist with the belief that one is "sick," that such treatment was somehow deserved or justified. In consciousness raising, ex-patients find that mistreatment was not an individual error, but is built into the system. The depersonalization experienced by the investigators in the Rosenhan study (in which "normal" volunteers had themselves admitted to mental institutions) is an experience common to all mental patients. People struggling to define themselves and their lives face a hostile environment in the mental hospital, where staff is apt to define only the most conventional attitudes as healthy.

Consciousness raising is an ongoing process. Negative stereotypes of the "mentally ill" are everywhere and are difficult not to internalize, no matter how sensitive one becomes. This stereotyping has been termed "sane chauvinism" or "mentalism" by mental patients' liberation groups. Like sexism, mentalism is built into the language—*sick* and *crazy* are widely used to refer to behavior of which the speaker disapproves. The struggle against mentalism is one of the long-range activities of mental patients' liberation.

I can perhaps best describe the effects of the consciousness-raising process by relating what it did for me. For several years before getting involved in mental patients' liberation, I had become increasingly angry about my hospitalization. There was no one to share these perceptions with. I knew no other ex-patients, and nonpatients seldom wanted to hear very much about it, even in those cases where they were sympathetic. In any case, I didn't dare confide in most people that I was an ex-patient. My anger existed side by side with my acceptance of my own "mental illness." I thought that my story was an isolated example of poor treatment, rather than a representative case of the damaging effects of mental institutionalization.

My feelings began to change when I discovered the existence of the Mental Patients' Liberation Project in New York, one of the earliest mental patients' liberation groups. We talked about our experiences and discovered how similar they were. Whether we had been in grim state hospitals or expensive private ones, whether we were there voluntarily or involuntarily, whether we had been called schizophrenic, manic-depressive, or whatever, our histories had been extraordinarily similar. We had experienced depersonalization, the stupefying effects of drugs, the contempt of those who supposedly "cared" for us. Out of this growing awareness came a deeper understanding of the true purpose of the mental health system. It is primarily a method of social control.

We also began to talk about the kinds of help troubled people need. Having experienced the dehumanizing effects of mental institutions, we saw that large facilities with rigid hierarchies could never be the kind of places we had in mind. It quickly became clear that there was no way to fix up the current mental hospital system. What was needed was an entirely new model. People who had been in places with carpets on the floors told the same stories of indifference and cruelty as those who had been in dingy, barren state hospitals. Institutions with lots of staff members (expensive hospitals with good reputations) were particularly oppressive, because they were able to control virtually every move patients made.

David was a patient in one of these highly regarded hospitals.[2] He had been taken there at the request of his parents (he was a teen-ager at the time) because they considered his interest in religion sick. David was also a vegetarian, and the hospital considered it therapeutic that he become a meat eater, which he resisted. David began to eat a lot of peanut butter at every meal, because he was concerned about getting enough protein in his diet. It was decreed that he be limited to one ounce of peanut butter per meal, a ruling that was enforced by a staff member assigned to be there to watch him eat.

It is clear that many of the things that are done to mental patients "for their own good," in the view of staff, are experienced as harmful by patients themselves. Mental patients' liberation groups believe that it is the patient's own assessment that is the most valid measure of whether a particular treatment is helpful or harmful. Once again, the semantic confusion caused by the medical model makes this simple fact difficult to see. In medicine, it is sometimes necessary to undergo a painful procedure in order to restore health. But psychiatric treatments are not analogous to medical ones. It was not in order to restore healthy physical functioning that David was being forced to starve. He was being starved into submission. It should be an individual's decision—not a psychiatrist's—whether or not to be a vegetarian. Defining meat eating as mentally healthy does not make forced meat eating a medical treatment.

In the past six years of activity in the mental patients' liberation movement, I have gotten to know literally hundreds of ex-patients. As we have told our stories to one another, it has been truly amazing how the same themes, often the same words, occur again and again.

In answer to the question, How did you get out of a mental institution? I have heard many ex-patients use the identical phrases I once used. "You tell them what they want to hear. You learn to play the game."

One common route into the mental hospital occurs when a person experiences a number of life crises at the same time. It can be truly frightening to find oneself suddenly without friends, money, or a place to live, which is what happened to eighteen-year-old Nancy.[3]

> I was involved in a painful and mutually destructive relationship with a woman whose life-style was very different from mine. Finally, I managed to break it off. We were oppressing each other—it was awful. Just as I was leaving her, leaving New York, she got sick. She couldn't go to a doctor because she didn't have any money. I felt so guilty, but at the same time I knew I had to leave. I came back to Boston, but I had no place to live except with two men that I hated. I thought I had a job, but I lost it. I didn't have any money. I began to hear my lover's voice; she was asking me for help. I thought I was going crazy. I went out for a walk and ended up at Cambridge City Hospital—I guess I was heading there without realizing it. I told them I was afraid—there were so many thoughts going around in my head that it was almost impossible to talk.
>
> What they did—all they really did—was to give me a lot of Stelazine. I was afraid of the other patients, and I hardly came out of my room. The hospital was an awful place to be. After a month, I escaped.

One way to look at Nancy's voices, the psychiatric way, is to see them as symptoms of illness, requiring hospitalization and drug treatment. But is it really that abnormal, unusual, or "sick" to react to such overwhelming stress so dramatically? Nancy's "treatment," which continued with three other hospitalizations within a short period, resulted in her thinking of herself as a chronic patient.

> By the time of the third hospitalization, I felt comfortable in hospitals. When I wasn't inside, I was scared. Everything was frightening. During the periods when I was home, my parents were very tense. They were watching me differently—no one believed I could make it on the outside. I thought I would spend the rest of my life in hospitals. I would look at people on the street and wonder what they had that I didn't. It was such a mystery to me.

Mystification is one of the characteristics of institutional psychiatric treatment. Nancy believed she was "different" because the treatment she received brought that message along with it. Being a mental patient meant that her problems were somehow different from other people's, since she seemed to require drugs and institutionalization. Instead of helping her to deal with the reality of her feelings, the hospital mystified them into symptoms of illness. It is realistic to feel guilt at the breakup of a difficult love relationship—guilt that Nancy experienced as "hearing" her lover's voice calling her. It is realistic to be frightened at finding oneself penniless and alone. Nancy's hospitalizations only added to her real-life problems. She began to believe that she was incapable of finding any solutions, and her family and friends turned away from her.

> For a long time after I got out, I stayed home all the time, except when I was at school. I stopped going to feminist meetings, although I had been very active before. Women in the women's movement, in the lesbian movement, women I had known for a long time and worked with, started treating me differently after I had been in the hospital. They were oppressing me. They wouldn't tell me things, wouldn't ask me to do any work, because they thought I couldn't handle stuff. They had been my friends, but now they would look at me as if I was crazy. When I tried to talk about it, I was afraid I was being paranoid.

Nancy's experience is a common one among ex-patients. People have so many stereotypes of mental illness that they and find it almost impossible to react normally to the ex-patient. When they see an ex-patient get angry or annoyed or express virtually any emotion, they become afraid that the patient is becoming "sick" again. The ex-patient, who is usually demoralized by the whole hospitalization experience, finds this stancing by old friends discouraging, just one more obstacle resuming a "normal" life.

What changed things for Nancy was her discovery of the mental patients' movement.

I came to the conference not knowing what to expect. What I found were people I could talk to, relate to, people who thought it was all right to be different. There was no one standard of behavior, except that we all hated hospitals. I would listen to people speak and then find myself thinking, not; "That's what I think too." I kept getting happier and happier. I stayed up all night talking, which is unusual for me: I was elated, but it wasn't like a manic high. I felt calm at the same time. What was happening was that I was finding a direction I could take and people I could take it with. People have to start fighting oppression by fighting their own oppression, and I saw that I was oppressed as a mental patient even more than I was as a woman or a lesbian.

I used to feel that it was important to fight oppression, but since I was one of the weak ones, I had to let others fight for me. I would always be one of the helpers, not a participant. Now I'm fighting—for myself and others. I found a place I could plug in, where I could address myself to my most immediate oppression. It made me so happy.

After the conference, I had the strength to confront my father about his attitudes toward me, his belief that I was sick. And he's been trying to change. It felt really good when he said to me, "It's been a privilege to watch you grow and change." I feel strong now. I feel good about myself.

The intensive consciousness raising experience of participating in an ex-patients' conference caused Nancy to change her attitudes about herself. She was able to change from feeling weak to feeling strong because she suddenly discovered support for ideas that she had thought were hers alone, ideas that had made her feel "paranoid" when she tried to discuss them with her old friends. Suddenly her feelings about herself—and about hospitals—underwent drastic revision.

> A few days after the conference I went back to Human Resource Institute [the place of her second psychiatric hospitalization]. I guess it was my old way of thinking showing itself for the last time. But suddenly I realized that what I got there—the medication, the constant put-downs—it was no good. I left calmly, knowing I would not be back. The hospital had ceased to be an alternative for me.

Frequently ex-patients are afraid to face their real feelings about the experience of mental institutionalization. Family and friends tend to react negatively to expressions of anger and hatred toward the hospital and staff, seeing these as indications of illness. Patients often feel the same way and may try desperately to believe that the hospital was a basically helpful and positive place. That was my experience, and Nancy's—it is a common one. Ex-patients need support in order to express the outrage they may never have admitted even to themselves. Being with other people who have gone through the same experience can be exhilarating, as it was for Nancy.

This change—from viewing the hospital experience as a positive one to seeing it as basically unhelpful—is crucial. During their institutionalization patients must believe (or appear to believe) that the hospital is a helpful place in order to be considered "well" by the staff. To be discharged, a patient must confirm the psychiatric version of reality, including an acknowledgment that hospitalization has been necessary and beneficial. Patients who maintain that the hospital is a prison and express this opinion to staff do not get discharged, as sociologist Robert Perrucci found when he studied discharge procedures. In one of the discharge interviews he observed, the patient gave a series of "appropriate" answers to staff questions, until the doctor asked her if she thought she had been helped.

PATIENT: No, I don't.

DOCTOR: What kind of treatment have you had here?

PATIENT: Lobotomy and shock.

DOCTOR: Do you think it's helped you or tortured you?

PATIENT: I think it's tortured me.[4]

The interview continued, with the patient presenting a reasonable explanation of why she preferred to leave the hospital and get a laboratory job rather than take a work-release placement while remaining a patient.

PATIENT: I'd do much better if the hospital would free me.

DOCTOR: What do you mean, "free you"?

PATIENT: Well, it would be just like the other work placements I've had. You're never really free.

DOCTOR: But if you stayed here on a work placement, you'd be free to come and go on your own time. It would be just like a job

PATIENT: No. You would still be controlling me if I stayed here.

DOCTOR: Do you mean we control your mind here?

PATIENT: You may not control my mind, but I really don't have a mind of my own.

DOCTOR: How about if we gave you a work placement in _____; would you be free then? That's far away from here.

PATIENT: Anyplace I went it would be the same setup as it is here. You're never really free; you're still a patient, and everyone you work with knows it. It's tough to get away from the hospital's control.

DOCTOR: That's *the most paranoid statement I ever* heard.[5]

Obviously, the patient did not get her discharge. When Perrucci interviewed her afterward on the ward, she remarked, "I did learn something from that staff [interview], though. If I ever get a chance to go again, I'll keep my big mouth shut, and I'll lie like hell. This time I said what I really felt, and look what happened."[6] Unfortunately, Perrucci does not tell us what ultimately happened to this patient.

The recognition that the hospital has not been a helpful place can lead to many new realizations, as it did for Nancy, who suddenly began to think of herself as strong, as capable of taking action, because she had freed herself from accepting the hospital's image of her.

While I was at Human Resource Institute in a sense I could see that it was a lot of game playing—having to talk about yourself at the meetings every day—but in a sense I went along with it too. I hated all the talking—but I didn't trust my own perceptions that it was all nonsense. It was much easier just to go along and do what they wanted me to do, say what they wanted me to say. But a part of me, even then, recognized that the talks the patients had in the kitchen in the evening, without staff, were much more helpful.

This kind of attitude change can lead to a person's making real changes in his or her life. It is not that an illness has suddenly been cured, but that a crippling belief has suddenly been proven false. The belief in one's own inferiority makes taking action impossible; the discovery that the inferiority doesn't really exist is liberating.

In the hospital, a lot of things seemed designed to make you feel lousy about yourself. Once, a group of patients were taken on an outing to the circus. It was fun, except during the intermission, when the nurse handed out pills to everyone.

Another activity that would have been fun, except for the staff's attitude, was cooking. When the staff member praised me for doing something well, she said, "Oh, you did it all by yourself," the way one would praise a small child.

> At Newton-Wellesley Hospital, the doctor who ran group therapy would be really sarcastic to the patients. When I would speak up in the group, he would say, "Do you want to be the star?" At the same time, we would be criticized if we didn't participate.

Not every ex-patient becomes demoralized by the experience of institutionalization. Leonard Roy Frank (whose story was told in Chapter 1) is one person who never doubted the wrongness of what was done to him.

> I never doubted my own sanity. Soon after awakening from the last shock treatment, I almost immediately perceived the situation as one in which I was being imprisoned. I knew something dreadful had been done to me, even though I had no recollection of the immediate past [an effect of ECT]. As soon as I had sufficiently recovered from the confusion caused by the shocks and the drugs, as soon as I had recuperated from the aftereffects of the tortures, I decided I would play along with the doctors in order to get out of there. I lied to them. When you lie to psychiatrists in this way, they accept it as the truth. But when you tell the truth—that the treatments are harmful, that you're not sick—that's regarded as "hostility," and as further evidence of the fact that the disease has persisted, or that you have "lack of insight."[7]

But few people have the strength to stand up for what they believe in the face of almost unanimous opposition, especially when their opponents control their lives and their freedom. Most people need a supportive atmosphere in order to recognize and express their negative feelings about hospitalization.

Not all ex-patients are angry about what was done to them. Some feel it was a valuable experience, even that it has saved their life. There are patients who feel better when they take Thorazine (or other psychiatric drugs). But it is impossible to know how common feelings of anger are, since ex-patients seldom are given the opportunity to express that anger without negative consequences. The positive values attached to psychiatric treatment by the general public often lead to the assumption that ex-patients who speak badly of their experiences are still "sick"—and the feelings, thoughts, and beliefs of many people believed to be "mentally ill" are simply not taken seriously. Books written by ex-patients in praise of their psychiatric treatment, on the other hand, find ready acceptance.[8]

The movement to set up true alternatives to the mental hospitals that many ex-patients have found so debilitating provides not only an opportunity for ex-patients to recognize their anger but also the chance to use what they have learned from their own experiences to shape alternatives that will meet real needs. From such experiences I and many others have learned the importance of emotional support from caring people, support that is difficult to find in rigidly structured mental institutions. Yet, it is in search of such support that many people have gone voluntarily into mental hospitals, only to discover that hospitals make true human contact between patient and staff nearly impossible.

Psychologist D. L. Rosenhan and his colleagues mimicked the symptoms of mental illness (they claimed to be hearing voices) and were admitted as patients to various mental institutions, where they experienced how rare support from staff members is. Rosenhan gives two reasons to explain this lack of contact:

> First are attitudes held by all of us toward the mentally ill—including those who treat them— attitudes characterized by fear, distrust, and horrible expectations on the one hand, and benevolent intentions on the other. Our ambivalence leads, in this instance as in others, to avoidance.
>
> Second, and not entirely separate, the hierarchical structure of the psychiatric hospital facilitates depersonalization. Those who are at the top have least to do with patients, and their behavior inspires the rest of the staff.[9]

The pseudopatients kept records of how much time they spent with professional members of the staff (psychiatrists, psychologists, and clinical residents)—it averaged

6.8 minutes per day.[10] "Clearly," Rosenhan concludes, "patients do not spend much time in interpersonal contact with doctoral staff. And doctoral staff serve as models for nurses and attendants."[11]

The hierarchical organization of the psychiatric hospital [leads to] those with the most power hav[ing] least to do with patients, and those with the least power [being] most involved with them. Recall, however, that the acquisition of role-appropriate behaviors occurs mainly through the observation of others, with the most powerful having the most influence. Consequently, it is understandable that attendants not only spend more time with patients than do any other members of the staff—that is required by their station in the hierarchy—but also, insofar as they learn from their superiors' behavior, spend as little time with patients as they can.[12]

The mental health establishment frequently claims that increased funding will lead to increased staffing and better patient care. Rosenhan doubts this:

> I have the impression that the psychological forces that result in depersonalization are much stronger than the fiscal ones and that the addition of more staff would not correspondingly improve patient care in this regard. The incidence of staff meetings and the enormous amount of record-keeping on patients, for example, have not been as substantially reduced [by fiscal pressures] as has patient contact. Priorities exist, even during hard times. Patient contact is not a significant priority in the traditional psychiatric hospital.[13]

I have given this lengthy account of Rosenhan's opinions to illustrate that it is not only angry ex-patients who have come to these conclusions. Rosenhan's study was published in early 1973, and his opinions were widely publicized. When a psychologist said what ex-patients had known for years, the ideas suddenly became credible. Rosenhan, however, qualified his conclusions by stating that he did "not pretend to describe the subjective experiences of true patients," whose experiences might have been different, "particularly with the passage of time and the necessary process of adaptation to one's environment."[14] It is unfortunate that the Rosenhan experimenters, living side by side with "real" patients, did not discuss their findings with them and find out whether or not the "real" patients perceived things differently.

It is important for ex-patients to practice consciousness raising with other ex-patients in order to develop their real feelings about themselves and their experiences. Often patients have accurate assessments of the problems that led them into the hospital, which are far different than the official, psychiatric opinion of what is wrong with them, an opinion that they must accept in order to be seen by the staff as well. This leads to incredible confusion and anger. Arlene Sen of the Mental Patients' Liberation Front in Boston recalls an incident:

> One thing I used to hate was when we had to answer questions about ourselves in front of a lot of doctors and other patients. Once they asked me what I thought my major problem was, and I said, "I think I'm too dependent on men." They really ridiculed that—here I was, this sick person, who did all these crazy things, that's the way they saw me, the way they wanted me to see myself. Of course, now, years later, after being in the women's movement and the mental patients' movement, I can see that I was right. But the institution was working against that realization, which was something I really needed in order to change my life in a good direction.[15]

By experiencing consciousness raising together, ex-patients can learn a new trust in their own strengths and abilities. The consciousness-raising process can lead a group in many different directions. One possibility that can arise is a joint effort to work toward alternative facilities. Along with the recognition of the antitherapeutic nature of much psychiatric treatment comes the formulation of what does make a good place for a person to come to in times of emotional distress.

In early 1971 a group of ex-patients in Vancouver, British Columbia, called a public meeting to discuss dissatisfaction with the psychiatric system. The organizers had been patients together in a psychiatric day hospital, a supposedly progressive arrangement that treats patients during the day and permits them to go home evenings and weekends. This group of patients, however, did not find the setup supportive, since they discovered that crises frequently arose precisely during the times when staff was unavailable (evenings and weekends), and it was against the rules for patients to see one another or talk on the phone outside the institution. One Monday morning the patients arrived on the ward and learned that over the weekend one of their number had committed suicide. Many strong emotions were expressed, and one immediate result was the clandestine circulation of a patients' phone list.

As time went on, some of the patients discovered that they were relying on these "illegal" phone calls far more than on the therapy they were receiving during day hospital hours, and they began to talk among themselves about the kinds of "help" that were truly useful. By the time all of them had been discharged from the hospital, and they felt that their informal network was the one form of real support they had. They decided to try to find more people who had similar feelings about psychiatric treatment and to discuss with this larger group what could be done.

A sympathetic newspaper columnist wrote a story about the group, publicizing the open meeting they were planning. More than seventy-five people came to the meeting, most of them ex-patients who had equally negative feelings about their treatment. Some had suffered truly horrifying mistreatment—one woman had received more than a hundred shock treatments and had spent years on the "back wards" of the province's public mental hospital. Out of the enthusiasm of finding one another and discovering that they shared similar feelings, the participants decided immediately to provide the services they had been unable to find through mental health agencies. One man offered the use of his house, and the group soon found itself operating a drop-in center. The question of what to call themselves arose, and after considering several ambiguous names, the group decided on the straightforward Mental Patients' Association.

Today the Mental Patients' Association operates a seven-day-a-week drop-in center and five cooperative residences—all on the principles of participatory democracy. Paid staff members are members of the association, not professionals, and are elected by the membership for six-month terms. All decision-making power is in the hands of the membership, expressed by votes taken at weekly business meetings and at general membership meetings held every three weeks. The Mental Patients' Association (which will be discussed in detail in Chapter 6) is living proof that ex-patients can formulate and run services in which the needs of the clients shape the direction and structure of the organization.

The origins of the Mental Patients' Association clearly show the process of consciousness raising at work. Originally, the day hospital patients went along with the rules, ignoring their own perceptions that their crises did not fit into the nine-to-five, Monday-to-Friday availability of the staff. They accepted the rule that they not have outside communications with one another, a rule that implied that only "experts" (and certainly not mental patients) could help people with their problems. The suicide led to a realization that they needed one another. Many of the patients wished they had reached out to the dead man and wanted to make sure that if they felt desperate themselves, they would be able to get support from one another. Gradually, as they saw how much they used the phone list and how helpful it was, they saw that the official psychiatric view was wrong and that patients could help one another as well as or better than the staff. From feeling weak and powerless, they had moved toward feeling strong.

At about the same time the Mental Patients' Association was being organized in Vancouver, a group of ex-patients in New York City began meeting together to discuss their dissatisfaction with psychiatric treatment. The two groups were unknown to each other, but their overall outlook was remarkably similar. The New York group called itself the Mental Patients' Liberation Project. Over the first few weeks of their existence, their discussions led to the writing of a mental patients' bill of rights. The production of this document is another example of the consciousness raising process at work. The membership of MPLP recognized that the abuses each of them had experienced were not isolated examples of mistreatment but were built into the system. The rights they listed were fundamental human rights, yet they were routinely denied to mental patients. "Because these rights are not now legally ours, we are now going to fight to make them a reality," they stated in the preamble.[16] The rights listed were:

1. You are a human being and are entitled to be treated as such with as much decency and respect as is accorded to any other human being.
2. You are an American citizen and are entitled to every right established by the Declaration of Independence and guaranteed by the Constitution of the United States of America.
3. You have the right to the integrity of your own mind and the integrity of your own body.
4. Treatment and medication can be administered only with your consent and, in the event you give your consent, you have the right to know all relevant information regarding said treatment and/or medication.
5. You have the right to access to your own legal and medical counsel.
6. You have the right to refuse to work in a mental hospital and/or to choose what work you will do; and you have the right to receive the usual wage for such work as is set by the state labor laws.
7. You have the right to decent medical attention when you feel you need it, just as any other human being has that right.
8. You have the right to uncensored communication by phone, letter, and in person with whomever you wish and at any time you wish.
9. You have the right not to be treated like a criminal; not to be locked up against your will; not to be committed involuntarily; not to be fingerprinted or "mugged" (photographed).
10. You have the right to decent living conditions. You're paying for it, and the taxpayers are paying for it.
11. You have the right to retain your own personal property. No one has the right to confiscate what is legally yours, no matter what reason is given. That is commonly known as theft.
12. You have the right to bring grievance against those who have mistreated you and the right to counsel and a court hearing. You are entitled to protection by the law against retaliation.
13. You have the right to refuse to be a guinea pig for experimental drugs and treatments and to refuse to be used as learning material for students. You have the right to reimbursement if you are so used.
14. You have the right to request an alternative to legal commitment or incarceration in a mental hospital.

The "Mental Patients' Bill of Rights" was drawn up in response to specific abuses that had been experienced by members of the group. The popular myth that holds that mental hospitals have improved dramatically since tranquilizers were introduced in the mid-1950s is belied by the existence of these abuses. The members of MPLP found strength in their united outlook and their sense of outrage. Providing an alternative to mental hospitals was a goal of MPLP, but money was not available, and the group turned to distribution of the bill of rights as a means of publicizing conditions inside mental hospitals. Later MPLP (which is no longer in existence) was able to obtain a storefront headquarters and ran a crisis center staffed by members.

Consciousness raising was one of the main activities of the Central Patients' Liberation Front in Boston, which was also founded in 1971. MPLF began with two ex-patients, each of whom had the dream of starting an organization of mental patients who wanted to fight back. Meeting first at the offices of *The Radical Therapist* (an antipsychiatry journal now called *State and Mind*) and then in the apartment of one of the members, the group focused on consciousness raising because, as Bette Maher, one of the founders, recalls:

> We needed it. Many patients were still into the head-trip of feeling that they deserved what happened to them—they were "psychologized" into believing it. At consciousness-raising meetings, we would talk about how people ended up in hospitals—it was because their lives had become intolerable. But hospitals made people worse off than they were to begin with.
>
> We had strategy meetings, too, but we alternated them with consciousness raising. And if someone came to a strategy meeting and ws really upset, the way we dealt with it was that one of us would volunteer to go into another room and talk to that person. We didn't want to turn the person off, but we needed to have strategy meetings, too.
>
> A lot of people stopped coming to strategy meetings because they didn't want to be involved in anything political. But they kept coming to the consciousness-raising meetings because they said that the meetings helped them to feel self-respect which they never had before.[17]

At MPLF, consciousness raising led the group toward the writing of a patients' rights handbook. "Because patients had so few rights, we didn't think the handbook would give patients that much actual help, but we saw it as a tool for consciousness raising among patients," Bette Maher says now. The handbook took months to write. A small group of ex-patients, although untrained in the law, thoroughly researched the mental health laws in Massachusetts. They had the help of a lawyer as a consultant, but they did all the research and writing themselves. When it was finished, they made the rounds of activist groups in Boston and got a number of small donations that enabled them to have the handbook printed at the New England Free Press, a nonprofit printing collective.

Your Rights As a Mental Patient in Massachusetts is a remarkable fifty-six-page document that covers the laws concerning commitment, voluntary and involuntary hospitalization, the special situation of minors, patients' civil rights and treatment, as well as providing an overall strategy for fighting back. The handbook also contains a bill of rights, which, while it contains many parallels with the one written by the Mental Patients' Liberation Project in New York, also contains many differences of emphasis. The final right listed in the handbook is especially significant:

> You have the right to patient-run facilities where the decisions that are made and work that is done are your responsibility and under your control.[18]

The handbook also contains a chapter on the special difficulties of ex-patients, such as problems of child custody, government access to psychiatric records, job discrimination, difficulty in getting driver's licenses, discrimination in admission to colleges and graduate schools, and the fear and distrust people feel toward ex-patients. And, the section concludes, "you probably won't be Vice President of the United States."[19]

This survey of some of the early mental patients' liberation groups has shown several of the directions in which consciousness raising can lead. There is no one single direction for ex-patient groups to take. The needs of members are what has shaped these and other groups, not adherence to any formula. Local conditions may differ, as may the energies and specific interests of members. Consciousness raising (which may not be specifically called that) helps groups to clarify what they want and what they need, as well as what is possible. Consciousness raising is a process that ensures that the needs of members are met, because everyone participates by contributing his or her own thoughts, feelings, and opinions, and because there is no one right way of doing things.

Mental patient consciousness raising may lead to many different kinds of action. As we have seen from these brief looks at groups in Vancouver, New York, and Boston, it can lead to the setting up of drop-in centers and communal residences, to action projects that publicize conditions inside mental hospitals, or to focusing on patients' rights. Other possible directions include the setting up of crisis centers (sometimes called "freak-out centers"), the establishment of new kinds of member-controlled social service centers (such as job-finding services), or the operating of nonprofit businesses to provide nonalienating work for members.

Whatever a group may decide to do as an outgrowth of consciousness raising will be enhanced by members' growing awareness that they can be strong and competent people. As the group proceeds with its chosen work, ongoing consciousness raising will help to ensure that members never lose sight of their ability to help one another and will be a constant reminder that there are no real "experts."

Notes

1. Frank M. Ochberg, "Community Mental Health Center Legislation: Flight of the Phoenix," *American Journal of Psychiatry* 133, no. 1 (January 1976): 56–61. This figure is broken down into $8 billion in the public sphere, ($4–5 billion for state and county hospitals, $1 billion for community mental health centers, and $2 billion spent by the military) and $5 billion in the private sphere ($1 billion for private hospitals and health maintenance organizations, and $4 billion for private practitioners).
2. David and I were in the same consciousness-raising group in 1972.
3. All quotes from Nancy from personal interview, October 26, 1976.
4. Robert Perrucci, *Circle of Madness* (Englewood Cliffs, N.J.: Prentice-Hall, 1974), p. 157.
5. Ibid., pp. 157–158 (emphasis added).
6. Ibid., p. 159.
7. Personal interview with Leonard Roy Frank, December 7, 1976.
8. See, for example, Clifford W. Beers, *A Mind That Found Itself* (Garden City, N.Y.: Doubleday, 1953); Barbara Field Benziger, *The Prison of My* Mind (New York: Walker & Company, 1969); Hannah Green, *I Never Promised You a Rose Garden* (New York: Holt, Rinehart and Winston, 1964); Nancy Covert Smith, *Journey Out of Nowhere* (Waco, Texas: Word Books, 1973); Ellen Wolfe, *Aftershock* (New York: G. P. Putnam's Sons, 1969). All were written by people who have been psychiatrically hospitalized. I exclude the large number of books written by grateful ex-patients who received office psychotherapy.
9. D. L. Rosenhan, "On Being Sane in Insane Places," Science 179 (January 19, 1973):256.
10. Ibid.
11. Ibid.
12. Ibid., pp. 254–255.

13. Ibid., p. 256 (emphasis added).
14. Ibid., p. 257.
15. Personal interview with Arlene Sen, January 11,1977.
16. Mental Patients' Liberation Project, "Bill of Rights," n.d.
17. All quotes from Bette Maher, from personal interview, March 17, 1997.
18. Your Rights as a Mental Patient in Massachusetts (West Somerville,Mass.: Legal Project/ Mental Patients' Liberation Front, 1974), p. 41.
19. Ibid, p. 39.

20

Leete, E. (1989). How I perceive and manage my illness. *Schizophrenia Bulletin,* *15* (2), 197–200

First person accounts of mental illness had been written before Leete, but few had been published in academic-research journals. In three articles published between 1987 and 1989, Leete, who had been diagnosed with schizophrenia about 25 years earlier, writes about her personal experience of mental illness and treatment. She discusses a number of personal coping strategies and offers recommendations for the range of services that community-based mental health programs should provide to persons with serious mental illnesses. These include consumer education about mental illness, supportive psychotherapy, pharmacotherapy, ongoing support, and access to meaningful and fulfilling activities such as education and work. Here, we include her account in *Schizophrenia Bulletin* about her experience of schizophrenia and the recovery process as she lived it, with practical suggestions for patients and their service providers about concrete instances of problems associated with schizophrenia. Leete discusses her experience of paranoia, for example, specifically her fear of being surprised by the presence of police who will come to harass her. Her method of coping with and managing her paranoia is to choose a chair that faces the door at home or in other places. The internal impetus that prompts the paranoia did not disappear, she writes, but a simple behavioral strategy helps her cope with it personally and, by enabling her to remain at her table in public helps her cope with it socially, as well.

How I Perceive and Manage My Illness

Abstract: The article describes some of the ongoing problems psychiatric patients encounter on a daily basis as perceived" by an individual who has lived with schizophrenia for more than 25 years. Specific carefully planned coping strategies which are seen as critical to the recovery process are presented.

More than by any other one thing, my life has been changed by schizophrenia. For the past 20 years I have lived with it and in spite of it—struggling to come to terms with it without giving in to it. Although I have fought a daily battle, it is only now that I have some sense of confidence that I will survive my ordeal. Taking responsibility for my life and developing coping mechanisms has been crucial to my recovery. I would like to share some of these with the reader now.

To maintain my mental health, I found I had to change my priorities and take better care of myself. I modified my attitudes, becoming more accepting and nonjudgmental of others. In addition, I altered my behavior and response to symptoms. I have also had to plan for the use of my time. When one has a chaotic inner existence, the structure of a predictable daily schedule makes life easier. Now, obviously structured activity can be anything, but for me it is work—a paying job, the ultimate goal. It gives me something to look forward to every day and a skill to learn and to improve. It is my motivation for getting up each morning. In addition, my hours are passed therapeutically as well as productively. As I work, I become increasingly self-confident, and my self-image is bolstered. I feel important and grownup, which replaces my usual sense of vulnerability, weakness, and incompetence. Being a member of the work force decreases stigma and contributes to acceptance by my community, which in turn makes my life easier.

Research continues to show that one of the differences between the brain of a "normal" person and one who has schizophrenia is a major difficulty filtering or screening out background noises. I am hyperalert, acutely aware of every sound or movement in my environment. I am often confused by repetitive noises or multiple stimuli and become nervous, impatient, and irritable. To deal with this, I make a deliberate effort to reduce distractions as much as possible.

I often have difficulty interacting with others socially and tend to withdraw. I have found I feel more comfortable, however, if I socialize with others who have similar interests or experiences to my own. To counteract my problem with poor eye contact, I force myself to look up from time to time, even if I have to look a little past the person with whom I am speaking. If I do become overwhelmed in a social situation, I may temporarily withdraw by going into another room (even the restroom) to be alone for a while.

I attempt to keep in touch with my feelings and to attend immediately to difficulties, including symptoms like paranoia. For example, instead of constantly worrying about the police surprising me, I always choose a seat where I can face the door, preferably with my back to a wall instead of to other people. In general, instead of working myself up emotionally over some threatening possibility, I will check out reality by asking the people I am with questions like who they are calling, where they are going, or whatever. It clears the air immediately, and usually I am satisfied with their answer and can go on about my business. In other words, I cope by recognizing and confronting my paranoid fears immediately and then moving on with my life, freeing my mind for other things. Also, I have learned to suppress paranoid responses, and I make an effort not to talk to myself or to my voices when others are nearby. It can be done through self-discipline and practice.

In addition, I suffer from feelings of isolation, alienation, and loneliness. This is difficult to deal with because on the one hand I need to be with people, but on the other hand I am frightened of it. I have come to realize my own diminished capacity for really close friendships, but also my need for many acquaintances. An ongoing and reliable support system has been extremely important. I have gained much practical information, insight, and support from my peer-run support group, a very comfortable means of coming to accept and deal with mental illness. Also, it has been invaluable to have someone I trust (often my husband) with whom I can "test reality." I let him know my perceptions and he gives me feedback. I am then able to consider the possibility that my perceptions may not be accurate, and I modify my response accordingly if I wish. In this way I can usually acknowledge more conventional ways of thinking, instead of automatically incorporating outside informtion into my delusional system.

A common complaint from persons with a mental illness is that of impaired concentration and memory. This can make holding a job or even completing a thought very difficult. To overcome the effects of a poor memory, I make lists and write down all information of importance. Through years of effort I have managed to develop an incredible amount of concentration, although I am only able to sustain this for relatively brief periods of time.

Sometimes I still find it difficult to keep my thoughts together. I therefore request that communication be simple, clear, and unambiguous. It helps me if the information is specific, as vague or diffuse responses only confuse me. When speaking to someone, I may need more time to think and understand before responding, and I take this time. Likewise, I have learned when working on a task to be careful, perhaps taking more time than others, and to concentrate fiercely on what I am doing. And I must be persistent.

Many times when becoming acutely ill, I am frightened of everything, feeling small and vulnerable. When I am in distress, I do whatever makes me feel better. This may be pacing, curling up into a ball, or rocking back and forth. I have found that most of these behaviors can be accomplished without appearing too strange, believe it or not. For example, I can pace by taking a walk, I can curl up when I sleep, and I can rock in a rocking chair or hammock or even by going to an amusement park. I am often able to relax by physically exercising, reading, or watching a movie. In general, then, I think I am discovering, how to appear less bizarre.

I find it crucial to schedule time between events rigidly. For example, I will not agree to give two talks on the same day. I find I must also give myself as much time as I can in which to make decisions; I have an enormous amount of ambivalence, and pressure to come to a decision quickly can immobilize me. (It is not a pretty picture.) Too much free time is also detrimental. Therefore, I find it useful to structure my leisure time and to limit it. Perhaps someday I will be able to handle it in greater increments, but for now I find it best to keep very busy, with minimal amounts of leisure time.

Perhaps the coping strategy I use the most is compulsive organizing. I think a controlled environment is probably so important to me because my brain is not always manageable. Making lists organizes my thoughts. It also increases self-esteem, because when I have accomplished something and crossed it off my list, it is a very concrete indication to me that I am capable of setting a goal, working toward it, and actually accomplishing it. These "small" successes build my confidence to go out and try other things. As a part of this process, I break down tasks into small steps, taking them one at a time. Perhaps organizing and giving speeches about my illness is another coping skill—and the audience response is a type of reality-testing.

In general, then, I believe I do have an irritable brain. I am super-sensitive to any stimulus. My behavior is sometimes erratic, and I am easily frustrated and extremely impulsive. I regret that I still have times of uncontrollable angry outbursts. I cope with these and other symptoms by taking low doses of medication. Before I came to realize the role medications could play in my illness, I was caught in a vicious circle. When I was off the medication, I couldn't remember how much better I had felt on it, and when I was taking the medication, I felt so good that I was convinced I did not need it. Fortunately, through many years of trial and error, I have learned what medication works best for me and when to take it to minimize side effects based on my daily schedule. Increasing my medication periodically is one means I often use for stabilization during a particularly stressful period.

I want to emphasize that stress does play a major role in my illness. There are enormous pressures that come with any new experience or new environment, and any change, positive or negative, is extremely difficult. Whatever I can do to decrease or avoid high-stress situations or environments is helpful in controlling my symptoms. In general terms, all of my coping strategies largely consist of four steps: (1) recognizing when I am feeling stressed, which is harder than it may sound; (2) identifying the stressor; (3) remembering from past experience what action helped in the same situation or a similar one; and (4) taking that action as quickly as possible. After I have identified a potential source of stress, I prepare mentally for the situation by anticipating problems. Knowing what to expect in a new situation considerably lowers my anxiety about it. In addition, I try to recognize my own particular limitations and plan in advance, setting reasonable goals.

Please understand that these are the kinds of obstacles that confront individuals with a psychiatric disorder every day. Yet we are perceived as weak. On the contrary, I believe we are among the most courageous. We struggle constantly with our raging fears and the brutality of our thoughts, and then we are subjected as well to the misunderstanding, distrust, and ongoing stigma we experience from the community. Believe me, there is nothing more devastating, discrediting, and disabling to an individual recovering from mental illness than stigma.

Life is hard with a diagnosis of schizophrenia. I can talk, but I may not be heard. I can make suggestions, but they may not be taken seriously. I can report my thoughts, but they may be seen as delusions. I can recite experiences, but they may be interpreted as fantasies. To be a patient or even ex-client is to be discounted. Your label is a reality that never leaves you; it gradually shapes an identity that is hard to shed. We must transform public attitudes and current stereotypes. Until we eliminate stigma, we will have prejudice, which will inevitably be expressed as discrimination against, persons with mental illness.

We rarely read about people who have successfully dealt with their emotional problems and are making it, and they will not usually identify themselves to us because they are all too aware of the general attitude. The current image the public has of the mentally ill must be changed, not to mention that of the individual himself. We have grown up in the same society and have the same feelings about mental illness, but we must also live with the label.

Ultimately we must conquer stigma from within. As a first step—and a crucial one—it is imperative for us as clients to look within ourselves for our strengths. These strengths are the tools for rebuilding our self-image and thus our self-esteem. I found that I first had to convince myself of my worthiness, then worry about others. Each time I am successful at a task it serves to reinforce my own capabilities and boost my confidence. Just this way, persons with mental illness can and must change the views and expectations of others.

Obviously, education about mental illness is critical for all parties involved, especially for the patient. I have made an extensive study of my disorder and have found education invaluable in understanding my illness, coming to terms with it, and dealing with it. We must conscientiously and continually study our illnesses and learn for ourselves what we can do to cope with the individual disabilities we experience.

Many of us have learned to monitor symptoms to determine the status of our illness, using our coping mechanisms to prevent psychotic relapse or to seek treatment earlier, thereby reducing the number of acute episodes and hospitalizations. My own personal warning signs of decompensation include fatigue or decreased sleep; difficulty with concentration and memory; increased paranoia, delusions, and hallucinations; tenseness and irritability; agitation; and being more easily overwhelmed by my surroundings. Coping mechanisms may include withdrawing and being alone for a while; obtaining support from a friend; socializing or otherwise distracting myself from stressor; organizing my thoughts through lists; problem-solving around specific issues; or temporarily increasing my medication.

Yet too many times our efforts to cope go unnoticed or are seen as symptoms themselves. If others understood us better, perhaps they would be more tolerant. We did not choose to be ill, but we can choose to deal with it and learn to live with it. By learning to modulate stress, we will more effectively manage our illness, thus endowing ourselves with an ongoing sense of mastery and control. I find my vulnerability to stress, anxiety, and accompanying symptoms decreases the more I am in control of my own life. Unfortunately, our progress continues to be measured by professionals with concepts like "consent" and "cooperate" and "comply" instead of "choose," insinuating that we are incapable of taking an active role as partners in our own recovery.

I see my schizophrenia as a mental disorder with a genetic predisposition, predictably expressing itself in times of extreme stress but often exacerbated by rather ordinary fluctuations in my environment. Mental illness is a handicap with biological, psychological, and social ramifications, making it a formidable obstacle to be overcome. I understand that life may be more difficult for me than for others and that I must preside over it more attentively for this reason. As with other chronic illnesses, it has demanded that I work harder than most. I know to expect good and bad times and to make the most of the good. I take my life very seriously and do as much with it as I can when I am feeling well, because I know that I will have difficult times again and will likely lose some of my gains.

Although there is no magic answer to the tragedy of mental illness, I contend that we need not be at its mercy. Appropriate treatment can help us understand our disease and we can learn to function in spite of it. We can overcome our illness and the myths surrounding it. We can successfully compensate for our disabilities. We can overcome the stigma, prejudice, discrimination, and rejection we have experienced and reclaim our personal validity, our dignity as individuals, and our autonomy. To do this, we must change the image of who we are and who we can become, first for ourselves and then for the public. If we do acknowledge and seriously study our illnesses; if we build on our assets: if we work to minimize our vulnerabilities by developing coping skills; if we confront our illnesses with courage and struggle with our symptoms persistently—we will successfully manage our lives and bestow our talents on society, the society that has traditionally abandoned us.

Clinical and Systems Theory, Conceptual, and Historical Texts

21

Gronfein, W. (1985). Psychotropic drugs and the origin of deinstitutionalization. *Social Problems, 32* (5), 437–454

Gronfein engages the debate over the impact of the new psychotropic drugs on deinstitutionalization, taking a position against that of those who claimed that the introduction of these drugs was a determining factor in reducing the patient population in state hospitals starting in the mid 1950s. Gronfein reviews historical data on aggregate changes in discharge rates from state and county mental hospitals before and after the introduction of psychoactive drugs. He argues they did not have a significant effect on discharge rates during the mid-1950s, in part because there was no community infrastructure in place at this time to accept putatively manageable patients. He concludes that the phenothiazines won over clinicians, staff, and policy makers to hope for a "new era in the treatment of mental illness" (p. 449), but that the seeming influence of these drugs on deinstitutionalization was tied more to the environment—a time of philosophical, public, and fiscal movement away from a reliance on institutionalization and an openness to, and demand for, different approaches—than to the biochemical properties of the drugs themselves. Gronfein also notes that from 1965 on, deinstitutionalization was strongly influenced by civil libertarian approaches that led to changes in hospital admission and discharge procedures favoring decreased admissions and shorter lengths of stay. The author has abridged his original article somewhat for this volume.

Psychotropic Drugs and the Origins of Deinstitutionalization

The deinstitutionalization of the mentally ill represents an important set of changes in the provision of mental health services. These changes involved the movement of patients out of state hospitals and the formulation of policies designed to promote community-based treatment alternatives. This paper examines the impact of psychotropic drugs on both population shifts and policy development. Using data on changes in discharge rates before and after the drugs were introduced in the mid 1950s, I find that the drugs did not affect movement out of the hospital significantly. I conclude that the introduction of psychotropic drugs encouraged policy changes that hastened the process of deinstitutionalization in the 1960s.

The treatment of the seriously mentally ill in the United States has undergone a series of radical transformations over the past 25 years. One of the principal changes was a marked reduction in the importance of state and county mental hospitals. In 1955 these institutions contained approximately 560,000 patients and accounted for almost half of all mental health patient care episodes; by 1977 they contained but 160,000 inmates and accounted for less than 10 percent of all mental health patient care episodes (Goldman et al., 1983; Kramer, 1977).

These sharp decreases in inpatient populations are one element in the complex of policies, philosophies, intentions, and facts which define the deinstitutionalization of the mentally ill. Deinstitutionalization has two goals. The first is the depopulation of state and county mental hospitals and other traditional institutions charged with the care of the mentally ill, and the second is the substitution of a network of community-based institutions to provide such care (Bachrach, 1978; General Accounting Office, 1977; Goldman et al., 1983). Deinstitutionalization has been sharply criticized for failing to implement its second goal, and much research has examined the problems created for patients, families, and communities (e.g., Arnhoff, 1975; Aviram and Segal, 1973; Aviram et al., 1976; Bachrach, 1976, 1978; Bassuk and Gerson, 1978; Becker and Schulberg, 1976; Braun et al., 1981; Freedman and Moran, 1983; Kirk and Therrien, 1975; Lerman, 1982; Morrissey, 1982; Rose, 1979; Segal and Aviram, 1978; Segal et al., 1974).

Deinstitutionalization is also grist for mills more explicitly analytic and sociological in character (e.g., Cohen, 1979; Estroff, 1981; Scull, 1977; Warren, 1981). The state hospital has been one of the densest symbols of disorder, estrangement, and exclusion to trouble the popular imagination, and has provided the central image for some of sociology's most influential treatments of social control. Goffman's (1961) delineation of total institutions, for instance, is based in part on his field work from 1955 to 1957 in St. Elizabeths, the public mental hospital serving the District of Columbia. Erikson's (1966) discussion of the persistence of exclusionary and segregative "deployment patterns" in the treatment accorded deviants in the United States likewise draws on the character of state hospitals prior to deinstitutionalization. The breakup of these models of social control is clearly a matter of both theoretical and practical importance.

Both the abrupt decline in state hospital populations which began in 1955, and the administrative, legislative, and judicial rulings at the state and federal levels which began in the late 1950s and early 1960s (Morrissey, 1982; Segal and Aviram, 1978) represented reversals of longstanding trends. Given the long domination of state and county mental hospitals over mental health services available to the seriously mentally ill (Pollack and Taube, 1975; Redick et al., 1973), a crucial question is why this institutional dominance ended when it did.

Since the turn of the century, state hospital populations had grown steadily, increasing fourfold from 1903 to 1955 (Council of State Governments, 1950; Kramer, 1977). During this period they were reviled as "bedlams," "snake pits," and "houses of horror" (American Psychiatric Association, 1949; Deutsch, 1948; Ward, 1946). The same critics who denounced these institutions urged that they be more generously funded, rather than depopulated (American Psychiatric Association, 1949, 1950, 1951, 1952, 1953, 1954; Beers, 1981; Deutsch, 1948). The Joint Commission on Mental Illness and Health (1961:190; emphasis in original) described publicly supported insane asylums with evident frustration as *"hospitals that seem to have no defenders but endure despite all attacks."*

The timing of deinstitutionalization raises many questions regarding the relative roles played by such factors as intraprofessional rivalry (Morrissey, 1982), ideological change (Bachrach, 1976, 1978), the expansion of the welfare state (Lerman, 1982), and fiscal crisis (Rose, 1979; Scull, 1977). This paper examines the impact of psychotropic drugs on the decline of state and county mental hospital populations and on the evolution of a mental health policy which espouses as one of its principal aims the "eschewal, shunning, and avoidance" (Bachrach, 1978:573) of such institutions.

I examine the impact of the introduction of psychtropic drugs on state hospitals for several reasons. First, the move away from state and county hospitals is a crucial element in the deinstitutionalization of the mentally ill. While deinstitutionalization calls for the creation of community-based facilities to provide mental health care, a reduction in the importance of state and county hospitals is an essential prerequisite for this kind of substitution. Second, as noted above, state and county mental hospitals were institutional responses to deviance that had great practical and symbolic importance (Bucher and Schatzman, 1962; Council of State Governments, 1950; Deutsch, 1948; Dunham and Weinberg, 1960; Erikson, 1966; Goffman, 1961).

Third, the psychotropic drugs have been the subject of intense interest and controversy ever since their introduction in 1954 (Brill and Patton, 1957, 1959; Clark, 1956; Joint Commission on Mental Illness and Health, 1961; Kinross-Wright, 1955; Morrissey, 1982; Rose, 1979; Scull, 1977; Sedgwick, 1982). Two opposing positions have emerged with respect to their effects on state hospitals. The more orthodox view holds with Pollack and Taube (1975:49) that "there appears to be no question that the sudden decrease in the state mental hospital population in 1956 ... was due to the widespread introduction of the psychoactive drugs into the mental hospitals" (see also Bachrach, 1976; General Accounting Office, 1977; Joint Commission on Mental Illness and Health, 1961; Pasamanick et al., 1967; Swazey, 1974). A number of "revisionist" authors (e.g., Aviram et al., 1976; Lerman, 1982; Rose, 1979; Scull, 1977; Segal and Aviram, 1978) downplay the importance of the drugs as a cause of deinstitutionalization and conclude with Sedgwick (1982:198) that this "straightforward 'pharmacological' explanation for the desegregation of patients ... is ... fatally flawed." These authors base their position on the methodological weaknesses of earlier studies that claimed to have demonstrated a drug effect on state hospital populations and on recent retrospective case studies showing that the expansion of federal health and welfare programs was more consequential in reducing state hospital populations than were the drugs (Aviram et al., 1976; Lerman, 1982; Scull, 1977; Segal and Aviram, 1978).

My analysis of the impact of the psychotropic drugs on the state hospitals is divided into five major sections. Deinstitutionalization refers to a number of processes and has proceeded quite differently at various times and in different places (Aviram et al., 1976; Bachrach, 1976; Lerman, 1982; Morrissey, 1982; Segal and Aviram, 1978). Therefore, I first analyze the conceptual, temporal, and geographic variations which have characterized deinstitutionalization. The second section discusses the consequences of the psychotropic medications for state hospital inmates, staffs, and administrations at the time of their introduction in 1954. The third section reviews evidence concerning the effects of drugs on state hospital populations in the aggregate. Here I supplement existing data with an analysis of changes in discharge rates at the level of individual states. The fourth section assesses the impact of the drugs on the development of mental health policy. In the fifth and final section, I summarize the changes in inpatient behavior, state and county hospital populations, and mental health policy which were stimulated by the introduction of the drugs.

Aspects of Deinstitutionalization

Although no terms are employed more routinely in contemporary discussions of mental health policy than "deinstitutionalization" and "the deinstitutionalization of the mentally ill," their precise definition is often left unstated (Lerman, 1982). Deinstitutionalization has multiple referents whose specification is a prerequisite for the examination of drug effects. Therefore, in the following discussion I outline the important conceptual, temporal, and geographic variations which have affected the meaning and content of the deinstitutionalization process.

The Conceptual Components of Deinstitutionalization

Deinstitutionalization is typically thought of as "a formal policy of the federal government ... [whose] numerical results to date are evident in a rapid decline in the inpatient populations of state and county hospitals" (Rose, 1979:430–31; see also Bassuk and Gerson, 1978; General Accounting Office, 1977; Kramer, 1977; Scull, 1977). Such a conception, in which population declines are taken as a straightforward reflection of policy directives, overstates the connection between changes in policy and changes in inpatient censuses. Although the first federal mental health initiative dates from 1963 (General Accounting Office, 1977; Kramer, 1977), national inpatient totals began to decline after 1955, some eight years earlier (Kramer, 1977). Further, 17 states began to experience consistent decreases in their state hospital censuses in the nine years from 1946 through 1954 (Gronfein, 1983). Once enacted, formal deinstitutionalization policy, at least as it was embodied in President Kennedy's Community Mental Health Center (CMHC) program, had but minimal impact on state hospital populations (Glasscote et al., 1969; Gronfein, 1983).

These observations suggest that changes in inpatient populations are only loosely coupled to the promulgation of programs and policies. Loose coupling between these two aspects of deinstitutionalization has an important consequence. Reductions in inpatient populations define deinstitutionalization in operational terms, and will therefore be referred to as *operational deinstitutionalization*. Operational deinstitutionalization and the programs, policies, laws, and judicial decisions which have such reductions as their aim may, however, develop independently of one another. The drugs could have contributed to the emergence of one aspect of deinstitutionalization but not the other; they could have influenced the formulation of mental health policy but not have been responsible for population changes. Thus, any discussion of the determinants of deinstitutionalization must treat *operational* deinstitutionalization and *policy* deinstitutionalization as relatively independent phenomena.

Temporal and Geographic Variation in Deinstitutionalization

Morrissey (1982:149) describes two distinct phases in the development of deinstitutionalization.

The first was characterized by relatively small and uneven declines in inpatient populations, was driven by an increase in discharges (while admissions were increasing simultaneously), and lasted until the middle to late 1960s. The second phase, which lasted from the late 1960s until the late 1970s, was characterized by much sharper and more consistent decreases in state hospital populations and involved a tightening of admissions as well as the maintenance of high discharge rates.

The data summarizing changes in inpatient populations from 1946 to 1980 in Table 21.1 are in accord with Morrissey's (1982) description. With the exception of the national totals for 1980, these data are drawn from annual censuses conducted by the U.S. Public Health Service and the National Institute of Mental Health from 1946 to 1975 on patients in mental institutions. These data include all the state and county mental hospitals which responded in each year, but do not include either private mental hospitals or Veterans Administration hospitals. The 1980 data are drawn from Goldman et al. (1983).

From 1956 to 1965, the annual rate of change in the size of the inpatient populations of state and county mental hospitals at the national level was approximately—1.5 percent, but from 1966 to 1975, the annual rate of change was close to −6.4 percent per year. The extent

Table 21.1. Changes in Inpatient Populations of State and County Mental Hospitals, 1946–1980

	National		State		
	Absolute Change	*Percent Change*	*Mean Change Per State (S.D.)*	*Coefficient[a] of Variation*	*Number[b] Against*
1946–1955	90,211	19.3%	16.3% (14.0)	.86	5
1946–1950	43,790	9.3	8.5 (6.7)	.79	3
1951–1955	38,596	7.4	5.4 (8.8)	1.63	8
1956–1965	−76,188	−13.8	−14.4 (15.0)	1.32	11
1956–1960	−15,850	−2.9	−3.5 (8.7)	2.49	15
1961–1965	−52,254	−9.9	−12.3 (13.1)	1.07	6
1966–1975	−258,653	−57.2	−54.2 (14.8)	.27	0
1966–1970	−114,470	−25.3	−25.2 (14.3)	.57	0
1971–1975	−115,547	−37.4	−32.2 (20.1)	.62	3
1976–1980	−32,809	−19.2	c	c	c

Notes:
a. Computed by dividing standard deviation by mean.
b. Number of states whose direction of inpatient change differs from mean.
c. Individual state data not available for 1980.

of change (i.e., the net decrease in the number of patients) from 1966 to 1975 was more than three times as great as the extent of change from 1956 to 1965.

Studies by Aviram et al. (1976) and Morrissey (1982) have shown that deinstitution-alization proceeded quite differently at different times and in different states. The state level data in Table 21.1 also show a substantial variation in inpatient change across states, particularly from 1956 to 1965. The mean percent decreases by state from 1966 to 1970 and from 1971 to 1975 are more than twice as large as those evident from 1956 to 1960 and from 1961 to 1965. Perhaps more important, from 1956 to 1965 states were much more dissimilar in the changes which they experienced in their state and county hospital popu-lations than was true from 1966 to 1975. This difference in variability is indexed by the coefficient of variation, which provides a measure of the degree of dispersion of individual observations about the mean for distributions with unequal means. This coefficient was nearly five times as large from 1956 to 1965 as it was from 1966 to 1975. The last column in Table 21.1 contains the number of states whose inpatient populations changed in a direc-tion opposite to the direction of the mean change across all states. More than 20 percent of the states experienced *increases* in inpatient populations from 1956 to 1965, although in general these populations were decreasing through this period.

There are, then, two distinct phases of operational deinstitutionalization: one lasting from the mid 1950s to approximately 1965 and another extending from 1965 to the present. Morrissey (1982:157) characterizes the earlier period as one in which the hospitals began to "open their back doors" and describes the later period as one in which they began to "close their front doors." Hereafter I focus on the period from 1955 to 1965, when dein-stitutionalization in both operational and policy senses was just beginning. Because the drugs were used more often in hospital settings than on an outpatient basis, we can expect whatever effects they may have had to contribute more to "opening the back door" (by increasing discharges) than to "closing the front door" (by decreasing admissions). Since inpatient changes at the state level were highly variable from 1955 to 1965, data drawn across all states are the most appropriate index of whatever impact the drugs might have had on deinstitutionalization as conceived operationally, and I will use such data when discussing the effects of the drugs on patient populations in the aggregate. First, I turn to an examination of the most immediate kind of drug effects—the impact they had on the state hospitals and their residents.

The Psychotropic Drugs and the Problem of Order

The Introduction of the Drugs

In 1953 Smith, Kline and French Labs began testing chlorpromazine, a new tranquilizing drug developed by the French firm of Rhone-Poulenc; in 1954 the American company received the approval of the Food and Drug Administration (FDA) to begin marketing the drug under the trade name Thorazine (Swazey, 1974). From the first, chlorpromazine was received with enthusiasm by the state hospitals. By 1956, two years after chlorprom-azine had received the imprimatur of the FDA, at least 37 states were using chlorprom-azine, reserpine—another psychoactive drug—or both (California State Senate Interim Committee on Treatment of Mental Illness, 1956), and 2000 articles had been written about the drugs (Kinross-Wright, 1956).

Such rapid diffusion was due in part to the efforts of the drug companies themselves. Smith, Kline and French Labs reorganized its entire sales force in order to market the drug, and lobbied state legislatures intensively in efforts to secure acceptance for Thorazine

(Swazey, 1974). Both Smith, Kline and French and Ciba-Geigy (which marketed reserpine) underwrote conferences in 1955 to discuss the results of administering the drugs to state hospital inmates (Lhamonn, 1955; Smith, Kline and French, 1955).

These investments in public relations were profitable, particularly for Smith, Kline and French. In 1952 and 1953, the two years prior to the official introduction of Thorazine, Smith, Kline and French reported total earnings of $23,440,000 on $99,972,000 in sales. In the two years subsequent to the introduction of Thorazine, earnings totaled $75,560,000 on $196,280,000 in sales, an increase of over 300 percent (Smith, Kline and French, 1956).

Social Problems and the State Hospital

While entrepreneurial initiative may have aided the process of drug diffusion, the perceived properties of the drugs themselves were an important factor as well. As described in a number of clinical reports, the drugs appeared to offer a solution to one of the problems which perennially plagued the state hospitals: the maintenance of order. Publicly supported insane asylums in the 1950s were, and long had been, an uneasy marriage of hospital and prison (Fox, 1978; Rock et al., 1968; Rothman, 1971). These facilities had a clear carceral function which at times overrode any purely therapeutic mandate (Stanton and Schwartz, 1954). They were depositories as well as hospitals, receptacles into which the community could place those individuals whose presence in civil society had become intolerable (Fox, 1978; Grab, 1983; Rothman, 1971). The mechanism of involuntary commitment, which was by far the most common admissions procedure until the 1960s, guaranteed that the community could maintain civil order by using legal procedures to compel patients to accept treatment, whatever wishes the patients may have had in this regard (Fox, 1978; Rock et al., 1968).

Involuntary commitment placed the state hospitals under compulsion as well as the patient. Hospitals were constrained to accept all those persons who had been committed for treatment, and thus lost the ability to regulate either the size or composition of its population (Greenley and Kirk, 1973; Rock et al., 1968). Just as the hospital's admissions decisions were shaped by community imperatives as well as by therapeutic desiderata, so too were its discharge decisions, since hospital administrators had to be sensitive to the anxieties of local communities (American Psychiatric Association, 1952; Stanton and Schwartz, 1954). While families and the police used the state hospital as a "last resort" for dealing with troubled individuals (Bittner, 1967; Sampson et al., 1962; Yarrow, et al., 1955), the hospital itself had no analogous option—the individuals who had been a problem of order for the outside community became a problem of order for the hospital's internal regime. Chronically short of resources and unable to regulate either inputs or outputs, the state hospitals accumulated large concentrations of very disturbed, psychotic, long-stay patients (Bucher and Schatzman, 1962; Council of State Governments, 1950; Deutsch, 1948; Kramer, 1957), who transformed these institutions into the "bedlams" described earlier.

Where Id Was, There Let Ego Be

State hospital physicians were genuinely impressed with what they saw when the drugs were introduced. As one review of drug-related research commented, "Reference to the psychiatric literature of the past year leaves one in no doubt that the chemotherapy of mental diseases has come of age ..." (Kinross-Wright, 1956:187). The general level of enthusiasm was so high that one observer commented disapprovingly, "I have attended conferences on these drugs where the atmosphere approached that of a revivalist meeting" (Bowes, 1956:530).

Descriptions of the clinical trials of chlorpromazine, reserpine, and the other newly-synthesized psychotropics consistently emphasized their ability to control even the most disturbed and dangerous patients. For instance,

> Robert W. was admitted to the state hospital in a highly excited, homicidal state. His eyes were red and bulging, face suffused, restraint required. This patient was loud, screamed that he would kill someone, and communicated his sincerity in this purpose to attendants ... CPZ [chlorpromazine] administration was begun soon after admission .... In the course of two more weeks of hospitalization, this patient had quieted down, had lost his anxiety almost altogether, and was able to discuss his illness and his future plans in an objective and rational manner (Goldman, 1955a:73).
>
> Within two months, Robert W. was discharged (Goldman, 1955b).

The drugs were particularly impressive in producing acceptable social behavior in chronic patients, some of whom had extensive experience with older somatic therapies.

> [A] 48 year old paranoid schizophrenic had spent most of the past two years in private and state mental institutions. She received electroshock, insulin treatment, and two prefrontal lobotomies without significant benefit. On admission, she was bellicose, sloppy in appearance, and actively hallucinating ... . Improvement continued for three months on a maintenance dose of 75 mg. [of thorazine] daily. For the past four months, she has been symptom free, manages her home, goes to bridge parties, dresses well, and amazes her husband and friends with her affectionate friendliness (Kinross-Wright, 1955:56).

The new drugs were effective at the group level, too; entire wards were transformed. A study of the effects of reserpine on chronic, back ward patients in California's Modesto State Hospital commented that:

> Prior to this study, these wards presented the usual picture of wards of this type, namely 10 to 12 patients in seclusion, some also in camisoles or other types of restraint ... . Owing to the raucous, hyperactive, combative, sarcastic, resistive, uncooperative patients, the ward was in a constant turmoil ... . Patients have undergone a metamorphosis from raging, combative, unsociable persons to cooperative, cheerful, sociable, relatively quiet persons who are amenable to psychotherapy (California State Senate Interim Committee on Treatment of Mental Illness, 1956:31).

A report from the chronic disturbed ward of a large Canadian hospital details a similar transformation:

> Within two weeks of commencing treatment, a striking change had taken place. The patients on Frenqual had become more sociable, they were neater, cleaner, and tidier ... . For the first time, the patients would read books and magazines instead of tearing them apart. Curtains could be left up instead of being pulled down. [The patients] appeared much more sociable ... . Some who had previously banged their heads against the walls and covered their heads with their overcoats stopped responding to their hallucinations. It was most impressive (Bowes, 1956:532).

Modest gains were greeted with enthusiasm, since they were viewed against such dark and disturbing backdrops. Progress was measured by bridge parties and the ability to converse intelligently. As an official in the Maryland state hospital system remarked, "It is a distinct pleasure to think of these patients ... going to the general dining room and eating with silverware" (California State Senate Interim Committee on Treatment of Mental Illness, 1956:134).

These startling improvements in the behavior of patients led to changes in the attitudes of staff. The possibility of instituting active therapy in place of a merely custodial regime led to the types of effects noted by Winfred Overholser (1958:214):

> A far greater interest [on the part of staff] has been developed. The morale has been increased. A hopeful attitude has come about as patients who had been previously troublesome were noted to be cooperative and helpful, and to show other signs of improvement.

These salutary effects were thought to extend outside the hospital:

> Legislative bodies have shown a greater interest in the problems of mental illness now that a positive and easily administered therapy appears to be available ... . Families have not only become more helpful but more demanding ... . It seems not too much to say that the community is at last developing an attitude of far greater tolerance toward the discharged mental patient, a greater readiness to accept him back into the community ... (Overholser, 1958:215)

Soon after they were introduced, the drugs began to appear indispensable in some quarters. In response to a California survey, Missouri officials wrote, "Attendants here stated emphatically that if the institution discontinues the use of the drugs, they will refuse to work" (California State Senate Interim Committee on Treatment of Mental Illness, 1956:170).

The drugs had a marked impact on state hospital patients and on state hospital staffs. Previous therapies (electroconvulsive therapy, insulin shock, lobotomy) had produced more tractable patients, but these measures were sometimes dangerous and were difficult to use outside the hospital. The drugs produced compliant patients and also had the advantage of being easily used in extramural settings.

The Effect of Psychotropic Drugs on Discharge Rates

The fact that psychoactive drugs could ameliorate disordered behavior at the individual level did not ensure that they would produce significant changes in patterns of patient movement. Even though use of the drugs resulted in more manageable patients and prompted more favorable attitudes towards the release of patients among the general public, state hospital officials faced the problem of where to place patients newly ready for discharge. There were few facilities available for aftercare, and many of the patients had been hospitalized for so long that their families were reluctant to take them back (Brooks, 1958; Pennington, 1955). [10] The critical question of whether use of the drugs led to actual decreases in inpatient populations was addressed in a number of reports, although their results were sometimes contradictory (Boudwin and Kline, 1955; Brill and Patton, 1957; Epstein et al., 1962; Joint Commission on Mental Illness and Health, 1961). In the next section, I review historical evidence on aggregate changes in discharge rates before and after the drugs were introduced.

Historical Studies of Drug Effects

At the time of the drugs' introduction, opinions as to their effects on inpatient population movement patterns varied widely. Even collaborators disagreed about their impact. A paper jointly authored by James Boudwin and Nathan Kline (1955:77) stated that "Allowing for some relapse, it appears that a minimum of five percent of the chronic mental hospital population of the country could be discharged if adequately treated with chlorpromazine and/or reserpine," but Boudwin took the unusual step of explicitly disassociating himself from this estimate. Although the California State Senate survey (1956) did not inquire directly about the effects of the drugs on population size or discharge rates, 18 of the 37 states responding volunteered such information. The officials of ten states thought the drugs had increased discharge rates, decreased population size, or both, while the officials of the other eight states were of the opinion that the drugs had not had a noticeable effect.

A similar variability marks three major state-specific studies undertaken specifically to investigate the effects of the drugs on mental patients in the aggregate. They were done in New York (Brill and Patton, 1957, 1959), Michigan (Michigan Department of Mental Health, 1956), and California (Epstein et al., 1962). In New York, Brill and Patton (1959:495) concluded "that the abrupt population fall [from 1955 to 1956] was in material degree due to the introduction of the new drugs." However, their study was methodologically flawed—Brill and Patton appear to have inferred causation from correlation. That is, they assumed that because the drugs were introduced just prior to the population declines, the drugs must have been responsible for these unprecedented decreases. However, since they did not compare the release rates of treated and untreated patients, they could not determine whether it was the drugs or some other development which was linked to the population decreases.[11]

Studies conducted in Michigan and California which did compare the release or retention rates of treated and untreated patients found that the drugs did not exercise a significant effect on discharge rates. The Michigan report stated that the "data indicate that ... the use of chlorpromazine and reserpine does *not* influence movement of patients out of the hospital" (Michigan Department of Mental Health, 1956:16, emphasis added), while the California study, which used data collected in 1956 and 1957 concluded that

> ... where a difference is found between the retention rate of ataraxic drug treated patients and those not so treated, the untreated patients consistently show a somewhat *lower* retention rate (Epstein et al., 1962:44, emphasis in original).

More recent retrospective studies (Aviram et al., 1976; Lerman, 1982; Morrissey, 1982) have found that in states such as California the drugs were less important in generating decreases in inpatient populations than was the expansion of federal health and welfare programs in the 1960s.

International data also cast doubt on the strength of the relationship between the introduction of the psychotropic drugs and declines in hospital populations. In England, inpatient populations began to decline before the drugs were introduced (Brown et al., 1966; Mechanic, 1969; Scull, 1977) and, in France, inpatient populations increased for 20 years after the drugs were introduced (Sedgwick, 1982).

The evidence from the United States suggests that the impact of the introduction of the psychotropic medications on discharge rates across states was variable. The more careful studies done in California and Michigan indicate that the drug impact was minimal in these states. However, as we have seen, changes in inpatient populations from 1956 to 1965 were characterized by a high level of interstate variability. It is therefore possible that the studies done in Michigan and California, while well-executed, reflected conditions which were not representative of those occurring in other states.

Interstate Data on Discharge Rates

In order to investigate the impact of the drugs across a larger sample of states, I used the data described in Table 21.1. Again, these data were drawn from annual censuses conducted by the Public Health Service and the National Institutes of Mental Health, and include information on the 48 states of the continental United States and the District of Columbia. I compared the extent of operational deinstitutionalization —as indexed by discharge rates from state and county hospitals—before and after the drugs were introduced in 1954. Discharge rates were used as a proxy for operational deinstitutionalization for two reasons. First, if the drugs were to have an effect on any component of patient movement, it would most likely be through an increase in discharge rates, since they were employed mainly in hospital settings (see footnote 4). Second, although the changes in inpatient population size are of primary interest, to use such changes as a measure of the drugs' effectiveness would be misleading. That is, if admissions also continued to increase, then increases in discharges might not be reflected in net population changes.

Discharge rates were computed using the method of Moon and Patton (1965). The number of live discharges from a state's hospitals in a given year was divided by the sum of the number of patients resident in those hospitals at the beginning of the year and the total number of admissions during the year. This quotient is multiplied by 100.

The state-level data I have assembled begin in 1946. Since the drugs were introduced in 1954, I have defined the period from 1946 to 1954 as the "predrug" period, and the period from 1955 to 1963 as the "postdrug" period. These periods are of equal length, and are long enough (nine years each) that the changes observed within them are not likely to be due to random fluctuations. The postdrug period ends in the year that John F. Kennedy declared his aim to reduce the inpatient loads of the nation's state and county mental hospitals by 50 percent (Foley and Sharfstein, 1983:160).

Two questions are of interest. First, were discharge rates subsequent to drug introduction higher than discharge rates prior to the introduction of the drugs? This question is crucial, since if there is no significant difference—or if "predrug" rates are actually higher than "postdrug" rates—then the drugs cannot be said to have exercised any significant influence on patient movement. Even if discharge rates in the 1955–1963 period were higher than those of the 1946–1954 period, it need not be the case that the drugs were responsible for the change. If discharge rates were already increasing prior to the introduction of the drugs, then any observed increase after 1954 could simply be a continuation of an existing trend. Thus, the second question is, were rates of change in discharge rates higher in the postdrug period than in the predrug period? If so, we have some support for the argument that the drugs did contribute to operational deinstitutionalization. If not, the contribution of psychotropic drugs to higher postdrug rates becomes questionable.

Table 21.2 shows the mean discharge rate per state from 1946 to 1963, and the mean yearly percentage change in discharge rates over the same period. With a single exception (1948) the mean discharge rate in each year in the series was higher than in the previous year. Also, the standard deviation in each year was small relative to the mean, indicating that the distribution of individual discharge rates was not highly dispersed.

Mean yearly percentage *changes* in discharge rates behaved quite differently from the mean rates. There was little consistency in increases or decreases—the magnitude of the mean changed sharply at several points—and the large standard deviations relative to the mean indicate that individual states differed appreciably in their degree of yearly change. Thus, although states tended to have similar discharge rates in any given year, the degree to which these discharge rates changed from year to year was highly variable.

To compare discharge rates in the predrug and postdrug periods more exactly, I computed the mean discharge rate for each state for the total periods from 1946 to 1954 and from 1955 to 1963, and used these nine-year means to index each state's discharge rate within each period. The mean discharge rate within each period (over all states) is shown in Table 21.3, as is the mean percentage change within each period.

Table 21.2. Discharge Rates and Mean Yearly Percentage
Change in Discharge Rates, 1946–1963

Mean Discharge Rate (S.D.)		Mean yearly Percentage Change in Discharge Rates (S.D.)	
1946	4.8 (4.1)		
1947	5.9 (4.3)	1946–1947	22.6 (60.1)
1948	5.7 (4.0)	1947–1948	13.8 (55.0)
1949	6.1 (4.1)	1948–1949	13.9 (38.4)
1950	6.7 (4.3)	1949–1950	17.3 (47.6)
1951	7.3 (4.9)	1950–1951	12.0 (35.7)
1952	7.8 (5.3)	1951–1952	8.8 (29.7)
1953	8.6 (5.3)	1952–1953	16.4 (33.2)
1954	9.0 (5.7)	1953–1954	9.4 (26.7)
1955	9.8 (6.7)	1954–1955	9.9 (28.6)
1956	10.7 (6.3)	1955–1956	18.2 (36.1)
1957	11.5 (6.5)	1956–1957	9.1 (18.9)
1958	13.3 (6.8)	1957–1958	19.1 (23.3)
1959	14.1 (7.2)	1958–1959	7.4 (12.7)
1960	14.7 (7.5)	1959–1960	7.8 (18.1)
1961	16.9 (7.8)	1960–1961	22.4 (36.7)
1962	18.6 (8.2)	1961–1962	9.2 (13.6)
1963	20.4 (8.7)	1962–1963	13.0 (19.0)

Table 21.3. Mean Discharge Rates and Mean Percentage Change
in Discharge Rates, 1946–1954 and 1955–1963

	1946–1954	1955–1963
Mean Discharge Rate	6.84	14.44
(S.D.)	(3.93)	(6.14)
Mean Percentage Change in Discharge Rates	172.39	164.19
(S.D.)	(264.10)	(165.64)

The mean discharge rate per state was clearly higher from 1955 to 1963 (14.64) than it was from 1946 to 1954 (6.84). The difference between these two means (7.60) is statistically significant at the .001 level. Every state except the District of Columbia had a higher mean discharge rate from 1955 to 1963 than it did from 1946 to 1954.

Table 21.3 also presents a comparison of the percentage change in discharge rates between the predrug and the postdrug periods. This comparison shows that the overall percentage change in discharge rates was greater *before* the drugs were introduced than afterwards. From 1946 to 1954 the mean increase per state was 172.39 percent, while from 1955 to 1963 the mean increase was 164.19 percent. The mean difference per state between the percentage increase from 1955 to 1963 and the percentage increase from 1946 to 1954 was - 8.20, indicating that on the average states showed a slightly greater relative increase in discharge rates *before* the drugs were introduced than they did afterwards. The difference between the two means was not statistically significant, however. Although the mean difference between the two periods was negative, 28 states showed a greater percentage increase in discharge rates from 1955 to 1963 than they did from 1946 to 1954, while the reverse was true for 17 states.

Overall, these data do not provide strong support for the position that the introduction of the drugs in 1954 *produced* an increase in discharge rates. Table 21.2 shows quite clearly that discharge rates increased steadily from 1946 to 1954, a period in which the drugs had not yet been introduced. While it is true that discharge rates were higher after the drugs were introduced than they were before, the mean percentage increase in discharge rates from 1946 to 1954 was greater than the mean percentage increase from 1955 to 1963. Also, while a majority of the states did experience a greater increase in discharge rates after drug introduction than before, fully 40 percent of the states showed the reverse pattern.

Thus, increases in discharge rates which took place after the psychotropic drugs were introduced did not arise *de novo,* but represented an extension of a trend which had been in evidence for some time. These results are consistent with earlier findings (Chittick et al., 1961; Kramer, 1959). A retrospective study done in Vermont's state hospital concluded that "no dramatic upswing in discharge rates is apparent with the advent of drug therapy in late 1954. Rather the picture for discharges in this period [1947 to 1958] is one of relatively smooth increases" (Chittick et al., 1961:20).

The fact that discharge rates were increasing *before* the advent of the drugs is itself an interesting finding. These early increases in discharge rates may have resulted from an acceleration of discharge rates for acute, short-stay patients, while chronic patients may have been affected more by the later increases. This possibility is suggested by the fact that one year release rates for first admissions in the predrug period were often quite high, while release rates for patients hospitalized for more than one year were quite low (Council of State Governments, 1950; Kramer, 1957; Pollack et al., 1959). Also, in Vermont chronic patients began to be discharged at an increasing rate only after the drugs were introduced, and the retention rate of schizophrenic first admissions (who were likely candidates for chronicity) was much lower after 1954 than it had been before (Chittick et al., 1961).

Drugs and Mental Health Policy

Reform and the State Hospital

From 1949 to 1954, the American Psychiatric Association (APA) sponsored a series of Mental Health Institutes. Attended largely by the superintendents of state and county hospitals, the proceedings of these Institutes provide a valuable picture of how the state hospitals were viewed by those who ran them.

Dr. Mesrop Tarumianz, superintendent of Delaware's single state hospital and a prominent member of the American Psychiatric Association, expressed the superintendents' general sentiments when he said, "I think that we should realize that conditions are abominable and obnoxious. There are no words in the dictionary that you can use to describe the conditions in mental hospitals" (American Psychiatric Association, 1949:12). Like other citizens concerned with the "abominable and obnoxious" conditions in the nation's mental hospitals, the superintendents' reform agenda gave demands for more money, more buildings, and more staff pride of place (American Psychiatric Association, 1952, 1953, 1954). A survey done at the 1949 meeting showed that 65 percent of the superintendents were engaged in construction projects (American Psychiatric Association, 1949:48). The 1951 Institute featured a session entitled "Appropriations: How Can Mental Hospitals Justify

Requests for Increased Appropriations and Charges" (American Psychiatric Association, 1951), and every meeting from 1949 to 1954 featured seminars on how to convince state legislatures and budget officers to allocate more money.

Hospital growth seemed inevitable. Dr. Granville Jones, a Virginia superintendent, commented that "It is nice to plan rooms to meet the demand, but if you make the room too large, *sooner or later you are going to be overcrowded, and you are going to put two patients in a room designed for one*" (American Psychiatric Association, 1950:15, emphasis added). Confronted with an apparently inelastic demand for services, the superintendents felt that lobbying state legislatures for increased appropriations to expand the supply of hospital beds and personnel was eminently reasonable. Given the security burden which the hospital had to shoulder and the relatively ineffective means available for resocializing chronic psychotics prior to the introduction of the drugs, it is not surprising that most reform efforts turned to improvement rather than abolition.

The introduction of the drugs changed this situation markedly. They sparked intense clinical excitement and produced significant improvements in staff morale (Bowes, 1956; Ferguson, 1956; Overholser, 1958). The drugs also exerted a favorable effect (albeit indirectly) on outside audiences such as state legislatures, which became more interested in the problem of mental health care generally after psychoactive medications were introduced (Overholser, 1958).

The drugs were even given credit where credit was not their due, particularly in the matter of their effects on aggregate populations. The upward trend in discharge rates, for instance, had been in effect for a number of years, but was "noticed more frequently since the tranquilizing drugs came upon the scene" (Kramer, 1959:118). The Joint Commission on Mental Illness and Health (1961) credited psychotropics with reversing the "upward spiral" of state hospital populations. This assertion was based on the Brill and Patton studies (1957, 1959). Interestingly, the better designed Michigan study—which showed that the drugs did not increase discharge rates—was not mentioned by the Joint Commission even though it was available. Further, some observers in the middle 1950s (e.g., Clark, 1956) questioned the clinical results obtained with the drugs, since the clinical trials were seldom run under blinded conditions (cf. Scull, 1977).

Policy makers believed the psychotropic drugs could potentially launch a new era in the treatment of mental illness (Lyons, 1984). A recent report by the American Psychiatric Association on deinstitutionalization cited the psychotropic drugs as one of the four principal causes of the development of deinstitutionalization policy (Boffey, 1984). The Joint Commission on Mental Illness and Health, commissioned by the Congress to investigate mental health problems, wrote that "Drugs have revolutionized the management of psychotic patients in American mental hospitals, and probably deserve primary credit for the reversal of the upward trend of the upward spiral in the state hospital inpatient load" (Joint Commission on Mental Illness and Health, 1961:39). A National Institute of Mental Health (NIMH) sponsored investigation of the feasibility of treating schizophrenics in the community stated that "with tranquilizers, fewer patients need to be hospitalized ... and patients [can be] more easily discharged .... [A]t all levels and in nearly all respects, tranquilizers have altered our hospitals and provided the impetus for community care" (Pasamanick et al., 1967:17).

A series of recent interviews with psychiatrists involved in the formulation of mental health policy in the 1950s and early 1960s shows a heavy reliance on the drugs, and former NIMH officials such as Robert Felix and Bertram Brown admit having "oversold" the drugs to the president and the Congress (Lyons, 1984). Most important, the drugs played a crucial role in President Kennedy's 1963 message to Congress. That speech is widely held to have ushered in the era of deinstitutionalization and community mental health (Bachrach, 1976; Bassuk and Gerson, 1978; General Accounting Office, 1977; Kramer, 1977). Kennedy gave the drugs credit for making his "bold new approach" possible:

> This approach rests primarily on the new knowledge and the new drugs acquired and developed in recent years which make it possible for most of the mentally ill to be successfully and quickly treated in their own communities and returned to a useful place in society (cited in Foley and Sharfstein, 1983:165).

It should be emphasized that the drugs were much more influential in the early period of deinstitutionalization than they were in the latter. As Morrissey (1982:148) has written, the drugs made the move away from the state hospital "plausible." While they did help "open the back door" of the state hospital, developments from 1965 onward—when deinstitutionalization accelerated markedly—were dependent on a number of other factors including: the emergence of a civil libertarian reform movement which transformed admission and discharge procedures (California Assembly Ways and Means Subcommittee on Mental Health Services, 1967; Morrissey, 1982); the expansion of federal health and welfare programs and the growth in nursing home capacity (Segal and Aviram, 1978; Shadish and Bootzin, 1981); and the development of fiscal crises in many states (Scull, 1977; Warren, 1981).

Conclusions

The effects of the psychotropic drugs on state and county hospitals and on deinstitutionalization lie somewhere between the "orthodox" and "revisionist" described earlier. The weight of the evidence presented here does not support the position that the introduction of the drugs was responsible for the increases in discharge rates that occurred after 1955. However, testimony from a number of sources does indicate that the advent of psychotropic medications was linked to the emergence of a new philosophy regarding what was possible and desirable in the provision of mental health care for the seriously mentally ill (Boffey, 1984; General Accounting Office, 1977; Joint Commission on Mental Illness and Health, 1961; Lyons, 1984).

The influences of the drugs on operational and policy deinstitutionalization were more a function of the environment into which they were introduced than a straightforward expression of their pharmacological properties. The reason discharge rates did not increase more sharply or inpatient censuses fall more dramatically after drug introduction in the United States may have had more to do with the short supply of alternative facilities in the community for state hospital inpatients than it had to do with any weakness in the drugs' capacities to influence behavior. By the same token, the contribution that the drugs made to the development of a policy of state and county hospital depopulation was not dictated by their pharmacology, since they could have been used as therapies which would promote inhospital adjustment as had electroconvulsive therapy, insulin shock, and lobotomy. To the extent that the drugs "led" to a policy of deinstitutionalization, they did so because they converged with the interests and needs of several different groups, including fiscal conservatives determined to save money and civil libertarian lawyers intent on attacking what they viewed as a repressive institution (Morrissey, 1982; Shadish and Bootzin, 1981).

The drugs, then, were an opportunity, not an imperative. That they stimulated deinstitutionalization does not mean that they had to do so. In an era in which institutional solutions to social problems were in favor, they might well have been used to buttress the internal order of the state hospital. Alone, psychotropic drugs could have had little impact on the actual size of patient populations, and the great acceleration in deinstitutionalization which occurred after 1965 owed much more to changes in the hospital's external environment than to the pacifying effects of these drugs on the internal environment of hospital wards.

References

American Psychiatric Association
  1949   First Mental Hospital Institute–Better Care in Mental Hospitals. Washington, DC: American Psychiatric Association.
  1950   Second Mental Hospital Institute–Mental Hospitals. Washington, DC: American Psychiatric Association.
  1951   Third Mental Hospital Institute–Working Programs in Mental Hospitals. Washington, DC: American Psychiatric Association.
  1952   Fourth Mental Hospital Institute–Steps Forward. Washington, DC: American Psychiatric Association.
  1953   Fifth Mental Hospital Institute–Progress and Problems in Mental Hospitals. Washington, DC: American Psychiatric Association.
  1954   Sixth Mental Hospital Institute–The Psychiatric Hospital: A Community Resource. Washington, DC: American Psychiatric Association.
Arnhoff, Franklin W.
  1975   "Social consequences of policy toward mental illness." Science 188:1277–84.
  Aviram, Uri and Steven Segal
  1973   "Exclusion of the mentally ill." Archives of General Psychiatry 27:126–31.
Aviram, Uri, S. Leonard Syme and Judith B. Cohen
  1976   "The effects of policies and programs on reductions of mental hospitalization." Social Science and Medicine 10:571–78.
Bachrach, Leona
  1976   Deinstitutionalization: An Analytical Review and Sociological Perspective. DHEW Publication No. (ADM)76–351. Washington, DC: U.S. Government Printing Office.
  1978   "A conceptual approach to deinstitutionalization." Hospital and Community Psychiatry 29:573–78.
Bassuk, Ellen and Samuel Gerson
  1978   "Deinstitutionalization and mental health services." Scientific American 238:46–53.
Beers, Clifford Whittingham
  [1908]   A Mind That Found Itself. Pittsburgh: University of Pittsburgh Press.
  1981   Becker, Alvin and Herbert D. Schulberg
  1976   "Phasing out state hospitals: a psychiatric dilemma." New England Journal of Medicine 294:255–61.
Bittner, Egon
  1967   "Police discretion in emergency apprehension of mentally ill persons." Social Problems 14:278–92.
Boffey, Phillip K.
  1984   "Community care for mentally ill termed a failure." New York Times Sept. 13: Al; B2.
Boudwin, James and Nathan Kline
  1955   "Use of reserpine in chronic non-disturbed psychotics." Pp. 71–78 in Jacques S. Gottlieb (ed.), An Evaluation of the Newer Psychopharmacologic Agents and their Role in Current Psychiatric Practice. Washington, DC: American Psychiatric Association.
Bowes, Angus H.
  1956   "The ataractic drugs: the present position of chlorpromazine, frenqual, pacatal, and reserpine in the psychiatric hospital." American Journal of Psychiatry 113:530–39.
Braun, Peter, Gerald Kochansky, Robert Shapiro, Susan Greenberg, Jon Gudeman, Sylvia Johnson, and Miles F. Shore

1981   "Overview: deinstitutionalization of psychiatric patients, a critical review of outcome studies." American Journal of Psychiatry 138:736–49.

Brill, Henry and Robert E. Patton
1957   "Analysis of 1955–1956 population fall in New York state hospitals in first year of large scale use of tranquilizing drugs." American Journal of Psychiatry 114:509–17.
1959   "Analysis of population reductions in New York state mental hospitals during the first four years of large scale use of tranquilizing drugs." American Journal of Psychiatry 116:495–508.

Brooks, George W.
1958   "Experience with the use of chlorpromazine and reserpine in psychiatry." Pp. 375–81 in Hirsch L. Gordon (ed.), The New Chemotherapy in Mental Illness. New York: Philosophical Library.

Brown, George W., Margaret Bone, Bridget Dalison, and John K. Wing
1966   Schizophrenia and Social Care. London: Oxford University Press.

Bucher, Rue and Leonard Schatzman
1962   "The logic of the state mental hospital." Social Problems 9:337–49.

California Assembly Ways and Means Subcommittee on Mental Health Services
1967   The Dilemma of Mental Commitment in California: A Background Document. Sacramento, CA: California State Assembly.

California State Senate Interim Committee on Treatment of Mental Illness
1956   First Partial Report. Sacramento, CA: California State Senate.

Chittick, R. A., G. W. Brooks, F. S. Irons, and W. W. Deare
1961   The Vermont Story-Rehabilitation of Chronic Schizophrenic Patients. Burlington, VT: n.p.

Chu, Franklin and Sharland Trotter
1974   The Madness Establishment. New York: Grossman.

Clark, Lincoln N.
1956   "Evaluation of the therapeutic effect of drugs on psychiatric patients." Diseases of the Nervous System 17:282–86.

Cohen, Stanley
1979   "The punitive city: notes on the dispersal of social control." Contemporary Crises 3:339–67.

Council of State Governments
1950   The Mental Health Programs of the Forty-Eight States. Chicago: Council of State Governments.

Deutsch, Albert
1948   The Shame of the States. New York: Harcourt, Brace.

Dunham, H. Warren and S. Kirson Weinberg
1960   The Culture of the State Mental Hospital. Detroit: Wayne State University Press.

Epstein, Leon J., Richard P. Morgan, and Lynn Reynolds
1962   "An approach to the effect of ataraxic drugs on hospital release rates." American Journal of Psychiatry 119:36–47.

Erikson, Kai T.
1966   Wayward Puritans. New York: John Wiley.

Estroff, Sue E.
1981   Making It Crazy. Berkeley, CA: University of California Press.

Ferguson, John
1956   "Improved behavior patterns in the hospitalized mentally ill with reserpine and methyl-phenidylacetate." Pp. 35–43 in Jacques S. Gottlieb (ed.), An Evaluation of the Newer Psychopharmacologic Agents and Their Role in Current Psychiatric Practice. Washington, DC: American Psychiatric Association.

Foley, Henry and Steven Sharfstein
1983   Madness and Government. Washington, DC: American Psychiatric Association.

Fox, Richard W.
    1978   So Far Disordered in Mind: Insanity in California, 1870–1930. Berkeley, CA: University
            of California Press.
Freedman, Ruth and Ann Moran
    1983   Wanderers in a Promised Land: The Chronically Mentally Ill and Deinstitutionalization.
            Unpublished report, Harvard Working Group on Mental Illness.
General Accounting Office
    1977   Returning the Mentally Disabled to the Community: Government Needs to Do More.
            Washington, DC: U.S. Government Printing Office.
Glasscote, Raymond, James W. Sussex, Elaine Cumming, and Lauren Smith
    1969   The Community Mental Health Center: An Interim Appraisal. Washington, DC:
            American Psychiatric Association.
Goffman, Erving
    1961   Asylums. Garden City, NY.: Doubleday.
Goldman, Douglas
    1955a   "The effect of chlorpromazine on severe mental and emotional disturbances." Pp.
             19–40 in Chlorpromazine and Mental Health: Proceedings of a Symposium Held
             Under the Auspices of Smith, Kline and French. Philadelphia: Lea and Fabiger.
    1955b   "The influence of chlorpromazine on psychotic thought content." Pp. 72–77 in William
             E. Lhamonn (ed.), Pharmacologic Products Recently Introduced in the Treatment of
             Psychiatric Disorders." Washington, DC: American Psychiatric Association.
Goldman, Howard H., Neal Adams, and Carl Taube
    1983   "Deinstitutionalization: the data demythologized." Hospital and Community Psychiatry
            34:129–34.
Greenley, James and Stuart Kirk
    1973   "Organizational characteristics of agencies and the distribution of services to appli-
            cants." Journal of Health and Social Behavior 14:70–79.
Grob, Gerald
    1983   Mental Illness and American Society: 1875 to 1940. Princeton, NJ: Princeton University
            Press.
Gronfein, William
    1983   From Madhouse to Main Street: The Changing Place of Mental Illness in Post-World
            War II America. Unpublished Ph.D. dissertation, State University of New York at Stony
            Brook.
Joint Commission on Mental Illness and Health
    1961   Action for Mental Health. New York: Basic Books.
Kinross-Wright, Vernon
    1955   "The intensive chlorpromazine treatment of schizophrenia." Pp. 53–62 in William
            E. Lhamonn (ed.), Pharmacologic Products Recently Introduced in the Treatment of
            Psychiatric Disorders. Washington, DC: American Psychiatric Association.
    1956   "A review of the newer drug therapies in psychiatry." Diseases of the Nervous System
            17:187–90.
Kirk, Stuart A. and Mark Therrien
    1975   "Community mental health myths and the fate of former hospitalized patients."
            Psychiatry 38:209–17.
Kramer, Morton
    1957   "Problems of research on the population dynamics and therapeutic effectiveness of
            mental hospitals." Pp. 145–72 in Milton Greenblatt, Daniel Levinson, and Richard H.
            Williams (eds.), The Patient and the Mental Hospital. Glencoe, IL: Free Press.
    1959   "Public health and social problems in the use of tranquilizing drugs." Pp. 108–43
            in Jonathan O. Cole and Ralph W. Gerard (eds.), Psychopharmacology: Problems in
            Evaluation. Publication No. 583, National Academy of Sciences. Washington, DC:
            National Research Council.

1977   Psychiatric Services and the Changing Institutional Scene: 1950–1985. DHEW
        Publication No. (ADM) 77–433. Washington, DC: US. Government Printing Office.
Lerman, Paul
    1982   Deinstitutionalization and the Welfare State. New Brunswick, NJ: Rutgers University
        Press.
Lhamonn, William E. (ed.)
    1955   Pharmacologic Products Recently Introduced in the Treatment of Psychiatric Disorders.
        Washington, DC: American Psychiatric Association.
Litteral, Emmet B. and William E. Wilkinson
    1955   "The advantages, disadvantages, and limitations of the use of chlorpromazine as a
        substitute for certain somatic treatment methods in psychiatry." Pp. 63–72 in William
        E. Lhamonn (ed.), Pharmacologic Products Recently Introduced in the Treatment of
        Psychiatric Disorders. Washington, DC: American Psychiatric Association.
Lyons, Richard D.
    1984   "How release of mental patients began." New York Times October 30:Cl,C4.
Mechanic, David
    1969   Mental Health and Social Policy. Englewood Cliffs, NJ: Prentice-Hall.
Michigan Department of Mental Health
    1956   A Summary of Behavioral Changes in Patients and Changes in Hospital Ward
        Management Associated with the Use of Chlorpromazine and Reserpine Therapy in
        Michigan State Hospitals: Research Report 23. Lansing, MI: Michigan Department of
        Mental Health.
Miller, Dorothy
    1966   Worlds That Fail: Part II. Disbanded Worlds—A Study of Returns to the Mental
        Hospital. Sacramento, CA: California Department of Mental Hygiene.
Moon, Louis E. and Robert E. Patton
    1965   "First admissions and readmissions to New York State mental hospitals —a statistical
        evaluation." The Psychiatric Quarterly 39:476–86.
Morrissey, Joseph
    1982   "Deinstitutionalizing the mentally ill: processes, outcomes, and new directions. Pp.
        147–76 in Walter Gove (ed.), Deviance and Mental Illness. Beverly Hills, CA: Sage
        Publications.
National Institute of Mental Health—Survey and Reports Section
    1974   Legal Status of Inpatient Admissions to State and County Mental Hospitals, 1972.
        Statistical Note No. 105. Washington, DC: U.S. Government Printing Office.
Overholser, Winfred
    1958   "Has chlorpromazine inaugurated a new era in mental hospitals?" Pp. 212–17 in Hirsch
        L. Gordon (ed.), The New Chemotherapy in Mental Illness. New York: Philosophical
        Library.
Pasamanick, Benjamin, Frank Scarpitti, and Simon Dinitz
    1967   Schizophrenics in the Community. New York: Appleton-Century Crofts.
Patton, Robert E. and Abbott S. Weinstein
    1960   "First admissions to New York civil state mental hospitals, 1911–1958." The Psychiatric
        Quarterly 34:245–74.
Pennington, Veronica M.
    1955   "The use of reserpine (serpasil) in three hundred and fifty neuropsychiatric cases."
        Pp. 105–11 in William E. Lhamonn (ed.), Pharmacologic Products Recently Introduced
        in the Treatment of Psychiatric Disorders. Washington, DC: American Psychiatric
        Association.
Pollack, Earl, Philip H. Person, Morton B. Kramer, and Hyman Goldstein
    1959   Patterns of Retention, Release, and Death of First Admissions to State Mental Hospitals.
        DHEW Public Health Monograph No. 38. Washington, DC: U.S. Government Printing
        Office.

Pollack, Earl and Carl A. Taube
  1975   "Trends and projections in state hospital use." Pp. 31–55 in Jack Zusman and Elmer
         Bertsch (eds.), The Future Role of the State Hospital. Lexington, MA: D.C. Heath.
Redick, Richard V., Morton Kramer, and Carl A. Taube
  1973   "Epidemiology of mental illness and utilization of facilities among older persons."
         Pp. 199–232 in Ewald W. Busse and Eric Pfeiffer (eds.), Mental Illness in Later Life.
         Washington, DC: American Psychiatric Association.
Rock, Richard, Marcus A. Jacobson, and Richard M. Janopaul
  1968   Hospitalization and Discharge of the Mentally Ill. Chicago: University of Chicago
         Press.
Rose, Stephen
  1979   "Deciphering deinstitutionalization: complexities in policy and program analysis."
         Milbank Memorial Fund 57:429–60.
Rothman, David
  1971   The Discovery of the Asylum. Boston: Little, Brown.
Sampson, Harold, Sheldon Messinger and Robert A. Towne
  1962   "Family processes and becoming a mental patient." American Journal of Sociology
         68:88–96.
Scull, Andrew
  1977   Decarceration: Community Treatment and the Deviant—A Radical View. Englewood
         Cliffs, NJ: Prentice-Hall.
Sedgwick, Peter
  1982   Psychopolitics. New York: Harper and Row.
Segal, Steven and Uri Aviram
  1978   The Mentally Ill in Community-Based Sheltered Care. New York: Wiley.
Segal, Steven, Jim Baumohl, and Elsie A. Johnson
  1974   "Falling through the cracks: mental disorder and social margin in a young vagrant
         population." Social Problems 24:387–400.
Shadish, William and Richard Bootzin
  1981   "Nursing homes and chronic mental patients." Schizophrenia Bulletin 7:488–98.
Smith, Kline and French
  1955   Chlorpromazine and Mental Health: Proceedings of a Symposium Held Under the
         Auspices of Smith, Kline and French. Philadelphia: Lea and Fabiger.
  1957   [1956]Annual Report. Philadelphia: Smith, Kline and French.
Stanton, Alfred and Morris Schwartz 1954 The Mental Hospital. New York: Basic.
Swazey, Judith
  1974   Chlorpromazine in Psychiatry. Cambridge, MA: MIT Press.
van der Vaart, H. Robert
  1978   "Variances, statistical study of." Pp. 1215–25 in William H. Kruskal and Judith M.
         Tanur (eds.), International Encyclopedia of Statistics. New York: Free Press.
Ward, Mary J.
  1946   Snake Pit. New York: H. Wolff.
Warren, Carol A. B.
  1981   "New forms of social control: the myth of deinstitutionalization." American Behavioral
         Scientist 24:724–46.
Weinstein, Abbott and Albert Maiwald
  1974   "Trends in New York state mental hospital
         admissions and length of stay." Pp. 11–21 in The State Hospital-Past and Present.
         Hanover, NJ: Sandoz Pharmaceuticals.
Yarrow, Marion R., Charlotte G. Schwartz, Harriet J. Murphy, and Leila C. Deasy
  1955   "The psychological meaning of mental illness in the family." Journal of Social Issues
         11:12–28.

22

Goldman, H. H., & Morrissey, J. P. (1985). The alchemy of mental health policy: Homelessness and the fourth cycle of reform. *American Journal of Public Health, 75 (7), 727–731*

Goldman and Morrissey's article starts with the premise that previous approaches to public mental health policy have erred in promising to prevent chronic mental illness through two linked approaches. The first involves individual treatment and institutional care. The second involves the alchemy of turning the lead of the social problems of persons with serious mental illness—poverty, racism, criminality, and others—into the gold of mental health problems with mental health solutions. In the new era, or cycle, of mental health reform, the authors argue, social problems will be treated as social problems and community mental health systems of care will be coordinated with public health and social welfare programs. Their article is, in part, a plea to save the Community Support Systems approach that began in the late 1970s and was declining in the early to mid 1980s due to shrinking public resources and the unrealistic expectation that it would be able to respond adequately to the problem of widespread homelessness. Goldman and Morrissey argue that homelessness is a social problem that extends far beyond the reach of the Community Support System movement. It is worth noting that the authors were leading researchers for the ACCESS (Access to Community Care and Effective Services and Supports) program of the federal Substance Abuse and Mental Health Services Administration of the 1990s, a nine-state, 18-site project designed to enhance and test the effectiveness of integrated systems of care, at both administrative and service levels, in improving clinical and social outcomes for persons with mentally illness who are homeless.

The Alchemy of Mental Health Policy: Homelessness and the Fourth Cycle of Reform

Introduction

As noted in the literature[1-3] the history of public mental health policy is characterized by a cyclical pattern of institutional reforms. Each cycle was marked by public support for a new environmental approach to treatment and an innovative type of facility or locus of care. The first cycle of reform in the early 19th century introduced moral treatment and the asylum[4-7]; the second cycle in the early 20th century was associated with the mental hygiene movement and the psychopathic hospital[8-12]; and the third in the mid 20th century developed out of the community mental health movement and its support for community mental health centers.[13-16] Each of these reforms promised that early treatment of acute cases would prevent chronic mental illness. Each innovation proved successful with acute and milder—not chronic— forms of mental disorder, yet failed to eliminate chronicity or to fundamentally alter the care of the severely mentally ill. In each cycle, the optimism of reform gave way to pessimism and therapeutic nihilism toward the increasing numbers of incurable chronic mental patients. In the face of an expanding population of needy patients, public support turned to neglect.

The reform movements that stimulated these cycles often gained momentum by transforming social problems (e.g., dependency, senility, criminality, poverty, and racism) into mental health issues. Failure to address the basic social problems themselves has resulted in a repeating cycle of policies which only partly accomplish the goals of their activist proponents.

This paper examines a fourth cycle of reform emerging in the past decade in response to the failures of community mental health and deinstitutionalization. The new reform advocates creating community support systems, a broad network of mental health and social welfare services for care of the chronically mentally ill in noninstitutional settings. This reform movement is different because it directly addresses the needs of the chronically mentally ill rather than promising to prevent chronicity through the early treatment of acute cases and because it recognizes the problem of the chronically mentally ill as a public health and social welfare problem. The breadth of this mandate, however, is threatened by shrinking health and welfare resources and by a growing expectation that it will solve the problem of homelessness.[3]

The Community Mental Health Movement

World War II marked the turning point from the mental hygiene reform to the community mental health movement. In its return to advocacy for a new type of treatment facility—the

296

community mental health center (CMHC)—the community mental health movement initiated a third cycle of reform devoted to the early treatment of acute cases and the hope that chronicity would be prevented.[13–16] Like mental hygiene, the main thrust of community mental health reform in America generally ignored chronic patients and embraced broader social issues.

Activities became involved in civil libertarian reform, and the community mental health movement took on poverty, racism, civil unrest, violence, and criminality. Data on the relationship between mental illness and low social class and racial minority status[17,18] justified the involvement with the war on poverty and the civil rights movements. Decades of mental health study of violent and criminal behavior[19,20] seemed to justify community mental health practice with police and court agencies, in jails and prisons, and in the streets in times of civil disturbance.

Several models of community mental health centers emerged in the post-World War II era. Some, like Lindemann's original center, Human Relations Service in Wellesley, Massachusetts (1948) were devoted principally to consultation and education with community agencies.[21] Only later did the center offer outpatients services and develop inpatient agreements with community hospitals. Others, often sponsored by state mental hospitals (as early as the 1950s), focused on ambulatory services, especially "after-care" and crisis intervention for a mix of disadvantaged acute and chronic patients in the public sector. The federal model of the community mental health center, which emerged in the 1960s and spread through the United States, was an anomalous combination of the two earlier models.[14–16]

In the late 1940s and early 1950s, psychiatrists like Erich Lindemann[23] and Gerald Caplan[24] adapted brief treatment methods and consultation techniques for use in outpatient settings and in community agencies. The first community mental health centers were developed, in part, to provide these services. Mental health professionals offered treatment to new populations of previously untreated, acutely ill, and emotionally troubled patients. Relatively few chronic patients were treated and public mental hospitals were largely ignored. Instead, these few early centers provided consultation to schools, religious organizations, police departments, welfare and other community agencies on specific mental health problems, environmental stress, and broader social issues.

As early as the 1930s, depression-poor public mental hospitals considered reducing the patient population in an effort to save resources. According to Grob,[10] the term "deinstitutionalization" was used to describe this process in a 1934 report sponsored by the American Medical Association.[25] Abraham Myerson described his "total push" program for discharging chronic patients in 1939.[26] Throughout the 1930s, state hospital superintendents worked hard to reduce the length of stay of newly admitted patients.[27] The process did not gain momentum, however, until psychiatrists returning from World War II introduced rapid treatment techniques and an attitude of therapeutic optimism.[28] The resultant declines in length of stay were accelerated by the introduction of the antipsychotic and antidepressant medications in the 1950s. State mental hospitals developed ambulatory service departments, offering crisis intervention, partial hospitalization, and after-care. Several state hospital systems had elaborate networks of decentralized services for acute and chronic patients by the early 1960s.[22] Not all states supported the decentralized service approach, a point of controversy among hospital superintendents since the mid-19th century.[1–4] Many hospital directors feared a loss of control over their fiefdoms. Other professional leaders mistrusted the state mental hospitals, often viewed as the root of the problem and an unseemly, unlikely change agent.

Indeed, by the late 1950s and 1960s, institutions and institutional care had become anathema to be avoided at all costs. Exposes,[29] sociological treatises,[30] public commissions,[13] and even organized psychiatry[31] deplored asylum conditions and advocated change. State mental hospitals were described as isolated, dehumanizing "warehouses"—"snake pits" where unfortunate deviants were sequestered, neglected, or abused. Mental institutions were transformed in the public's mind from medical treatment centers into factories for the manufacture of madness.[32] Clinical evidence of social and functional deterioration following long-term institutional care[33-35] reinforced the notion that institutions were the cause of chronic mental disorder. Community mental health reformers advocated for mental health centers to make institutions obsolete. *Action for Mental Health,* the final report of the Joint Commission on Mental Illness and Health,[13] called for federal support; President John F. Kennedy promised a "bold new approach," and the Congress passed the Community Mental Health Centers Act in 1963.

The federally funded community mental health centers merged the prevention ideology and acute treatment/consultation philosophy of the early community-based centers with the service mix of the state hospital-based centers. The federal model required five essential services: inpatient, outpatient, partial hospitalization, emergency, and consultation-education services. The approach was predicated on an integrated services model, promoting continuity of care for patients throughout an episode of illness. There was no clear mandate, however, for the community mental health centers to coordinate their efforts with state mental hospitals or to care for chronic patients. In fact, federal policy makers intentionally created a program granting federal resources to local agencies, bypassing state mental health authorities.[36] As a result, mental health centers primarily served new populations in need of acute services and failed to meet the needs of acute and chronic patients discharged in increasing numbers from public hospitals. Furthermore, centers were not required to provide for housing or income support for discharged mental patients. Homelessness and indigency were predictable outcomes for many.

Deinstitutionalization and Its Aftermath

Advocates of the federal community mental health center program often took credit for dramatic changes in the delivery of mental health services in the US. Data, however, do not support a direct relationship between the expansion of community mental health centers and deinstitutionalization. The decline in the resident census of many states preceded the community mental health center program by more than a decade, and catchment areas with community mental health centers did not uniformly experience decreased use of the state mental hospital.[36]

The community mental health movement, as a reform, did change the delivery of mental health services dramatically—for acute and chronic patients. Between 1950 and 1980, for example, the resident population of state mental hospitals was reduced from approximately 560,000 to less than 140,000; admissions to psychiatric inpatient facilities increased dramatically, and outpatient services expanded twelve-fold. Since the mid 1960s, more than 700 community mental health centers have been created, serving catchment areas representing 50 per cent of the US population.[37,38] Nursing homes became the residence and long-term care facility for approximately 700,000 chronically mentally ill Americans.[39-46] [Each year tens of thousands of elderly state mental hospital residents were transferred to nursing homes, reversing the aging trend in public psychiatric institutions that began at the turn of this century when the senile were transferred from local almshouses to state hospitals.[10] Hundreds of thousands of elderly and chronic mental patients were diverted from hospitals directly into nursing homes. As of 1977, about half of the 1.3 million nursing home residents had a mental disorder, especially organic mental disorder, making nursing homes the single most commonly used psychiatric long-term care facility.[39,40] As the population ages this phenomenon is expected to grow. Changing the locus of care, however, did not solve the problem of chronic mental illness and, in fact, may have made matters worse.

Community mental health reform in America generally ignored chronic patients and embraced broader social issues.

Deinstitutionalization, the policy of releasing mental patients into the community, often without adequate mental health and social welfare supports, was reinforced by the expectation that communities and their community mental health centers could handle the problem. It was believed, naively, that chronicity was a function of institutional care and that release from the hospital would eliminate the problem. Institutions were regarded as harmful, or at least undesirable, and they were a major item in state budgets. To sustain the movement, the civil libertarian/community mental health reformers joined forces with fiscal conservatives, who viewed deinstitutionalization as a way to save state resources and shift fiscal responsibility onto federal programs, [i.e., CMHCs, Medicare, Medicaid, Supplemental Security Income (SSI), and Social Security Disability Insurance (SSDI)]. Together, they propelled the community mental health reform into serious trouble.[41-53]

By the mid 1970s, the policy of deinstitutionalization was being criticized for its neglect of the chronically mentally ill. Eloquent criticism came from professional journals,[41-43] government publications,[44-46] political white papers,[47-49] newspapers,[50-52] and popular literature.[53] The zeal of the community mental health activists for trying to solve social problems without also focusing on the need for the humane care of the chronically mentally ill had, in part, contributed to the new set of social problems associated with deinstitutionalization. Even the 1975 revisions of the Community Mental Health Centers Act, which mandated cooperation with state mental hospitals and encouraged care for chronic patients, did not address the social welfare and housing needs of the mentally disabled. The expansion of Social Security disability to the indigent (Supplemental Security Income) provided some assistance but was not equal to the growing problems of deinstitutionalization. The over-promise of community mental health to relieve widespread social distress and disenfranchisement and to prevent chronicity, in fact, left thousands of former patients homeless or living in substandard housing, often without treatment, supervision, or social support. By the late 1970s, the General Accounting Office[46] deplored the lack of federal support for a rational deinstitutionalization policy, and the President's Commission on Mental Health[49] called for a national mental health policy focused on the chronically mentally ill.

The Community Support Movement

The Community Support Program was the National Institute of Mental Health (NIMH) response to the criticism of the federal role in deinstitutionalization.[54,55] A total of $3.5 million was allocated annually for contracts with 19 states for three-year pilot demonstration programs designed "to provide services for one particularly vulnerable population—adult psychiatric patients whose disabilities are severe and persistent but for whom long-termed skilled or semiskilled nursing care is inappropriate."[54] The Community Support Program responded to "a much needed social reform" by championing "community support systems"—a community network of crises care services, psychosocial rehabilitation services, supportive living and working arrangements, medical and mental health care, and case management for the chronically mentally ill.[54] The federal program became a model for states throughout the United States,[55]

Mental health centers failed to meet the needs of acute and chronic patients discharged in increasing numbers from public hospitals. Homelessness and indigency were predictable outcomes for many.

In some respects, the community support movement has been only a mid-course correction in the community mental health movement, an adminstrative fix for the problems of deinstitutionalization.[56] However, the community support movement may be viewed as a fourth cycle of reform in that it advocates a new approach to treatment, in this case, a whole system of care.[3,55] It also proposes a fundamental change in attitude and approach to the chronically mentally ill. Rather than prevent chronicity, the community support reformers offer direct care and rehabilitation for the chronic mentally ill.

The systemic approach to the care of the chronic mentally ill also marks a shift in the tendency to transform social problems into mental health policies and to ignore the chronic mentally ill. In a sense, the advocates of community supports have recognized that the problem of chronic mental illness is first and foremost a social welfare problem. They do not recommend mental health solutions to social problems; instead, they propose social welfare solutions to mental health problems. A community support system includes health and mental health services but also recognizes entitlement programs, income supports, transportation, and housing as critical elements.

Recent fiscal policy and resource constraints have threatened the community support reform movement: the repeal of the Mental Health Systems Act, the termination of disability benefits to tens of thousands of mentally ill beneficiaries of SSI and SSDI, and prospective payments systems that may increase admissions to state mental hospitals have all compromised the care of the chronic mentally ill in the community.[3] In addition, the Community Support Program, each year, struggles to maintain its appropriation.

Homelessness: a New Social Problem Beckons

Community mental health brought mental patients "home"; deinstitutionalization left them homeless.

Deinstitutionalization without community support and adequate housing has contributed to the problem of homelessness in America[57–59] but it is not the whole story. Although studies demonstrate that there are mentally ill individuals among the homeless, not all (or even most) of the homeless are chronically mentally ill. Those who are mentally ill focus on their housing and welfare needs rather than on mental health treatment needs.[60] Do the homeless mentally ill need more mental health treatment or a return to the asylum, as some have suggested?[61] Or is the problem more fundamental, a lack of adequate community-based housing, jobs, and other services?[62]

At this critical juncture in its short history, the community support reform is faced with a sensitive issue: How to handle its involvement and define a role for mental health in the national problem of homelessness? Having declared chronic mental illness in the community as a social welfare problem and advocated for housing reform for deinstitutionalized mental patients, mental health advocates now find themselves once again confronted with the dangers and opportunities associated with offering a mental health solution to a larger social problem.

Changing the locus of care did not solve the problem of chronic mental illness and, in fact, may have made matters worse.

The problem of the homeless mentally ill is complex and may be defined from two perspectives: Who among the homeless are mentally ill, and who among the mentally ill are homeless?[63] Both are important questions relevant to mental health policy. Mental health activitists, however, must protect against offering a mental health solution to the problem of all of the homeless, but also must not allow social welfare activists to forget the psychopathology of the homeless mentally ill. Bachrach[65] recalls Susan Sontag's description of illness as a metaphor[66] in her warning not to blame the homeless victims of deinstitutionalization by ignoring their mental illness. Bachrach and Sontag suggest that mental illness may serve as a metaphor for personal failings. We suggest that labeling problems as "mental" may also be used metaphorically to avoid having to deal fundamentally with social problems. A recent American Psychiatric Association Task Force on the homeless mentally ill[64] recognizes these problems and points a middle course for mental health policy, recognizing the mental health *and* social welfare needs of the chronic mentally ill homeless.The community support activists may have found a balance between specialized mental health and basic social welfare needs of chronic patients. They have learned the importance of caring as well as curing but their reform is frail and in danger of failing, due to resource limitations, frustration dealing with chronic patients, and exaggerated expectations. They must resist the temptation of the alchemy of past reforms for fear of turning the base metals of social welfare into the fool's gold of overly optimistic mental health policy. The base metals are dull and heavy but solid and dependable; fool's gold glitters but serves no useful purpose.

Beyond Alchemy in Mental Health Policy

Hopefully, this community support reform will avoid fiscal threats to its existence and will not be diluted by the expectations that community support systems will solve the generic problem of homelessness in America. For the reform to persist, however, will take more than sailing the narrow course between this Scylla and Charybdis. The dichotomy between caring and curing, between chronic and acute patients, that evolved over the four cycles of reform is deeply rooted in the ideology of the mental health professionals who practice in community settings. A new professional, a nonclinician case manager has been offered as a partial solution to the problem of prevailing professional attitude. This approach, however, may create new problems related to nonclinicians' insensitivity to psychopathology and their inability to provide needed treatment.

Changes in the diagnostic nomenclature in psychiatry, reflected in the advent of the Third Edition of the Diagnostic and Statistical Manual (DSM-III) of the American Psychiatric Association,[67] narrow the focus of psychopathology to more reliably defined disorders with specific criteria. This marks a change away from a broad labeling of distress and deviance as pathology that was common from the 1950s into the 1970s. It reinforces the more biomedical aspects of mental disorder, de-emphasizing individual moral and psychosocial responsibility. Hopefully, DSM-III will reduce confusion between the disorders and their social context without ignoring either one. Although potentially destigmatizing, this approach must also be accompanied by acceptance of the social welfare needs of chronic mental patients, if it is to contribute to better care. Disorders need treatment and medical intervention; social dependence and homelessness demand social welfare solutions. Both are required for the chronically mentally ill.

Community support advocates recognize that chronic mental illness is first and foremost a social welfare problem.

Public attitudes, too, must change if there is to be progress. Recent advances in biological psychiatry offer a redefinition of mental illness as "an illness like any other"— not a moral issue. However, the psychoactive drug "revolution" that accompanied the third cycle of community mental health reform did not succeed in overcoming the stigma of mental illness.

Another hopeful sign in the process of changing attitudes is the current reintroduction of lay leadership into mental health activism, not seen since Clifford Beers in mental hygiene and Horace Mann and Dorothea Dix in the moral treatment era. Self-help and family groups are growing. A new, popular movement may revitalize the fledgling community support reform, if it can gain political strength. Such a movement would be new in the sense of being led by patients and their families rather than by professionals. It would be a democratic movement rather than a social reform fueled by guilt and noblesse oblige.

The history of public policy on behalf of the mentally ill has been a search for the proper balance between professionalism and lay leadership, between caring and curing, and between social welfare and mental health needs and services. The next decade will tell us if the fourth cycle of reform is more successful in achieving this balance than its predecessors.

References

1. Morrissey JP, Goldman HH, Klerman LV: The Enduring Asylum: Cycles of Institutional Reform at Worcester State Hospital. New York: Grune and Stratton, 1980.
2. Dain N: The chronic mental patient in 19th-century America. Psychiatric Annals 1980; 10:323–327.
3. Morrissey JP, Goldman HH: Cycles of reform in the care of the chronically mentally ill. Hosp Community Psychiatry 1984; 35:785–793.
4. Grob GN: The State and the Mentally Ill: A History of Worcester State Hospital in Massachusetts, 1830–1920. Chapel Hill: University of North Carolina Press, 1966.
5. Caplan RB, Caplan G: Psychiatry and the Community in Nineteenth-Century America. New York: Basic Books, 1969.
6. Rothman DJ: The Discovery of the Asylum. Boston: Little, Brown, 1971.
7. Grob GN: Mental Institutions in America: Social Policy to 1875. New York: Free Press, 1973.
8. Deutsch A: The history of mental hygiene. *In:* Hall JK, Zilboorg G, Bunker HA (eds): One Hundred Years of American Psychiatry. New York: Columbia University Press, 1944.
9. Rothman DJ: Conscience and Convenience: The Asylum and Its Alternatives in Progressive America. Boston: Little, Brown, 1980.
10. Grob GN: Mental Illness and American Society, 1875–1940. Princeton, NJ: Princeton University Press, 1983.
11. Quen JM: Asylum psychiatry, neurology, social work, and mental hygiene: an exploratory study in interprofessional history. J Hist Behav Sci 1977;13:3–11.
12. Sicherman B: The Quest for Mental Health in America, 1880–1917. New York: Arno Press, 1980.
13. Joint Commission on Mental Illness and Health: Action for Mental Health. New York: Basic Books, 1961.
14. Levinson A, Brown B: Some implications of the community mental health center concept. *In* Hoch P, Zubin J (eds): Social Psychiatry. New York: Grune and Stratton, 1967.
15. Musto D: Whatever happened to community mental health? Public Interest 1975; 39:53–79.
16. Foley HA, Sharfstein SS: Madness and Government: Who Cares for the Mentally Ill? Washington, DC: American Psychiatric Press, 1983.
17. Faris REL, Dunham HW: Mental Disorders in Urban Areas. Chicago: University of Chicago Press, 1939.
18. Hollingshead A, Redlich F: Social Class and Mental Illness. New York: Wiley, 1958.
19. Menninger K: The Human Mind. New York: Knopf, 1945.
20. Karpman B: Criminality, insanity, and the law. J Criminal Law Criminal Policy Sci 1949; 39:586–604.
21. Mora G: The history of psychiatry. *In:* Freedman AM, Kaplan HI (eds): Comprehensive Textbook of Psychiatry, 1st Ed. Baltimore: Williams & Wilkins, 1967.

22. Decentralization of Psychiatric Services and Continuity of Care. New York, Milbank Memorial Fund, 1962.
23. Lindemann E: Symptomatology and management of acute grief. Am J Psychiatry 1944; 101:141–148.
24. Caplan G: Principles of Preventive Psychiatry. New York: Basic Books, 1964.
25. Grimes JM: Institutional Care of Mental Patients in the United States. Chicago; AMA, 1934.
26. Myerson A: Theory and principles of the "total push" method in the treatment of chronic schizophrenia. Am J Psychiatry 1939; 95:1197–1204.
27. Bryan WA: Administrative Psychiatry. New York: Norton, 1936.
28. Spiegel J, Grinker R: Men under Stress. Philadelphia: Blakiston, 1945.
29. Deutsch A: The Shame of the States. New York: Harcourt, Brace, 1948.
30. Goffman E: Asylums. New York: Doubleday, 1961.
31. Solomon HC: The American Psychiatric Association in relation to American psychiatry. Am J Psychiatry 1958; 115:1–9.
32. Szasz T: Manufacture of Madness. New York: Harper and Row, 1970.
33. Gruenberg E: The social breakdown syndrome and its prevention. *In:* Arieti S (ed): American Handbook of Psychiatry, 2nd Ed, Vol 2. NewYork: Basic Books, 1974.
34. Wing J: Institutionalism in mental hospitals. J Soc Clin Psychol 1962; 1:38–51.
35. Barton R: Institutional Neurosis, 2nd Ed. Baltimore: Williams and Wilkins, 1966.
36. Windle C, Scully D: Community mental health centers and the decreasing use of state mental hospitals. Commun Mental Health J 1976; 12:239–243.
37. Goldman HH, Adams NH, Taube CA: Deinstitulionalization: the data demythologized. Hosp Community Psychiatry 1983; 34:129–134.
38. Morrissey J: Deinstitutionalization the mentally ill: process, outcomes, and new directions. *In:* Gove W (ed): Deviance and Mental Illness. Beverly Hills: Sage, 1982.
39. Goldman HH, Gattozzi AA, Taube CA: Defining and counting the chronically mentally ill. Hosp Community Psychiatry 1981; 32:21–27.
40. Goldman HH: Longterm Care for the Chronically Mentally Ill. Washington DC: Urban Institute (working paper) 1983.
41. Bassuk E, Gerson J: Deinstitutionalization and mental health services. Sci American 1978; 238:46–53.
42. Rose S: Deciphering deinstitutionalization: complexities in policy and program analysis. Milbank Mem Fund Q 1979; 57:429–460.
43. Gruenberg E, Archer J: Abandonment of responsibility for the seriously mentally ill. Milbank Mem Fund Q 1979; 57:485–506.
44. Bachrach LL: Deinstitutionalization: An Analytical Review and Sociological Perspective. Rockville, MD, National Institute of Mental Health, 1976.
45. National Institute of Mental Health: Where Is My Home? Proceedings of a Conference on the Closing of State Mental Hospitals, Scottsdale, AZ, 1974, Stanford Research Institute, 1974.
46. General Accounting Office: Returning the Mentally Disabled to the Community: Government Needs to Do More. Washington, DC: General Accounting Office, 1977.
47. Chu F, Trotter S: The Madness Establishment. New York: Grossman, 1974.
48. Santiestevan H: Deinstitutionalization: Out of Their Beds and Into the Streets. Washington, DC: American Federation of State, County, and Municipal Employees, 1975.
49. President's Commission on Mental Health: Final Report. Washington, DC: Govt Printing Office, 1978.
50. Koenig P: The problem that can't be tranquilized: 40,000 mental patients dumped in city neighborhoods. *New York Times Magazine,* May 21, 1978.
51. Drake D: The forsaken: how America has abandoned troubled thousands in the name of social progress. *Philadelphia Inquirer, July 18–24, 1982.*
52. Trotter S, Kutner B: Back wards to back alleys. *Washington Post,* Feb. 24, 1974.
53. Sheehan S: Is There No Place on Earth for Me? Boston: Houghton Mifflin, 1982.
54. Turner J, TenHoor W: The NIMH community support program: pilot approach to a needed social reform. Schizophrenia Bull 1978; 4:319–348.

55. Tessler RC, Goldman HH: The Chronically Mentally Ill: Assessing Community Support Programs. Cambridge: Ballinger, 1982.
56. Lamb HR: What did we really expect from deinstitutionalization? Hosp Community Psychiatry 1981; 32:105–109.
57. Lamb HR: Deinstitutionalization and the homeless mentally ill. Hosp Community Psychiatry 1984; 35:899–907.
58. Arce AA, Vergare J: Identifying and characterizing the mentally ill among the homeless. *In:* Lamb HR (ed): The Homeless Mentally Ill. Washington, DC: American Psychiatric Press, 1984.
59. Bassuk EL, Rubin L, Lauriat A: Is homelessness a mental health problem? Am J Psychiatry 1984; 141:1546–1550.
60. Ball FLJ, Havassy BE: A survey of the problems and needs of homeless consumers of acute psychiatric services. Hosp Community Psychiatry 1984; 35:917–921.
61. Krauthammer C: For the homeless: asylum. *Washington Post,* Jan. 4, 1985, Section A15.
62. Rubenstein LS: The asylum will not help the homeless. *Washington Post,* Jan. 12, 1985.
63. Bachrach LL: Research on services for the homeless mentally ill. Hosp Community Psychiatry 1984; 35:910–913.
64. Lamb HR: The Homeless Mentally Ill. Washington, DC: American Psychiatric Press, 1984.
65. Bachrach LL: Interpreting research on the homeless mentally ill. Hosp Community Psychiatry 1984; 35:914–917.
66. Sontag S: Illness as Metaphor. New York: Vintage Books, 1979.
67. Diagnostic and Statistical Manual of the Mental Disorders, Third Ed. Washington DC: American Psychiatric Press, 1980.

23

Estroff, S. E. (1985). Medicalizing the margins: On being disgraced, disordered, and deserving. *Psychosocial Rehabilitation Journal, 8* (4), 34–38

This brief article begins with Estroff's response to the American Psychiatric Association's 1984 book-length report, *Homelessness and the Mentally Ill*, edited by Richard Lamb. Estroff criticizes the reports focus on serious mental illness and the individual pathology of homeless persons as causes of homelessness, as persons with mental illnesses constituted only a large subset of the homeless population at the time. She also critiques the report for its proposed professional and medical response to homelessness at the expense of addressing the socioeconomic forces that cause it. Related problems, she writes, are the report's emphasis on creating staff positions rather than low income housing and on the role of psychiatrists in responding to the needs of homeless persons with mental illness, given psychiatrists' lack of training for the job and the discipline's dismal record of coming to the aid of poor persons. Estroff also criticizes the report for its tendency to pit the categories of the deserving—mentally ill persons who are not responsible for their illness—against the undeserving—those who could help themselves if only they would. Estroff's article is a pivotal piece during this era for its attention to the questions of public psychiatry's responsibility, capability, and leadership or adjunct role in addressing the problems of poverty and socioeconomic disadvantage among homeless persons with mental illness.

Medicalizing the Margins:
On Being Disgraced,
Disordered, and Deserving

In our very suspicious society, losing one's home, like losing one's mind, raises questions about cause, usually among those who have lost neither. Space and sanity are possessions that all of us expect to have and expect others to have; why, then, do some apparently lack both? The answers are complicated. My purpose in raising this question is to question the question itself, and to suggest that the question itself is part of the problem.

Living space, social place, and membership in some sort of human group are such basic cultural necessities that, when violated, the handiest explanation is either deliberate cultural defiance or an inability because of illness to satisfy these basic needs. Dichotomizing the explanations as either willful refusal or inability due to illness emphasizes the importance of establishing presence or absence of mental disorder. Compassion, care, and resources, scant as they are, flow more benignly to victims than to those who consciously break rules. My point is that our preoccupation with discovering the causes of homelessness is perhaps not due to an overwhelming desire to prevent or eradicate this obscenity, but rather to the more urgent cultural requirement of determining if those who are living in public places *deserve* attention, care, and kind contribution.

The difference between being merely disgraced (and disgraceful) and being disgraced but deserving rests most often in our culture on the latter's being disordered or diseased, in this case, being severely or chronically mentally ill (Stone, 1979). The status of legitimate disorder is, of course, conferred primarily by physicians, and thus the APA report on homelessness takes on very special social and symbolic importance. The report seeks in part to delimit lines of responsibility for and responses to certain types of persons who are homeless. The very act of forming a task force of psychiatrists can be seen as a symbolic and public statement, indirectly and effectively diagnosing the people as well as the problem. (One notes, for example, that no similar effort was launched by cardiologists or pediatricians, thereby publicly absolving heart disease and infancy of contributing to homelessness.) My concern in this regard reverts back to the circuitry between disorder and being deserving. The report and its recommendations could inadvertently identify some homeless persons as more deserving of care than others because some are diseased and disordered and thus not at fault, while others who are not ill are thus more deserving of their wretched fate than of concern.

Hopper (1983) and Hopper & Hamberg (1984) argue convincingly and with eloquence that "something has gone grievously wrong with the fundamental needs-satisfying structures of our society." That thousands of persons who have serious problems in thinking and in relations with others are left to suffer in isolation and danger without shelter or subsistence should not distract our attention from others who suffer similarly, and who, because they live in such dire circumstances, are at predictably high risk for psychological turmoil, personal anguish, and further psychosocial disintegration. I am not suggesting that all homeless people are mentally ill or even want or need psychiatric care, nor am I suggesting that mental health systems or personnel be held responsible for causing homelessness or caring for all of the homeless. I am, however, wary of the unintentional designation of some people as diseased and deserving while others remain under scrutiny as perhaps willingly marginal and malfunctioning, potentially undeserving.

Despite this broader set of cultural concerns, one has to welcome this effort on the part of the American Psychiatric Association. Several extraordinarily compassionate and thoughtful psychiatrists (and staff), led by Talbott and Lamb, have produced a laudably thorough and useful document. The remarks that follow, while somewhat critical, should not be construed as unappreciative of the value and quality of the report.

The report acknowledges accurately that broad and confluent socioeconomic forces both increase and create homelessness, but then reverts to professionalizing and medicalizing the responses. The predictably heavy emphasis on provision of services and aggressive peddling of psychiatric and psychosocial treatment raises some concerns about medicalizing those on the margins. The report basically recommends providing more and better care for those able, in professional opinion, to navigate community life, locking up those who cannot, and exerting more control via case management or conservatorship over those whose functioning fluctuates over time. It is difficult, at times, to distinguish between designated case management and conservatorship in the report; both serve similar purposes of social and clinical control, albeit arguably in the client's interests.

One also has to raise the spectre of creating yet more jobs for mental health professionals and expending more money on staff positions, perhaps at the expense of commodities such as food and shelter. Even the most ingenious and dedicated case manager cannot locate low-cost housing that does not exist, or find temporary residence for clients in abandoned and deteriorated SRO hotels. One has to be skeptical of the prospect of creating more layers of service providers, who will of course need to have more meetings with each other and more time to deal with their own fatigue, despair, and righteous indignation. To be fair, the same reservations must apply to the calls for more research, resulting unavoidably in yet another group of domiciled and well-fed people depending on the plight of the destitute for their own subsistence. I am not recommending that there be no case management or research. I am, however, entering a plea for being mindful of the symbiosis between providers and clients, researchers and research subjects, and for constant vigilance in the setting and resetting of priorities in the expenditure of precious resources.

Again I have to question whether professionalization of the problem will accomplish more than protecting some precariously perched people from loss of shelter or succor. At present (and for at least the next four years) there simply are not enough resources or the public will to create them to carry out these urgent missions on a large scale. From a strictly utilitarian point of view, how many can reasonably benefit from such extensive and intensive services as are proposed here? And even more to the point, what of those who really do not want to be labelled, served, or treated, but who do want food, shelter, safety, and structure? Medicalizing those on the margins may be the best way at present to get them the resources they so desperately need, but what would be the long-term social consequences of such an action? We have already witnessed the dangers of heavy reliance on disability-contingent income support; are we about to bait the trap again?

I am a bit curious about the actual and potential roles of psychiatrists, who have not traditionally been extensively involved in obtaining or retaining housing for their patients. As has recently been reiterated by Mollica (1983), psychiatrists as a group have not rushed to care for the poor or the marginal members of our society, including many of those who are poor, marginal, and chronically mentally ill. Other mental health professionals carry the bulk of the burden of both planning for and providing hospital and community care for the lower social classes and for the most severely disabled. If this report signalled a change of heart or interest on the part of the psychiatric profession, one might see cause for both optimism and caution. Yet I do not see any evidence that psychiatrists in increasing numbers will sit on urban planning commissions or administer community mental health centers or programs. I do not see any indications that psychiatrists will spend the time required to assess a patient's living situation, help to improve or change it, or spend hours or weeks working with landlords and other tenants to improve the household relations of clients. I do not see, in these recommendations, a plan for doing anything new or different. The call is for more of what we already have.

I have to disagree that the underlying problem is a lack of comprehensive community support programs. The underlying problems go far deeper than that and have to do with why the resources required to provide for disabled and poor people are so grudgingly offered, so often reduced, so seldom adequate. The problem is in the legislatures, in the neighborhoods of housed people, in the chambers of commerce of annoyed businessmen, in the offices of social services departments, in the thinking and values of federal administrators. Where, indeed, do we see the most inexplicable behavior? Who, indeed, has done the most harm to whom? Who represents the most danger to whom? How many will have to suffer the dangers and disgraces of life in the margins of our society before we stop shrugging our shoulders, excusing ourselves from trying to influence social forces because they are too complex and out of our control?

This report and its recommendations are eminently reasonable, professional responses to professional conceptualizations of apparently "escalating cycles of disenfranchisement" (Hopper, 1982) in our society. As I and others write these essays in the comfort of our own homes and offices, I hope each of us is aware of how nearly unentitled we are to comment on that of which we know so very little. As an anthropologist who learns primarily via experiencing the worlds of others, I cannot even pretend to comprehend adequately what homelessness is for those who are. This ignorance, however, should not result in being unable to know what each and all of us must do. In reference to medicine, Hauerwas has said what I think also applies to mental health professionals regarding persons who are homeless: "It is the burden of those who care for the suffering ... to teach the suffering that they are not thereby excluded from the human community. In this sense, medicine's primary moral role is to bind the suffering and the non-suffering into the same community." There are, in my opinion, no acceptable excuses, professional or fiscal, for failing in this task.

References

Hauerwas, S. Reflections on suffering, death and medicine. *Ethics in Science and Medicine,* 1979, 6(4), 230.

Hopper, K. Deinstitutionalization in 1984: Prospects for the homeless mentally disabled. Paper presented at the American Orthopsychiatric Association Annual Meeting. Boston, Mass., April 7, 1983.

Hopper, K., & Hamberg, J. *The making of America's homeless: from Skid Row to New Poor, 1945–1984.* Unpublished ms., 1984.

Mollica, R. F. From asylum to community: The threatened disintegration of public psychiatry. *New England Journal of Medicine,* 1983, 308(7), 365–173.

Stone, D. Diagnosis and the dole: The function of illness in American distributive politics. *Journal of Health Politics. Policy and Law,* 1979, 4, 507–521.

24

Anthony, W. A., and Liberman, R. P. (1986). The practice of psychiatric rehabilitation: Historical, conceptual, and research base. *Schizophrenia Bulletin, 12* (4), 542–559

William Anthony, a leading researcher on psychiatric rehabilitation starting in the 1980s and of the mental health recovery movement of the 1990s to the present, presents in this article with Robert Liberman a foundational document on the field of psychiatric rehabilitation. The discipline emerged from the community mental health movement as practitioners, administrators, and researchers came to understand that the movement was missing essential tools for helping persons with serious mental illness to function and prosper in the community. Treatment alone did not fill a gap in social and occupational skills that had wasted away from years of institutionalization or that had never been strong in some. Internal challenges of mental illness and external stigma that accompanied it complicate the task of developing skills, or acquiring and using the right tools, for "making it" in the community. Psychiatric rehabilitation emerged as the leading social arm of community psychiatry, allied with and seen as essential, if still serving as a secondary partner to it. As the mental health recovery movement picked up steam in the late 1990s and into the twenty-first century, psychiatric rehabilitation would both inspire and be seen, by some, as a compromised approach to community integration and empowerment of persons with mental illness. Here, in a shorter version of the original, Anthony and Liberman review the concepts and practices of psychiatric rehabilitation and its status in the community mental health field in the mid-1980s.

The Practice of Psychiatric Rehabilitation: Historical, Conceptual, and Research Base

With the recognition that most psychiatric disorders are associated with severe and persisting disability and the development of effective procedures for improving the long-term outcome of patients, the term "psychiatric rehabilitation" is becoming routinely used in the mental health field. Psychiatric rehabilitation has begun to take its place as a viable, credible intervention approach, even infiltrating professionals' jargon and administrators' program descriptions. The field of psychiatric rehabilitation has progressed to the stage where its history can be traced; its conceptual base and treatment strategies described; its practice observed, monitored, and replicated; and its future growth anchored in a research foundation.

> How many times it thundered before Franklin took the hint! How many apples fell on Newton's head before he took the hint! Nature is always hinting at us. It hints over and over again. And suddenly we take the hint.
>
> —*Robert Frost*

The essential elements of a psychiatric rehabilitation approach have been hinted at for well over a century. Different elements of a psychiatric rehabilitation approach have periodically moved in and out of favor, highlighted almost serendipitously as the mental health field progressed through various developmental phases. Currently there is a consensus developing as to what constitutes the field of psychiatric rehabilitation. The overall goal of psychiatric rehabilitation is to assure that the person with a psychiatric disability can perform those physical, emotional, social, and intellectual skills needed to live, learn, and work in the community, with the least amount of support necessary from agents of the helping professions (Anthony 1979). The major methods by which this goal is accomplished involve either teaching persons the specific skills needed to function effectively or developing the community and environmental resources needed to support or strengthen their present levels of functioning (Anthony, Cohen, and Cohen 1983; Livneh 1984; Liberman and Evans 1985).

The work of current researchers and practitioners will determine whether psychiatric rehabilitation becomes an evolving field of study and practice, or merely a historical footnote. At present it seems that many mental health professionals recognize the need for rehabilitation interventions to complement existing treatment approaches (Anthony 1977; Liberman and Foy 1983). However, this recognition of need does not mean that psychiatric rehabilitation is a well-understood field of study. Because all types of mental health disciplines practice psychiatric rehabilitation, and because relevant research and conceptual articles appear in a wide range of professional journals, psychiatric rehabilitation is a field that until recently has been difficult to define.

310

Historical Context

The origins of the psychiatric rehabilitation field are rooted in several historical developments: (1) the moral therapy era; (2) the inclusion of the psychiatrically disabled into public-supported vocational rehabilitation programs; (3) the development of community mental health ideology; (4) the psychosocial rehabilitation center movement; and (5) the development of skills training techniques as an effective mental health intervention.

Moral Therapy Era. The 19th century reformists for more humane care of the mentally ill aimed "to treat the patients as far as their condition would possibly admit, as if they were still in the enjoyment of the healthy exercise of their mental faculties...and to make their condition as comfortable as possible" (Bockoven 1963, p. 26). Moral treatment stressed a comprehensive assessment of the psychiatrically disabled, examining the person's work, play, and social activities. For example, a chaplain at a British asylum recognized the importance of patients' reentry into social life "by obtaining for them a change of scene and air and assisting them to obtain suitable employment" (Hawkins 1871, p. 107). Consistent with present-day rehabilitation practice, moral treatment recognized that structured activity can have therapeutic value. Today the goal of psychiatric rehabilitation practice is to have the person *do* something differently.

Vocational Rehabilitation Programs. While initial governmental programs for employment of the disabled, sparked by the end of World War I, focused on the physically handicapped, they did demonstrate that rehabilitation principles could be effectively implemented and won public support for rehabilitation as a societal responsibility. The 1943 amendments to the United States Vocational Rehabilitation Act extended financial support and vocational rehabilitation services to the psychiatrically disabled, with similar legislation appearing at the same time in England. These governmental actions provided legitimacy to the idea of training and rehabilitating people with psychiatric disabilities and grounded the practice of psychiatric rehabilitation in the vocational arena. The discovery of the capacity of the mentally retarded for gainful employment (O'Connor and Tizard 1956) led to studies on the effects of psychiatric disability on work and to the introduction of paid industrial subcontract work into large mental hospitals (Carstairs, O'Connor, and Rawnsley 1956).

The last three decades have seen the scope of rehabilitation move beyond a singular concern with vocational functioning to additional arenas of social and community functioning, but vocational activity has remained a preeminent ingredient in current rehabilitation practices (Beard, Propst, and Malamud 1982; Grob 1983). For example, Lamb (1982) has written that "work therapy geared to the capability of the individual patient should be a cornerstone of community treatment of the long-term patient" (p. 176).

Community Mental Health. The legislation that established community-based treatment for the mentally ill and retarded in the late 1950s and early 1960s endorsed the parity between physical and psychiatric disorders and their treatment. Mental illness and retardation no longer merited removal from society to large institutions; thus, the British Mental Health Act of 1959 supported "forms of training and social services which can be given without bringing patients into hospital as inpatients, or which make it possible to discharge them from hospital sooner" (Royal Commission 1957, p. 76). A new basic assumption prevailed—namely, people with major mental illness should be helped to maintain themselves in the community in as normal a manner as possible. Unfortunately, community mental health centers (CMHCs) failed to provide the comprehensive services needed by the severely psychiatrically disabled (Braun et al. 1981), who were not a high priority population for the CMHCs, perhaps because their interdisciplinary staff members were ill-equipped with techniques for effective work with chronic psychotics (Liberman, King, and DeRisi 1976).

The deinstitutionalization movement, which accompanied the opening of the CMHCs, fostered an appreciation of the value of work training in the preparation of patients for resettlement in the community. Psychiatrists were forced to match their view of the patient's abilities and disabilities against the realities of adaptation in the "real world." Studies were carried out in industrial therapy programs that showed the benefits and hazards of work for the mentally ill, changed the attitudes of citizens and professionals about the employability of mentally ill persons, and led to job placement programs (Bennett 1983).

Consistent with modern concepts of rehabilitation are those additional elements of community mental health ideology—accessibility to and comprehensiveness of services, and continuity of care. The emphasis on treating patients in proximity to their natural families and work settings has now been extended by the initiative of the National Institute of Mental Health for community support programs, which has encouraged State and local investments in a spectrum of services for the chronically mentally ill. In turn, this has meant an infusion of key operating principles for psychiatric rehabilitation, including case management, coordination, and advocacy with a variety of agencies capable of meeting the full range of needs of persons with severe psychiatric disabilities; involvement of patients and relatives in self-help; and assertive outreach.

Psychosocial Rehabilitation Centers. The realization that severely and chronically mentally ill persons would rarely experience a full return of psychosocial functioning in the community led to a movement emphasizing accommodation to the needs of these persons in sustaining some semblance of normalization. With mental health professionals' neglect of the chronic mentally ill, nonprofessionals and patients themselves initiated psychosocial self-help clubs located in cities where the mentally ill congregated in large numbers. The early clubs, such as Fountain House and Horizon House, were founded by groups of ex-patients for the purpose of mutual aid and support. These early social clubs gave birth to comprehensive, multiservice psychosocial rehabilitation centers such as Thresholds in Chicago; the Social Rehabilitation Center in Fairfax, Virginia; Center Club in Boston; Fellowship House in Miami; Hill House in Cleveland; and Portals House in Los Angeles. The psychosocial centers assist patients to deal with their "real life" problems by providing opportunities for acceptable role performance and successful mutually interdependent relationships with others, by buffering stressors, and by making available a range of housing and employment options. From the very beginning, these centers have emphasized (1) strategies to help people *cope* with the environment rather than *succumb* to it, (2) health induction rather than symptom reduction, and (3) belief in the potential productivity of the most severely psychiatrically disabled client (Beard, Propst, and Malamud 1982).

Psychosocial centers have not valued the development of therapeutic insight (Dincin 1981). Their orientation has been on reality factors rather than intrapsychic factors, and on improving the person's ability to do something in a specific environment, even in the presence of residual disability (Grob 1983).

Psychosocial centers have played a significant role in the development of the psychiatric rehabilitation field. Their influence in the foreseeable future should be even greater since Fountain House has been conducting a training program to assist CMHCs and other types of mental health settings to establish rehabilitation services based on the psychosocial center model. In a 5-year period, individuals from agencies located in 38 states, the District of Columbia, Sweden, and Canada have been trained. During that time the number of rehabilitation programs has increased from 18 to 148. As the number of psychosocial rehabilitation centers continues to grow, this serves to ensure the presence of settings in which future research can be conducted and new rehabilitation techniques tested.

Skills Training. The most recent development in shaping psychiatric rehabilitation has been the introduction of skills training methods derived from social learning principles, human resource development training, and vocational rehabilitation. Effective coping with life stressors requires skills to promote problem solving, engage others in successful affiliative and instrumental relationships, mobilize supportive networks, and engage in work. Rehabilitation techniques that use active-directive learning principles—behavioral practice and role playing, social and tangible reinforcement, shaping, coaching, and prompting, and generalization activities—strengthen an individual problem-solving capacities and convey protection against exacerbations of psychiatric symptoms (Cohen, Ridley, and Cohen 1983; Wallace and Liberman 1985).

Skills training has been found effective in group and individual therapy, family therapy, milieu therapy, and vocational settings (Anthony, Howell, and Danley 1984; Liberman et al., this issue; Strachar this issue). The point of training interpersonal skills is to improve the individual's ability to master the challenges and problems inherent in daily life. It is assumed that, within genetic and constitutional constraints, each patient tries to do his or her best, so that the problem lies not in resistance or lack of motivation, but in a deficit of some sort. The source of deficit is regarded as less important than using remedial training methods to enhance the individual's ability to cope. Successful coping leads to attainment of social and emotional goals that define competence and adjustment. While skills-training approaches have shown much promise and empirical efficacy (Carkhuff 1972; Paul and Lentz 1977; Carkhuff 1983; Liberman 1984), they have been adopted by practitioners very slowly because of the demanding competencies required of those who seek to do such training (Backer, Liberman, and Kuehnel 1986; Cohen et al., this issue).

Conceptual Model for Rehabilitation

Within the last several decades, a consensus has developed about what constitutes a conceptual model for rehabilitation and its underlying philosophy, as well as what constitutes appropriate rehabilitation practice (see Table 24.1). The conceptual model was introduced

Table 24.1. Stages in the Rehabilitation of Chronic Mental Patients, with Examples of the Elements in Each Stage

Stage	Pathology	Impairment	Disability	Handicap
Definition	Lesions or abnormalities in the central nervous system caused by agents or processes responsible for the etiology and maintenance of the biobehavioral disorder	Any loss or abnormality of *psychological, physiological,* or *anatomical structure* or *function* (resulting from underlying pathology)	Any restriction or lack (resulting from an impairment) of *ability to perform an activity* in the manner or within the range considered normal for a human being	A disadvantage for a given individual (resulting from an impairment or a disability) that limits or prevents *the fulfillment of a role* that is normal *(depending on age, sex, social, cultural factors)* for that individual
Example	Brain tumors or infections etiologically linked to psychotic symptoms	Positive and negative symptoms of schizophrenia (delusions, anhedonia)	Deficient social skills	Unemployment, homelessness
Interventions	Laboratory and radiographic tests	Syndromal diagnosis, pharmacotherapy, hospitalization	Functional assessment, skills training, social support	National and state vocational rehabilitation policies, community support programs

by leaders in physical medicine and rehabilitation and later extended the mental health disciplines (Anthony 1980, 1982). Both physically and psychiatrically disabled persons exhibit disabilities in social function; handicaps in role performance; needs for a wide range of services, often for a long period of time; and frequent failure to experience total recovery. Rehabilitation of psychiatric disorders, as with physical illnesses, begins when the *pathology* and *impairments* of the acute stage stabilize. In cardiac rehabilitation, then, intervention begins after the myocardial infarction and its associated pain and stress have resolved. Similarly, rehabilitation for a person with schizophrenia begins when the acute and florid psychotic symptoms recede or stabilize. Even if symptoms persist, rehabilitation can proceed within the limits of the individual's capability to respond to training and supportive interventions. The focus of the rehabilitation practitioner is on remediating *disabilities* and compensating for *handicaps* (Wood 1980; Frey 1984).

The *vulnerability-stress-coping-competence* model of major mental disorders explains the onset, course, and outcome of symptoms and social functioning as a complex interaction among biological, environmental, and behavioral factors (Liberman 1982b; Nuechterlein and Dawson 1984), and is congruent with the rehabilitation conceptualization. Psychobiological vulnerability may result in psychotic symptoms when stressful life events or ambient tensions in the family or work setting overwhelm coping skills.

Vulnerability and stressors (Figure 24.1) are moderated in their impact on impairment, disability, and handicap by the presence and action of protective and potentiating factors. Prime among protective factors are coping and competence exercised by individuals, families, natural support systems, and professional treatment. Examples of protective factors

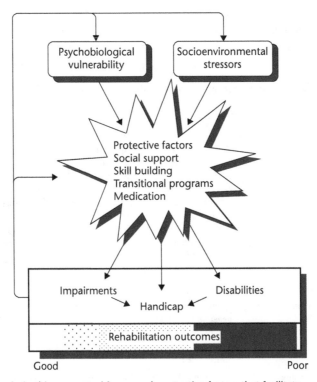

In this conceptual framework protective factors that facilitate coping and competence can modulate the deleterious affects of psychobiological vulnerability and socioenvironmental stressors. Coping and competence confer protection against impairment, disability, and handicap

include rehabilitation programs that offer skill building, social support, or transitional employment. Coping and competence can be attributes of the individual or of the social environment. From this point of view, an exacerbation or relapse of schizophrenic symptoms that accompanied use of street drugs of abuse (e.g., PCP, amphetamines) would result from the stressful action of these drugs on the individual's underlying biological diathesis for schizophrenia. In like manner, stressful life events (e.g., loss of a trusted therapist or discharge from long-term hospitalization) that overwhelm the protective effects of medication, personal coping, and social support can also lead to symptomatic exacerbation. Even in the absence of a time-limited stressor, vulnerable individuals can succumb to ambient levels of challenge, tension, or conflict in their environment if they lack the protection conferred by medication, coping abilities, and social support.

The *vulnerability-stress-coping-competence* model highlights the role of specific psychosocial interventions in developing personal and familial coping skills, and interpersonal and vocational competence as protective factors in the course of mental disorders. Psychosocial protective factors buffer the impact of potentiators and stressors, and thereby reduce the probability of symptomatic relapse. Socially learned coping helps individuals to obtain their instrumental and social-emotional needs by meeting the challenges and solving the problems of everyday life. Coping and competence protect an individual with a given level of vulnerability to schizophrenia from stressful life events and ambient levels of environmental tension. At any level of psychopathology, coping can reduce the social, occupational, and self-care impairments that are associated with the disorder.

The model also encourages investigators to design optimal psychopharmacological interventions to modify the effect of psychobiological vulnerability factors. For example, antipsychotic medication serves as a personal protective factor against biological vulnerability; it thereby decreases relapse rates and improves the course of schizophrenic disorders. Antipsychotic medication also raises the threshold at which environmental potentiators and stressors precipitate psychotic symptoms in an individual with a given level of vulnerability to schizophrenic episodes (Leff et al. 1973; Vaughn and Leff 1976a, 1976b). However, the modulation of biological vulnerability by antipsychotic medication cannot fully remediate a vulnerable individual's susceptibility to relapse when faced with severe stressors, loss of social support, or diminution in personal problem-solving skills. Even with reliable ingestion of neuroleptics, for example, upwards of 30–40 percent of schizophrenic patients relapse within a year (Liberman 1984).

In this *vulnerability-stress-coping-competence* model, the appearance or exacerbation of characteristic schizophrenic symptoms and associated disabilities may occur in susceptible individuals when:

- Underlying psychobiological vulnerability factors are triggered, which is more likely in the absence of optimal antipsychotic medication.
- Stressful life events intervene that exceed the individual's coping skills and competencies in social and instrumental roles.
- The social support network weakens or diminishes;
- Coping and problem-solving skills atrophy as a result of disuse, reinforcement of the sick role, or loss of motivation.

Psychiatric Impairment, Disability, and Handicap

From the point of view of rehabilitation professionals, the psychobiological abnormalities in the nervous system that produce deficiencies in cognitive, attentional, and autonomic functions, and in regulation of arousal and information processing, represent the active *pathology* or *disease* state. The neurosciences are just beginning to develop instruments and techniques that can sensitively measure these abnormalities. However, they can be inferred through assessment of *impairments* that presumably index the more basic disturbances in brain function.

While impairments in physical rehabilitation include vision or hearing loss, reduced range of motion in an extremity, and loss of strength in a muscle group, *psychiatric impairments* can include thought disorder and speech incoherence, delusions, hallucinations, anxiety, depression, loss of concentration or memory, distractibility, and apathy and anhedonia. Thus, psychiatric symptoms and cognitive-emotional deficits are both correlates of the course and outcome of psychiatric illnesses and of the pathological processes in the nervous system. Presumably, these impairments are somewhat specific for each of the major mental disorders and vary with the severity of the underlying psychobiological vulnerability. The specificity of the impairments enables diagnosticians to categorize psychiatric disorders reliably (e.g., *DSM-III);* however, there is considerable overlap between disorders as evidenced by the presence of delusions and hallucinations in a variety of psychotic disorders (Pfohl and Andreasen 1986).

When functional limitations imposed by psychiatric *impairments* result in decrements in the ability to perform certain activities, the individual is said to have a *disability*. *Disabilities* are defined as inability or limitation to perform tasks expected of an individual within a social environment (Frey 1984). Among individuals with severe psychiatric disorders such as schizophrenia, *disabilities* include poor self-care skills (e.g., cooking, cleaning, grooming, and teeth care), social withdrawal and seclusiveness, abandonment of family responsibilities, and work incapacity. *DSM-III* (American Psychiatric Association 1980) has highlighted the importance of these disabilities by including them as criteria for many diagnosable psychiatric conditions. To be diagnosed as having schizophrenia, for example, it is not sufficient to experience the characteristic symptoms of thought disorder, delusions and hallucinations, but the person also must evince a "deterioration from a previous level of functioning in such areas as work, social relations, and self-care" (American Psychiatric Association, 1980, p. 189).

The *disabilities* shown by persons with psychiatric disorders are influenced by the same protective and risk factors that influence the appearance, exacerbation, and remission of symptoms or *impairments*. Thus, correlations between symptoms and disabilities would be expected; however, not every impairment results in a disability. Furthermore, similar patterns of disability can result from different disorders and impairments. Persons with mental retardation or affective disorders may have the same profile of disabilities as those with schizophrenia. Social and vocational disabilities form a major cluster of behaviors that both reflect and influence the course and outcome of a psychiatric disorder.

Research data substantiate a consistent relationship between a person's abilities and vocational outcome. For example, in every study in which work adjustment skills were assessed, they were found to be significantly related to future work performance (Anthony and Jansen 1984). Similar to these data on work adjustment skills, ratings of interpersonal or social skills have been found to predict vocational performance even though social functioning was measured differently in the various studies (Anthony, Cohen, and Cohen 1984).

A final element in the rehabilitation model is *handicap,* which occurs when *disabilities* place the individual at a disadvantage relative to others in society. This can occur through stigma and discrimination, as when employers are reluctant to hire persons with mental illnesses. Handicap also occurs because society does not provide settings where mentally ill persons can find accommodation and compensation for their *impairments* and *disabilities*.

Wheelchairs and ramps have enabled paraplegics to overcome their impairments and disabilities to find remunerative work and fulfilling recreation; hence, their handicaps are compensated. Because mentally ill persons require special *social environments* to compensate for their problems, overcoming handicap is much more difficult. Long-term institutional care in state and county mental hospitals was formerly society's method of dealing with the *impairments* and *disabilities* of psychiatric patients; unfortunately, institutionalization also created its own set of secondary disabilities and handicaps. That society has not yet succeeded in compensating for the impairments and disabilities of psychiatric patients is reflected in the extraordinarily high rates of unemployment and homelessness among this population (Anthony, Cohen, and Vitalo 1978; Farr and Koegel 1986).

Psychiatric Rehabilitation

The conceptual framework elucidated above, joined with the rehabilitation view of disability, provides a coherent set of strategies for rehabilitation interventions with the psychiatrically disabled. The clinical practice of psychiatric rehabilitation, just like its counterpart in physical rehabilitation, comprises two intervention strategies: (1) patient skill development and (2) environmental resource development. In developing these intervention techniques, psychiatric rehabilitation practice is guided by the basic philosophy of rehabilitation; that is, disabled persons need *skills* and *environmental supports* to fulfill the role demands of various living, learning, and working environments. The assumption of clinical rehabilitation is that if psychiatrically disabled persons' skills and/or the supports in their immediate environment are augmented, they will be more able to perform those activities necessary to function in specific roles of their choice. In other words, interventions designed to lessen or compensate for the disability are assumed to lead to a decrease in the handicap.

Interventions begin with a comprehensive medical-psychiatric diagnosis and a functional and resource assessment. This enables mental health and rehabilitation professionals to describe individuals by diagnostic disorder, level of behavioral functioning, and amount of environmental supports, key to identifying their impairments and disabilities. Identification of impairments and disabilities permits the mental health and rehabilitation practitioner to prioritize problems, formulate specific goals, and organize and implement treatment and rehabilitation plans. Medical-psychiatric diagnosis and a functional and resource assessment are necessary to match patients to drug and psychosocial treatments and rehabilitation programs that will be effective (Taylor, Liberman, and Agras 1982). Furthermore, knowing the patient's diagnosis aids the clinician in providing the patient and family members with a reasonable prognosis and in determining the degree to which environmental support vs. remedial skills training can be provided to overcome handicaps.

Reduction of Impairments. Rehabilitation interventions with psychiatric patients require reduction or elimination of the symptomatic and cognitive impairments that interfere with social and vocational performance. Interventions for reducing impairments are fortunately available from psychopharmacology. The past 20 years has seen major accomplishments in both treatment and prevention of morbidity from psychopathology through the use of antipsychotic, antidepressant, and anxiolytic drugs. Note that these psychotropic drugs are not panaceas. Even when taken regularly, they are frequently only able to reduce rather than abolish symptoms, and delay rather than prevent relapse. Psychotropic drugs are also associated with unpleasant side effects which at times can interfere with skills-training activities. However, they are usually helpful in reducing impairments to the point where psychosocial strategies can be used effectively to remediate disabilities and handicap.

While a patient's symptoms and syndromal diagnosis clearly impair social and vocational performance, as is highlighted by the mixed symptomatic and functional criteria in *DSM-III*, the remitting and exacerbating nature of most major mental disorders obscures the relationship between psychopathology at time A and behavioral functioning at time B. The changing character of the symptomatic impairments of psychiatric disorders with the passage of time accounts for the insubstantial correlations often found between psychopathology measured during an acute episode and future work performance (for a review, see Anthony and Jansen 1984).

The disappointing failure of research studies to find correlations between impairments and disabilities might be a result of their having been conducted in an era preceding the availability of objective and reliable instruments for eliciting and rating psychopathology. Research using the standardization in diagnosis brought about by *DSM-III* should yield studies that suggest a stronger relationship between syndromes and long-term outcome (Tsuang, Wooson, and Fleming 1979; Pfohl and Andreasen 1986).

Remediation of Disabilities Through Skills Training. Once a patient has benefited optimally from psychotropic drugs and the therapeutic effects of brief hospitalization, rehabilitation strategies use skills training to remediate disabilities in social, family, and vocational functioning. Skills training as a principal strategy in psychiatric rehabilitation starts from the assumption that many patients will suffer persisting disabilities despite the best efforts at pharmacotherapy and hospitalization. A relatively new field, training of social and vocational skills has relevance for a wide variety of psychiatric patients and for the professionals who serve them.

The psychiatric disorders with the greatest chronicity—schizophrenia, major depression, and organic syndromes—are those most in need of a skills-training focus. While appropriate drug treatment significantly reduces symptoms in most schizophrenics and depressives, many are refractory to drugs and others experience continuing social and vocational handicaps even with symptomatic improvement. The negative or deficit symptoms of schizophrenia, for example, pose a largely unanswered challenge to the pharmacopeia. Social withdrawal, apathy, energy, slovenliness, and anhedonia do not respond as well to neuroleptic drugs as do hallucinations, delusions, and thought disorder. Neither do drugs teach life and coping skills, except indirectly through removal or reduction of symptoms. Most schizophrenic persons need to learn or relearn social and personal skills for surviving in the community.

Skills training can begin immediately after the stabilization of an acute episode or exacerbation of a psychiatric disorder—which usually results in the loss of social and role functioning. The goals of rehabilitation professionals are to sustain symptomatic improvement over the long haul; establish or reestablish interpersonal and independent living skills; and help the individual reach a satisfactory quality of life.

Because the goals of rehabilitation center on adjustment to everyday life, it is vital for the schizophrenic individual to participate maximally in the choice of objectives, and in the learning process. Comprehensive rehabilitation involves assessment, training, and modification of living environments in those areas relevant to personal and community life—self care, including medication and symptom management; family relations; peer and friendship relations; avocational and employment pursuits; money management and consumerism; residential living; recreational activities; transportation; food preparation; and choice and use of public agencies. Specific goal setting, within these generic areas, should actively involve the patient, his or her family, and significant others.

Remediating Disabilities Through Supportive Interventions. When restoration of social and vocational functioning through skills training is limited by continuing deficits and refractory symptoms, rehabilitation strategies aim at helping the individual compensate for the disability by (1) locating living, learning, and working environments that can accommodate to the residual deficits and symptoms; and (2) adjusting the individual's and family's expectations to a level of functioning that is realistically attainable. Thus, environmental modification and supportive-prosthetic social and vocational environments are complementary approaches to skills training in the reconstitution of social roles for patients with severe and chronic psychiatric disorders.

Environmental interventions attempt to provide the patient with supportive persons, supportive settings, or both. A "support person" might reduce a person's disability and handicap through a number of different roles (e.g., advocate, companion, counselor, and advisor). Attempts at making the setting more supportive focus on the programs or resources within the environment rather than on support persons, per se (e.g., sheltered work and living settings, and special discharge programs). The distinction between supportive persons and supportive settings simply highlights the different ways in which environmental modifications occur. In practice, these modifications often occur simultaneously.

The main identifying feature of both types of supportive interventions, as distinguished from skill-development interventions, is that they do not attempt to change the patient's behavior systematically and directly. Rather, the attempt is simply to support and accommodate the patient's present level of functioning. The early studies by Katkin (1971, 1973) and a more recent study by Cannady (1982) have clearly demonstrated the positive impact on patient outcome of a support person. Cannady (1982) used citizens from the discharged patients' rural neighborhood to function as "supportive case workers." Over a 12-month period, inpatient days were decreased by as much as 92 percent.

Remediation of Handicap. In addition to clinical rehabilitation interventions of skill and support development, psychiatrically disabled persons can be helped to overcome their handicaps through societal rehabilitation interventions (Anthony 1972). Societal rehabilitation is designed to change the system in which psychiatrically disabled persons must function. Unlike clinical rehabilitation, its focus is neither on the skills of specific psychiatrically disabled individuals nor on their unique environments. Rather, the focus is on system changes that can help many psychiatrically disabled persons overcome their handicaps. Examples of this type of system intervention are the Targeted Job Tax Credit legislation, changes in the length of the trial work period in the Social Security Disability program, and the development of a European-type quota system for the employment of disabled workers. The importance of these system-type interventions cannot be overemphasized. Obstacles in overcoming a handicap may be more a function of a nonaccommodating and discriminating social and economic system than of the person's impairment and disability. Community support programs are another example of a system-wide response to the problems of persons who are severely psychiatrically disabled (Turner and TenHoor 1978).

Clinical and societal rehabilitation interventions are not mutually exclusive. As a matter of fact, the 1973 amendments to the Vocational Rehabilitation Act recognize the value of societal rehabilitation efforts. The amendments established the principle of affirmative action by contractors who do business with the Federal Government and also attempted to establish the Government as a model employer with respect to architectural access (Stubbins 1982).

Integrating Rehabilitation Strategies

In view of the pervasive impairments, disabilities, and handicaps of most persons with chronic mental disorders, a combined approach to psychiatric rehabilitation, employing skills training and environmental modification strategies, is most often required. As the following case vignette illustrates, the rehabilitation practitioner or team needs to integrate skills training, social support, and governmental incentives and regulations to bring about an optimal outcome.

> A 30-year-old male with a 15-year history of being in and out of private and state psychiatric hospitals decided he would like to get a job in the community after being in a psychosocial work adjustment program for 1 year. He did not have a good work history; for example, 6 months was the longest he had ever been able to hold a job. Using the targeted job tax credit legislation as an incentive to the employer, the psychiatric rehabilitation team was able to find the disabled person a job working in a video repair shop, a job consistent with the client's interests and talents. To keep his job at the repair shop, the patient needed to learn the skills of taking orders from authority figures (showing understanding of what others say and expressing his own thoughts and feelings to others). The team also made the environment more supportive to the patient by educating the employer to the patient's needs and obtained employer agreement on reducing the initial work load/time until the disabled person became comfortable with the new environment.

In general, all available interventions are used in combination—psychotropic medication; partial and full hospitalization; case management; skills training; social self-help clubs; and environmental support initiatives—to achieve the maximum degree of adaptation that is feasible. The emphasis on each of the types of intervention varies with the nature of the disorder, the premorbid level of competence of the patient, and the phase of illness.

Historically, mental health treatment has tried to develop interventions aimed at the patient's impairments. Somatic and psychological treatment efforts have attempted to alleviate the signs and symptoms of psychopathology. Leitner and Drasgow (1972), in analyzing the differences between treatment and rehabilitation, point out that treatment attempts are directed more toward minimizing sickness, whereas rehabilitation aims more toward maximizing health. Eliminating or suppressing impairments does not lead automatically to more functional behaviors. Likewise, a decrease in disability does not always lead to reductions in impairment. Note that a chronic or severe impairment (e.g., diabetes, schizophrenia, and stroke) does *not* always result in chronic disability or handicap. What the impairment does is increase the risk of chronic disability and handicap.

Conclusion

With an emerging consensus that major psychiatric disorders are stress-linked biomedical disorders, rehabilitation approaches have grown out of eclectic and empirical traditions emphasizing the development of patients' skills or supportive environments for coping with the enduring disabilities and handicaps of illnesses such as schizophrenia and affective disorders. Psychiatric rehabilitation uses assessment and intervention techniques based on such orientations as social learning and behavior therapy (Paul and Lentz 1977; Liberman and Foy 1983; Liberman and Evans 1985); client-centered therapy and human resource development (Rogers 1957; Carkhuff 1972, 1983; Carkhuff and Berenson 1976); and lifespan developmental psychology (Strauss and Carpenter 1981; Pepper 1985).

The psychiatrically disabled person must be involved as much as possible in setting rehabilitation goals—a process that necessitates the development of a trusting, mutually respectful, and empathic relationship with service providers. The preferred mode of intervention combines judicious and rational psychopharmacology with an educational approach that trains patients directly in the knowledge and skills they need to function in society. "Teaching as treatment" (Carkhuff and Berenson 1976) is supplemented by interventions at the level of the person's immediate environment, as well as at the community support system and societal level.

The rehabilitation process encompasses three overlapping stages that recur for as long as the patient requires professional services (Anthony, Cohen, and Cohen 1983). *Assessment* at the symptomatic, functional, and resource levels initiates the patient and professional in a collaborative *planning phase*. Through diagnostic and assessment interviews, inventories, informants, historical data, role plays, and direct behavioral observation, the assessment yields information about the psychiatrically disabled person's current deficits, psychopathology, skills, and supports, as well as the skill level demanded by the living, learning, or working environments in which the patient wishes to function. The assessment information enables the rehabilitation practitioner to work with the patient and family member in the *planning phase* to develop a rehabilitation plan that specifies how the person or the person's environment must change to achieve the goals of rehabilitation. With respect to changes in the person, the plan develops the skill steps the person needs to raise his or her level of functioning to the level required by the environment. With respect to changes in the person's environment, a sequential plan describes what and how the necessary coordination, advocacy, and modifications are to be made. The rehabilitation plan also identifies the persons (e.g., practitioner, patient, agency, and family member) responsible for implementing the various parts of the plan.

In the *intervention phase,* the rehabilitation plan is implemented to increase the person's skills and to make the environment more supportive of the person's functioning. These interventions can lead to the achievement of the rehabilitation goals, first identified during the assessment phase. Repeated and regular monitoring of the change process informs all concerned about goal attainment and enables clinical decisions to be made about continuation or change of interventions and goals.

Psychiatric rehabilitation is the recovery of social and instrumental role functioning to the fullest extent possible through learning procedures and environmental supports. When restoration of functioning is limited by continuing deficits and symptoms, rehabilitation efforts aim at helping the individual (1) acquire living, learning, and working environments that are compensatory; and (2) adjust to the level of functioning that is realistically attainable. Because of the limitations of currently available training methods, patients with more chronically disabling disorders, such as schizophrenia or organic brain disorders, may be unable to reestablish specific impaired or lost skills. In such cases, alternate compensatory skills and environments, such as learning to function in sheltered employment and residential settings, would be the focus of rehabilitative efforts.

Research conducted by a large number of investigators in the United States and Europe supports the following conclusions:

- Severely psychiatrically disabled persons can learn skills.
- The psychiatrically disabled person's skills are positively related to measures of rehabilitation outcome.
- Skill development interventions improve the psychiatrically disabled person's rehabilitation outcome.
- Environmental resource development improves the psychiatrically disabled person's rehabilitation outcome.

In our attempts to conceptualize psychiatric rehabilitation, the "key and lock" analogy might be apt. While it is desirable to maximize an individual's social and instrumental role functioning through training and reeducative procedures, persistent deficits are likely to plague the patient, the family, and the rehabilitation team. Endeavors to upgrade the patient's repertoire of skills hone the "key," but it is often necessary to modify the "lock"— the patient's environment. Recent interventions aimed at modification of the family environment have led to dramatic reductions in relapse, exacerbation, and rehospitalization of patients with schizophrenia (Strachan, this issue). Other examples of environmental prostheses are sheltered workshops, transitional employment, halfway houses, and psychosocial clubs.

Guiding the rehabilitation professional is:

- Optimism that desirable change is possible if principles of human learning can be harnessed to the needs of the patient.
- Belief that motivation for change can come from special arrangements of the patient's rehabilitation and natural environments, as well as from within the patient.
- Confidence that by building upon the patient's assets and interests, including supportive treatment and family environments, even small improvements can lead to significant functional changes and uplift the patient's quality of life.

The principles of rehabilitation have the potential to tie researchers and professionals engaged in psychiatric rehabilitation into a cohesive, empirically based field. Rehabilitation practice has taken root in a variety of settings, including mental health centers and clinics, mental hospitals, general hospitals, psychosocial centers, and community support programs. More than ever before, psychiatric rehabilitation is perceived as a legitimate and credible field of practice, education, and research; as complementary to the existing fields of prevention and treatment; and as a necessary component of mental health system planning and policy-making.

References

American Psychiatric Association. *DSM-III: Diagnostic and Statistical Manual of Mental Disorders.* 3rd ed. Washington, DC: The Association, 1980.

Anthony, W.A. Societal rehabilitation: Changing society's attitudes toward the physically and mentally disabled. *Rehabilitation Psychology,* 19:117–126, 1972.

Anthony, W.A. Psychological rehabilitation: A concept in need of a method. *American Psychologist,* 32:658–662, 1977.

Anthony, W.A. *Principles of Psychiatric Rehabilitation.* Baltimore: University Park Press, 1979.

Anthony, W.A. A rehabilitation model for rehabilitating the psychiatrically disabled. *Rehabilitation Counseling Bulletin,* 24:6–21, 1980.

Anthony, W.A. Explaining "psychiatric rehabilitation" by an analogy to "physical rehabilitation." *Psychosocial Rehabilitation Journal,* 5:61–65, 1982.

Anthony, W.A., and Buell, G.J. Predicting psychiatric rehabilitation outcome using demographic characteristics: A replication. *Journal of Counseling Psychology,* 21:421–422, 1974.

Anthony, W.A., Buell, G.J., Sharratt, S., and Althoff, M.E. Efficacy of psychiatric rehabilitation. *Psychological Bulletin,* 78:447–456, 1972.

Anthony, W.A., Cohen, M., and Cohen, B. The philosophy, treatment process and principles of the psychiatric rehabilitation approach. *New Directions in Mental Health,* 17:67–79, 1983.

Anthony, W.A., Cohen, M.R., and Cohen, B. Psychiatric rehabilitation. In: Talbott, J., ed. *The Chronic Mental Patient: Five Years Later.* New York: Grune & Stratton, 1984. pp. 213–252.

Anthony, W.A., Cohen, M.R., and Vitalo, R. The measurement of rehabilitation outcome. *Schizophrenia Bulletin,* 4:365–383, 1978.

Anthony, W.A., Howell, J., and Danley, K. The vocational rehabilitation of the psychiatrically disabled. In: Mirabi, M., ed. *The Chronically Mentally Ill: Research and Services.* New York: SP Medical & Scientific Books, 1984. pp. 215–237.

Anthony, W.A., and Jansen, M. Predicting the vocational capacity of the chronically mentally ill: Research and policy implications. *American Psychologist,* 39:537–544, 1984.

Anthony, W.A., and Margules, A. Toward improving the efficacy of psychiatric rehabilitation: A skills training approach. *Rehabilitation Psychology,* 21:101–105, 1974.

Backer, T.E., Liberman, R.P., and Kuehnel, T.G. Dissemination and adoption of innovative psychosocial interventions. *Journal of Consulting & Clinical Psychology,* 54:111–118, 1986.

Ballantyne, R. Community rehabilitation services: A new approach to aftercare. *Network,* 3:4–6, 1983.

Beard, J.H., Propst, R.N., and Malamud, T.J. The Fountain House model of psychiatric rehabilitation. *Psychosocial Rehabilitation Journal,* 5:47–59, 1982.

Bennett, D.H. The historical development of rehabilitation services. In: Watts, F.N., and Bennett, D.H., eds. *Theory and Practice of Psychiatric Rehabilitation.* New York: John Wiley & Sons, Inc., 1983. pp. 15–42.

Bockoven, J.S. *Moral Treatment in American Psychiatry.* New York: Springer, 1963.

Braun, P., Kochansky, G., Shapiro, R., Greenberg, S., Gudeman, J.E., Johnson, S., and Shore, M.F. Overview: Deinstitutionalization of psychiatric patients. *American Journal of Psychiatry,* 131:736–749, 1981.

Buell, G.J., and Anthony, W.A. The relationship between patient demographic characteristics and psychiatric rehabilitation outcome. *Community Mental Health Journal,* 11:208–214, 1976.

Cannady, D. Chronics and cleaning ladies. *Psychosocial Rehabilitation Journal* 5:13–16, 1982.

Carkhuff, R.R. New directions in training for helping professionals: Towards a technology for human and community resource development. *The Counseling Psychologist,* 3:12–20, 1972.

Carkhuff, R.R. *Interpersonal Skills and Human Productivity.* Amherst, MA: Human Resource Development Press, 1983.

Carkhuff, R.R., and Berenson, B.C. *Teaching as Treatment.* Amherst, MA: Human Resource Development Press, 1976.

Carstairs, G.M.; O'Connor, N.; and Rawnsley, K. *Organization of a hospital workshop for chronic psychotic patients.* British Journal of Preventive and Social Medicine, 10:136–140

Cohen, M.R., Danley, K., and Nemec, P. *Psychiatric rehabilitation trainer packages: Direct skills teaching.* Center for Psychiatric Rehabilitation, Boston University, Boston, MA, 1986.

Cohen, B.F., Ridley, D., and Cohen, M.R. Teaching skills to severely psychiatrically disabled persons. In: Marlowe, H.A., ed. *Developing Competence.* Tampa, FL: University of South Florida Press, 1983. pp. 96–115.

Dincin, J. A community agency model. In: Talbot, J.A., ed. *The Chronic Mentally Ill.* New York: Human Sciences Press, 1981. pp. 212–226.

Eisenberg, M.G., and Cole, H.W. A behavioral approach to job seeking for psychiatrically impaired persons. *Journal of Rehabilitation,* April/May/June, 46–49, 1986.

Falloon, I., Boyd, J., and McGill, C. *Family Care of Schizophrenia.* New York: Guilford Press, 1984.

Falloon, I.R.H., Doane, J.A., and Pederson, J. Family versus individual management in prevention of morbidity of schizophrenia: III. Family functioning. *Archives of General Psychiatry,* 42:887–896, 1985.

Farkas, M., Cohen, M.R., and Nemec, P. *Psychiatric Rehabilitation Programs: Putting Concepts Into Practice?* Center for Psychiatric Rehabilitation, Boston University, Boston, MA, 1986.

Farkas, M., Rogers, S., and Thurer, S. *Rehabilitation Outcome for the Recently* Deinstitutionalized *Client: The Ones We Left Behind.* Center for Psychiatric Rehabilitation, Boston University, Boston, MA, 1986.

Farr, R.K., and Koegel, P. *A Study of Homelessness and Mental Illness in the Skid Row Area of Los Angeles.* Project Report available from Los Angeles Dept. of Mental Health, 2415 W. 6th Street, Los Angeles, CA 90057, March 1986.

Foy, D.W., Wallace, C.J., and Liberman, R.P. Advances in social skills training for chronic mental patients. In: Craig, K.D., and McMahon, R.J., eds. *Advances in Clinical Behavior Therapy.* New York: Brunner/Mazel, 1983. pp. 153–172.

Frey, W.D. Functional assessment in the 80's: A conceptual enigma, a technical challenge. In: Halpern, A., and Fuhrer, M., eds. *Functional Assessment in Rehabilitation.* New York: Brooke Publishing Co., 1984. pp. 11–43.

Goldstrom, I., and Manderscheid, R. The chronically mentally ill: A descriptive analysis from the uniform client data instrument. *Community Support Services Journal,* 2:4–9, 1982.

Grob, S. Psychosocial rehabilitation centers: Old wine in a new bottle. In: Barofsky, I., and Budson, R., eds. *The Chronic Psychiatric Patient in the Community.* Jamaica, NY: SP Medical and Scientific Books, 1983. pp. 265–280.

Harding, CM., and Brooks, G.W. Life assessment of a cohort of chronic schizophrenics discharged 20 years ago. In: Mednick, I.S., Harway, S.M., and Finello, K., eds. *The Handbook of Longitudinal Research.* New York: Praeger Press, 1984. pp. 375–393.

Harrow, M., Grinker, R.R., Silverstein, M.L., and Holzman, P. Is modern-day schizophrenic outcome still negative? *American Journal of Psychiatry,* 135:1156–1162, 1978.

Hawkins, H. A plea for convalescent homes in connection with asylums for the insane poor. *Journal of Mental Science,* 17:107–116, 1871.

Hirschfeld, R.M.A., Klerman, G.L., Clayton, P.J., Keller, M., McDonald-Scott, P., and Larkin, B. Assessing personality: Effects of the depressive state on trait measurement. *American Journal of Psychiatry,* 140:695–699, 1983.

Jacobs, H.E., Kardashian, S., Kreinbring, R.K., Ponder, R., and Simpson, A.R. A skills-oriented model for facilitating employment among psychiatrically disabled persons. *Rehabilitation Counseling Bulletin,* 28:87–96, 1984.

Katkin, S., Ginsburg, M., Rifkin, J.J., and Scott, J.T. Effectiveness of female volunteers in the treatment of outpatients. *Journal of Counseling Psychology,* 18:97–100, 1971.

Katkin, S., Zimmerman, U., Rosenthal, T., and Ginsburg, M. Using volunteer therapists to reduce hospital readmissions. *Hospital & Community Psychiatry,* 26:151–153, 1975.

Kelly, J.A., and Lampariski, D.M. Outpatient treatment of schizophrenics: Social skills and problem-solving training. In: Hessen, M., and Bellack, A.S., eds. *Handbook of Clinical Behavior Therapy With Adults.* New York: Plenum Press, 1985. pp. 485–508.

Lamb, H.R. *Treating the Long-term Mentally Ill.* San Francisco: Jossey-Bass, 1982.

Leff, J.P., Hirsch, S.R., Gaind, R., Rhode, P.D., and Stevens, B.C. Life events and maintenance therapy in schizophrenic relapse. *British Journal of Psychiatry,* 123:659–668, 1973.

Leitner, L., and Drasgow, J. Battling recidivism. *Journal of Rehabilitation,* July-August, 29–31, 1972.

Liberman, R.P. Social factors in schizophrenia. In: Grinspoon, L., ed. *The American Psychiatric Association Annual Review.* Washington, DC: American Psychiatric Press, 1982a. pp. 97–111.

Liberman, R.P. What is schizophrenia? *Schizophrenia Bulletin,* 8:435–437, 1982b.

Liberman, R.P. Psychosocial therapies for schizophrenia. In: Kaplan, H.I., and Sadock, B.J., eds. *Comprehensive Textbook of Psychiatry.* 4th ed. Baltimore: Williams and Wilkins, 1984. pp. 724–734.

Liberman, R.P., and Evans, C.C. Behavioral rehabilitation for chronic mental patients. *Journal of Clinical Psychopharmacology,* 5:8S–14S, 1985.

Liberman, R.P., Falloon, I.R.H., and Wallace, C.J. Drug-psychosocial interventions in the treatment of schizophrenia. In: Mirabi, M., ed. *The Chronically Mentally Ill: Research and Services.* New York: SP Medical & Scientific Books, 1984. pp. 175–212.

Liberman, R.P., and Foy, D.W. Psychiatric rehabilitation for chronic mental patients. *Psychiatric Annals,* 13:539–545, 1983.

Liberman, R.P., King, L.W., and DeRisi, WJ. Behavior analysis and therapy in community mental health. In: Leitenberg, H., ed. *Handbook of Behavior Analysis and Modification.* Englewood Cliffs, NJ: Prentice Hall, 1976. pp. 566–603.

Liberman, R.P., King, L.W., DeRisi, W.J., and McCann, M. *Personal Effectiveness: Guiding People to Assert Themselves and Improve Their Social Skills.* Champaign, IL: Research Press, 1975.

Liberman, R.P., Massell, H.K., Mosk, M., and Wong, S.E. Social skills training for chronic mental patients. *Hospital & Community Psychiatry,* 36:396–403, 1985.

Linn, M.W., Klett, C.J., and Caffey, E.M. Foster home characteristics and psychiatric patient outcome. *Archives of General Psychiatry,* 41:157–161, 1980.

Livneh, H. Psychiatric rehabilitation: A dialogue with Bill Anthony. *Journal of Counseling and Development,* 63:86–90, 1984.

Medication Management Module. *A Skills Training Program to Teach Patients Reliable Use of Neuroleptic Drugs.* Available from the UCLA Research Center, Box A, Camarillo, CA 93011, 1986.

Monti, P.M., Corriveau, D.P., and Curran, J.P. Social skills training for psychiatric patients: Treatment and outcome. In: Curran, J.P., and Monti, P.M., eds. *Social Skills Training: A Practical Handbook for Assessment and Treatment.* New York: Guilford Press, 1982. pp. 185–223.

Monti, P.M., Fink, E., Norman, W., Curran, J.P., Hayes, S., and Caldwell, A. The effect of social skills training groups and social skills bibliotherapy with psychiatric patients. *Journal of Consulting and Clinical Psychology,* 47:189–191, 1979.

Nelson, G.L., and Cone, J.D. Multiple baseline analysis of token economy for psychiatric inpatients. *Journal of Applied Behavior Analysis,* 12:255–271, 1979.

Nuechterlein, K., and Dawson, M. A heuristic vulnerability/stress model of schizophrenic episodes. *Schizophrenia Bulletin,* 10:300–312, 1984.

O'Connor, R.N., and Tizard, J. *The Social Problems of Mental Deficiency.* London: Pergamon Press, 1956.

Paul, G.L., and Lentz, R. *Psychosocial Treatment of Chronic Mental Patients.* Cambridge, MA: Harvard University Press, 1977.

Pepper, B. The young adult chronic patient: Population overview. *Journal of Clinical Psychopharmacology,* 5:5S–8S, 1985.

Pfohl, B., and Andreasen, N.C. Schizophrenia: Diagnosis and classification. In: Frances, A.J., and Hales, R.F., eds. *Psychiatry Update: The American Psychiatric Association Annual Review.* Vol. 5. Washington, DC: American Psychiatric Press, 1986. pp. 7–24.

Presly, A.J., Grubb, A.B., and Semple, D. Predictors of successful rehabilitation in long stay patients. *Acta Psychiatrica Scandinavica,* 66:83–88, 1982.

Rogers, C.R. The necessary and sufficient conditions of therapeutic personality change. *Journal of Consulting and Clinical Psychology,* 21:95–103, 1957.

Royal Commission on the Law *Relating to Mental Illness and Mental Deficiency 1954–1957.* London: Her Majesty's Stationery Office, 1957.

Stein, L.I., and Test, M.A. *Alternatives to Mental Hospital Treatment.* New York: Plenum Press, 1978.

Stickney, S.K., Hall, R.L., and Gardner, E.R. The effect of referral procedures on aftercare compliance. *Hospital & Community Psychiatry,* 31:567–569, 1980.

Stockdill, J. *Definition of Psychosocial Rehabilitation.* Technical Assistance Transmittal No. 1—NIMH Office of State & Community Liaison to State Mental Health Directors. Rockville, MD: National Institute of Mental Health, 1985.

Strauss, J.S., and Carpenter, W.T., Jr. *Schizophrenia.* New York: Plenum Press, 1981.

Stubbins, J. *The Clinical Attitude in Rehabilitation: A Cross-Cultural View.* World Rehabilitation Fund Monograph #16. New York: World Rehabilitation Fund, 1982.

Sylph, J.A., Ross, H.E., and Kedward, H.B. Social disability in chronic psychiatric patients. *American Journal of Psychiatry,* 134:1391–1394, 1977.

Taylor, C.B., Liberman, R.P., and Agras, W.S. Treatment evaluation and behavior therapy. In: Lewis, J., and Usdin, G., eds, *Treatment Planning in Psychiatry.* Washington, DC: American Psychiatric Press, 1982. pp. 151–224.

Tsuang, M.T., Woolson, R.F., and Fleming, J.A. Long term outcome of major psychoses. *Archives of General Psychiatry,* 36:1295–1301, 1979.

Turner, J., and TenHoor, W. The NIMH Community Support Program: Pilot approach to a needed social reform. *Schizophrenia Bulletin,* 4:319–348, 1978.

Vaughn, C.E., and Leff, J.P. The influences of family and social factors on the course of psychiatric illness. *British Journal of Psychiatry,* 129:125–137, 1976a.

Vaughn, C.E., and Leff, J.P. The measurement of expressed emotion in the families of psychiatric patients. *British Journal of Social and Clinical Psychology,* 15:157–165, 1976b.

Vaughn, C.E., Snyder, K.S., Freeman, W.E., Jones, S., Falloon, I.R.H., and Liberman, R.P. Family factors in schizophrenic relapse: A replication. *Schizophrenia Bulletin,* 8:425–426, 1982.

Wallace, C.J., and Liberman, R.P. Social skills training for patients with schizophrenia: A controlled clinical trial. *Psychiatry Research,* 15:239–247, 1985.

Wallace, C.J., Nelson, C.J., Liberman, R.P., Aitchinson, R.H., Lukoff, D., Elder, J.P., and Ferris, C. A review and critique of social skills training with schizophrenic patients. *Schizophrenia Bulletin,* 6:42–63, 1980.

Wasylenski, D.A., Goering, P.N., Lancee, W.J., Ballantyne, R., and Farkas, M. Impact of a case manager program on psychiatric aftercare. *Journal of Nervous Mental Disease,* 173:303–308, 1985.

Weinberger, D.R., and Kleinman, J.E. Observations on the brain in schizophrenia. In: Frances, A.J., and Hales, R.E., eds. *Psychiatry Update: The American Psychiatric Association Annual Review.* Washington, DC: American Psychiatric Press, 1986. pp. 42–67.

Weinman, B., and Kleiner, R.J. The impact of community living and community member intervention on the adjustment of the chronic psychiatric patient. In: Stein, L.I., and Test, M.A., eds. *Alternatives to Mental Hospital Treatment.* New York: Plenum Press, Inc., 1978. pp. 139–159.

Witheridge, T.F., Dincin, J., and Appleby, L. Working with the most frequent recidivists: A total team approach to assertive resource management. *Psychosocial Rehabilitation Journal,* 5:9–11, 1982.

Wood, P.H.N. Appreciating the consequences of disease—The classification of impairments, disability, and handicaps. *The WHO Chronicle,* 34:376–380, 1980.

25

Scheper-Hughes, N., and Lovell, A. M. (1986). Breaking the circuit of social control: Lessons in public psychiatry from Italy and Franco Basaglia. *Social Science and Medicine, 23* (2), 159–178

Our readers may wonder why the longest article in a volume devoted to 50-plus years of community psychiatry in the United States concerns a mental health movement in Italy. The influence of this movement has, arguably, been limited mainly to ultraliberal and radical reformers in research, academic, and consumer circles in the United States. In addition, the article also goes into detail on the influence of German phenomenology, Marx, and the French Resistance on a psychiatrist-politician who produced little clinically informed work on community mental health care. Perhaps the best answer to these rhetorical questions is that the work of Franco Basaglia and his colleagues on mental health reform at disciplinary, institutional, and political levels in Italy during the 1960s and 1970s embodies a dramatic challenge to the U.S. approach to deinstitutionalization and community mental health. Or perhaps an even better answer is to pose another set of questions that suggest a way to pry open Scheper-Hughes and Lovell's rich account of mental health reform outside the United States: "What is 'democratic psychiatry' [the name of an organization Basaglia founded and a term that Scheper-Hughes and Lovell use in this article]? Does it make sense to combine a political term and the name of a medical discipline? Are they not separate domains?" Whatever the reader's answers to these questions, the historical, social, and political contexts of its setting must, in part, qualify the potential lessons that the Italian experience has for the United States. But only in part.

Breaking the Circuit of Social Control: Lessons in Public Psychiatry from Italy and Franco Basaglia

Abstract—Much public discourse in the United States and in Canada acknowledges the dismal failure of the policy to "deinstitutionalize" mental patients and to return them to some semblance of community living. The American Psychiatric Association has recently called for a reassessment of institutional alternatives—a call for a return to the asylum—in response to the needs of the new population of so-called homeless mentally ill. Here we contrast the failures of North American deinstitutionalization with the relative successes achieved in those regions of Italy where deinstitutionalization was grounded in a grassroots alternative psychiatry movement and professional and political coalition, *Psichiatria Democratica*. Democratic psychiatry challenged both the medical and the legal justifications for the segregative control of the "mentally ill": madness as disease, and the constant over-prediction of the dangerousness of the mental patient. In addition, the movement challenged traditional cultural stereotypes about the meanings of madness, and was successful in gaining broad-based community support from political parties, labor unions, student groups, and artist collectives that were enlisted in the task of reintegrating the ex-mental patient. The Italian experiment, although flawed and riddled with its own inconsistencies and contradictions, offers evidence that deinstitutionalization can work without recreating in the community setting the same exclusionary logic that was the foundation of the asylum system.

Key words—deinstitutionalization, community psychiatry, madness, social control

A plague upon you if you are deceiving us, and if among these madmen you are hiding enemies of the people [1].

With these harsh words the president of the Paris Commune rejected Philippe Pinel's proposal to free the 'lunatics' of Bicétre asylum during the aftermath of the French Revolution. Central to the revolutionary fervor of 1789 was the attack upon the old penal institutions of violence and confinement that symbolized the tyranny of the *ancien regime*. Even the famed l'Hôpital Général in Paris came to be viewed as a less than benevolent institution, as a kind of prison for the containment and correction of sick paupers, a means of controlling dissent while, simultaneously, aiding the production of clinical knowledge [2]. Hence, during this period, legislation was proposed to extend home-based medical care and treatment to the sick-poor, freeing these unfortunates from their dread of public hospitalization. But the revolutionary spirit of the times came crashing down, finally, with respect to the treatment of the mad. Even the progressives of the Paris Commune were not quite prepared to extend the revolutionary intent to madmen and lunatics, perceived as a class "who cause[d] horrible suffering to humanity" [3]. Instead, under the revolution, and later continuing under the Empire, the old institutions of punishment and confinement were gradually reopened and used for the internment of the mad, and for the mad alone, one social group totally abandoned by the revolutionary philanthropy of the times.

Consequently, the proposals of Pinel (1745–1826) in France and of Chiarugi (1759–1820) in Italy [4] that had originally attacked the very idea of institutional segregation of the insane, were recast as the more palatable proposals to reform and humanize those same institutions. This meant, in both instances, a movement to unchain mental patients within the walls of the institutions that continued to exclude and confine them. In place of torture and punishment a new regime of 'moralizing sadism' [3, p. 197] transformed the mental asylum into a new kind of court of law in which the madman was continually judged guilty of the crime of Unreason. The reforms of Pinel and Chiarugi, by leaving intact the whole psychiatric institutional apparatus, allowed the old contradictions between *madness* and *badness,* and between *custody* and *treatment* to be reproduced, and allowed the question of the humane treatment of mental patients to depend, precariously, on the temperament and treatment philosophy of the individual superintendent of each institution.

With the incipient psychiatric revolution of the late 18th and early 19th centuries aborted, for the next 150 years mental health reformers would continue to propose changes in the institutional treatment of lunatics, the insane, mental defectives, psychopaths, psychotics, the chronically mentally ill, etc. as each new generation of professionals would redefine them according to their treatment programs and agenda. Moral treatment, vocational rehabilitation, behavior modification, psychosurgery, therapeutic community, milieux therapy, institutional analysis, psychosocial treatment, etc. each represented a new gambit in the continuing search to legitimate the involuntary commitment of the psychologically different or distraught.

The more radical proposal to transform psychiatry outside the walls of the institution as part of a larger social movement to transform society as a whole waited to be taken up in Italy, once again on the forefront of psychiatric reform, in the early 1960s. The protagonist this time was Franco Basaglia, a brilliant, young Venetian psychiatrist who had assumed the directorship of an old, traditional asylum *(manicomio)* on the Italian-Yugoslav border. Basaglia, like many reformers before him, was revolted by what he observed as the traditional regime of institutional 'care': keys and locked doors only partially successful in muffling the screams and weeping of the patients, many of them lying naked and helpless in their own excreta. And he observed, with repugnance, the institutional response to human suffering: strait jackets, physical abuse, bed ties, ice packs, ECT and insulin-coma shock therapies to 'soothe' the terrified and the melancholy, and to strike terror in the difficult and the agitated.

A patient at Gorizia described the conditions there in the years before Basaglia arrived as follows, but he might have been describing almost any one of the provincial (public) hospitals in Italy at the time [5]:

> Those who were here prayed to be the next to die. Each time the bells tolled each one would say, "God, if only they tolled for me. I am so tired of this life in here". How many died who could have been alive and healthy! But humiliated and deprived of their humanity they refused to eat. Then the food would be forced down their nose with a tube. There was nothing else to do, locked up inside here with no hope of getting free. We were like scorched plants with leaves withered from drought.

The first time he entered the mental hospital, Basaglia later recalled, he was struck by a terrible odor—an odor redolent of death and defecation. It was not unlike the fetid odor of the prison cell where he had experienced his first institutional encounter when, as a medical student active in the Italian resistance, he was arrested and held prisoner under the German occupation. This formative experience provided Basaglia with the materials for his evocative equation of asylum, prison and concentration camp, as well as with a single-minded passion to *negate,* to destroy once and for all, the institution itself. Hence, his subsequent transformation and negation of the asylum at Gorizia shared intellectual roots, stemming from the Second World War, with the Saint Alban group in France that had provided health care for their companions in the French Resistance, while continuing to practice psychiatry. Under the leadership of Francois Tosquelles, a psychiatrist and a hero of the Spanish Civil War, the group went on to humanize the mental hospital by uniting insights from Marx and Freudian psychoanalysis. The Saint Alban experience culminated in a movement known as French Institutional Psychotherapy, which interpreted the dynamics of the mental hospital as the manifestations of a kind of collective unconscious, but which also took into account the social origins of psychological suffering. Institutional psychotherapy became the dominant alternative psychiatry in France, but it fell short in its ability to draw connections between the sources of oppression *inside* and *outside* the asylum, a task that Basaglia and his co-workers in Italy would accomplish later. Nor did institutional psychotherapy either challenge or change the fact of the mental hospital and its controlling functions. Nonetheless, several off-shoots and variants of institutional psychotherapy evolved, each with a distinct ideological commitment, among these Lourau's 'institutional analysis' and Mandel's 'socio-psychoanalysis'. Likewise, Franz Fanon, Felix Guattari and M. Mannoni had each, at some point in their careers, been affiliated with the institutional psychotherapy movement, and Basaglia often acknowledged the affinity of some of his proposals with ideas generated by these radicals and reformers of psychiatry. Franz Fanon, in particular, who like Basaglia, was a psychiatrist influenced by Sartre and existentialism, was one who also made the connections between oppression within the asylum and oppression outside [6]. Although disfavorable political circumstances forced Fanon out of favor before he could accomplish as much in the area of psychiatric reform as did Basaglia, Fanon's thought and evolving praxis went through many of the same stages.

Basaglia's intellectual roots also include an early commitment to German phenomenology. When Basaglia first assumed the directorship at Gorizia in 1961, he brought with him 13 years of experience as a research scientist at the neuropsychiatric clinic at the University of Padua. At that time existential phenomenology offered the only real alternative to the organicist schools that then dominated Italian psychiatry. Psychoanalysis, which also questioned the way in which biological psychiatry objectified the individual, did not really surface as a significant intellectual tradition in Italy until the 1970s. Basaglia then, became one of a score of younger Italian psychiatrists who embraced phenomenology, strongly influenced by the writings of Eugene Minowski, Ludwig Binswager and Erwin Strauss. The phenomenologist psychiatrists, reacting against the vast dehumanization wrought by the Second World War, sought to understand individuals through an appreciation of the diverse possibilities of their existence. This necessarily precluded enclosing individual patients within any system of fixed psychiatric categories.

Essential to Basaglia's analysis of psychiatric situations was Husserl's concept of 'bracketing': the suspension of judgements in the first encounter with the reality of the immediately given. It was Basaglia's 'bracketing' of mental illness as medical disease that provided ammunition to the critics who for many years falsely accused Basaglia of denying the existence of mental illness. Basaglia meant only to imply that we could not know what was the reality of the illness until we could first strip away the many layers created by poverty, stigma, segregation, confinement that covered and concealed it. He made this point very clearly in an interview:

> It is not that we put illness aside, but rather that we believe in order to have a relationship with an individual it is necessary to establish it independent of the label by which the patient has been defined. I have a relationship with someone not because of the diagnosis he or she carries but for what he or she is. So, in the moment in which I say: this individual is a *schizophrenic* (with all that is implied, for social reasons, by this term) I behave toward her in a very unique way, knowing full well that schizophrenia, as we know it, is an illness for which nothing can be done. My relationship will be that of someone who expects only 'schizophrenicity' from the person. Now we can see how, on this basis, the old psychiatry had discarded, imprisoned, and excluded this ill person for whom it is believed there was no recourse, no tools for treatment. This is why it is so very necessary to draw closer to her, bracketing the illness, because the diagnostic label has taken on the weight of a moral judgement that passes for the reality of the illness itself [5, pp. 32–33].

In his day-to-day work at Gorizia, bracketing meant paying little attention to 'the diagnosis', and listening closely to what the patient had to say. Suspending the most general labels—psychotic, alcoholic, depressive- was difficult, for the trained clinician was then left without any other language. It was noted that often it was only the lay persons—the *'voluntari'* who later came to the hospital from the outside—who (innocent of psychiatric jargon and terminology) were able to break from the traditional and stagnating way of relating to patients. Basaglia's suspension of psychiatric knowledge also implied leaving behind the batteries of psychological tests, the mental status exam, diagnostic and statistical manuals in order that he and those who worked with him could see the patient in a new, evolving manner.

At Gorizia as elsewhere, Basaglia would always search to restore a subjectivity to patients, not only in individual therapy, not only in his writings, but through praxis—the collective effort to change, to verify the new ideas that emerged. But it was at Gorizia, too, that Basaglia came to realize the limitations of phenomenology, especially its inability to cast light on the class dimensions of psychiatric illness and the larger social and political forces that shaped its modes of expression. "Like psychoanalysis", Basaglia wrote in 1967,

> [Phenomenology] has yet to modify the nature of the relationship with the object of its inquiry. It keeps [the person who is ill] at a distance, in the same objective and a-dialectical dimension to which classical psychiatry has already relegated it. Both theories have penetrated institutional practices only very marginally [7].

Once he began turning away from phenomenology, Basaglia's emerging praxis was most influenced by the Italian Marxists who were developing a language to describe the changes and the emergence of a new social consciousness brought about by the 'Hot Autumn' of 1969 [8]. During this period the writings of Antonio Gramsci were rediscovered, and the concepts of hegemony, the role of the bourgeois intellectual and the development of critical consciousness were applied to the current context—in Basaglia's case, they were applied to a relentless criticism of the psychiatric institution, its logic and its professional and patient roles.

In this way Basaglia was able to confront, finally, the ultimate reality of the *manicomio* that would hereafter transform the nature of his psychiatric practice. This was the realization that the *manicomio* was not a hospital at all, but a prison:

> There are the doctors, white gowns, orderlies and nurses, just as in a general hospital, but in reality a psychiatric hospital is a custodial institution where medical ideology is an alibi for the legalization of violence [9].

At the heart of institutional psychiatry, then, was a lie, a gross deception: the institution existed not to answer the real physical, social and psychological needs of the patients, but rather to serve its own needs and those of the social order whose interests it represented. If the hospital was, in reality, a prison, and the hospital workers were prison guards, then reasoned Basaglia, there must have been a crime. But what crime had these unfortunate inmates committed? Unlike ordinary criminals, he concluded, psychiatric inmates were confined not for what they had *actually* done, but rather for the 'phantom' of what it was they *might* do, for what was presumed *could* happen. Institutional psychiatry was justified, in the final analysis, by the constant over-prediction of the dangerousness of the common mental patient, recruited from the marginalized, asocial and potentially unruly Italian underclass. This anxiety was clearly articulated in the existing mental health legislation (see below). In addition to the problem of potential dangerousness there were also the frequent violations of probity associated with the underclass—the public disgrace and scandals occasioned by the 'disorderly conduct' of the impoverished and working class 'mentally ill'. Here lies the core of Basaglia's class analysis of psychiatry. Basaglia recognized that psychiatric diagnoses were not independent of the prevailing moral and social order which tended to define normality and abnormality in its own class-based terms. There was, of course, the observation that the Italian public institutions—mental hospitals, orphanages, and reform schools—were crowded with the poorest and most marginalized classes of Italian society. Many of the inmates were aggressive adolescents and unemployed young men; many were women who deviated from the rigid gender norms of Italian society, the demands imposed by lower class marriage and family life. The presumed and intuited 'dangerousness' of these inmates could be linked to their ambivalent relations to societal norms, especially those related to conventional productivity and reproductivity. We could interpret their 'passive refusal' to participate in the commonsense but highly exploitative terms of productive and reproductive labor as a wildcat strike, thus explaining the need to remove them (forcibly if necessary), lest the strike spread to the rest of society.

Psychiatry, then, provided an ideology to cover over the layers of contradiction underlying the medical rationale for institutionalized violence against the classes of alienated poor found in the back wards of most public mental institutions. Basaglia concluded:

> Once the medical pretenses are gone, we can see the misery and the poverty that are the true nature of the asylum. The specificity of madness is also gone. The deception is obvious: it is one thing to say that an institution locks up fifty 'sick' people. It is quite another to say that fifty 'poor' people have been locked up because there is no other solution to their problems [10].

If institutional psychiatry was a lie and a whitewash for what was, in reality, a covert apparatus of brutal social control, then asylum psychiatrists were the original masters of deceit, or in Basaglian terms, 'special agents of public consensus', masquerading as men and women of science, and as caring and compassionate physicians. Institutional psychiatrists acted in the capacity of traditional bourgeois intellectuals, as defined by Gramsci, to swallow and ruminate any new type of thought, including even the most indigestible ideologies, in order to preserve the hegemony of the dominant social classes, whose interests they are paid to protect and to represent. Above all, it was the function of the psychiatric technicians to deny, to fail to see the reality of human needs expressed through psychiatric symptoms, especially the poverty and the exclusion of the mental patient both inside and outside the asylum. For Basaglia the psychiatric technicians diagnosed, with greater and greater precision and specificity, thus fragmenting the problem of 'mental illness' into a multitude of diseases so as to avoid confronting its *wholeness*, its unifying dimensions as a shared experience of alienated human needs.

Consequently, psychiatric knowledge is used, perversely, against the mental patient. Basaglia opens his essay, 'Institutions of Violence' with the evocative image of mental patients herded together into large day rooms where they are not able to leave, even to use the toilet [11]. If the patient soils herself, she is chastized for 'acting out' against the staff, or 'incontinence' (a symptom of regression) is written in on the patient's chart. The inhuman regulations of the institution produce signs and symptoms that justify locking up the inmate. Here deception is further confounded with self-deception, as one imagines the defenses necessary to maintain the legitimacy of this virulent and destructive social order. In the same piece Basaglia notes that hospital orderlies sometimes take advantage of the passivity and immobility of so-called catatonic schizophrenics by assigning two to a bed when the wards are overcrowded. The transformation of *patient* into *object* is almost literal, as in the note left by a ward nurse when she went off duty for the evening: "Before leaving all *locks* and *patients* were checked". In recounting this incident, anecdotal though it is, Basaglia captures the dehumanizing nature of asylum logic. Basaglia's critique goes far beyond what now pales by comparison as a limited and almost benign analysis of 'total institutions' (and of patients' methods of 'working the system') in Erwin Goffman's *ASYLUMS,* published in 1961, the year that Basaglia took over the institution at Gorizia. But how to proceed? What to do next? How to transform psychiatry as part of a larger program of transforming the society that produced both psychiatrists and mental patients?

The Theory and Practice of Democratic Psychiatry

The corpus of Basaglia's writings, collected in two volumes published after his death and running to more than a thousand pages [12], is of a theoretical, sometimes philosophical, often rhetorical nature, with only tantalizing and passing references to his own revolutionizing practice in the asylums of Gorizia, Parma and Trieste, and in the region of Rome. The history of his work and that of his followers in the Democratic Psychiatry Movement *(Psichiatria Democratica),* the powerful force behind Italy's radical deinstitutionalization movement and its sweeping and innovative mental health reform of 1978 (Law 180), must be reconstructed from the numerous Italian books and articles that capture the debates and controversies, and from newspaper clippings and journalistic writings [13].

As an individual Basaglia was charismatic, direct and uncondescending, explaining, in part, his enormous appeal to many segments of Italian society and his effectiveness even outside the country. Whether talking to factory workers outside Venice or to students at the University of Paris, or to psychiatrists in São Paulo, Brazil, Basaglia avoided the presentation of prescriptions, rules, models, or recipes for action. Rather, he offered a critical way of seeing, of spurning surface interpretations and easy solutions, and of experiencing the conditions of one's life. While he recognized that a sprawling city in a 'developing' country in Latin America was not analogous to Gorizia or Trieste, he empathized without restraint, and he stimulated and energized others, spurring them on to analyze their particular situation with their own cultural tools.

Mario Tommasini, the communist city councilman and health commissioner who eventually brought Basaglia to Parma, described some of these qualities in discussing his first meeting with the founder of democratic psychiatry:

> ... I found myself before a person who expressed a large, cultural openness, but who could relate this larger vision to everyday life, translating it into understandable behaviors and practical initiatives which—even if seemingly insignificant—were a stimulus to peoples' participation in social change [14].

But in his writings Basaglia left behind no famous case histories, no specific therapeutic techniques or practices. This was, of course, consistent with his epistemology of psychiatry as politics, with his rejection of the idea of scientific neutrality, with his suspiciousness of the traditional bourgeois intellectual. His brief, published 'excerpts' concerning the dramatic events and radical changes initiated at the asylum of Gorizia were

> not intended to be a description of a technique, or of a system that is more efficient or more positive than any other. The reality of today will differ from tomorrow's reality, and in trying to freeze it, it either becomes distorted or irrelevant [5].

Here Basaglia is taking up Sartre's conception of ideology that runs throughout his work: i.e. that ideologies can be liberating while they are still in formation and oppressive once they become institutionalized [15]. Instead of a technique or a system, then, Basaglia offers the dialectical method of negation, or negative thinking, a means of working through paradoxes to reveal the contradictions underlying traditional practice and logic. The 'negative worker' continually raises the questions: "What is *wrong* here?", "What is the *real* problem?", "Whose needs are being served—whose are being *neglected?*' Once the contradictions are exposed, and the group thrown into crisis, old roles and institutional arrangements and solutions are rejected, destroyed, negated, allowing new forms to appear. The work of negation could be devastating, for it entailed a refusal to allow the efficiency and well-functioning of the hospital to interfere with the unmasking of patients' real and unmet needs. In the case of Basaglia's anti-institutional movement the process of negation—pursued through open community meetings (the *assemblea,* to be explored below)—led to a denial of the custodial functions of the institution and a denial of professional roles and statuses in psychiatry, including a refusal of the power to name the illness, to define the norm, and to control through punishment or by over-medication. When you point out contradictions, wrote Basaglia,

> you are opening up a crack. For example, when we demonstrate that psychiatric institutions only exist as an apparatus of social control, the state is forced to create something else to replace it. From the time when the contradiction first explodes into consciousness, to the time when it is inevitably covered up, there is a moment, a chance for people to realize that the health system does not correspond to their needs because society itself is not organized to meet those needs [16].

It was in this tiny crevice, this fragile space that Basaglia and his co-workers tried to reconstruct psychiatry as a critical practice of freedom, a truly alternative psychiatry that would help resituate the marginal, the excluded, the scapegoated and help them reclaim their buried history. Through Basaglia's series of challenges to the false consciousness of individuals and of groups, and through the development of a collective practice, Basaglia, like Antonio Gramsci, merged theory and practice. He removed revolutionary praxis from the abstract domain of 'historical necessity' and returned it to the hands of real, active, critical human beings.

What made Basaglia's radical anti-institutional alternative possible was a confluence of factors obtaining in Italy in the early 1960s. The backwardness of Italian psychiatric institutions was anachronistic for a rapidly expanding capitalist society. There was as yet no bourgeois, liberal or humanist social psychiatry to compete with the prevailing bio-deterministic and other positivist models of mental illness, as existed for example in France, England and the United States and which spawned in those countries institutional psychotherapy, therapeutic community, the *politique du secteur,* and the community mental health movements. An attempt to import the French model of institutional psychotherapy by the Bologna Provincial Administration in 1964 had failed miserably.

Second, the existing mental health legislation in Italy was archaic, blatantly concerned with the control of social deviance and with anti-social behaviors (sociopathy). The mental health code of 1904 (with slight modifications in 1968) established the precedent of linking psychiatry to the Italian criminal justice system, and assigned it a function of control and custody *(custodia)* over that of care and treatment *(cura)*. The special relationship between psychiatry and the courts was, to an extent, overdetermined by the high proportion of young, "unsocialized aggressive", 'psychopathic' patients represented in the Italian mental hospital censuses. Italy's *manicomios* were filled with poor, working-class, and immigrant people, as well as with 'delinquents' and young social 'misfits'. In all they represented individuals who could not keep up with school, factories, or other institutions that reproduced 'normal' behavior.

Third, the sociopolitical context of Italy, with its strong labor movement and later, its student and feminist movements, offered the possibility of broad-based alliances and coalitions. Leftist trade unions and political parties were willing to give their support to the struggle against institutions that abused their constituents. University students and feminists were able to empathize with the most miserable and abandoned segment of the Italian underclass—mental patients—and to draw parallels between their situation and aspects of their own.

In 1961 when Basaglia began his work at Gorizia there were 800 patients in that asylum and nearly 100,000 in all of Italy. Despite the introduction and widespread use of neuroleptic drugs, psychiatric hospital censuses were continuing to rise. At the time of Basaglia's death in August of 1980, however, there were less than 50,000 mental patients in Italy and several traditional *manicomios* had all but closed down, and Italy had passed a revolutionary piece of legislation—mental health law No. 180, that effectively decriminalized madness, and which proposed to completely dismantle the old system of public asylums. As the principal architect behind these events, Basaglia's experiments at Gorizia, Parma and Trieste are instructive.

Stage One: Destroying the Mental Hospital (Gorizia)

As a first moment, Basaglia and his colleagues (including his wife, Franca Ongaro Basaglia) recognized the *manicomio* as a micro-social archetectural space that reproduced perversions in human relationships that were not only counter-therapeutic, but which created an illness specific to itself. British and American researchers had already recognized and named this phenomenon: institutional psychosis or hospitalism. The *manicomio,* wrote Basaglia during this period, was

> ... an enormous shell filled with bodies that cannot experience themselves and who sit there, waiting for someone to seize them and make them live as they see fit, that is, as schizophrenics, manic-depressives, hysterics, finally transformed into things [5].

And elsewhere he would state about the locus of his practice:

> Within its four walls, the pulse of history ceases to beat, the social identity of the individual contained therein is suppressed, and the process of total identification of the individual with its psychic dimensions takes place. The conditions of his life may be offered as proof of his innate inferiority, his culture disregarded as the expression of his irrational deviation. The silence which thus sets in, in the asylum, becomes both typical of it and the guarantee that from it no other message will reach the outside world [17].

The immediate milieux that he encountered was so inhumane that, like Philippe Pinel, Dorothea Dix and other psychiatric reformers before him, Basaglia sought first simply to unshackle the patients, to end the more violent institutional practices of physical restraint, seclusion and shock treatments. He maintained chemotherapy as an intermediate measure, making it possible to eliminate the more immediately violent forms of treatment, and enabling him to begin to distinguish the damages produced by the illness from the damages produced by the institution. Chemotherapy, however, produced the first of many paradoxical situations that forced Basaglia to look for alternatives. Psychotropic drugs adversely affected the anxieties of both doctor and patient. They calmed the doctor's anxieties about his inability to relate to the patient as a human being, to find a shared language. On the other hand, the drugs increased the patient's level of awareness of his situation, convincing him that he was utterly lost and without appeal (why else would he be in a back ward?). Eventually, Basaglia came to the conclusion that medication could be used appropriately, and that there was a significant difference between using chemotherapy to suppress a 'symptom', and using it to establish a relationship. Medication could be used to put an anguished person to sleep, or they could be used to calm the patient down enough to talk with the doctor. But here another contradiction emerged. How to 'talk' with a patient who has lost all her subjectivity, whose only body is the body of the institution? In an early piece, while still heavily influenced by his phenomenological training, Basaglia challenged the clinician to search for meaning in the silences, in the stillness before the words, where the assaulted, battered psychiatric inmate could slowly regain her ego, recover her buried subjectivity, experience her sense of self, her ability to *be with* another, without fear of being annihilated [18]. Later on, the words might come more easily.

Similarly, the task of creating a more beautiful, more humane hospital environment also produced a contradiction. Basaglia recognized that the asylum could be transformed into a kind of 'gilded cage' where basic physical needs could be met (food, safety, shelter) but where more profoundly human needs (for autonomy, liberty, love) would be forever stifled. It was with respect to the failure of the 'open door' policy to radically alter the inmates' condition that allowed Basaglia to see the limitations of the therapeutic community model and which caused him to search for a more global solution that bridged the gap between *inside* and *outside* the asylum.

Where initially Basaglia considered the 'open door' the unifying symbol of psychiatric liberation, and he referred to it as the 'holy terror of our legislators', he soon discovered that the 'open door' merely reminded the patients of the fact of their exclusion and rejection by the world outside. Instead of taking the cue to freedom and autonomy offered by the open door, the newly 'liberated' inmates at Gorizia remained passive and imprisoned by an internalized image of the asylum that was part of their new sense of self. Basaglia would write with marked frustration:

> They sit quietly by and wait for someone to tell them what to do next, to decide for them, because they no longer know how to appeal to their own efforts, their own responsibility, their own freedom. As long as they accept liberty as a gift from the doctor they remain submissively dominated [9].

And so, the open door produced the third paradox: fewer escapes, less 'acting out', and the great quagmire of patient gratitude to the benevolent doctor/father. Basaglia drew on an ancient Chinese parable to explain the inmate's dilemma:

> An Asian fable tells of a serpent that crawled into the mouth of a sleeping man. It slid down his stomach and settled there, imposing its will on him and depriving him of his freedom. The man now lived at the mercy of the snake, and no longer had mastery over himself. One morning the man noticed that the snake had left, and he was once again a free man. But he no longer knew what to do with his freedom. During the long period of domination the man had

become so accustomed to submitting his will to the serpent, and giving over all his impulses to the creature, that he had lost the capacity to desire, to strive, to act autonomously. Instead of his freedom, the man found only the emptiness of the void ... [5].

The analogy with the situation of his 'newly liberated' mental patients was startling to Basaglia, for they were still very much slaves of the institutional serpent.

Basaglia's immediate solution to prevent his newly emerging 'therapeutic community' from rapidly deteriorating into a 'cheerful haven for grateful slaves' was to engage his patients in a relationship of reciprocal tension, to challenge their mortified humanity, using as leverage each inmate's potential aggressivity. Basaglia encouraged even his most regressed patients to participate actively and aggressively in what he later referred to as the "destruction" of the hospital: first, to destroy, with their own hands, the more noxious barriers that had confined and excluded them: doors, bars, window gratings. An entire hospital wall was dismantled in a collective expression of what Basaglia later referred to as 'institutional rage'. On another occasion patients and nurses destroyed backward furnishings and equipment that were ugly, archaic, or symbolic of punishment.

The process of destroying the 'internalized' hospital—the negative logic of the institution—was more gradual, and took place through two main instances. The first was the task of opening up the wards by creating paid work in the hospital. To be able to work, and at Gorizia this could mean in the kitchen, maintaining the grounds, caning chairs or farming, gave patients a reason to leave the ward. It stirred the general stagnation and the emptiness of lives where all temporality and all contact with the external world had stopped.

By instituting fair standards of wage labor for employed inmates, Basaglia and his coworkers were able to expose the sham of previous models of so-called 'work therapy' through which unpaid labor was extracted from patients, a labor upon which the general maintenance of the psychiatric jail depended. As paid wages came to replace token cigarettes (the rewards for 'good behavior'), work in the hospital came more to resemble the social reality of labor on the outside, allowing inmates to feel more in common with ordinary working people.

By 1967 over half of Gorizia's patients were working, three times as many as when Basaglia had arrived. But this situation opened up new dilemmas such as whether equal compensation should be given to inmates of very differing competencies and commitment. Meanwhile, paid labor to inmates was introduced during a period of severe budget cuts. Lively discussions among patients and staff on these issues influenced the development of work cooperatives as a non-exploitative alternative.

The second instance of transformation was the meetings, and in particular the daily *assemblea,* a general gathering of patients and staff with a rotating chairman, elected from among the patients. This was a spontaneous event to which one could come and go, and no one was required to attend. No formal distinctions separated nurses, doctors and patients, and the topics for discussion came from the floor, centering on patients' needs, which they were beginning to express, both collectively, and as individuals. The *assemblea* are not to be confused with the general meetings that are part of the therapeutic community model of Maxwell Jones and his followers. Basaglia's *assembleas* were disorganized, uncontrolled, and open to anger, passion and unreason. They were anything *other* than 'safe' places for the 'controlled' venting of interpersonal or intra-psychic problems. A co-worker of Basaglia described the meetings as follows:

The first *assembleas* were chaotic. They suffocated in a passionate struggle for power, the bitterness and hostility breaking through in both verbal and physical attacks. Certain administrators would scorn this event where everybody had a right to speak their mind, where the first stammering phrases of the most repressed and regressed patients were encouraged, where even delirious speech was accepted without stigmatization [19].

For some patients the *assembleas* represented the first public occasion at which their angry complaints were recognized for what they were—legitimate demands for unmet human needs—rather than suppressed as essentially meaningless symptoms of psychiatric disease. The recognition was both gradual and collective. For example, initially the meetings were disrupted by a patient who refused to enter the room, but who insisted on yelling through the window. What was first dismissed as the annoying interruptions of a disoriented patient, gradually came to be viewed differently by the group. The patient was not yelling through the window because he was crazy. Rather, the man was protesting. He, too, had found a way to use the *assemblea* to take power through speech, and his protest was henceforth recognized as a legitimate demonstration, an exercise of his civil rights.

What began to emerge at the *assembleas* was the collectivization of responsibility for the consequences of behavior. Individual problems were analyzed and translated into institutional terms. The dialectical method of negation, mentioned previously, is perhaps best exemplified in the way that problems were solved in the *assembleas*. One woman at Gorizia was using the *assemblea* as a vehicle to express her demand for electroshock treatments. Finally, the current president of the meeting—a patient—said: "Why do you feel guilty? Why do you want to be punished?" In the heated discussion that resulted, participants interpreted the woman's guilt in *institutional* rather than in *psychoanalytic* terms. That is, all the patients had, at one time or another, sought an explanation for their confinement. If they had been locked up, they *must* have committed a crime. Therefore, perhaps they *should* be punished. This perverse institutional logic, now finally brought out and uncovered for the sham that it was, provoked a crisis as the patients' long suppressed anger for their unjust commitment was allowed expression. The hospital as prison had to be negated.

There was a gradual evolution from the use of the *assemblea* as a place to vent personal problems toward using it as a vehicle for translating the personal into the collective and the political. If an alcoholic, for example, now free to leave the hospital grounds, went off on a drinking binge, his 'failure' was discussed as a shared responsibility. It became a crisis for the whole ward, not just for the individual, and a collective explanation was sought.

The new freedom to make choices, including the freedom to come and go on the wards, left open many possibilities for disruption and crisis that had previously been suppressed under the hospital-as-prison regime. For example, the *assemblea* might address what was to be done about a ruckus and free-for-all caused by an alcoholic who returned from town with a bottle of spirits in his jacket. The patient's action might provoke a collective decision to force another choice. Either the disruptive patient would have to leave the hospital, or he would have to act more decorously and responsibly.

Without a doubt, the most poignant expression of empowerment, collectivization of responsibility, and anti-institutional practice to have emerged at an *assemblea* took place in 1968, when Basaglia was indicted for manslaughter after a patient who was released into the community murdered his wife. According to a quirk of Italian law in effect at that time, the asylum director was responsible for the actions of patients committed to the mental hospital. There was an attempt to close down the asylum until a new director could be found, and the patients were to be transferred. Student and other community activists arrived and stayed at the hospital to keep it open. For 15 days there was no mention of 'the incident' at the *assemblea*, until finally, one patient exploded:

> Why can't we talk about this terrible thing? How can we keep silent when *he* [Basaglia] has to pay dearly for something we are all responsible for?

During the anguished discussion that followed, it emerged that everyone felt guilty for what the 'bad' patient had done. To both hospital workers and patients 'the incident' represented the frontline, symbolizing everything they had worked for. It was at the *assemblea* where most of the decisions regarding deinstitutionalization were made, including the timing of individual discharges, community and work placements, role of family members, etc. The decisions were not made by a panel of experts using psychiatric criteria. Rather, they were made collectively, largely on the basis of commonsense and lay criteria. If there had been a mistake in judgement, it should be acknowledged, but the responsibility for the error should be shared. It was a moment of crisis, but also a moment of breakthrough in the anti-institutional struggle. People wanted to stay together, to experience the trauma collectively, and so hospital and community workers started living in the hospital. As a result, for the first time real efforts were made to reach the most regressed, back ward patients, using play, gymnastics where possible, or any simple gesture that might come to mind.

The *assemblea* was one of about fifty meetings held each week by nurses, by other staff, and by smaller groups of patients. Visitors to the hospital were invited to attend and to participate. These meetings became instances of critical consciousness-raising through which 'new subjects' were created and collectively empowered. But the meetings represented only one of the collective movements that was to run through all Italian anti-institutional practice. Consciousness-raising and the creation and exchange of new knowledge also went on in the hospital cafe, in the spontaneous meetings with visiting family members and townspeople, as well as in more formal political forums. It is essential to understand how democratic psychiatry evolved as a practice.

While Basaglia's method of 'negative thinking' was used to confront contradictions and to pierce through the false consciousness of psychiatric and institutional ideologies, power-sharing was expressed symbolically as staff and patients gave up their traditional uniforms and with these their former role identities. And, with the 'open door' rendering it superfluous in any case, staff members relinquished their primary symbol of authority: the large ring of heavy, institutional keys. Yet, Basaglia and his co-workers never glossed over the fact that as long as the institution existed at all, nurses and doctors would continue to maintain control over the inmates, just as the doctors would control the nurses within a hierarchy that mimicked the division of labor in the larger society. Therefore, Basaglia and his equipe relentlessly examined the sources and the nature of their professional power, how it was delegated, and in the name of what objectives it was maintained.

The experiences at Gorizia went far beyond the techniques—such as therapeutic community—which had been borrowed. The meetings, as we have seen, bore no resemblance to group psychotherapy. Traditional therapeutic communities, as even the American sociological studies of the 1960s were revealing, never questioned the structure of power relations. At Gorizia authority, power and status were constantly rendered explicit, as problems to be challenged. Moreover, the contradictions within the hospital were linked to larger social ones. Basaglia and his co-workers gave priority to an analysis of the global and political economy dimensions of psychiatric problems in place of the more traditional micro-analysis of intrapsychic and interpersonal psychodynamics.

Finally, once doors were opened, new services appeared: a community mental health center for patient after-care; a school, a day hospital all on the grounds of the old institution. These were preparatory to the more difficult task of social reintegration that lay ahead.

Stage Two: Community Praxis at Parma: "Everyone or No One"...

In 1970 the Provincial Administration of Parma invited Basaglia to take over the direction of its psychiatric hospital. By now the word about events at Gorizia had spread throughout Italy and elsewhere in Europe. The anti-institutional, anti-authoritarian nature of the Gorizian experiment resonated with the new values then being expressed in the student and worker protest movements of 1968. The currents of European marxism (in which both Sartre and the critical theorists of the Frankfort School participated) focused the struggle on groups and institutions that mediate between the individual and the means of production. Hence, the major unions, especially the GCIL, were turning to issues such as public schools and health care facilities, and they demanded a series of major reforms that would become central in the 1970s, as will be discussed at length further on.

Mario Tommasini, the provincial director of health for Parma, and other public officials had long been aware of the terrible conditions existing in the institutions of Parma and its surrounds, where neglected children, juvenile delinquents, unwanted elderly and mental patients were warehoused. In 1967, nurses had demonstrated against the 'instruments of torture' routinely used in the mental asylum by marching through the streets of Parma in strait-jackets, while the hospital itself (the former horse stables of Napolean's wife, Marie-Louise) was occupied in protest by medical students and the Parma Student Movement. Similar actions took place in other Italian cities: in Turin, for example, students demonstrated against the construction of a new psychiatric hospital. Meanwhile, the patients themselves went on strike in their sheltered workshops demanding higher wages and better work and living conditions. Many different popular and political organizations to respond to the problem of 'mental illness' and its treatments were spawned. Furthermore, political alliances were beginning to be formed between labor unions and the more progressive political parties. In the process of these linkages psychiatric issues were addressed as part of a general denunciation of segregation of all kinds and a new, critical examination of the social and political functions of medicine. Meanwhile, Basaglia was actively involved in attempts by workers to gain control of their health care and to change the many threats to health and safety at the workplace.

1970 also marked the diaspora of the original Gorizia group, for several years providing the only alternative to conventional institutional psychiatry. The publication of *The Institution Denied* in 1968, a collective product of the Gorizia equipe, made available the first synthesis and articulation of the anti-institutional practice (that Basaglia and his co-workers were developing) to a large public throughout Italy and abroad in Europe and Latin America. Members of the original group were invited to other cities and regions of Italy. Others, stymied by political barriers against the extension of the anti-institutional movement into the community of Gorizia, resigned in protest and sought to apply their practice elsewhere. In tracing the lines of dispersion outward from Gorizia, like the roots of a tree, we can begin to reconstruct the evolution of the movement. Of the original Gorizia equipe, Giovanni Jarvis went to Reggio Emilia where he by-passed the hospital entirely in order to set up community alternatives to hospitalization and to develop new forms of family therapy in public clinics. Agostino Pirella assumed directorship of the hospital at Arezzo which was to become a model deinstitutionalization experiment in Italy. Others came to Parma with Basaglia, and from there went on to Ferrara, Naples and Genoa. During this same period of growth and fission, an independent anti-institutional movement evolved in Perugia, which soon split along two fault lines: one developed a model for community psychiatry, with psychoanalytic overtones; the other developed a political practice which, nonetheless, emphasized *madness* rather than *marginality,* a departure from Basaglia's original approach.

In 1973 the various approaches and models would converge within a formal organization, *Psichiatria Democratica*, founded by Franco and Franca Basaglia and other members of the original Gorizia group. In their original founding document the group made the following pledges: (1) to continue the fight against exclusion by examining both its structural aspects in relations of production, and its ideological aspects in cultural norms and values; (2) to struggle against the asylum as the most obvious and violent paradigm of exclusion; (3) to avoid reproducing institutional mechanisms for exclusion in the community; and (4) to make a clear link between health and mental health care, especially through the reform of the Italian health care system.

It had been evident to Basaglia and his followers from the very outset that mental patients should not simply be returned to the same hostile families and antagonistic communities that had originally rejected them. He recognized that provisions had to be made for them: alternative social and medical services; adequate housing; and employment that was neither exploitative nor demanding. In short, the job of 'destroying' and, ultimately, closing down the wards of the *manicomio* had to be accompanied by the far more radical and difficult task of 'opening up' communities, making them more receptive and responsive, and more than just passively and indifferently 'tolerant' of the psychologically different, troubled, or suffering individuals who would be returned to their midst.

The work of Basaglia with Tommasini at Parma involved the first attempts both to go into the community, with the patients, and to work side by side with other organizations, such as unions, for broader structural changes. Basaglia did not entertain naive misconceptions about the readiness and willingness of Italian communities to accept the released 'madmen' and women. He recognized that his was a deeply cultural as well as political task, and that his co-workers had to confront and do battle with the demons of archaic superstitions and negative stereotypes about the 'mentally ill'. Italy did not differ from other Western countries in which 'mental illness' is a highly stigmatized condition, popularly viewed as incurable, even contagious, sometimes fatal and strongly hereditary. The stigma, therefore, attaches to family members of the patient, and is destructive to social relations in a society that is still, to a large extent, defined in terms of family ties. Basaglia was sympathetic to these families and their community relations:

> In our constant struggle against false consciousness and the dominant ideology, our work inevitably involves a certain violence to the community. When we release the mentally ill into the community in a real sense this is a violation of that community and it provokes a crisis [16].

First, there was the labor crisis: the problem of convincing unions and factory owners and managers of small firms to accept as workers a new class of social marginals who had either never worked before, or who had been institutionalized for so long that they had lost whatever work skills they once had. In this task Basaglia was greatly aided by the work of Mario Tommasini who, himself an ex-plumber, worked very effectively with the unions. His passionate humanism and commitment to the reintegration of ex-mental patients, especially troubled adolescents and the mentally retarded, was infectious. Once Basaglia had moved on to Trieste, Tommasini continued the anti-institutional work they had started together, particularly the work with labor unions and factory workers.

A deeply moving documentary film, produced in the late 1970s by the March 11th Film Collective and entitled 'Fit To Be United', captured the Parma experiment in process. In one segment of the film a group of metal workers discuss with some pride how they succeeded in integrating a dozen seriously mentally handicapped people into their factory, and how these people are now accepted as ordinary workers. A middle-aged man with Down's syndrome, flanked on either side by his co-workers, tells of his first, anxious day at the factory, and how he now tears out the pages of his calendar for Saturday and Sunday because these are his least favorite days, the days away from work and from his co-workers. This is followed by a candid, cinema verité sequence in which a militant union organizer apologizes to the camera and film crew for not being 'prepared', but he says that it seems to him that the way he and his workers have approached the problems of those called 'crazy' and 'retarded' is perhaps more useful than the methods and techniques of the psychiatrists. He adds that the relationships and the rewards are reciprocal, and that the presence of former psychiatric inmates on the factory floor—their pride and pleasure in work and in the company of others—deeply changed something at the factory: "Until their arrival we had lost a certain dimension, a certain way of being human".

The second crisis provoked by deinstitutionalization is to the families of the ex-patients, many of them ill-prepared to receive back into the bosom of the hearth family members who had proved troublesome in the past. This was especially so in the case of returning 'troubled adolescents' and so-called juvenile delinquents to their over-wrought parents who often lacked the skills and the resources to cope with behaviors that sometimes brought in the police. This dilemma was, again, captured in 'Fit To Be United' where a prematurely aged and worn mother of a young delinquent, Paolo (a boy filled with mischievous wit, charm and boundless energy), tried to explain why her son ran into so many problems with school authorities and with the law: "The problems were ours; we were poor, no? I've always had rotten luck". The return of her prodigal son from a mental institution closed by Tommasini was interpreted as just one more stroke of bad luck. One's sympathy is with the harried mother of eight other children, as well as with the difficult, but altogether winsome, Paolo.

Although Basaglia and his followers understood that the crises provoked by the return of the mental patient to be part of the necessary dialectic that made radical change possible, he also recognized the needs of the families for empathy and social and material support. "It is our duty", he wrote,

> to work with those we have violated. We must be present with them throughout their crisis [16].

Despite these words, in retrospect, a major shortcoming of Basaglia's work was his failure to develop any real praxis with respect to the special needs of those families to whom a deinstitutionalized member had been returned. Nonetheless, other co-workers in Democratic Psychiatry did develop new forms of family therapy and support in the community; Cancrini, for example, adapted aspects of Palazoli's 'paradoxical encounter' [20] (i.e. the Milan School) for work among families of the deinstitutionalized in Rome.

Central to Basaglia's community praxis was the work of a new species of mental health worker. The community presence that he envisioned implied a far more active and more political role for the worker than any that had previously been proposed. The work would require a clear rejection of the old psychiatric control apparatus. She could not serve simply as a go-between in revolving door relationships between the ex-patient and the mental hospital (so common among community psychiatrists in the United States) now that the institution no longer existed as a back-up social control apparatus. Without the threat of punishment and confinement lurking in the wings to extort conformity from the ex-patient, as crises arose they had to be dealt with on the spot. Nor were the new mental health workers to base themselves in community mental health centers and day hospitals which Basaglia always feared for their potential as 'involvement shields', barriers to community participation, and worse, for their potential of developing over time into micro-mental hospitals *in* the community. Rather, the new community health worker had to be fully present and available to the ex-patients in their daily conflicts in the real world, wherever these occurred: at home, on the job, at the marketplace, in bars and restaurants, at social welfare agencies, and in the streets and piazzas of the city. These represented new arenas of struggle, for it was absolutely necessary that the former 'private' troubles of the patient be turned back into *public* issues, and that people's problems be understood as political and economic in nature, as well as psychological. The old 'false neutrality' and 'impartiality' of the 'objective' psychiatrist had to give way to situated and positioned community workers who were willing to take sides, and to put themselves squarely on the side of the ex-patients and their families.

Stage Three: 'Freedom is Therapeutic' The Hospital and the Piazza as Loci of Cultural Revolution (Trieste)

When he became director of the Psychiatric Hospital at Trieste in 1971, Basaglia was finally able to carry through to fruition the total elimination of the asylum, and venture forth fully into the unexplored terrain of the community. Trieste presented still a new situation: once part of the Austrian-Hungarian Empire, this magnificent city on the Adriatic Sea is home to a large number of marginal people, including many elderly and recent refugees from the Istrian Peninsula of Yugoslavia next door. Despite a 'white', or Christian Democrat administration, in addition to neo-fascist groups and political parties, the province's administrator, Michele Zangetti, was willing to promote the transformation of the mental hospital where 1200 patients were interned.

Trieste quickly became a crucible of innovations, experiments, actions. Young people, radicalized by the demonstrations of 1968, and the new political movements of the seventies, came to work as volunteers, or on student fellowships. Hence, non-professionals were a constant presence at the asylum, and the anti-institutional slogan, 'Freedom is Therapeutic', scrawled with other political graffiti on the hospital walls, captured the drama and the youth and the excitement of the early phase of deconstructing the hospital, as it were.

However, as the lessons learned through Gorizia and Parma indicated, one could not simply destroy the inner space of the hospital, leaving those once confined there at the mercy of the outside world. Alternative solutions had to be worked out, links re-established with the community; ex-patients had to develop new personal and social identities and to regain contractual power within the community.

The movement at Trieste, therefore, took place simultaneously on two fronts: in the hospital and in the community. Soon after his arrival, Basaglia restructured the hospital into 'open communities', corresponding to geographical sections of the province. But of primary concern was the reversal of the institutional logic that made the hospital a guardian and the patients its wards through the establishment of patient rights. Another step entailed reaching out to the community, enlisting the support of ordinary citizens, those for whom the *manicomio* represented 'protection' against the threat of chaos, disorder and dangerousness presumed to be contained within its walls. Popular stereotypes had to be confronted and challenged *before* and *throughout* the gradual process of returning inmates to the community.

In the asylum at Gorizia there had been the problem of that minority of inmates who were either too old or too senile, too physically frail or too deeply institutionalized, to return to community living. Three hundred of these still remained in the institution by 1968. Of these, approximately 100 were senile, infirm and bedridden, requiring constant care by the nursing staff. Another 100 were elderly and senile, but ambulatory, patients for whom the hospital was, for better or worse, their only home and they refused to leave. The final 100 inmates were chronically and actively psychotic individuals who were unable to function in the community or for whom no alternative placements could be found outside the hospital. And some of these, as well, preferred to remain living at the hospital.

At Trieste, on the contrary, even before most of the patients had left the hospital, a new legal status was created: that of *ospite,* or guest. Some of these could not yet find housing. Others, like some of the remaining patients at Gorizia, were either too elderly or too ill. But as *ospites* their full civil liberties were restored. They were free to come and go as they wished, with meals and lodging provided on the hospital grounds. Some worked even in the city. This was a *demedicalized* solution to the thorny problem of 'chronicity': neither medication nor psychotherapy was mandated.

But more than that, the creation of the legal status of *ospite* was part of a whole series of changes

> around the organization and disciplinary pillars of the therapeutic universe. Work therapy was replaced by the creation of a cooperative of workers; the ospites' lack of money set in motion a large machine to abolish interdiction and guardianship and to obtain pensions; the criteria for entitlements were modified through successive struggles and vindications; play therapy was ridiculed; art therapies were turned on their heads by experiments with animation, through which the city began to come into the asylum [21].

As the wards were unlocked and replaced with smaller units and by autonomous housing, such as the apartments where guests lived, the 'Basagliani' encouraged the flow of traffic through the doors to go both ways: inmates into the city, the citizens into the asylum. Staff went out to talk with families, officials and administrators. But for the latter to come inside the asylum, there had to be strong inducements, and these were provided in the form of film-festivals, and shows, plays by traveling repertory companies, performances by musicians, actors, artists. Naturally interspersed among the patients, townspeople could begin to recognize in the distress and suffering of former inmates some of the problems in living that plagued their own lives.

Basaglia and his co-workers had a particular affinity for the Italian artists' community, seeing in the works of the surrealists and post-impressionists, in cinema verité, street theatre, compatible metaphors of the sick-making contradictions of contemporary society. Through the vehicle of art there existed yet another way of sensitizing the public at large to the violence of segregative control. At Trieste, local and visiting artists were invited to participate in the anti-institutional movement, and some even moved into vacant wards and buildings. The best known group was the Rainbow Collective. With the inmates they painted colorful and outrageous murals, psycho-political graffiti, and ironic cartoons with captions such as: "Come and get your electroshocks with us; signed Pinochet". Sculptures created by Ugo Guarino and put on display in a former back ward gave mute but terrifying testimony to the suffering of the patients once imprisoned there. The collages were created out of the debris left from the stage of 'destroying' the hospital: bits of decaying wood, paint peelings, broken furniture stained with blood, sweat, urine and feces.

Outside the hospital grounds a group of actors and ex-inmates formed a company that performed puppet shows and guerrilla theatre on the streets and piazzas of the town. They enacted the history of the asylum and its inmates, and they celebrated the victory of its demise. In 1975 a group of artists worked with the inmates of Trieste in building a unifying symbol of the anti-institutional movement: *Marco Cavallo,* a giant, blue, paper-mache horse on wheels. Artists and ex-inmates paraded Marco through the streets and squares of the city, as a symbol—reminiscent of the Trojan Horse—of the freeing of the captive inmates.

Marco Cavallo, 'the large theatrical machine', the horse of the patients' desires, became a symbol, in schools, at fairs, in the marketplaces throughout Italy and elsewhere in Europe as well. But it brought out another, and darker side to the transformation of Trieste. The day of its triumphant exit into the city, the nurses went on strike, protesting the archaic conditions in which they worked, the long hours, impossible shifts, the paltry salaries. They complained both of the present reality in which the mental patients lived, and of the poverty that awaited them outside. They were joined in the strike by all employees of the province.

The strike assumed a key significance for the anti-institutional movement at Trieste: it reminded movement workers that every extra lire for entitlements, every new room for a community center, had to be fought for. Basaglia was to reflect on the uses of power several years later:

> The problem of power and its pedagogy isn't about the empty attributions of power, but rather how it is conquered, and how we can change things through this conquest [5].

Eventually, Basaglia and his co-workers were able to open six alternative community mental health centers in Trieste, through their ability to build a power base of sometimes shifting alliances with the Provincial Administrator, political parties and labor unions. But when political constellations changed and became less supportive, or when funds dried up, the Trieste workers went directly to the townspeople, and began to collaborate with other institutions, such as the prison and the general hospital.

By the mid-seventies the foray into the community had produced a new phenomenon: poverty from the asylum now joined the poverty outside, that of chronic unemployment and housing shortages. There was also the poverty of human contact, that of loneliness, exclusion and abandonment. With no existing type of social services, a new response had to be created: a kind of arsenal of emergency assistance and welfare. By obtaining money for ex-inmates—and Basaglia and his staff continually badgered the provincial administration for higher entitlements—they broadened their possibilities and choices for community existence.

By the time Basaglia left Trieste to take over the psychiatric services in Rome in early 1980, the hospital was completely emptied. In Gorizia and other cities where Democratic Psychiatry had been active, the hospital walls and fences were literally torn down. In Trieste the buildings had been reconverted and reassimilated into the definition and parameters of community life. A beauty shop, dormitories for college students, the local pirate (alternative) radio station, and a cooperative day care center for children now occupied the emptied wards and buildings. The buildings, including those where the *ospites* still resided, were given municipal street numbers, symbolizing the rites of reincorporation. The effect of the blurring of the lines between 'inside' and 'outside' was described by one woman who worked at the child care center at Trieste:

> The significance of the presence of children in a mental hospital lies ... in the hope that one day we will stop building mental hospitals in and on the heads of children. The contradiction lies in the fact that "normal" children are in a space for "crazy" people. Hope lies in the possibility that this space could be used by the adult to learn to live with children [22].

Had Basaglia simply stopped with the destruction of the asylum, had he abandoned the physical space of the institution, he would have left intact the very *idea* of segregative control as a possibility to be rediscovered by other, newer agents of social consensus yet to come. Perhaps Basaglia was mindful of Michel Foucault's history of the total institution in Europe, with which we began this essay, by which each successive generation, each new episteme, recreated the old segregative and penal institutions to incarcerate, in turn, a new category of social outcasts. In this way, the leper was replaced by the witch and the heretic, who were in turn replaced by the debtors and paupers of the 18th century, and still later by prostitutes and defrocked priests, and finally all of these by the madman. In destroying the hospital as a locus of discipline and punishment, and by redefining and resocializing the shell that remained as a positive social space, Basaglia chipped steadily away at the cultural foundations of exclusionary logic. Instead of excluding the contradictions, isolating and hiding them away, Basaglia's work returned them to our social space so that we might once again recognize that part of ourselves we have for so long denied as madness, as folly, as delirium. Having successfully challenged the special expertise of medicine and psychiatry in the management of human misery, Basaglia went on to confront the old and uneasy alliance between psychiatry and the law. Demedicalizing and decriminalizing madness went hand in glove.

Psychiatry and the Law: 'The 180'

The mental health reform bill, or Law 180, marks a final turning point in Basaglia's anti-institutional itinerary. It was an off-shoot of the anti-institutional movement's concern with breaking the circuit of social control that defined normal and abnormal behavior and which punished and excluded that which could not be domesticated or neutralized.

Law 180 begins from the premise that all psychiatric evaluation and treatment should be voluntary. It put a freeze on all new admissions to psychiatric asylums, and demanded that all current and 'chronic' patients be gradually discharged and reintegrated into community life through a network of new outpatient services. Meanwhile, all existing psychiatric hospitals were to be unlocked and patients' civil liberties returned to them. The law prohibited the construction of new psychiatric hospitals or the upgrading of all existing ones. 'New' patients were to be evaluated and treated in the community. If necessary, during an acute phase of illness or distress, a person could be admitted to psychiatric wards of general, district hospitals. These wards could not contain more than 15 beds, and in no case could compulsory hospitalization last for more than 15 days, with independent judicial reviews required at 2 and 7 days.

The significance of the law is apparent. Its unambiguous goal is the total abolition of the state mental hospital system. More important, the law recasts the relationship between law and psychiatry; 'dangerousness' is no longer the rationale for compulsory treatment and segregation. Nor is the law concerned with the definition and classification of the various types of 'mental diseases' (and the degree of threat each is presumed to pose to society). Rather, 'the 180' establishes the State's only interest in psychiatry as the supervision of the *forms* and *reasons* for treatment, both voluntary and compulsory. The law destigmatizes the psychiatric patient: mental illness is no longer treated as a special case of illness that allowed for special violations of the patient's civil rights. Instead, 'mental illness' becomes, under the law, one of many conditions (some infectious diseases are another example) which *might* require compulsory treatment or brief hospitalization. Gone in Law 180 are allusions to the 'irrationality', the 'mental incompetence', and the 'presumed dangerousness' of the mentally afflicted. Furthermore, the commitment process itself is politicized by assigning responsibility for compulsory commitment to the Mayor, an elected public official, in addition to two doctors. In other words, the delegation of responsibility to a 'gatekeeper' who is directly accountable to the public is made explicit. Commitment is no longer hidden behind a medical mask and confounding psychiatric language and false expertise.

Basaglia was the principal architect throughout the many phases of drafting the Law 180. In order to understand how he had reached such a level of political influence it is necessary to backtrack and explore the social conditions which aided passage of the legislation. In a fertile climate of change and experimentation—in the period between the student and worker revolts of 1968 and the end of the left-center coalition in the 1980s—Italians largely redefined the meaning of 'political'. Women, school children, parents, neighbors, workers, youth were the protagonists of the transformation, the 'new subjects' united by a common denominator that ran throughout their demands and projects: subjectivity, personal needs, diversity, autonomy. The women's movement expressed this new current most clearly, perhaps, in their insistence of control over their reproductive system and the demedicalizing of pregnancy, birth and the female life-cycle. The labor movement claimed not only a right to occupational safety and health, but also control over health services so as to lessen their dependency on factory and company physicians. Similarly, Basaglia's incessant questioning of the parameters of normality and of reason resonated with women, youth and intellectuals. In this sense, health was central to the agendas of all these movements.

Health issues, including the questioning of psychiatric power, were taken up by the labor movement very early on. At a landmark congress on 'Psychology, Psychiatry, and Power Relationships' in 1969, health professionals, progressive intellectuals and representatives from the unions discussed concrete proposals, and the Italian Communist Party presented the first joint health-psychiatric care platform. Democratic psychiatry, too, had solidified its political base since it first brought together 2500 people at Gorizia in 1974. Although schisms rocked the organization (especially around the use of specific techniques), members united around the issue of much needed mental health reform. Gradually, local administrations had begun to develop programs outside the hospital except in the South where few such initiatives existed beyond Naples. Then in 1976, the heavy gains made by Left parties in the legislative elections boosted democratic psychiatry's influence, especially in the shaping of national health reform.

Basaglia, himself, became more politically focused following the *en masse* resignation of the Gorizia staff in 1972. Although he continued to work within his professional sphere as a clinician and psychiatrist, he also practiced beyond it, illustrated in his 6-year relationship with the Trieste administration, under Michele Zanetti, who translated Basaglia's concepts and ideas into political platforms and programs. In Western countries, the model of a psychiatrist who simultaneously operates on the local level, as director of a transformed psychiatric hospital, while actively negotiating the political system, from a global perspective, is altogether rare. Basaglia, also the archetypal *homme politique,* in his ability to maintain the double relationship to popular social movements and to established politics, was able to influence directly the sweeping mental health reforms of 1978.

During 1977, most of the political parties drafted and introduced proposals into the Italian Parliament for a national health service. The parties of the Parliamentary Left introduced legislation on psychiatric reform that incorporated many changes the anti-institutional movement had been advocating for several years: closure of the asylums, and of other total institutions (such as orphanages, special schools, etc); abolition of the 1904 law; establishment of community mental health as the core of psychiatric care; use of the general hospital for acute psychiatric uses; and overhaul of involuntary commitment and guarantee of a maximum of patient rights.

Shortly thereafter, members of the Radical Party, a champion of constitutional and civil rights in Italy, took to the piazzas with petitions calling for a referendum on a constitutional amendment that would totally abolish the commitment procedures and the public mental hospitals that were established by the 1904 law—but without any provisions for community-based alternatives. Due to general frustration with the pace with which the mental health reforms were taking shape in Parliament, they very nearly amassed the required number of signatures. It was largely out of fear that the Radical Party might succeed, and massive dumping of mental patients result, that Law 180 was quickly drafted and passed through the efforts of a Christian-Democrat and Communist Party coalition. Basaglia was consulted by the Law's sponsors throughout the period of its passage. The Radical Party initiative had separated psychiatric reform from the general health reform by limiting it to a constitutional amendment. To the contrary, the proposal that emerged as Law 180 was later incorporated into the National Health Services Act (Law 833). The expediency with which Law 180 was drafted and passed had serious consequences to be explored below.

Although a compromise measure, the law reflected some basic tenets of Basaglia's work, especially the dismantling of the asylum system and the de-criminalization and depsychiatrization of 'mental illness'. The law, however, did maintain a form of involuntary commitment, and neither forensic hospitals nor private hospitals, nor university clinics fell under its jurisdiction.

In 1979, Basaglia moved to Rome to become Director of Mental Health Services for the Lazio region. Before his untimely death in August 1980, he was able to witness the rather striking immediate impact of 'the 180': the large decrease in public hospital patient censuses (from 54,000 in 1978 to 42,000) and the 60% decrease in compulsory admissions. In addition, National Research Center Statistics had indicated no corresponding increase in admissions to private facilities or evidence of dumping. Definitive studies and evaluations of the effects of the law are yet to come, and up-to-date reliable statistics have not been published. After an initial wave of enthusiasm, however, its supporters became aware of the problems involved in implementation, including direct sabotage.

Opposition to the so-called 'Basaglia method', which its detractors eventually identified with the 'Basaglia law', came from various sources. Already in the seventies, Basaglia's work had been contested in lawsuits and other types of harassment. Meanwhile, traditional, biodeterministic psychiatrists had been gaining strength with a resurgence and reformulation of positivist psychiatric models beginning in the late seventies, while classical psychotherapies were enjoying their first broad support. Hospital nursing staff had gone on strike against 'open door' policies, on the grounds that *they* would have to take the brunt of patient aggressivity 'unleashed', once inmates were free to move about. And although no jobs were lost when wards or buildings of the mental hospitals closed down, many hospital staff rejected the alternative of working in the community. Like chronic patients, these psychiatric workers were often 'over-institutionalized'. And some of them joined the backlash.

Furthermore, every Minister of Health since 1978 has consistently avoided providing leadership or support for nationwide application of the law. First, the Minister postponed the date for prohibiting re-admissions to psychiatric hospitals by three years, while appointing several commissions to examine the question. Then, although no funds were allocated over a 5-year period to implement the '180' (as it was called), ample funds were promised to implement proposals that would move Italy back toward a hospital-based system. But there were other obstacles as well.

Five years after its passage, it was possible to venture a typology of regions according to degree of implementation of the law. Those areas where the anti-institutional movement had been most active before 1978 (e.g. Trieste, Arezzo, Ferrara, Perugia) acted most in accordance with the spirit of the law.There, hospital populations were successfully reduced, and a network of alternative services, from work cooperatives to free-standing clinics to supervised apartments to group homes, continued to grow. In other areas, deinstitutionalization efforts were underway, but success still limited. This was true mainly in Northern cities such as Genoa, Turin, and Venice.

Finally, there were areas (especially in the South of Italy) where implementation of the law was practically absent, or worse, where it was applied in a negative way, guaranteed to provoke a crisis. In some provinces of the South of Italy patient censuses in large hospitals had been maintained or even increased, with special regional decrees postponing the date after which readmission would no longer be possible. Elsewhere in the South, deliberate misapplication of the law resulted in a form of 'dumping' that Italians call 'wild discharges'—i.e. patients literally bused off hospital grounds without any discharge plans or material or social resources. As a result, homelessness seems to have increased in several cities.

The particular situation obtaining in the South of Italy deserves special attention, for the region has always remained locked into a kind of hostile, economic vassalage to the more 'economically developed' and politically progressive North. Non-compliance to national laws and programs has been one way in which provincial administrators have maintained their hegemony. So, for example, although the mental health law of 1904 had required each province to establish an asylum, in 1973 only three of seventeen Southern provinces had a mental hospital. Likewise, the 1968 Law ('Legge Mariotti') which called for the reduction of hospital populations to a maximum of 677 beds and which established community mental health centers, was barely followed. Some hospitals simply subdivided, creating 'two' hospitals as a way of circumventing the reduced bed criterion ruling.

In place of provincial public mental hospitals, the Southern regions had always favored an alternative: a system of private hospitals under religious auspices to which patients were taken from cities and towns all over the South, and where they were warehoused under minimal public supervision. Hence there should be no surprise that after 1978 funds for psychiatric hospitals were rarely converted into support for alternative, community-based services.

However, regional differences go beyond the North-South division. The law decentralizes the administrative level of psychiatric assistance, holding the regions responsible for planning. As of 1983, however, nine of the twenty regions in Italy had not yet designated preventive, rehabilitative, and treatment services outside the hospital (in the *'territorio'*).

Neglect, sabotage and incompetency in carrying out the law's intent can explain only part of the problem. It should be recalled that the law was a compromise measure and at least two structural aspects render it vulnerable to misapplication.

First, the only service that is specifically required is the Diagnosis and Treatment Unit (SDC), a ward of no more than 15 beds attached to a general hospital. Generally, such units are locked and rely heavily upon psychopharmacology as the treatment of (staff's) choice. By locating the service in hospitals, the very space determines their medicalized character. This certainly defeats the spirit and purpose behind Basaglia's and his colleagues' work in democratic psychiatry. And, because community services, which are not specifically mandated, have either not been funded or else are extremely limited in staff and in hours of operation, the SDC is the only facility in most places that people (or their families) can fall back on when they are in an acute phase of distress. Meanwhile, the 15-day limitation (originally intended as a protection to patients' civil liberties) has been subverted by the technique of multiple readmissions. In other words, the SDC has become a new 'revolving door' facility.

Second, the absence of adequate regulations, mechanisms and funding for community alternatives has tended to produce the distortion pictured above. Perhaps Rome exemplifies this situation the best. Plagued by typical problems of metropolises everywhere— unemployment and a large underground economy, immigration, shortage of public services, etc.—it has few community mental health centers for a population of almost four million. Members of democratic psychiatry would challenge the explanation that cost factors prevent the Italian community 'model' from being carried out on a wide scale, contending instead that community care and hospital care cost approximately the same. Nonetheless, the entitlements that allow an ex-patient to obtain housing and the minimum money needed to live outside the hospital are still provided primarily and unsystematically by the provinces. As a result, a major incentive to an adequate level of community living is limited by the lack of a universal entitlement, such as Supplemental Security Income in the United States.

By the early mid-eighties, a new block had arisen in opposition to the law. On radio talk programs and in the newspapers, families of patients pleaded their cause. Some asked for the public mental hospitals to be reopened; others joined with Democratic Psychiatry to push for an 'honest' implementation of 'the 180'. Family associations are most vocal in Rome. There, with a ratio of SDC beds to general population on the order of 2 per 100,000 and scarcely any other services, patients are either abandoned or left as a burden for the family to deal with, most often a wife or mother. Thus in a span of a few years, a visible segment of the general public has become a new force to which psychiatrists and administrators must respond.

Franco Basaglia: Legacies and Utopias

In part the legacy of Basaglia is with Democratic Psychiatry and with those community workers in cities where anti-institutional work continues. In part, his legacy is with alternative psychiatric workers throughout Europe, North America and Latin America who identify with the spirit of collective human decency, radical tolerance and deestrangement that were the hallmarks of Basaglia's vision.

Although conditions in the Italy of the eighties (as elsewhere in much of the West) are not the most conducive to a demedicalized and alternative practice of community psychiatry, as the economic crisis has taken its toll on jobs and housing, and as cutbacks threaten social services and the new health system, there are still grounds for guarded optimism, Basaglia, himself, had warned against the anti-institutional movement being nipped in the bud; yet he also grasped new possibilities emerging. With respect to the passage of law 180 he said:

> Even though it is the fruit of a struggle, a law can only be the result of the rationalization of a revolt. But it can also succeed in diffusing the message of a practice, rendering it a collective heritage ... it can diffuse and homogenize a discourse, creating the common bases for subsequent action ... [23].

Certainly the gains made by all the Italian social movements in the decade following 1968 were nothing short of astounding: a national health service, anti-pollution laws, the gradual elimination of asylums, free continuing education (the '150 Hour'), and a long list of victories attained mostly by the feminist movement: legitimization of divorce and abortion, publicly-funded day care, reform of family law and women's health clinics. New forms of protest and politics had won nothing less than an expansion of citizen's rights, an increased participation in government, and a multiplication of social services. Italy had moved from an old system of charity toward a more modern welfare state model guaranteeing universal rights, not only to the traditional groups linked to production (workers and their families), but to the various marginal groups—the 'emarginati'—that had appeared.

Once stereotyped as a 'backward' and 'backwater' European nation, a second class citizen in the world economy, and stigmatized by the persistence of some archaic social forms, Italy in the last decades of the 20th century has emerged as a truly modern, humane and cosmopolitan society, a world leader in progressive social reform, of which Basaglia's anti-institutional movement represents its most daring and dangerously fragile creation. Paulo Freyre once remarked mischievously that North Americans have had to turn increasingly to the materially depressed Third World for spiritual inspiration, specifically to Brazil and Central America, to discover a rejuvenated and vital theology of hope and liberation. So, too, dispirited community psychiatrists in the United States, Canada and Great Britain might question their ethnocentric assumption that progressive social movements always originate at the core of the industrialized world. Instead of prematurely declaring deinstitutionalization policy a failure, they might well pause for a moment and turn their attention to the semi-periphery—to Italy—for a rejuvenated psychiatry, a psychiatry of hope, a psychiatry turned *inside-out*.

As we conclude this essay (Anne Lovell in New York City, and Nancy Scheper-Hughes in Berkeley), we would be altogether remiss were we not to reflect, finally, on the status of deinstitutionalization in the United States, and on the plight of the homeless—many of them ex-psychiatric inmates—who are sometimes *quite literally* at our doorsteps. With respect to Basaglia's legacy, what message, what lessons are there for an enlightened practice of psychiatry outside asylum walls in our own embattled cities?

Lessons for the United States

No possible alternative to the institution exists unless it is a constant and practical critique of every form of institution: the mental hospital to the mental health system, from the center to the neighborhood [24].

At approximately the same time that Basaglia and his co-workers were 'destroying' the institution at Gorizia and 'deconstructing' the logic behind institutional psychiatry, Governor Ronald Reagan was blithely closing down state mental hospitals in California, preparatory to a total 'pull-out' of public responsibility for, and commitment to, the plight of the 'chronically mentally ill'. Although there were many different rationales behind the policy of 'deinstitutionalization' in the United States (medical, social scientific, ideological) [25], what motivated Governor Reagan (and other public officials elsewhere) was a concern to save his tax-paying constituency money. He was quite prepared to increase the public coffers by consigning public mental patients to the streets. This particular American social tragedy, then, begins and ends here, with a policy founded on a distortion—a promise to 'humanize' and 'communitize' care for the mentally ill by reducing the State's financial commitment to them.

American deinstitutionalization was the result of several factors converging from the mid-1950s on. For one, the existing physical plant of the public asylum system—a legacy of the 19th century—was rapidly approaching a state of total decrepitude that made their renovation or replacement mandatory [26]. Then, during the next two decades, civil libertarians and patients rights activists would gain landmark legal cases to push their cause against the conditions of psychiatric institutions, if not the very nature of confinement and psychiatric treatment itself. Wyatt *v.* Stickney, in 1972, established guidelines for upgrading Alabama's notoriously punitive and repressive mental hospitals—from improving patient-ratio staff to the purchase of bed sheets to the building of new toilet and shower facilities. A few years later, a case won by a long-time hospitalized patient Kenneth Donaldson, made involuntary commitment and treatment more difficult to enforce. Regardless of the political climate in which these battles were fought, judicial decisions were implemented in such a way as to favor deinstitutionalization, as both a humane *and* a cost-saving policy of reform. The availability of new forms of income maintenance that could be used in the community and in other types of institutions, such as nursing homes and adult residency programs, gave further impetus to the transfer of patients from mental hospitals to the community. Medicaid, which could not be used in psychiatric hospitals, had a similar effect.

Beyond these basic fiscal considerations, however, lies even more potent political issues, especially those concerning the control of social deviance. It has been suggested that the mental asylum had outlived its usefulness to the State and that it represented an archaic institution of social control, inappropriate to the needs of an advanced capitalist society such as the United States in the late 20th century [26]. Although North American psychiatrists had readily taken up the task of managing the huge state-run 'monasteries for the mad' (as Andrew Scull calls them), they were never, as a profession, totally committed to this particular psychiatric practice. The mental asylum has coexisted for at least half a century with 'softer' forms of intervention and control- -psychotherapies, mental hygiene programs, community-based care. But it persisted for the control of the less tractable and the more hopeless psychiatric cases. American psychiatrists were among the first to suggest that the advent of modern psychotropic drugs in the 1950s rendered long-term institutionalization superfluous [27]. With new outpatient compulsory treatment laws replacing earlier involuntary commitment laws, deviance and madness could now be controlled where they first occurred: in the community. And, given the proliferation of 'psychologies' and medical and social work professionals operating at street-level, the circuit of social control could be further extended and diffused throughout the city. It could be said that we have exchanged tranquilized wards for tranquilized ghettos filled with poor and homeless psychotics whose only resource is a weekly shot of Prolixin at a storefront clinic.

In Foucauldian terms we have entered a new episteme in the long history of the (mis) treatment of the mad in which punishment and seclusion have given way to regulation and surveillance—or even to self-regulation and self-colonization. This is certainly *one* interpretation we might give of the new population of so-called 'Young Adult Chronics' who learn to survive by 'making it crazy', as Estroff writes of her sample of drug-dependent 'street crazies' who bounce off and between day hospital and night shelter, between drop-in clinic and drop-out training programs [28]. With their only form of dependable subsistence (SSI) tied to a damaging and chronic diagnosis, it is little wonder that in the bustling, impersonal marketplace of life on American streets, ex-mental patients now 'traffic' in illicit symptoms, trading their illness for the semblance of economic security through welfare for the 'totally and permanently disabled'. And so we have chronicity born of economic necessity, a new possibility for existence determined by the social welfare bureaucracy.

An alternative Basaglian view might lead us to explore the forms of resistance that also occur within this homeless street population where alcohol and street drugs are often used defensively in place of tranquilizing neuroleptics and psychotropics, where an intimate knowledge of the city and its surrounds can sometimes provide a protective camouflage that defies even the most experienced police and other street-level agents of social consensus, and where welfare 'abuse' can be understood as a rare act of autonomy in an otherwise altogether desperate situation. We realize, of course, that these are marginal and often self-defeating survival strategies, and we would not want to fall into the easy trap of romanticizing the 'culture' of the streets or minimizing the suffering of the chronically afflicted and disoriented.

Indeed, the very *public* nature of madness and vagrancy on our public streets—as the poverty of the asylum joins the poverty of the streets—recreates a modern substitute for Jeremy Bentham's Panopticon. Bentham's design for the perfect nineteenth century total institution was one able to induce in the inmate a sense of conscious and permanent visibility, an arrangement of space that rendered him a perfect object of continual surveillance. In his *Discipline and Punish* Foucault describes the Panopticon as a

> machine for dissociating the see/being seen dyad: in the peripheral ring, one is totally seen, without ever seeing; in the central tower, one sees everything without ever being seen [19].

Visibility has become a trap, a new metaphor of powerlessness. Likewise, if the new population of so-called homeless mentally ill is said to be an 'eye-sore', this of course implies that they are rendered the objects of our discriminating, incriminating, hostile gaze. Surveillance is no longer contained within a perfectly rationalized architectural space; its gaze is polyvalent, its viewers a multiple public, the colonizers of those street people who transgress a newly privatized terrain. Deinstitutionalization has occurred in the United States during a period of rapid gentrification and privatization of the commons. By this we are referring to the transformation of once public domains—churches, subways, parks, squares—into extensions of private space, so that neighborhood 'homeowners' can express a kind of righteous indignation at the very presence of 'vagrants' and 'derelicts', as if the homeless were violating their own living rooms when they pass time in public. It is as if there were no longer any neutral ground. In New York City the renovation of Times Square, of the grounds behind the New York Public Library, of Union Square are designed to make these public spaces inhospitable to vagrants, the homeless, the propertyless. In San Francisco the construction of new city parks is likewise designed to discourage the homeless from thinking of themselves as part of the public. For example, Boedekker Park, created out of the corner rubble in a section of the run-down Tenderloin district, is said to "demonstrate the gentle art of landscape architecture ... in taming the urban jungle" [30]. Its special 'safety features' include high visibility (it can be seen entirely from the street—there are no trees or shrubbery that might conceal 'derelicts, drug dealers and low life'): 175-W bulbs stationed every 40 ft; a 6-ft high fence and gates to keep out night visitors; and short benches with arm rests to prevent 'anyone but a midget' from sleeping there. Finally, a Recreation and Park Department staff member will be on constant 24-hour surveillance duty.

Despite the perhaps only partially recognized possibilities for new forms of social control implied in the harboring of a vulnerable and exposed psychiatric street population, both professional and lay public discourse now descries the 'failure' of deinstitutionalization. A new 'humanitarian' rhetoric has arisen that condemns the 'dumping' of asylum wreckage on city streets, and that calls for a reexamination of the old institutional solutions for managing those who seem unable to manage themselves. The APA task force report on the *Homeless Mentally Ill,* released in the fall of 1984, refers to deinstitutionalization as a 'major social tragedy' and the group reached "... agreement on the need to change the laws in order to facilitate involuntary treatment" [31]. Similarly, letters to the editor and opinion columns in newspapers throughout the country increasingly carry calls for the 'clean sweep' of bag ladies and grate gentlemen, and for a return to long-term, custodial care. New legislation recently introduced in California would make compulsory treatment easier and would create the legal status of 'involuntary' out-patient, i.e. the coercively tranquilized.

There remain, however, a small but persistent group of social scientists, community psychiatrists and patients' rights activists who believe that deinstitutionalization has not failed, because it was never really attempted. Insofar as the closure of state hospitals was never accompanied by the 'opening up' of communities, and in the absence of any redefinition of the meanings of 'mental illness', or any redefinition of psychiatry as a social practice, deinstitutionalization merely reproduced in the local setting the same exclusionary, institutional logic that was the very foundation of the public asylum system.

The myth is that U.S. mental patients were returned to community life; the reality is that 'community' was defined as *any* setting outside the grounds of the state mental hospital. What really occurred was a transfer of mental patients from state-run hospitals to federally supported or privately financed community-level institutions. Locked, skilled nursing facilities—the most common alternative placement for the elderly, senile or incontinent ex-mental patient—constitute, in many cases, a more restrictive and punitive environment than the often spacious 'campuses' of state asylums.

The myth is that mental patients have been returned to their families; the reality is that few ex-inmates have been taken in by their relations. In fact, American families have grown more vocally opposed to deinstitutionalization, and some have formed their own parent or family support groups to block plans that would return their needy and dependent relations to their care. With the demise of state responsibility for the 'chronically mentally ill', and as American families of ex-patients have refused to take up the burden of their parents and children, fertile ground has been created for a 'new trade in lunacy', as Andrew Scull refers to the modern scandal of private 'Board-and-Care Homes'. Ex-patients, alone, disoriented and needy, are unable to make informed choices and so fall easy prey to a host of new and enterprising 'penny capitalists', speculating in human misery. The Board-and-Care Homes operators offer food, shelter and a promise of protection for the ex-inmates often thrown into a hostile and rejecting inner city or working class neighborhood. Many of these so-called 'homes' are, in fact, full-blown, but largely unregulated institutions warehousing as many as two or three hundred ex-patients as cheaply as possible. One can only speculate as to the 'quality of life' offered in these new community-based madhouses, and whether they offer any improvement over life in the back wards of the state asylums. Today, in San Jose, Calif., for example, there are more than 1000 board-and-care homes in the dense and deteriorated downtown section alone.

Among the 55 middle-aged chronically distraught psychiatric patients who had been released from Boston State Hospital and returned to their white, ethnic, working class community in south Boston, studied by one of us (N.S-H.), many were living in non-institutional settings, but their daily lives were highly regimented through their daily attendance at a day hospital, rehabilitation programs or sheltered workshops. In fact, these ex-patients functioned almost entirely within the decentralized mental health system, punctuated by occasional readmissions to the state hospital. Rather than a toe-hold in the difficult transition from hospital to community, the day hospital and sheltered workshops had become a *permanent placement* in the community, their only 'ecological niche'. In this traditionally Irish-American neighborhood of south Boston, the transfer of care for the chronically disoriented passed, in part, from State to Church as the Boston Archdiocese began to reopen only recently closed convents and rectories as half-way houses and community residences for the deinstitutionalized, in some cases supervised by the few remaining religious Sisters. As one parish priest wryly summed up the current situation: "The Good Lord must have known when he had us building all those Catholic schools, and parish houses and convents in the 1950s, that they were meant to house all the drifters, and crazies, and drunkards of the 1970s". These Church-affiliated community placements (although often austerely and monastically run) were, in fact, highly valued by the ex-patients of Boston State. As one said:

> All my life I've been poor and needy and sick. I have to keep it in mind that whenever my relatives see me, they're going to think, 'here comes trouble'. I always cost them money. But living here, under the protection of the Catholic Church, I'm *somebody* for the first time.

Another, and much less benevolent 'community' institution that has taken up the slack created by the State's massive pull-out from the Mental Health Industry is the criminal justice system—i.e. the prison. In the last decade the prison population in the United States has risen by 80% to an unprecedented national census of 350,000 prison inmates. Several prison surveys have reported the appalling increase in the numbers of psychiatrically disturbed inmates. An earlier phase in the history of the treatment of the insane seems to have returned, full-circle, as 'madness' once again is recast as 'badness' and as prisons are accepted as appropriate institutions for housing the disturbing and 'presumed to be dangerous' social deviant.

In the states of New York, Massachusetts and California where 'wild discharges' and casual dumping have been most pronounced, a new, particularly jail-prone population has emerged: the young adult, male, transient, destitute and desperate, as well as angry and disoriented (psychiatric) street person, 'space-cases' in Berkeley street parlance. To mental health professionals they are the so-called new Young Adult Chronics [32], the bane of social workers and psychiatrists alike. What makes this population difficult is, in part, the historical context in which they came of age:

> Their relationships with institutions have been formed in an era of civil rights and consumerism. Few have experienced long-term hospitalization, and few exhibit the apathy, lack of initiative, or the resignation that numerous studies found to characterize the long-term mental hospital resident. These 'new' chronic patients *have not been socialized to docility, to the role of acquiescent* mental patient; they do not use services in the tractable fashion of their predecessors but rather as wary, often angry consumers demanding response to their broad needs for social and economic support [33] *(editors' italics)*.

Worse, to add insult to injury, the authors note that today's younger chronic patients "... tend to resist the contention that they are mentally ill". In short, we have a population not yet destroyed by institutional treatment and logic, but without an alternative community psychiatry—such as Basaglia's democratic psychiatry—to recognize the legitimacy of their complaints and to channel productively and politically their anger and aggressivity. The result is tragic. Prison, asylum, board and care home, shelter, street—these are the components of the new circuit of control. In this case, surveillance is often the only response given to human suffering and need.

In 'liberal' Berkeley the huge psychiatric street population of 'space cases' are less than benignly neglected, while in nearby Santa Cruz, the street people are called 'trolls'—because of their tendency to seek shelter under bridges—and they are harassed and physically assaulted by college student vigilantes calling themselves 'troll busters'. They provoke street fights that often lead to the arrest of the more vulnerable group.

Before, however, the resounding failure of American deinstitutionalization is recognized as a foregone conclusion, and before plans for the reinstitutionalization of the 'mentally ill' are in place, we might consider the lack of planning and the absence of a unifying ideology that contributed to the current situation. At the very least we need to re-examine our operating assumptions and to (radically) reformulate our current practices.

The Italian experiment, although flawed and riddled with its own inconsistencies and contradictions, offers evidence that deinstitutionalization can be done differently and with considerable success. To what extent, however, the Basaglian program and ideology can be exported or imitated in other contexts is debatable insofar as the Italian experiment—where it succeeded—did so *exactly* because it was able to articulate with the vernacular culture, with the anti-authoritarian and communitarian ethos of large segments of the Italian working *and* professional classes.

What would it take to apply something analogous to the Italian experience in the United States? Certainly, many of the ingredients of success in Italy are lacking: a professional leadership committed to radical change; a cultural and political environment open to sweeping social reform; a political conception of madness as alienated human needs; a healthy mistrust of the objectivity of science and the neutrality of the social and medical professions; a popular consensus in sympathy with anti-institutional principles; a coherent and universal health insurance program covering both medical and social services. While Basaglia and his co-workers developed alternative solutions in politicized cities, such as Parma, with the help of communist party leaders and labor unions, such organized bases of support can hardly be expected to be forthcoming in middle-American cities and towns. Meanwhile, with few exceptions, charismatic leaders in psychiatry have yet to appear on behalf of the deinstitutionalized homeless and communityless in the United States and Canada. Yet, within the vacuum left by the absence of an enlightened and energetic psychiatric professional leadership, what *has* arisen is a plethora of citizen and self-help advocacy groups—patients' rights movements and grassroots coalitions for the homeless [34]. These are *our* special cultural legacy of the identity politics that emerged during the 1960s, and what these groups are demanding is no less radical than Basaglia's anti-institutional, demedicalized, and deprofessionalized response to the unmet needs of the alienated mad-poor.

In sympathy with these creative, if widely scattered, 'counter-psychiatry for the people' groups, we could at least see to it that our communities are organized so that the deinstitutionalized, but still distraught, could always find a place to sleep, meals, basic health care *without strings*—i.e. without obligatory and mind-altering chemotherapy, painfully intrusive psycho-therapies or degrading, menial sheltered work [35]. Our reading of the results of numerous outcome studies for deinstitutionalized individuals leads us to the conclusion that the safest, most protective environment for the deinstitutionalized, but still chronically psychologically afflicted, individual is one characterized by: a high tolerance for difference; a low expectation for *conventional* productivity, mutuality and reciprocity from the ex-psychiatric inmate; within a caring, but non-institutionalized setting. In other words, with Basaglia and his equipe, we agree that, above all, *'Freedom is therapeutic'*. Such a regime would require a transformation of cultural norms about the limits, the parameters of the 'normal', the 'acceptable.'

Insofar as a fundamental characteristic of madness is a refusal or an inability to participate according to the 'commonsense' ground rules of everyday living, this new spirit of tolerance would require an acceptance of some disorder, chaos, unreason in the speech, thoughts, actions of the so-called psychotic individual. It would mean a surrender of our reality-centric world view and an acceptance of the subjective experience of alternative realities. Following Michel Foucault's early analysis, a necessary requirement for social reintegration would be a willingness to 'give madness back its voice' [36]. In Basaglian terms, this means an empowerment through words, an understanding that even 'delusional' or 'delirious' speech may be a febrile voice of protest, the only possible act of resistance and autonomy available to a silenced and excluded population.

Perhaps the greatest existential problem faced by the population of psychiatrically distraught and homeless is that of finding a space where they can legitimately *be* during the day [37]. They are suspect in public parks and on city benches, unwanted in libraries and churches; the time they can 'hang out' in donut shops and cheap diners is limited. Many attend day hospital programs and conform to the medicalized regimes offered there only to participate in the free lunch program and to have a place where they can 'hang out' unharassed. The psychiatric policy of abandonment is expressed most flagrantly in the current wave of homeless persons who include among their ranks many who in an earlier era would have filled the wards of state hospitals.

In the current debate over housing vs mental health services for the mentally ill homeless (well documented in the American Psychiatric Association's Task Force Report) the side to choose should be clear. While housing alone can never suffice or substitute for the broad range of social, cultural, political and individual responses to human suffering and afflictions of various kinds, it is, at the most basic survival level, a mandatory requirement. And so we have in mind, as a *minimal* program, the establishment throughout the United States of a network of hostels where the homeless, the vagrant—especially those younger and more desperate populations set adrift, one way or another, by the closure of hospitals and by 'dumping'—might find a place to live, to participate in community life with a minimum of externally imposed or institutionalized structure. These permanent hostels would bear some resemblance to Basaglia's *ospite* or guest quarters at Gorizia and Trieste, implying a new legal status for an *autonomous* although perhaps economically dependent population. These hostels would come to replace the current and inadequate hodge-podge of 'emergency shelters' functioning unsystematically in most American cities.

The lack of housing faced by the current population of displaced and distraught homeless is a problem of chronic dimensions, not one that can be solved by recourse to makeshift, first come-first serve flop houses. Segal and Baumohl, who have been following the Berkeley street people for several years, have concluded that

> Like unemployment, 'unhousing' is a problem of political economy not amenable to simple tinkering with the victims ... Without [the building of low-income housing or residential hotel units], shelters will become long-term encampments of the poorest citizens regardless of social work interventions [33, p. 115].

And they have proposed, in addition to the provision of low-income housing, the creation of another kind of protected space for the 'young chronics': the 'community living room'. They envision a network of non-residential store-front living rooms that would offer street people refuge, companionship, and basic survival services: a place to 'hang out', to receive mail, make telephone calls, cash checks and get paralegal services and social casework management and advice. Finally, the community living room programs—a kind of indoor 'People's Park'—would offer daytime shelter and meals. We see this proposal as also participating in the collective spirit of Basaglia's anti-institutional program.

But beyond these basic survival needs, the deinstitutionalized homeless will eventually require some real economic contractual power within the community: the opportunity to work for fair wages in alternative and creative capacities that recognize not only the limitations and disabilities of the 'chronically mentally ill', but also their particular talents and abilities. This does not mean 'sheltered workshop/sweat shop' environments, but work through public and community programs in education and the arts, in construction and computer programming, in parks and recreation, wherever the individual talents lie.

In addition, the deinstitutionalized and displaced require someone who cares about them—not as a doctor or a social worker cares about a client—but as one family member, one friend, one colleague cares about another: freely and spontaneously. What is needed are the stream of '*Basagliani*'—the volunteer college students and housewives, artists and artisans, working people and the retired (those like the townspeople of Gorizia, Trieste and Parma)—who rose to the occasion and came out to welcome the ex-mental patients back into the human community. This entails a redefinition of community, meaning not merely any geographical location outside hospital grounds, but a Basaglian conception of community as gemein-schaft or 'communitas'—a community of mind and will and spirit, a physical, psychological and social space where the suffering and non-suffering, the conventional and the uniquely different, can both find a home. Finally, what is needed is an American variant of Marco Cavallo, a unifying cultural symbol that encompasses a new psychiatry of hope for ex-patients, their families, their co-workers and co-residents. We need to allow madness to emerge from behind the medical mask that has concealed its most social properties: the cumulative effects of rejection, exclusion, and stigmatization. We need to look madness in the face and to recognize ourselves in the play of contradictions that is revealed there.

Susan Sontag writes at the beginning of *Illness as Metaphor* that

Illness is the night-side of life, a more onerous citizenship. Everyone who is born holds dual citizenship, in the kingdom of the well, and in the kingdom of the sick. Although we prefer to use only the good passport, sooner or later each of us is obliged, at least for a spell, to identify ourselves as citizens of that other place.

She is expressing here the intense feelings of marginality, exclusion, experienced by the afflicted, especially by the stigmatized afflicted—those from whom it is all too easy to turn away in disgust, revulsion and pity. It is also, however, a sobering reminder that each of us ambulatory, sane, 'whole' individuals holds only a temporary truce against illness, madness, suffering, exclusion, and death. We are, as Sue Estroff likes to remind us—the temporarily able, the temporarily sane [38]. It is an essential truth that Basaglia and his co-workers were able to convey to a large populace in Italy. Another was the reminder that a person's differentness, her malaise or her suffering is not legitimate grounds for her ostracism, exclusion, and confinement. Democratic Psychiatry, as developed by Franco Basaglia and his co-workers, implies the creation of a social space in our communities where those who are the veterans of intra- and inter-personal conflicts, of mental prisons and of medical wards, can coexist with, and not apart from, the rest of us.

A member of the film collective that produced and distributed the documentary, 'Fit To Be Untied', summed up the anti-institutional movement when he explained [39].

What we were trying to say is just this: community life is like a banquet table. We wanted to make sure that everyone has a seat at the banquet.

References

1. "Malheur a toi si tu nous trompes, et si parmi tes fous caches des ennemis du peuple". Semelaigne R. *Philippe Pinel et son Oeuvre au Point de Vue de la Medicine Mentale.* Paris, 1888.
2. Foucalt M. *The Birth of the Clinic: An Archaeology of Medical Perception,* pp.84–85. Vantage, New York, 1975.
3. Foucault M. *Madness and Civilization,* p. 194. New American Library, New York, 1967.
4. Benaim S. The Italian experiment. *Bull. R. Coll. Physns* 7, 7–10, 1983.
5. Translations of Basaglia, unless otherwise indicated, are by Anne Lovell and Terry Shtob, from Scheper-Hughes N. and Lovell A. (Eds) *Psychiatry Inside Out: Selected Writings of Franco Basaglia.* Columbia University Press, New York/In press. The original Italian sources will also be given, as in the following. Basaglia F. (Ed.) *L'istituzione Negata.* Einaudi, Turin, 1967.
6. Fanon F. *Peau Noire, Masques Blancs.* Maspero, Paris, 1952. See also McCullough J, *Black Soul, White Artifact: Fanon's Clinical Psychology and Social Theory.* Cambridge University Press, Cambridge, 1983,
7. Basaglia F. Crisi Istituzionale o Crisi Psichiatrica? *Scritti,* Vol. I, p. 443. Einaudi, Torino, 1981.
8. A comparison is often made between the French 'May Events' of 1968 and Italy's 'Hot Autumn' of 1969. In Italy 1968 witnessed a handful of factory strikes, but the real conflict peaked during the more generalized worker and student strikes in the fall of 1969. Unique to the Italian events were two innovations: strikes and workers' councils that largely by-passed union structures, and grassroots forms of representation, such as the *assemblea,* or spontaneous general meeting, that had its counterpart in the Italian anti-institutional movement.
9. Basaglia F. La distruzione dell' ospedale psichiatrico. *Annali Neurol. Psichiat.* LIX, 1, 1965.
10. Basaglia F. Conversazione: a proposito della nuova legge 180. In *Dove va la psichiatria?* (Edited by Onnis L. and Lo Russo G.). Feltrinelli, Milano, 1980.

11. Le istituzione della violenza. *L'istituzione negata,* Einaudi, Torino, 1968.
12. Basaglia F. *Scritti,* Vols 1 and 2, Einaudi, Torino, 1981, 1982.
13. The best English sources on Italian democratic psychiatry and Franco Basaglia are: Crepet P. and De Plato G. Psychiatry without asylums: origins and prospects in Italy. *Int. J. Hlth Serv..* 13, No. 1, 119–129, 1983; Mosher L. Radical deinstitutionalization: the Italian experience. *Int. J, Ment.* 11, No. 4, 129–136, 1983; and Ramon S. Psichiatria democratica: a study of an Italian mental health service. *Int. J. Hlth Serv.* 13, No. 2, 307–324, 1983.
14. Tommasini M. and Ongaro-Basaglia F. Vocidi periferia: Parma 1965–1983. Unpublished manuscript.
15. Sartre J-P. *Situations II.* Gallinard, Paris, 1948.
16. Basaglia F. Conversazione: a proposito della nuova legge 180. In *Dove va la psichiatria?* (Edited by Onnis L. and Lo Russo G.). Feltrinelli, Milan, 1980.
17. Basaglia F. Problems of law and psychiatry: the Italian experience. *Int. J. Law Psychiat.* 3, 17–37, 1980.
18. Basaglia F. Silence in the dialogue with the psychotic. *J. Existentialism* 6, No. 21, 99–102, 1965.
19. Tranchina P. *Norma e Antinorma,* p. 169. Feltrinelli, Milan, 1979.
20. Palazzoli S. *Paradox and Counterparadox.* Jason Aronson, New York, 1978.
21. Gallic G. La Memoria del Manicomio. *In La Liberta e Terapeutica? L'Esperienza Psichiatrica di Trieste* (Edited by Mauri D.). Feltrinelli, Milan, 1983.
22. Lovell A. From confinement to community: the radical transformation of an Italian mental hospital. *State Mind Spring,* 10, 1978.
23. Basaglia F. Cited in Ergas Y. Allargamento della Cittadingaza del Conflitto: Le Politiche Social; Negli Anni Settanta in Italia. *State e Mercato* 6, 429, 1982.
24. From a document, 'Alternative alle Istituzione', prepared by Barcola Mental Health Center, 1977 (mimeographed). Cited and translated by Anne Lovell in Lovell [22, p. 7].)
25. See Scheper-Hughes, N. Dilemmas in Deinstitutionalization. *J. Opl Psychiat.* 12, No. 2, 1981.
26. Scull A. *Decarceration: Community Treatment and the Deviant,* p. 144. Rutgers University Press, New Brunswick, 1984.
27. See, for example, Brill H. and Patton R. Psychopharmacology and the current revolution in mental health services. *Proceedings of the Fourth World Congress of Psychiatry,* Part One, pp. 288–295. Exerpta Medical Foundation, Amsterdam, 1966.
28. Estroff S. *Making it Crazy.* University of California Press, Berkeley, 1981.
29. Foucault M. *Discipline and Punish: the Birth of the Prison,* p. 202. Vintage, New York, 1979.
30. Adams G. An urban oasis in tenderloin. *San Francisco Examiner,* 21 March, B8, 1985.
31. Lamb R. (Ed.) *The Homeless Mentally Ill,* p. xviii. A Task Force Report of the American Psychiatric Association. American Psychiatric Association, Washington, D.C., 1984.
32. See Bachrach L. Young adult chronic patients. *Hosp. Commun. Psychiat.* 33, 189–197, 1982; Lamb H. Young adult chronic patients: the new drifters. *Hosp. Commun. Psychiat.* 33, 464–468, 1982.
33. Segal S. and Baumohl J. The community living room. *Social Casework,* February, 112, 1985.
34. See, especially, Chamberlin J. *On Our Own: Patient Controlled Alternatives to the Mental Health System.* McGraw–Hill, New York, 1978.
35. The following four paragraphs are adapted from Scheper-Hughes N. Benevolent anarchy: workable model or Utopian vision? *Med. Anthrop. Q.* 14, 3, 11–15, 1983.
36. Foucault M. *Mental Illness and Psychology,* pp. 80–84. Harper & Row, New York, 1976.
37. See Duncan J. Men without property: the tramp's classification and use of urban space. *Antipode* 10, 24–33, 1978.
38. Estroff S. 'Who are you?' 'Why are you here'?: Anthropology and human suffering. *Hum. Org.* 43, 368–370.
39. Bruno-Bossiso G. Personal communication.

26

Mechanic, D., and Aiken, L. H. (1989). Improving the care of patients with chronic mental illness. *New England Journal of Medicine, 317* (26), 1634–1638

"The task for effective public mental health systems is one of recreating the functions and responsibilities of the mental hospital in a community context," Mechanic and Aiken write [p. 1635]. Some might object to what would appear to be an institutional mindset for community-based mental health services in the statement above, as the inpatient psychiatric hospital is hardly the obvious model for mental health care in the community. The authors are concerned with the functions of mental health care, however, and go on to note that community systems of care, in 1989, had not shone in these areas. They emphasize, in fact, the need for a wide range of social and support services as well as mental health treatment. In addition, 7 years after Steven Sharfstein's proposals for the establishment of mental health HMOs, another factor— homelessness for persons with mental illnesses— had come into play. The call for comprehensive and coordinated services in Mechanic and Aiken's article is not new, but their particular approach involves linking hospital and outpatient services both programmatically and fiscally. Given the risks of homelessness and substandard housing for persons with serious mental illness, they also argue that mental health authorities and agencies need to develop expertise in housing and should collaborate with public housing authorities, nonprofit developers, and landlords. Medicaid reform would loom large, they write, in efforts to create comprehensive and coordinated local systems of care that integrate medical management and social services and that span inpatient and outpatient settings.

Improving the Care of Patients with Chronic Mental Illness

The organization of community care for patients with the most severe chronic mental illnesses is seriously deficient. Most of these patients depend exclusively on underfinanced, fragmented, and often inaccessible public services. The difficulties of providing adequate medical and psychiatric services are compounded by homelessness, abuse of alcohol and drugs, and large gaps in the continuum of services necessary to meet the profound needs of these people. Patients lost to the system are commonly found in shelters or jails or on the streets.

Before 1955, when deinstitutionalization began, serious chronic mental illness was treated in public mental hospitals that had responsibility for, and control over, numerous aspects of patients' lives, including their shelter, nutrition, medical care, medication, and daily activities. Many public hospitals, which were substantially overcrowded and understaffed, developed a harsh custodialism that led to vigorous criticism and a devaluation of care in public mental hospitals. Critiques of those hospitals failed to differentiate between poor and good hospital care and confused common abuses with the important functions of appropriate hospital care.[1]

A variety of technological, cultural, legal, and financial influences reduced patient populations in public mental hospitals from 560,000 patients in 1955 to about 116,000 today. The introduction of neuroleptic drugs in large public hospitals in the middle 1950s controlled the most bizarre manifestations of psychotic illness, gave hospital staff and families hope and a greater sense of control, and increased administrative flexibility. The civil-rights and civil-liberties concerns of the 1960s contributed to activism and litigation that extended the rights of the mentally ill and constrained civil commitment. The abuses of the mental hospitals and the criticism of those abuses gave impetus to community care, which was furthered by ideologies of equality, personal autonomy, and environmental determinism. The growth of public welfare programs in 1960s and the opportunities they provided for states facing economic constraints to shift costs to federal budgets promoted deinstitutionalization. Between 1955 and 1965, the reduction of populations in public hospitals proceeded at a rate of about 1.5 percent per year; between 1965 and 1980, the rate accelerated to approximately 6 percent a year.[2]

Loss of control over the life circumstances of patients diminishes care. Deficiencies in housing, income, basic medical care and community participation are common and serious. Estimates of the amount of homelessness may vary as much as 10-fold, but studies agree that substantial numbers of homeless persons are psychiatrically impaired and constitute as much as one fourth to two fifths of the homeless population.[3,4] Many patients with chronic illness are impoverished and disoriented and lack basic coping skills, and they require assistance in obtaining disability benefits, Medicaid, and housing. Monitoring drug therapy to maintain necessary medication regimens and to limit severe adverse effects requires care sufficiently aggressive to achieve compliance and to prevent withdrawal and isolation within the community. The care of patients with chronic mental illness is substantially a task of maintenance and rehabilitation that requires longitudinal responsibility and the ability to maintain continuity of care.[5]

The task for effective public mental health systems is one of recreating the functions and responsibilities of the mental hospital in a community context, and this requires highly coordinated services of considerable complexity. Most community systems fail even to approximate this task. It may seem curious that we persist in seeking better organized systems of community care despite many obstacles when we have the alternative of creating good mental hospitals. The community alternative, however, is more consistent with our views of the preciousness of individual autonomy, our beliefs about providing care in the least restrictive setting, and the wishes of patients who prefer deprivations in the community to the restrictions of hospitalization. Moreover, there is much evidence that despite the difficulties, care and rehabilitation services suitable for most patients can be provided in the community and can achieve results superior to those attained in most mental hospitals.[6] Whether this can be done less expensively in the community is more debatable, but comparable funding buys more in the community context.[7]

Effective community care involves the ability to respond to needs ranging from appropriate housing to medical management of serious psychiatric illnesses (frequently compounded by other medical problems) requiring a wide range of medical and social services.[8] But psychiatric and medical leadership in community services for patients with chronic illnesses has seriously declined.[9] Initially, it was believed that Community Mental Health Centers (CMHCs), each of which was responsible for a particular catchment area, would provide after-care services for patients discharged from hospitals or serve in lieu of hospitals in the care of patients with acute psychotic episodes. In their early years, CMHCs failed to respond to these needs and served large numbers of new clients with less severe psychiatric problems. At first, there was considerable psychiatric leadership and involvement in CMHCs, but ironically, as these centers began to direct more of their efforts to the most impaired patients, medical involvement and responsibility eroded.

The CMHCs, particularly those serving patients receiving public assistance, face many difficulties. With the termination of direct federal funding, they now look to state and local government and third-party payers in order to survive, and these agencies push the CMHCs in conflicting directions. By assuming care for the most severely ill patients receiving public assistance, CMHCs create barriers in regard to the fee-for-service patients they would like to treat. Because they have limited funds, CMHCs depend predominantly on psychologists, social workers, nurses, and paraprofessional personnel, who can be recruited at relatively low salaries, limiting the role of psychiatrists to evaluation and supervision of medication use. Psychiatrists working in these centers have become increasingly isolated from responsibility for the patients' total care. When given competing and more remunerative opportunities, many have abandoned CMHCs that serve patients receiving public assistance. Many of the necessary services for the chronically mentally ill are psychosocial and are properly carried out by professionals other than psychiatrists, but there is no justification for the erosion of medical evaluation and supervision as a central component of care.

Case management is vaguely perceived as a solution to many of the tough issues that plague community care for patients with serious mental illnesses. This concept has a long tradition in social work, in which case workers identify and mobilize necessary services on behalf of clients and may use varying approaches, including street teams, crisis intervention, and brokering of services. One need only recall the intensive discussion in medicine of the role of primary care to appreciate the complexity of the tasks expected of case managers. Typically, case managers assigned to patients with severe mental illnesses are the lowest-ranking service personnel; they have limited training and experience and little control over the medical and community resources needed by patients. The pay is low, career ladders are nonexistent, and attrition is high. It is foolish to place so much hope on an intervention that is as weak as this one and has so little supporting structure. If case management is to be effective, it must be embedded in an organizational strategy that clearly defines who is responsible for care, that has in place the necessary service elements to provide the full spectrum of needed services, and that can control a range of resources so that balanced decisions can be made. The remainder of this discussion will address these strategies.

Community tolerance of the mentally ill has diminished in the absence of decent services. The public mental health sector must be revitalized if we are to avoid the recreation of public asylums. Building an effective public system will take dedicated professional commitment, a focused planning and organizational structure, and a new way of consolidating public financing. There is a compelling need for psychiatrists to become involved in the public sector and to provide the essential medical management.

Unlike public mental hospitals, or typical medical outpatient systems, public mental health services must reach patients in a variety of settings, including shelters, the streets, board and care facilities, and jails. Services have to be more aggressive than those typically provided and less dependent on the initiative and appreciation of those served. The service system, whether through direct services, contracts, or coordinating mechanisms, should have the capacity to negotiate needs for housing, social welfare benefits, medical evaluation, medication maintenance, rehabilitation services, and the like. In most urban areas, however, the responsibility for such services is divided among various levels of government, and service agencies are financed by diverse sources.

A key element in any effort to improve community services is to capture more hospital funds for programs of managed care at the local level that are responsible for both inpatient and outpatient services for defined populations. Some regions are establishing mental health boards, nonprofit mental health corporations, public authorities, and other types of legal entities that are responsible for receiving and disbursing mental health funds from diverse sources, including state and local governments, Medicaid, and private insurance (Walsh AH, Leigland J: unpublished data). Wisconsin, for example, provides state funding to local county mental health boards, which either directly provide or purchase all outpatient and inpatient care for mentally ill residents.[10] Savings achieved by preventing unnecessary hospitalization are available to finance innovative community care models for persons with severe mental illnesses. Ohio has developed a legal framework for strong local mental health boards and is considering legislation to divert funding traditionally allocated to state mental hospitals to these boards for more comprehensive management of care. Several areas, including Philadelphia, Rochester, New York, and South Carolina, are in varying stages of implementing limited capitation approaches for the chronically mentally ill. With the assistance of $100 million in resources from the Robert Wood Johnson Foundation and the U.S. Department of Housing and Urban Development, nine large cities are developing mental health authorities intended to have the capacity to cope with financial and organizational fragmentation.[11]

Consolidating resources across inpatient and outpatient services is particularly difficult in states with entrenched hospital systems, in communities that are economically dependent on such hospitals, and in areas with well-organized and unionized hospital employees. The need to maintain the stability of existing hospital services and to achieve necessary political support argues for transition strategies aimed at shifting funding directions over a certain period. A well-organized system diverts inappropriate admissions to suitable community programs and makes provision for discharge planning soon after hospital admission.

Except for state mental health budgets (67 percent of which are used to maintain hospitals[12]), Medicaid constitutes the largest potential funding source for reorganizing the financing of care for the severely mentally ill population. Federal Medicaid contributions represent more than two thirds of all federal funds received by state mental health agencies,[12] and in 1983, Medicaid contributed $991 million for care in state and county mental hospitals.[13] In addition, mostMedicaid funds for mental health services are spent outside the control of public mental health administrators or a managed system of mental health care. In 1980, Medicaid was the expected principal source of payment for 23 percent of all psychiatric admissions tononfederal general hospitals and for 7 percent of alladmissions to private psychiatric hospitals.[12] A rough estimate suggests that in 1980 Medicaid was the expected principal source of payment for 1.9 million bed-days in nonfederal general hospitals and private psychiatric institutions and that approximately two thirds of these bed-days were for patients with chronic mental illnesses. Patients with such illnesses come to or are brought by police to emergency rooms, where they are seen by physicians who are unfamiliar with them and who, because of the insecurities that uncertainty provokes, choose hospitalization, which is often financed by Medicaid. In a well-organized system, many of these admissions could be prevented and the patient referred to more appropriate community services.

Reforming Medicaid in this context would be complex, but managed care for Medicaid patients with chronic mental illnesses that is also supported by capitated state mental health funding holds considerable promise. Surles and McGurrin[14] found that in Philadelphia, persons who frequently use facilities providing emergency psychiatric services typically use the facilities as a point of entry to the mental health system. Moreover, although such patients account for only 20 percent of the unduplicated caseload, they use 60 percent of all service hours and constitute 55 percent of all admissions. These patients are not part of an organized program appropriate for their needs, and their unpredictable episodic use of services causes crises in the system and is extremely costly. Officials in Philadelphia are making efforts to negotiate a capitation program with state and federal Medicaid authorities to manage the care of such high-risk patients in order to provide appropriate psychiatric care in conjunction with sophisticated psychosocial services. They believe they can do so within the current range of expenditures for these patients.

There are many uncertainties in capitation, but careful demonstrations that allow better management of expenditures for defined populations of patients at high risk must go forward. In 1986, Congress made specific provisions for such managed-care waivers in Medicaid-financed mental health services. Unlike the situation in traditional managed-care systems (health maintenance organizations [HMOs]), which share risks among enrollees, the objective of the new systems is to provide meaningful trade-offs among types of care for a population of high-risk patients. Thus, the design of a managed-care system for these patients should not be confused with the inclusion of patients with chronic mental illnesses into mainstream HMOs, where such patients typically do not fare well.[15] The idea of capitated care targeted to patients with chronic mental illnesses requires a sophisticated and responsible mental health entity that has the authority and organizational capacity to balance community and inpatient care, as well as psychiatric and social services. In many communities, the framework and spectrum of necessary services are deficient, but managed care contributes to a resource base and incentive to develop the necessary components of service into a system.

Building a strong organizational structure that can give coherence to the system of services for the chronically mentally ill is central to the types of tasks that must be addressed if a true alternative for hospitalization is to be developed on a broad basis. The effectiveness of doing so has been demonstrated in selected programs and in some controlled clinical trials.[6,16,18] The Stein and Test "training in community living" model, which combines aggressive psychiatric community care with case management and training in psychosocial skills, has been partly or entirely adopted in a number of communities.[19] In the period 1979 to 1981, the model was replicated in Sydney, Australia, and evaluated in a randomized controlled trial. The outcomes were favorable as compared with those achieved with traditional care.[20] At the 12-month follow-up, for example, almost two thirds of the patients who had received the experimental treatment were very satisfied, as compared with less than one third of controls. Similarly, 83 percent of the relatives of patients in the experimental-treatment group with whom the patients lived were very satisfied with treatment, as compared with 26 percent of the controls.

The challenge is to learn how to adapt successful models developed in smaller communities to more complex urban, political, and professional environments. The Sydney experience suggests that such an effort is feasible. In a recent review, Kiesler and Sibulkin[21] identified 14 experimental studies, most of which incorporated random assignment, demonstrating that community alternatives were more effective than hospitalization across a wide range of patient populations and treatment strategies. Substantial organizational barriers persist. The catchment-area concept that has dominated community mental health services divides large cities into multiple relatively autonomous service units. Within a catchment-area framework, chronically ill patients are easily lost to follow-up, and the limited population base makes it difficult to organize specialized services, such as jail diversion and programs for patients with multiple illnesses and for homeless mentally ill persons. In addition, the mental health system typically is not in a position in the structure of local governments to allow it to influence non-health-related local services required to build an effective alternative to hospital care. Often, mental health services remain under the jurisdiction of the state government, whereas public housing, welfare, and police services necessary for effective psychiatric emergency response systems are controlled by the city or county government. The challenge is to integrate services at the local level without diminishing existing state financial obligations.

Since housing is a particularly critical element in developing an alternative to hospital care, it serves as an example of the gap between the present and potential opportunities. Mental health agencies in large cities have limited available housing placements, despite the facts that homelessness is an acute problem among mentally ill persons and that housing is an integral part of the therapeutic care plan. In many of our largest cities, as little as 5 to 10 percent of the estimated housing placements needed are available to the mental health services system. A range of housing options, from supervised group homes and apartments to scattered site locations, is essential. Many chronically mentally ill persons are eligible for housing assistance but receive little attention from city housing authorities who have no understanding of their special needs, or from mental health centers who have limited understanding of how to garner a larger share of public housing resources. A strong local mental health entity could develop sufficient expertise in housing to collaborate more effectively with the public housing authority and nonprofit developers in order to initiate joint ventures to provide suitable housing opportunities for this population. The availability of crisis support for landlords has been useful in achieving successful housing placements in the Training for Community Living Program in Dane County, Wisconsin,[19] and in community programs in Boston managed by the Massachusetts Mental Health Center.[22] In reality, this is not a large service burden, but the promise that help, if needed, is available on a 24-hour basis gives landlords, employers, police, and others sufficient confidence to cooperate. Such efforts have not been attempted in many larger cities, and the approach still requires evaluation.

The success of programs in each of the above areas has been demonstrated in one setting or another, but rarely do such programs come together in a single community. The difficulty of consolidating the necessary administrative authority, control over financing, and complex intraorganizational relations necessary is an important part of our present crisis and future challenge. An effectively constituted public organization with the ability to direct substantial resources and with credibility would make it possible to link components essential for maintenance of function and rehabilitation into a responsible and effective alternative to care in a mental hospital.

References

1. Mechanic D. Mental health and social policy. 2nd ed. Englewood Cliffs, N.J.: Prentice-Hall, 1980.
2. Gronfein W. Incentives and intentions in mental health policy: a comparison of the Medicaid and Community Mental Health programs. J Health Soc Behav 1985; 26:192–206.
3. Lamb HR, ed. The homeless mentally ill: a task force report of the American Psychiatric Association. Washington, D.C.: American Psychiatric Association, 1984.
4. Rossi PH, Wright JD, Fisher GA, Willis G. The urban homeless: estimating composition and size. Science 1987; 235:1336–41.
5. Mechanic D. The challenge of chronic mental illness: a retrospective and prospective view. Hosp Community Psychiatry 1986; 37:891–6.
6. Stein LI, Test MA, eds. Alternatives to mental hospital treatment. New York: Plenum Press, 1978.
7. Weisbrod BA, Test MA, Stein LI. Alternatives to mental hospital treatment. II. Economic benefit-cost analysis. Arch Gen Psychiatry 1980; 37:400–5.
8. Mechanic D. Correcting misconceptions in mental health policy: strategies for improved care of the seriously mentally ill. Milbank Q 1987; 65:203–30.
9. Faulkner LR, Bloom JD, Bray JD, Maricle R. Medical services in community mental health programs. Hosp Community Psychiatry 1986; 37: 1045–7.
10. Stein LI, Ganser LJ. Wisconsin system for funding mental health services. In: Talbott J, ed. New directions for mental health services: unified mental health systems. San Francisco: Jossey-Bass, 1983:25–32.
11. Aiken LH, Somers SA, Shore MF. Private foundations in health affairs: a case study of the development of a national initiative for the chronically mentally ill. Am Psychol 1986; 41:1290–5.
12. Taube CA, Barrett SA, eds. Mental health, United States, 1985. Washington, D.C.: Government Printing Office, 1985. DHHS publication no. (ADM) 85–1378.
13. Redick RW, Witkin MJ, Atay JE, Manderscheid BW. Specialty mental health organizations, United States, 1983–84. Washington, D.C.: Government Printing Office, 1986. DHHS publication no. (ADM) 86–1490.
14. Surles RC, McGurrin MC. Increased use of psychiatric emergency services by young chronic mentally ill patients. Hosp Community Psychiatry 1987; 38:401–5.
15. Schlesinger M. On the limits of expanding health care reform: chronic care in prepaid settings. Milbank Q 1986; 64:189–215.
16. Falloon IRH, Boyd JL, McGill CW, et al. Family management in the prevention of morbidity of schizophrenia: clinical outcomes of a two-year study. Arch Gen Psychiatry 1985; 42:887–96.
17. Stein LI, Test MA. Alternatives to mental hospital treatment. I. Conceptual model, treatment program, and clinical evaluation. Arch Gen Psychiatry 1980; 37:392–7.

18. Leff J, Kuipers L, Berkowitz R, Eberlein-Vries R, Sturgeon D. A controlled trial of social intervention in the families of schizophrenic patients. Br J Psychiatr 1982; 141:121–34.
19. Stein LI, Test MA, eds. Training in community living model: a decade of experience. New directions for mental health services, no. 26. San Francisco: Jossey-Bass, 1985.
20. New South Wales, Department of Health. Psychiatric hospital versus community treatment: a controlled study. Sydney, Australia: Department of Health, 1983. HSR 83–046.
21. Kiesler CA, Sibulkin AE. Mental hospitalization: myths and facts about a national crisis. Newbury Park, Calif.: Sage, 1987.
22. Gudeman JE, Shore MF. Beyond deinstitutionalization: a new class of facilities for the mentally ill. N Engl J Med 1984; 311:832–6.

27

Bachrach, L. L. (1988). Defining chronic mental illness: A concept paper. *Hospital and Community Psychiatry, 39* (4), 383–388

Leona Bachrach is the great "synthesizer" of community psychiatry. She has examined theories and practices of deinstitutionalization at multiple levels, including the meaning of "least restrictive environment," deinstitutionalization as a series of distinct but related strategies and policies, lessons learned about homelessness and mental illness (at a critical period of trying to understand the link between the two), and model public mental health programs. Bachrach sums up current understanding and progress at the time of her writing and proposes frameworks from which to approach the challenge of providing effective community-based treatment and social services to persons with serious mental illnesses. In this article Bachrach takes on a topic—chronic mental illness—that, like deinstitutionalization or least restrictive environment, is used freely but imprecisely, and asks the obvious but difficult question, "What do we really mean when we use this term?" She approaches the definition of chronic mental illness via the elements of diagnosis, duration, and disability, but notes that there is no consensus on the relative importance of these elements or quite what they are in the first place. In the end, she stops just this side of a definition of chronic mental illness but clarifies and provides guidance on how to approach its constitutive elements in service planning and research.

Defining Chronic Mental Illness: A Concept Paper

Three criteria—diagnosis, duration, and disability—are gaining currency in efforts through-out the United States to define the concept of chronic mental illness in a precise manner. However, there is presently no consensus on the specific character or relative importance of these criteria. Nor is there consensus on the nature of the interrelationships among these elements. These conceptual concerns must be resolved if uniformity in service planning and research on the chronic mentally ill is to be achieved.

He who speaks in favor of unclarity raises a justifiable suspicion that he merely seeks to attract attention; or worse, that he is promoting a subtle form of anti-intellectualism. To be accused of either is a serious matter, but every now and then, I think, someone must run the risk in hope of sensitizing us once more to the ever-present dangers of language. Language should periodically be put on trial, and when it is, even its accepted virtues, e.g., clarity, must be doubted.

—Garrett Hardin (1)

The adjective "chronic" is defined, according to Webster, as "lasting a long time or recur-ring often" or, alternatively, as "continuing indefinitely; perpetual, constant." Consistent with its Greek origins, the word implies a persistent longitudinal course. It is often used to describe the progress of a disease or an illness, and it is to be distinguished from the word "acute," which implies a course of more limited duration.

The definition provided in the dictionary seems simple enough. Yet the meaning of chronicity eludes mental health service planners and mental health service researchers, for the notion of persistence lacks a clear empirical referent. May persistence be inferred from certain specified diagnoses? Does it refer to an individual's experience of active symptoms associated with his or her illness? Or does it refer instead to the functional disabilities that result from having the illness?

These are important questions, for it is becoming increasingly clear that the two events, illness and disability, are neither synonymous nor coterminous (2). Several British authori-ties argue persuasively that disability may endure long after the primary symptoms of an illness have disappeared (3,4). They assert further that some sources of disability—the so-called tertiary disabilities or "social disablements"—are actually extrinsic to the individual and have their roots in societal reactions to the mentally ill rather than in the illness itself.

In addition to confusion about how to establish persistence, there is considerable dis-agreement over which psychiatric conditions or diagnoses might qualify an individual as being chronically mentally ill. Although psychotic disorders such as organic brain syn-drome, schizophrenia, major affective disorder, and paranoid and other psychoses gener-ally raise little question, there is less certainty about diagnoses such as personality disorder, alcohol and drug abuse disorders, and mental retardation (5).

Concern over our failure to delineate chronic mental illness in a precise manner is quite recent. In the days before deinstitutionalization, relatively little thought was given to the meaning of persistence in mental illness, to the distinction between major and minor diagnoses, or to the difference between illness and disability in establishing chronicity. Because most people identified as mentally ill were admitted to state mental hospitals, and because they usually stayed in those hospitals for very long times—often for life—illness and disability tended to be indistinguishable, and both tended to be defined in terms of the locus of care (6).

There was, in effect, a single criterion for chronicity: hospitalization. To be a patient in a state mental hospital was to be identified as having a chronic mental illness—a situation captured in a characterization of chronic mental patients as individuals who had previously been, who currently were, or who but for deinstitutionalization policies and practices might be state hospital residents (7). This description, while hardly operational, was considered to have face validity (8).

Moreover, it is likely that in the past, attempts to draw more precise distinctions among mental patients—at least those who were admitted to state mental hospitals—would have been futile. Protracted institutional residence tended to minimize observable individual differences among patients (9). Even if such distinctions were theoretically acknowledged, mental patients appeared to be more or less "all the same," and there was little need for a finer definition of chronicity.

With deinstitutionalization, however, the need for language that could acknowledge distinctions among mentally ill individuals became apparent. New directions in service planning and service delivery were focusing on the personal strengths of mentally ill people, and on the possibility of improving their functioning by matching treatment interventions to individual need. People with major mental disorders were no longer seen as static at best and immutably deteriorating at worst, and rehabilitation, the enhancement of each person's potential for living as a productive member of society (10), was increasingly viewed as an essential ingredient of treatment (11).

Criteria of Chronicity

This altered, more refined, view of the correlates of mental illness is reflected in official designations of chronic mental illness in use in several states. For example, the Arizona Checklist for Chronic Mental Illness Determination (12) uses the following definition:

> The chronically mentally ill are defined as those persons whose emotional or behavioral functioning is so impaired as to interfere grossly with their capacity to remain in the community without supportive treatment or services of a long-term or indefinite duration. The mental disability is severe and persistent, resulting in a long-term limitation of their functional capacities for primary activities of daily living such as interpersonal relationships, homemaking and self-care, employment, or recreation. The mental disability may limit their ability to seek or receive local, state, or federal assistance such as housing, medical and dental care, rehabilitation services, income assistance and food stamps, or protective services. Although persons with primary diagnoses of mental retardation or organic brain syndrome frequently have similar problems or limitations, they are not to be included in this definition.

"Prior hospitalization often is the standard for extending benefits and entitlements to the mentally ill. This approach has prejudicial effects on service accessibility for many patients."

This official document goes on to pinpoint diagnoses in the *DSM-III* 295 through 301 series—which includes such designations as schizophrenic disorders, affective disorders, and personality disorders—as qualifying conditions, and it defines specific medical and psychosocial criteria for their inclusion.

Thus the three criteria of diagnosis, duration, and disability—that is, impaired functioning associated with a major mental disorder over a long period of time—are used in the Arizona definition. Moreover, these same criteria are gaining currency throughout the nation (5,6,13,14) even though, as previously noted, there is little consensus about their specifics.

However, a growing acceptance of these criteria has also led to acknowledgment of how difficult it is to operationalize them—to give them precise dimensions. In addition to disagreement over which diagnoses to include and which kinds of disabilities to consider, there is uncertainty about the length of time that a person must be ill or impaired in order to qualify as chronically mentally ill. And the duration criterion is even further confounded by the periodic or episodic nature of many individuals' illnesses and related disabilities.

To complicate matters further, little consistent thought has been given to the matter of how to consider the *interactions* of the three criteria. How should the relationship between diagnosis and disability be viewed? Is major mental illness in the absence of severe functional disability sufficient to render an individual chronically mentally ill? Is severe functional disability in the absence of major mental illness sufficient? How much of each is necessary? Should disability supersede or be secondary to diagnosis? And, beyond this, should the duration criterion be applied to the illness itself, to the disability, or to both?

However, despite these very real problems, the disability criterion is emerging today as a strong contender for primacy in the definition of chronic mental illness. There appears to be growing consensus that disability should be given consideration at least equal to that of diagnosis, and probably more (15). Diagnosis is, in short, a necessary but not sufficient condition for defining chronic mental illness.

Hospitalization as a Criterion

There is, however, a disparity between these emerging academic views on mental illness and the actual practice of applying standards for chronicity in service planning and service delivery. Perhaps because the problems of operationalizing the three criteria of diagnosis, disability, and duration are so great, a fourth criterion, prior hospitalization—a survival from an earlier era—often takes precedence in the real world of mental health service delivery.

Despite growing recognition of its irrelevance, the criterion of prior hospitalization remains a strong official and de facto indicator of chronicity in many jurisdictions. To be sure, the hospitalization criterion has undergone a change. Whereas in the past, its informal use as an indicator of chronicity was largely limited to care in state mental hospital settings, the hospitalization criterion today generally allows for care in short-term community-based inpatient facilities as well. Thus the original guidelines for eligibility in the federally supported community support program (CSP) for the chronic mentally ill require an individual to have been enrolled in either long- or short-term inpatient programs, institutional or community based (16). Indeed, prior hospitalization is the only criterion used consistently among states to define CSP eligibility (17).

This approach is problematic, for prior hospitalization, whether inside or outside of state mental hospitals, is often an extremely flawed indicator of chronicity. In today's deinstitutionalized service systems, many individuals who might otherwise be regarded as chronically mentally ill receive all of their care, if any, in outpatient settings (5,11,15). The continued use of prior hospitalization thus effectively denies some basic realities about service delivery to the mentally ill in the 1980s.

Were this simply a matter of words, the issue might be of small consequence. However, prior hospitalization has in many instances become the standard for extending benefits and entitlements to the mentally ill, and this approach has had a prejudicial effect on service accessibility for many individuals. Pepper and Ryglewicz (18) report, for example, that a major segment of the chronic mentally ill population is systematically denied New York State community support system services because of their failure to fulfill a prior-hospitalization criterion for eligibility.

Freedman and Moran (19) echo this concern: "Often the chronically mentally ill are defined *de facto* in terms of their eligibility for existing governmental programs. For example, if persons meet the eligibility criteria of a specific entitlement, such as the Federal Supplemental Security Income Program, or a specific program, such as the National Institute of Mental Health's Community Support Program, then they might be considered chronically mentally ill. This *de facto* method serves as a pragmatic way to place boundaries or limits on a rather diffuse population. But as the political and fiscal climate of government changes over time, the eligibility criteria and program regulations of these programs might tighten or relax, which in turn affects the nature and scope of the population defined as chronically mentally ill."

The practical effects of this situation are extremely serious. As Freedman and Moran (19) state, "These fluctuations in definition pose problems for legislators and policymakers who require a specific, constant, operational definition of chronic mental illness to identify current and future members of this population, evaluate the needs of these individuals, and plan effective programs for them."

Not only is service delivery affected; the reliance on prior hospitalization as the major criterion for establishing chronicity has similarly had confounding effects on the conduct of research. Studies purporting to investigate the outcomes of deinstitutionalization sometimes evaluate only those individuals who have been treated in inpatient settings, particularly state mental hospitals (20), and overlook the effects of that policy on the mentally ill who have never been hospitalized (21).

This is a serious concern, for research results may be inappropriately skewed when measurements are limited exclusively to individuals who fulfill the gate-keeping requirements for admission to the system of care and overlook nonparticipating individuals (22). Indeed, this concern does not apply only to prior hospitalization as a criterion of chronicity; it also extends to prior treatment of any kind. Increasingly, large numbers of individuals who might otherwise be considered chronically mentally ill use no mental health services whatever; they are entirely outside the system of care (23–25).

Research is also generally limited by the fact that the failure to operationalize criteria for chronicity has made it extremely difficult to collate findings and to generalize from existing and ongoing studies. State and local definitions of chronicity vary widely. While many of them continue to rely on prior hospitalization, others are beginning to eschew this criterion. However, even when prior hospitalization is accepted as a valid criterion, the specifics about length of stay or number of admissions are highly inconsistent. One is tempted to paraphrase Humpty Dumpty to say that any research effort concerning the chronic mentally ill is free to proceed on the basis that the word chronic means "just what I choose it to mean, neither more nor less."

It is thus clear that the important criteria for establishing chronicity—diagnosis, disability, and duration—are difficult to operationalize, while the one that is easy to operationalize—prior hospitalization—survives despite its limited relevance.

Alternatively, research is often conducted in the absence of *any* definition of chronicity. For example, Harding and her colleagues (26), in an article summarizing their research on the chronic mentally ill, effectively take the research community to task for viewing chronicity in a biased manner. Yet, on closer examination, these investigators themselves fail to provide a working definition of chronicity and, in fact, implicitly and casually equate that term with a diagnosis of schizophrenia (27).

Chronicity as Forecasting

Three essential factors have thus far been discussed as major contributors to the problems associated with defining chronicity among the mentally ill. First, chronic mental illness is a composite designation in which some elements are more readily ascertained than others. Second, there is no consensus on the specific character or the relative importance of the composite elements. Third, there is no consensus on the interrelationships among the composite elements.

A fourth critical factor is the fact that ascertainment of the composite elements requires the employment of subtle forecasting techniques. It is essential to predict the duration of the diagnosis, the disability, or both in order to establish chronicity.

Mental illness is not alone in the use of forecasting to establish chronicity. Patients with somatic illnesses such as cancer or diabetes are similarly designated as chronic according to the likelihood of their improvement over time. There is, however, a major difference— one that has contributed to accusations of "labeling" with the use of the term chronic mentally ill. In characterizing a somatically ill person as chronically ill, the probability of improvement is largely calculated, formally or informally, on the basis of observable clinical, laboratory, or other findings related to the illness itself; considerations relating to functional disability do not enter as they do in the case of chronic mental illness. For example, for a cancer patient, the size, location, and histological type of the lesion are primary in the prediction of chronicity. That the patient may be more or less disabled as the result of his or her illness is typically a secondary consideration. By contrast, it is not enough to forecast the duration of illness for the chronic mental patient. Forecasts of the duration of disability are at least as important as, and perhaps are more important than, predictions of the course of illness per se.

The Issue of Labeling

In the definition of chronic mental illness, the relationship between forecasting and stigma is a major concern. Many advocates for the mentally ill have taken issue with the term chronic mental illness on the basis that it predicts continued, often life-term, disability. They perceive the label as negative, limiting, and profoundly stigmatizing. And they note that, with proper resources and treatment, many mentally ill individuals whose course might otherwise be considered chronic show substantial improvement and that labeling in this manner consigns them to a hopeless future.

The issue of labeling is perceived as particularly pernicious when it is applied to a special subgroup of chronic mentally ill individuals, those identified as "young adult chronic patients" (28). Generally described as being between the ages of 18 and 35 and having a wide variety of diagnoses and multiple disabilities, these patients are described by Pepper and associates (23) as a "new generation of persistently dysfunctional young adults..., requiring new programs in community care."

Wintersteen and Rapp (28) note that using such a label is "inherently stigmatizing, since it can become an epithet to be applied to all patients with a major psychiatric diagnosis in this age group. It is likely to set up a pattern of self-fulfilling prophecies, in which clinicians unconsciously give up before they even begin."

Like Wintersteen and Rapp, Estroff (29) asserts that such a designation is an inherently pejorative one that blames the victim: "So many intractable problems sadden the lives of these individuals that it seems unjustifiable to add a pessimistic, condemnatory label to their sorrows."

Thus, although the historical value of the concept of the young adult chronic patient is acknowledged, for it is a term that has uniquely alerted service planners and service providers to the changing needs of chronic mentally ill individuals (25), it has evoked considerable concern. And these criticisms of the concept of the young adult chronic patient may in fact be extended to more general use of the term chronic. On the other hand, on a pragmatic level, the failure to note persistence of disability, particularly when it is combined with periodicity, may prejudice the provision of disability benefits to many persons who require them.

Using Substitute Terminology

The very word chronic is thus a source of controversy, some of which potentially might be avoided through the adoption of alternate terminology (30). In fact, the literature contains some references that seek to substitute the word "severe" or "serious" for the word chronic (31–35). However, using such a substitute does not attack the very real methodological problems inherent in precisely defining and achieving consensus on the three basic criteria of diagnosis, disability, and duration or their complex interactions. Nor does using such a substitute alleviate the operational problem of weighting the relative contributions of these three criteria. Most important, using the word severe or serious does not attend sufficiently to the need to acknowledge the longitudinal nature of chronic mental illness and hence to make forecasts or predictions.

Some British investigators have overcome this problem by using the concepts of "old long-stay," "new long-stay," and "new long-term" mental patients. Old long-stay patients are those who were admitted to institutional care long ago and have remained institutionalized in spite of deinstitutionalization efforts. New long-stay patients constitute a group of long-term institutional residents building up from among recent admissions—patients who are unlikely to be considered good risks for community-based care and who will probably not be discharged.

New long-term patients, a recently added category (4), are those who "cannot be called 'long-stay' as they are not necessarily staying in hospital. Instead, they are moving between hospital admission wards, day services, hostels, family homes, etc." (3). By referring to these individuals, who are roughly similar in concept to young adult chronic patients (36), as new long-term patients, the British note their repeated and prolonged contact with the service system in the absence of long-term hospitalization.

While this British trichotomy conveys both duration and periodicity, and while it overcomes the disadvantages associated with using prior hospitalization as a criterion of chronicity, it fails to take into account the growing numbers of individuals who might be described as chronically mentally ill but who are essentially untreated in the mental health service system. As Goldman and associates (5) note, substantial numbers of such individuals—by some definitions, a majority of the chronic mentally ill—are treated outside the formal mental health service system (11). And, as indicated above, increasing numbers of individuals who might be considered chronically mentally ill receive no treatment at all.

Does it, then, make sense to discard the term chronically mentally ill in favor of a substitute concept? It is probable that dropping the word chronic altogether would have some immediate positive benefit in allaying the concerns of advocates. Labeling is, after all, deeply stigmatizing and itself imposes tertiary disabilities on the mentally ill (3,4). However, it is also probable that, in the long run, any terminology suggesting a long-term continuing course of illness or disability will take on stigma and will eventually be viewed as inappropriate. The word chronic at least has the advantage of familiarity.

"Dropping the term "chronic" might help allay the concerns of advocates. But in the long run, any language suggesting long-term continuing illness or disability likely will take on stigma."

Summary and Conclusions

Whether the term chronically mentally ill is endorsed, or whether substitute terminology is adopted, certain fundamental considerations must be observed in identifying the target population.

First, the definition must allow for a distinction between illness and functional disability, and consensus must be reached about whether one or the other of these criteria is to take primacy.

Second, consensus must be reached about which mental disorders, under what circumstances, are properly subsumed under the heading chronically mentally ill.

Third, the definition must allow for the duration-of-time factor implied in the word chronic, and consensus must be reached about how long a history of illness or disability is required. The definition must also allow for the possibility of periodicity. To expect persons who are called chronically mentally ill to be continuously ill, symptomatic, or disabled—to fail to acknowledge the possibility of episodic flare-ups or recurrences—is to deny clinical realities for some members of the target population.

Fourth, the definition must allow for forecasts of future illness or disability.

Fifth, the definition must minimize hospitalization and prior treatment as criteria for chronicity.

Sixth, the definition must allow for great heterogeneity within the target population. Unlike the target population of the predeinstitutionalization era, those who might be defined as chronically mentally ill today vary widely in their diagnoses, their treatment histories, their functional levels, and their treatment needs. Any definition that implies homogeneity in histories or treatment needs is flawed and potentially harmful to the target population.

Finally, the concept of disability to be employed in the definition of chronic mental illness must be operationalized so that a variety of classes of disability are tapped. Today's literature increasingly focuses on the idea that individuals who might be defined as chronically mentally ill suffer from more than one source of disability. Disabilities related to the illness itself, to the individual's unique responses to his or her illness, and to extrinsic societal influences (37) must all be considered.

New directions in service planning for the chronic mentally ill have introduced the need for more clarity and better precision in the use of concepts and terms (38). It is essential that the process of refining our language begin at the beginning: with the definition and description of the target population itself.

References

1. Hardin G: The threat of clarity. American Journal of Psychiatry 114:392–396, 1957
2. Gruenberg EM: Social breakdown in young adults: keeping crises from becoming chronic. New Directions for Mental Health Services, 14:43–50, 1982
3. Shepherd G: Institutional Care and Rehabilitation. London, Longman, 1984
4. Wing JK, Morris B: Clinical basis of rehabilitation, in Handbook of Psychiatric Rehabilitation Practice. Edited by Wing JK, Morris B. Oxford, England, Oxford University Press, 1981
5. Goldman HH, Gattozzi AA, Taube CA: Defining and counting the chronically mentally ill. Hospital and Community Psychiatry 32:21–27, 1981
6. Deitchman WS, French SD, Weerts TC: Defining chronic psychiatric disability: preliminary results. Community Support System Journal, 6:4–8, 1981
7. Bachrach LL: Deinstitutionalization: An Analytical Review and Sociological Perspective. Rockville, Md, National Institute of Mental Health, 1976
8. Talbott JA: A brief note concerning use of the term chronic mental patient, in The Chronic Mental Patient. Edited by Talbott JA. Washington, DC, American Psychiatric Association, 1978
9. Goffman E: Asylums: Essays on the Social Situation of Mental Patients and Other Inmates. Garden City, NY, Anchor, 1961
10. Anthony WA, Cohen MR, Cohen BF: Philosophy, treatment process, and principles of the psychiatric rehabilitation approach. New Directions for Mental Health Services, 17:67–79, 1983
11. Bachrach LL: A conceptual approach to deinstitutionalization. Hospital and Community Psychiatry 29:573–578, 1978
12. Checklist for Chronic Mental Illness Determination. Phoenix, Division of Behavioral Health Services, Arizona Department of Health Services, 1979
13. Minkoff K: A map of chronic mental patients, in The Chronic Mental Patient. Edited by Talbott JA. Washington, DC, American Psychiatric Association, 1978
14. President's Commission on Mental Health: Task Panel Reports Submitted to the President's Commission on Mental Health, vol 2. Washington, DC, 1978
15. Pepper B, Ryglewicz H: Treating the young adult chronic patient: an update. New Directions for Mental Health Services, 21:5–15, 1984
16. Goldman HH: Epidemiology, in The Chronic Mental Patient: Five Years Later. Edited by Talbott JA. Orlando, Fla, Grune & Stratton, 1984
17. Hoff MK, Ashbaugh JW, Schneider LC, et al: The chronically mentally ill: a descriptive analysis. Administration in Mental Health 10:171–180, 1983
18. Pepper B, Ryglewicz H: Concluding comments. New Directions for Mental Health Services, 14:121–124, 1982
19. Freedman RL, Moran A: Wanderers in a Promised Land: The Chronically Mentally Ill and Deinstitutionalization. Medical Care 22 (Dec suppl):Sl–S60, 1984
20. Solomon PL, Gordon BH, Davis JM: Community Services to Discharged Psychiatric Patients. Springfield, Ill, Thomas, 1984
21. Bachrach LL: Deinstitutionalization: What do the numbers mean? Hospital and Community Psychiatry 37:118–119,121, 1986
22. Rossi PH: Issues in the evaluation of human services delivery. Evaluation Quarterly 2:573–599, 1978
23. Pepper B, Kirshner MC, Ryglewicz H: The young adult chronic patient: overview of a population. Hospital and Community Psychiatry 32:463–469, 1981

24. Bachrach LL: Young adult chronic patients: an analytical review of the literature. Hospital and Community Psychiatry 33:189–197, 1982
25. Bachrach LL: The concept of young adult chronic psychiatric patients: questions from a research perspective. Hospital and Community Psychiatry 35:573–580, 1984
26. Harding CM, Zubin J, Strauss JS: Chronicity in schizophrenia: fact, partial fact, or artifact? Hospital and Community Psychiatry 38:477–486, 1987
27. Bachrach LL: Chronicity in schizophrenia (ltr). Hospital and Community Psychiatry 38:1226–1227, 1987
28. Wintersteen RT, Rapp CA: The young adult chronic patient: a dissenting view of an emerging concept. Psychiatric Rehabilitation Journal 9:3–13, 1986
29. Estroff SE: No more young adult chronic patients. Hospital and Community Psychiatry 38:5, 1987
30. Knisley MB: Watch your language: a call to abandon stigmatizing terms such as "the young adult chronic patient." Tie Lines (Information Exchange on Young Adult Chronic Patients, New York):5(Jan), 1986
31. California Lieutenant Governor's Task Force for the Seriously Mentally Ill: An Integrated Service System for People With Serious Mental Illness: A Preliminary Proposal. Sacramento, 1987
32. Denver, Colorado Division of Mental Health. Definitions for Chronic, Critical, and Serious. Denver, Colorado Division of Mental Health, 1987
33. Hargreaves WA, Legoullon M, Gaynor J, et al: Defining the severely disabled. Evaluation and Program Planning 7:219–277, 1984
34. Columbus, Ohio Department of Mental Health Counting Procedures for Severely Mentally Disabled Persons. Columbus, Ohio Department of Mental Health, 1985
35. Sullivan JP: Case management, in The Chronic Mentally Ill: Treatment, Programs, Systems. Edited by Talbott JA. New York, Human Sciences Press, 1981
36. Bachrach LL: The context of care for the chronic mental patient with substance abuse problems. Psychiatric Quarterly 58:3–14, 1987
37. Bachrach LL: Dimensions of disability in the chronic mentally ill. Hospital and Community Psychiatry 37:981–982, 1986
38. Bachrach LL: Slogans and Euphemisms: The Functions of Semantics in Mental Health and Mental Retardation Care. Austin, Tex, Hogg Foundation, 1985

28

Wing, J. K. (1990). The functions of asylum. *British Journal of Psychiatry, 157,* 822–827

Asylum carries mostly negative association across the 50-plus year span of community psychiatry, conjuring institutional noncare where people are warehoused with little treatment and no opportunity to live a life they could have lived in a more humane environment outside of institutions. Yet *asylum,* like refuge, is a beautiful word, rich in history and, paradoxically, in association with human freedom. In the Pentateuch, a man who has harmed another through no fault of his own, or whose brother has killed a man, finds safety from unjust vengeance in a city of refuge. In the Middle Ages and beyond, those being persecuted for political and other reasons sought asylum in the church. Wing writes of asylum that provides rest, refuge, and recuperation for people suffering from psychosis, difficult life circumstances, stigma, or inability to care for themselves at a given point. The availability of such services, Wing argues, is essential to a humane system of mental health care whether it is provided in a large psychiatric hospital or a community residence. If asylum is not available, he writes, then community care will fall short of providing a core component of comprehensive mental health, and ultimately will come to have a bad name, as asylum does today due to the failures of long-term state hospitalization for persons with serious mental illnesses.

The Functions of Asylum

Many of the functions of large psychiatric hospitals were those of asylum. As the structure of services has changed and the role of the large hospital has diminished, the necessity to continue to cover their functions has tended to be forgotten, partly because it has been thought that, even at best, they were purely protective. Such a point of view cannot be sustained. The functions of asylum have always been both refuge and recuperation. "Community care" will come to deserve the odium now attached to the worst practices of former times if the tradition of asylum practised in the best of the large hospitals is not (with appropriate modification) acknowledged, properly placed in the psychiatric curriculum, and given high priority in service planning.

When Mr Enoch Powell, then Minister of Health, made his famous speech to the National Association of Mental Health in 1961 he made the following central point:

"Building hospitals is not like building pyramids, the erection of memorials to endure to a remote posterity. We have to get into our heads that a hospital is like a shell, a framework to contain certain processes, and when the processes are superseded, the shell must, most probably, be scrapped and the framework dismantled." (Powell, 1961)

This serves as text for a commentary on community care in the 1990s, but for 'framework and process' I will substitute 'structure and function'

The functions that were being superseded were those of bad institutions - authoritarian, custodial and deadening. They were the reason for the reaction against the idea of institutions more generally. However, as Titmuss (1959) had earlier pointed out:

"No such swing of opinion away from the *good* institution can be discerned: the effective general hospital for the acutely ill, the public school and other socially approved forms of institutional care. But these have been experienced and remembered only by a minority; for most people institutional life has spelt little besides ugliness, cheapness and restricted liberties."

The Oxford English Dictionary (OED) definition of 'asylum' actually conjures up quite a warm and humanitarian image: "inviolable protection"; "a secure place of refuge, shelter or retreat". One of the illustrations given is a quote from 1728: "A port, where his ships might find an azylum". The functions of asylum are those of a haven: to provide a calm and peaceful environment, protection from violence outside, and a base for repair; and reprovision. These functions may be carried out in "a benevolent institution ... for some class of the afflicted, the unfortunate or destitute". The OED gives several examples of such classes, but adds a rider to that of the lunatic asylum, to the effect that the term 'asylum' is sometimes popularly restricted to this one type.

The labels we give to our concepts should be no more than a shorthand for a more extended description that others can check against their own observations. However, in everyday usage some words tend to take on a connotation that owes more to emotion than to reason. 'Asylum' is one of these. It is often popularly restricted in meaning, if not to an 18th-century madhouse, then to a 'total institution' as pictured by Goffman (1961)—Asylum with an upper case 'A'. The 'community', on the other hand, tends to be seen as a cohesive and caring neighbourhood, although there are very few such in industrialised societies. 'Asylum' then becomes a convenient Aunt Sally, while being in the 'community', by a process of tautology, becomes an administrative goal in itself. I propose to adopt the OED definitions, which allow an impartial examination of the extent to which asylum (lower case 'a') functions are being carried out, whatever the nature of the setting.

'Asylum' in the 18th and 19th Centuries

When William Tuke, in 1792, set up an establishment for the 'moral treatment' of the insane he did not wish to call it either an asylum or a hospital. "York already possessed an asylum, operating under conditions which made the use of the term a mockery, and the Retreat was not a hospital." William Tuke had a strong distrust of the medical profession and its methods. Daniel Hack Tuke states that 'The Retreat' was suggested by his grandmother, William's daughter-in-law, "to convey the idea of what such an institution should be, namely ... a quiet haven in which the shattered bark might find the means of reparation or of safety" (Jones, 1972, p. 47). The functions of asylum that Samuel Tuke described in his *Description of the Retreat,* published in 1813, were very similar to those put forward by Pinel in his *Traité Médico -Philosophique sur l'Aliénation Mentale* of 1801 (Pinel, 1806). Both regarded the functions as twofold—refuge and recuperation.

To John Conolly (1830) the lunatic asylums and madhouses with which he was acquainted were not fit for the care of the insane, whether acutely disturbed or convalescent: "so long as one lunatic associates with another lunatic, supposing the cases to be incurable, so long must the chances of restoration to sanity be very materially diminished." But in view of the squalour, disease and misery endured by the sane in larger towns, what was the alternative? Scull (1989) quotes MacGill, writing in 1810: "... the circumstances of the great body of mankind are of such a nature as to render every attempt to recover insane persons in their own houses extremely difficult, and generally hopeless."

Scull argues: "To improve the living conditions of lunatics living in the community would have entailed supplying relatively generous pension or welfare benefits to provide for their support, implying that the living standards of families with an insane member would have been raised above those of the working class generally ... something approximating a modern social welfare system, while their brethren were subjected to the rigours of a Poor Law based on the principle of less eligibility." This has a familiar ring to it.

Conolly's antipathy to asylums was restricted to their use for curable cases ("two-thirds, or I might say four-fifths of the cases of reception"), and he was particularly concerned about those "who have been accustomed to refined society" (Conolly, 1830). When he introduced the principle of non-restraint to the large asylum at Hanwell, following Gardiner Hill's demonstration at Lincoln, he seemed tacitly to accept that his earlier estimate of prognosis had been optimistic. Conolly's success at Hanwell provided an acceptable alternative both to the madhouses and to the community neglect of the time, and gave a much needed gloss to the public image of the asylum. In this way he contributed to the growth and systematisation of the asylum system during the next 100 years.

I am not here concerned with the merits and demerits of that system, except to point but that the structure within which the functions of asylum are carried out must, as Scull suggested, always be judged within the context of the social conditions of the time. I would add the context of medical and social knowledge to that. There must always be a balance between the protective and the rehabilitative functions. The reason for beginning with this brief historical sketch is to set the scene for the changes that have occurred since the 1920s, interrupted and then accelerated by World War II.

'Asylum' After World War II

During the late 1940s and the 1950s the foundations of the welfare state were laid in legislation that included every aspect of social life—pensions, family allowances, education, unemployment and sickness benefits, a complex of personal social services, a national health service and provisions for the disabled and the destitute. The 'community' that had looked so threatening and brutalising, especially for vulnerable people, during the earlier stages of the industrial revolution, now seemed more welcoming. Parallel changes, which Alexander Walk called "back to moral treatment", were made in the mental hospitals.

All the techniques of rehabilitation and resettlement now accepted as good psychiatric practice were introduced or reintroduced in hospitals like Glenside, Netherne and Warlingham well before the introduction of reserpine and chlorpromazine. The same is true of admission policies like that at Mapperley, where the emphasis on care outside hospital originated before the war when Duncan Macmillan was medical officer of mental health for Nottingham, as well as superintendent of the mental hospital. However, the success of the new medications, the first really effective physical treatments to be introduced, reinforced the optimism of the time and made it inevitable that the structure of the mental health service must change. Perhaps the most obvious reason for this was that the acute symptoms of psychosis often abated within a few weeks of admission, and, if patients wanted to leave hospital, it was their right to do so. What became known, often disparagingly, as "the early discharge policy" leading to the 'revolving door' system of care, was at many hospitals not a policy at all but an acceptance of the inevitable.

Two theory-driven studies of the clinical and social practice at Netherne, Mapperley and Severalls hospitals, carried out during the 1960s, illustrate the variation in standards at the time. One compared the quality of the care provided in the three hospitals for long-stay women under the age of 60 with a diagnosis of schizophrenia, in order to test the assumption that there would be an association with disability. In 1960, the environment at Netherne was socially rich in most respects, particularly by comparison with Severalls. One of the central factors seemed to be length of time doing nothing, which was strongly associated with severity of negative symptoms, and was least prominent at Netherne. As the environment of Severalls Hospital improved in this respect during the subsequent eight years so did the level of disability of many of the residents who had been admitted in 1960 (Wing & Brown, 1970).

The other study was a five-year follow-up of patients with schizophrenia admitted to the same three hospitals in 19S6 (Brown *et al,* 1956). Here the hypothesis was that shorter hospital stay and greater contact with community services in Nottingham would be associated with a more favourable clinical course and less family burden. Unlike the in-patient study, however, no significant differences could be demonstrated. This was partly due to refusals by patients or families to accept follow-up visits, partly because there were not enough agencies to undertake long-term domestic and industrial rehabilitation, and partly because the most severely disabled people did not necessarily receive the most community contact. Such problems were not solved in any of the three areas. In fact, the average amount of time spent doing nothing by patients who were unemployed was higher than that of long-term in-patients in the first study.

A feature of both studies was that the general trends in the results could, with hindsight, have been predicted from a knowledge of the personalities of the medical superintendents of the three hospitals.

The functions of asylum can be specified in some detail from comparative research into the practice, at that time, of the best hospitals and of the new facilities set up outside to supplement their services. The first function (refuge, shelter, retreat, sanctuary) included protection from: cruelty; exploitation; intolerable stress; competition (e.g. if unable to compete for housing or work on the open market, or unable to use ordinary amenities for recreation); pauperism (insufficiency of food, light, heat, clothing and basic personal possessions); social and intellectual poverty and isolation; and harming self or others, whether by self-neglect or violence. The second function, reparation, included: identification of the causes of social disablement, by skilled diagnosis and psychosocial assessment; treatment, within the limits of contemporary medical knowledge, of the physical and mental disorders responsible for admission; and provision, within the limits of local social attitudes and facilities, of the means of rehabilitation and resettlement. In addition, a place was usually rapidly available at times of emergency, however difficult the problem, and all services were provided free.

The most typical structure within which these functions were being carried out, sometimes very well by the standards of the time but often not well enough, was the mental hospital estate, with its limited apparatus of outreach into the community and links to the medical and welfare departments, now abolished, of local authorities. Early in the history of Sunnyside Royal Hospital, near Montrose, a superintendent who gave thought to the question of how much land was needed, suggested four acres per patient. When I attended its 200th anniversary, Sunnyside looked not much more suitable for people trying to recuperate from severe mental disorders than the factory buildings that form the present 'state of the art' district general hospitals. Nevertheless, when working well, the system did have the substantial advantages listed above, as well as two more that tend to be forgotten. There was a relatively limited and identifiable line of responsibility to a physician superintendent at the top, and there were the appreciable benefits of space, trees and grass.

The disadvantages were mainly those of size, cheapness and overprotection: having wards the size of aircraft hangars; the necessity of conforming to timetabled routines because of low supervisory staff ratios; the restriction of individual choice; and the distance (in some cases) from centres of ordinary social activity. Stigma was also attached to the buildings and perhaps amplified the odium that is always accorded to deviant behaviour, whatever the setting. Scandals were not uncommon, usually in some part of the hospital that had become isolated from the rest and was not under vigilant supervision.

How far these advantages and disadvantages were specific to large institutions was a matter for intense debate then as it is now. Two compilations of papers provide a good account of the arguments (Freeman & Farndale, 1963; Freeman, 1965). Since the functions carried out by mental hospitals had changed so radically, Enoch Powell's point about the need to dismantle the structure seemed apposite. He did not say, however, what structure should be put in its place (Powell, 1989).

Several major problems were foreseen. Many long-stay patients lacked the motivation and the skills to achieve their own resettlement. On the hospital estate, or within reach of it, all the steps and landings on the three stairways of residential, occupational and social rehabilitation (Wing, 1986) *could* be provided. The staff, who were needed to help people mount at their own pace or (just as important) descend without falling precipitously to the bottom, *could* be in easy communication with each other.

This is not to say that they were, only that the structure allowed such functions. If services became geographically fragmented, and responsibility diffused between different statutory, voluntary and commercial organisations, integration into a well planned and interconnected whole could be difficult. Co-ordination between dispersed day and residential units would be particularly problematic. Further problems concerned the extent to which professionals would and could be replaced by informal carers (Abrams, 1978) and how far professionals would wish to continue to serve the most disabled patients if a wider choice of work were on offer (Wooff *et al*, 1986).

In order to judge the success of any structure, it is not sufficient only to improve on the standards of an isolated and poverty-stricken 2000-bed Victorian hospital with a chronic staff shortage, poor facilities and a reputation for scandals and neglect. The standard by which to judge any new structure should be fourfold: (a) whether the functions of asylum are being carried out at least as successfully as in the *best* hospital-based services of the past; (b) whether any disadvantages thought to be inherent in the old structure were being avoided; (c) whether problems specific to the new service were being introduced; (d) whether extra advantages were being derived by people who might once have become: long-term residents because of an increased interaction with their families and with the general public. Chief of these latter might be enhanced enabling functions that would provide greater choice to handicapped people than could have been provided in hospital and thus lead to a better quality of life.

Very few such studies on new structures have been published. The most comprehensive attempt to provide a full and integrated structure that would allow the catchment hospital to be closed was the Worcester Development Project (WDP). Substantial central resources were put into the area in order to make the demonstration. In particular, new day services were provided in generous measure along with two new acute psychiatric hospital units. The proceedings of the conference called to mark the final closure of Powick are now published (Hall & Brockington, 1990)—the financial, administrative and clinical statements made there will be examined carefully.

There were critical comments at the conference about health authorities that were proposing to close hospitals even though no alternative structure based on the WDP model had been established. However, very few districts in fact have such a range of services. Even if there were, Worcester and Kidderminster are substantially more socially advantaged than the average across the country, and it would be unwise to generalise from them to average or below-average districts. That not all the problems had been solved even in the WDP area was indicated by a story on the front page of the *Malvem Courier,* published during the conference. It began: "Care agencies in Malvern have expressed fears about the lack of support for people who have been discharged into the community from mental institutions." Scandals featured in the press now occur in the 'community' rather than in the hospitals. Torrey (1988) has described experiences of people discharged from American hospitals to an uncaring and hostile 'community' that are as harrowing as any described two centuries ago. Scandals may not be typical of the general level of care but that was also true of the hospital cases featured in the 1960s. Torrey is complimentary about the safety net provided by our own health and social services, but we have no reason for complacency.

Who Needs Asylum?

Most of the patients who used to accumulate in the large psychiatric hospitals even though their need for long-term high-dependency care had ceased, have now left. Very few new admissions lead to such long-term care. Many of the functions of asylum can be served by a variety of geographically and administratively separated agencies, as long as all the units are in place and there is co-ordination and cooperation to ensure smooth movement and sharing of functions between them. On the other hand, a fragmentation of functions and lack of a strong overall management policy, particularly when added to a scarcity of resources, must lead to disasters. The Commons' Social Services Committee report (1985) and Griffiths' proposals (1988) were designed to prevent this, but it is not clear how the procedures recommended in the White Paper on community care will promote continuity and provide the tough leadership, on a defined geographical basis, that is required.

Whether the functions of asylum can be completely fulfilled without an 'Asylum' as one component of a district service is as hotly debated now as it was 25 years ago. The word itself has been devalued but there is a measure of agreement that, at the bottom of the three stairways that should form the main framework of a comprehensive district structure for people with high-dependency needs associated with long-term mental disabilities, there should be a strong foundation on which the rest of the edifice rests; a haven of needed refuge but also a harbour from which to set out again. The name 'community', in the sense of a small group of people sharing common aims and needs, is much more appropriate to a place that continues the tradition of Tuke's Retreat than to the modern localities that are usually given the name (Abrams & McCulloch, 1976).

Two groups of people, with relatively well defined dependency needs, those with severe mental handicap or dementia, will not be considered here. A third, more heterogeneous group is represented by people with a variety of mental disorders who still, in spite of everything that is done (deliberately or by default) to prevent it, accumulate as long-stay hospital patients. There are many like them who do not acquire this status, but are to be found at home with their families, in bedsits or lodgings, in National Health Service (NHS) or local authority or charitable hostels or homes, in Salvation Army shelters, or in prison on remand or sleeping rough on the streets. It seems much more difficult, therefore, to estimate numbers or to assess their current status than it was in the 1960s. A much larger part of the prevalence is invisible. As the large hospitals run down further, and the small ones focus only on acute episodes, this element of uncertainty will seem to grow.

However, because there has been no major breakthrough in treatment or in methods of rehabilitation since Robertson (1981) made some projections based on trends in hospital statistics up to 1981, his figures do still provide a reasonable estimate of the numbers of people on behalf of whom many (in some cases all) of the functions of asylum still need to be exercised. Because of differing levels of social deprivation across health and local authority districts, no single formula can be applied, but the average for England works out at about 50 per 100 000 population. The kinds of psychiatric and social problems experienced by the people concerned are discussed elsewhere (Wing, 1986; Wing & Furlong, 1986).

So vociferous has been the condemnation of Asylums, and so universal the identification of Enoch Powell's out-of-date structure with the functions that it served, that very little attention, and virtually no experiment, has been devoted to the alternative structures that might serve the functions of asylum. It is a classic case of the baby and the bath water.

Such new structures might take two forms, depending on the availability of sites. Where a large hospital estate is conveniently situated in relation to the population it serves, a section could be reserved for a sheltered community, organised on the core and cluster model, with close connections to other parts of the service. The rest of the estate should be used imaginatively, with sectors devoted to housing, shops and leisure and business facilities that would become part of the neighbourhood as well as being available to patients. Most of the former hospital functions could be served from buildings that merged into the new complex without being specially identified. In this way, the 'community' would be brought on to a site where a mental hospital had stood for a century or more and where local people were familiar with its presence. John Burrell has worked out the architectural basis of the idea in substantial detail (Burrell, 1986).

Another possibility is the free-standing core and cluster model, although this might be at greater risk of becoming isolated from the rest of the district services and from the locality as well. One health region (South East Regional Health Authority, SETRHA, 1988) has adopted the name 'haven' but equated it with the more limited hospital-hostel concept (Hyde *et al*, 1987). At the Maudsley this is developing into a core and cluster arrangement with the central house and most day care on the hospital site and other houses off it (Wykes, 1982; Garety *et al*, 1988). Comparative research has not been undertaken into the merits and demerits of more extensive contemporary forms of sheltered community. But whatever structure is found to be most effective, a comprehensive and integrated district service requires co-ordinated planning, management and finance and a clear-cut policy for caring for the most persistently disabled people. It is essential to understand that such havens must be an integral part of such a district service. If the rest of the system is not in place and working, the name is inappropriate and should not be used (Wing, 1990).

Conclusion

Parry-Jones (1988) is generally sympathetic to the aims and practice of asylum with a small 'a', and sensitive to the swing of the pendulum during the 19th century from neglect to reform to neglect again – and then back during this century as far as reform. On the basis of his analysis, he could have added that the pendulum could still be swinging towards further neglect. If so, a way to stop it is to insist that the functions of asylum be fully incorporated into all the new structures, and tested for their efficacy, as we dismantle the old ones. Although these functions have been elaborated and systematised, they remain much the same as in the time of Tuke and Pinel. We have more effective medical treatments at our disposal which make the task of rehabilitation and settlement easier, and there is beginning to be a respectable body of knowledge about how to help and sustain families. Our social security system, whatever its faults, is immeasurably better than in the time of the Poor Law. However, the needs of severely and chronically disabled people still have a low priority and there is little sign that 'the district' has any therapeutic function in itself.

References

Abrams, P. (1978) Community care. Some research problems and priorities. In *Social Care Research* (eds J. Barnes & C. Connelly). London: Bedford Square Press.

____ & McCulloch, A. (1976) *Communes, Sociology and Society*. London: Cambridge University Press.

Brown, G. W., Bone, M., Dalison, B., *et al* (1966) *Schizophrenia and Social Care,* London: Oxford University Press.

Burrell, J. (1985) The *Psychiatric Hospital as a new Community*. London: Burrell-Foley Associates.

Conolly, J. (1830) *The Indications of Insanity*. London: Taylor. Republished with introduction by R. Hunter and I. Macalpine (1964). London: Dawsons.

Freeman, H. (ed.) (1965) *Psychiatric Hospital Care*. London: Baillière, Tindall & Cassel.

____ & Farndale, J. (eds) (1963) *Trends in the Mental Health Services*. Oxford: Pergamon Press.

Garety, P. A., Afele, H. K. & Isaacs, A. D. (1988) A hostel-ward for new long-stay patients. *Bulletin of the Royal College of Psychiatrists*, 12, 183–187.

Goffman, E. (1961) On the character of total institutions. In *Asylums*, ch. 1. Harmondsworth: Penguin.

Griffiths , R. (1988) *Community Care, Agenda for Action*. A report to the Secretary of State for Social Services. London: HMSO.

Hall, P. & Brockington, I. F. (eds) (1990) *The Closure of Mental Hospitals*. London: Gaskell.

Hyde, C, Bridges, K., Goldberg, D., *et al* (1987) The evaluation of a hostel ward. *British Journal of Psychiatry*, 151, 805–812.

Jones, K. (1972) *A History of the Mental Health Services*. London: Routledge & Kegan Paul.

Parry-Jones, W. Ll. (1988) Asylum for the mentally ill in historical perspective. *Bulletin of the Royal College of Psychiatrists*, 12, 407–410.

Pinel, P. (1806) *A Treatise on Insanity* (trans. D. D. Davis). Sheffield: Cadell and Davies.

Powell, E. (1961) Address to National Society for Mental Health. In *Emerging Patterns for the Mental Health Services and the Public*. London: NAMH.

____ (1989) In conversation with Enoch Powell. *Bulletin of the Royal College of Psychiatrists*, 12, 402–406.

Robertson, G. (1981) *The Provision of Inpatient Facilities for the Mentally Ill*. A paper to assist NHS planners. London: DHSS (Unpublished).

Scull, A. (1989) *Social Order/Mental Disorder. Anglo-American Psychiatry in Historical Perspective*. London: Routledge.

Social Services Committee, House of Commons (1985) *Community Care with Special Reference to Adult Mentally Ill and Mentally Handicapped*. Second report of the Committee. London: HMSO.

South East Thames Regional Health Authority (1988) *Mental Illness Services. The Need for a Haven*. Bexhill: SETRHA.

Titmuss, R. M. (1959) Community care as a challenge. *The Times*, 12 May.

Torrey, E. F. (1988) *Nowhere to Go*. New York: Harper & Row.

Wing, J. K. (1986) The cycle of planning and evaluation. In *The Provision of Mental Health Services in Britain. The Way Ahead* (eds G. Wilkinson & H. Freeman). London: Gaskell.

____ (1990) Meeting the needs of people with psychiatric disorders. *Social Psychiatry*, 25, 2–8.

____ & Brown, G. W. (1970) *Institutionalism and Schizophrenia*. Cambridge: Cambridge University Press.

____ & Furlong, R. (1986) A HAVEN for the severely disabled within the context of a comprehensive psychiatric community service. *British Journal of Psychiatry*, 149, 449–457.

Wooff, K., Goldberg, D. P. & Fryers, T. (1986) Patients in receipt of community psychiatric nursing care in Salford, 1976–1982. *Psychological Medicine*, 16, 407–414.

Wykes, T. (1982) A hostel ward for 'new' long stay patients. An evaluative study of a ward in a house. In *Long-Term Community Care. Experience in a London Borough* (ed J. K. Wing). *Psychological Medicine* (suppl.), 41–45.

Practice and Research Texts

29

Estroff, S. E. (1981). *Making it crazy: An ethnography of psychiatric patients in an American community.* Berkeley: University of California Press

Estroff writes of "making it" as a designated crazy person and of the "making of" a community-based program that presupposes and requires the craziness of its service recipients. *Making it Crazy*, published in 1981 but based on research Estroff conducted in the early 1970s, provides an invaluable ethnographic counterbalance to randomized controlled trials of community-based programs during the early years of deinstitution-alization. For the ethnographer, the only given about mental illness is the fact that it is ascribed to some persons and that these persons are the objects of various interventions and other actions taken to address their diagnosed illness. Her job is to become immersed in the culture and lives of its inhabitants, to describe it, and to reflect on its lived meaning and significance for its actors. Estroff's book, based on her research with the Program for Assertive Community Treatment (PACT) in Madison, Wisconsin, the predecessor for today's Assertive Community Treatment programs, is a seminal work in community psychiatry as well as of ethnography. It also gained notoriety for her anthropological pushing of the envelope in taking the psychiatric drug, Prolixin, for 6 weeks in order to experience its effects on her and her interactions with others. The excerpt here from the chapter "Normals, Crazies, and Outsiders" concerns social categories that patients in the PACT intervention constructed.

Normals, Crazies, and Outsiders

Inside Crazies

An Inside Crazy is a person who not only knows that ego is crazy but who is crazy as well. Ego and the Inside Crazy share this information, and they share a special quality of knowledge through experience with medications, psychosis, and psychiatric treatment. The Inside Crazy does not reject or avoid ego because ego is crazy. S/He may, in fact, know and associate with ego because both ego and other are crazy. There are no formal or necessary restrictions in sharing time and space. Most of the limits that exist are negotiated relatively freely between ego and other. However, some temporal-spatial sharing is not controlled by either party. Staff decides, for example, which social-skills groups the clients may attend and which activities they may join, thus determining to some extent which clients are together at these times. Discharge, loss or change of job, and loss or change of living space are also somewhat out of ego's direct control and may affect the relationship with other. Ego and other have nearly equal control of and access to resources such as money, living space, employment, and medications. An Inside Crazy is or can be involved in the reciprocal exchange system described in the previous chapter.

With few exceptions, the clients in this group shared most of their time, space, and resources with Inside Crazies, both in treatment and nontreatment activities. This sharing included romantic heterosexual relationships, such as those among five client couples, living in the same apartment as with six sets of clients, living in the same hotel or rooming house, or among the multiple pairs and groups of same sex friends within the group. A dozen clients had known each other in high school and through rock band connections prior to their PACT encounter, and six clients had become acquainted during concurrent stays on various psychiatric wards. The remainder came to be friends through PACT activities, through living and working in the same places, and through various treatment-related factors. Toward the end of the fieldwork period, the PACT staff began to encourage companionship among clients.

These Inside Crazy relationships exhibited some interesting features. As a rule, client friends did not discuss emotional or psychiatric problems with one another. Often there was very little verbal communication of any subject. Practical problems such as lack of money, a job, or eviction were mentioned much more frequently. Part of this was owing to PACT encouragement to share psychiatric difficulties with the program staff. For example, one social-skills session focused on referring a friend who was hallucinating to staff instead of working on the problem within the client group. Clients seemed to follow this rule independently, probably because they believed that people experiencing the same problems and deficits could offer little objective advice. At times, clients might encourage one another to stay in the treatment program, to take medications, to follow staff advice, or to go to work. At another time, they might give the opposite counsel.

Clients who seemed to be friends, sharing much time away from treatment activities, often lost contact if one were discharged, or moved home, or left a common work or living situation. Dorothy and Alice shared an apartment at the three-quarter way house for nearly a year, but upon Dorothy's departure to live with a male friend, the relationship ceased to be active. Ben and Pogo worked together at MOC, regularly ate dinner together, and even planned a joint suicide. But when Ben left MOC and moved to his parents' home after discharge, their comradeship did not continue. Some clients who developed no outside relationships remained among PACT and Inside Crazy friends even after discharge. On occasion, a client would disappear from the scene. Usually his or her Inside Crazy friends did not know that the person had been hospitalized, but I could ascertain the person's whereabouts from PACT staff.

A curious pattern of sharing and relating emerged. Even if time, space, and resources had been generously exchanged among Inside Crazies, the contingencies of PACT treatment, of periodic psychotic episodes, and of exits from the interpersonal system could be accepted in unquestioning fashion. Inside Crazies apparently had much in common, including their mutual appraisal of their friendship as satisfactory but ineffectual and powerless in coping with life problems. CAS responses revealed that this satisfaction indeed existed even though clients felt more distant from friends than they perceived friends to feel toward them, and even though friends did not help them when they were in need. This pattern may have been owing to the fact that Inside Crazies, like ego, were not seen to possess the material or mental resources necessary to provide mutual assistance and to engender feelings of trust and reliance. Inside Normals were the ones who possessed these resources. Inside Crazies perceived one another as satisfactory and accessible companions who occupied similar dependent and incompetent positions vis-à-vis all other types of persons. Clients' ambivalence and negative estimations of themselves were reflected in their judgments about their Inside Crazy friends.

Inside Crazies were usually fellow PACT clients. Also in this group were fellow clients at the county mental health center, and relatives or high school friends who had psychiatric difficulties. Salient characteristics were a relatively high quality and a large quantity of shared time, space, resources, and information, and an equivalency with regard to the symmetry of the exchanges. For example, Doc and Cy were Inside Crazies in relation to each other. They voluntarily shared large amounts of time, space, and resources, and each knew the same amount of information about the other. They drank together, loaned each other money and cigarettes, and shared an apartment.

Outside Crazies

This group comprised those that ego knew to be crazy by virtue of their being in PACT, or seeing them at the county mental health center, or in a psychiatric ward, sheltered workshop, or therapist's office. This may have been the only information, time, and space exchanged between the subjects. Simply having been in these places concurrently told each a great deal about the other. Resources were probably equal, but were not customarily exchanged, except for an occasional cigarette. Equal control of time and space existed, but these were not shared on a voluntary, purposeful, or consistent basis. Even though these persons might be in therapy groups together, or got their medications at the same times, or crossed paths when they utilized the same social services, they did so only because of system-dictated factors, not because they chose to share time, space, or information.

Outside Crazies were usually PACT clients in another research group or phase, or PACT clients with whom ego did not associate beyond group activities and coincidental meetings at the PACT house. They were also co-workers at sheltered workshops or fellow residents at the hotels or Y's. For example, Morris and Rod were Outside Crazies in relation to each other. They saw each other occasionally during PACT activities, on the street, or at the county mental health center. But they did not know where the other lived. No meals were shared and money did not pass between them. They shared special knowledge, namely, the subjective experience of psychosis and medications, being in PACT, receiving SSI, and being periodically hospitalized.

Other Outside Crazies included those half dozen clients in the research group who were loners, who preferred solitude to companionship of any kind, or who actively avoided identifying with or being seen with other clients outside the treatment setting. Another type of Outside Crazy was the person whom ego might encounter in a public situation, who, because of his behavior or appearance, could be identified as a crazy person. For example, one evening during a social-skills group, five clients and I decided to take a walk for our assignment. Along the way, we found an older man sitting on some steps that were overgrown with greenery and almost hidden from view. As we approached, we could hear that he was talking. No one was with him, and a row of cough-syrup bottles were lined up in front of him. He was addressing God in directive and familiar fashion. Steven turned to the rest of us and said, "He's crazy!" After we all shared a good laugh about the irony of Steven's remark, we walked on. This man was an Outside Crazy.

Only by virtue of their experiences, diagnoses, and PACT patienthood did Outside Crazies qualify for inclusion in the "us" part of the distinction between "us" and "them." Relative to insiders, they shared with ego a lower quality and a smaller quantity of time, space, information, and resources. Relative to Outside Normals, they shared with ego a higher quality and a larger quantity of these commodities. With regard to symmetry, Outside Crazies had equal control of what was shared with ego. Being in PACT directly influenced what could be shared. In other words, a certain amount of sharing was involuntary, but negotiation as equals usually characterized the exchange beyond this level. Having psychiatric difficulties and being in the same treatment program entailed sharing powerful intimacies over which clients could exert little control.

Inside Normals

This category included persons who were not crazy, and who were aware that ego was crazy, but who did not refuse to interact with ego. Many Inside Normals had contact with ego *because* they were presumed normals and ego was crazy. Inside Normals included PACT staff, therapists, family, community volunteers, financial guardians, supervisors and counselors at the sheltered workshops, and the DVR counselor. Inside Normals shared resources, time, space and information with ego, but in asymmetrical fashion. That is, control of and access to these factors was held by Inside Normals in nearly all instances.

For example, space was controlled by PACT staff at the PACT house and at their own residences. They did not disclose their home addresses to clients, and clients did not visit them at their homes. In fact, they contracted with clients' parents to keep clients away from their homes. But staff persons knew clients' addresses, entered their places of residence, sometimes provided rent money for the spaces, and could exercise control by admitting clients to the hospital. The DVR counselor, another Inside Normal, controlled resources, such as subsidy for sheltered workshop employment, rent, and clothing. Further, he controlled time with clients in that they could see him only by appointment. Inside Normals also had much more information about clients than vice versa.

Nonprofessional Inside Normals (normal friends) were rare in the clients' interpersonal network. Only five clients had friends who (to my knowledge) were not in some way involved in psychiatric treatment. The client group as a whole did not have insider relationships with normals who were not part of the psychiatric treatment delivery system. Many clients had difficulty understanding why I would spend time with them, or would even like them, demonstrating how unaccustomed they were to interaction with Inside Normals who were not somehow treating or advising them. This observation was confirmed when I met several friends of clients. They were strangers to me, but they quickly revealed their Mendota Mental Health Institute alumni status or their current psychiatric difficulties. It was as if they were identifying themselves to me so that I could categorize them, as if they, too, recognized the same divisions.

Four female clients engaged in periodic, short-lived sexual relationships with normal males they had met in bars. Dorothy was an exception, having developed a long-lasting romantic involvement with a man she had met at Alcoholics Anonymous. But members of that group term themselves "sick people," and Dorothy's shared problem with alcohol abuse brought them together. Myrtle married while in the PACT program, but she had met her spouse at Mendota Mental Health Institute. He had a long history of psychiatric difficulties and abuse of cough syrup. Dennis was one of the few clients who lived with and had friendships with normals, and he also married while in PACT. The marriage ended in divorce after six months. Although his friends did not have formal psychiatric problems, most were heavily involved with street drugs and maintained a counter-culture stance toward the "liberals" of the community at large.

The clients as a group had few relationships with normals other than those who were involved with them as professional or volunteer helpers. Some clients avoided these contacts, expressing frustration with and painful awareness of their inadequacies when they compared themselves with normals. Steven, for example, disliked seeing old friends from high school because he was ashamed to say that he was not working and had spent much time just trying to cope with daily living. He also indicated that he was embarrassed to be seen with other clients, even his friends, if he ran into a normal acquaintance. The contacts with normals that did occur for clients outside the help-giving system seemed to be short-lived, negative experiences that highlighted differentness.

Mixed exceptions to this were provided by various landlords, co-workers, volunteers, and employers who took special and genuinely caring interest in some clients. The asymmetry in giving help remained in these relationships, as did discrepancies in access to resources, but these interactions had decidedly fewer boundaries and limits than did the professional ones. For example, the client women's group was run by women volunteers from the community. These women would go to bars with the group, would drink with clients, would talk about their jobs, their families, their personal lives, and would take no active evaluative or directive role with the clients. The clients perceived these women as "leaders" and depended upon them for transportation, ideas, and sometimes advice, but they did not talk to them about symptoms and current clinical problems, and they exhibited a sense of managing information and personal disclosure distinct from their interactions with staff. An occasional landlord or employer would take special interest in a client, offering meals, companionship, special consideration on rent or work hours, and cooperation with PACT staff in reaching treatment goals. Edgerton (1967) described a similar, although more frequently occurring, relationship among his adult mildly retarded subjects and their benefactors.

Outside Normals

Outside Normals were community members who usually were not aware that ego was crazy. If they were, they exhibited neutral, negative, avoidance, and perhaps punitive responses. These persons were not among those with whom ego voluntarily shared information, time, space, and resources. In fact, Outside Normals were avoided by ego. This category included landlords, employers, police, business persons, and other community members who were not formally or informally involved in the mental health care system.

Clients interacted with Outside Normals as infrequently as possible. When they did, it was usually for a formal or goal-oriented purpose. My observation was that the same held true for Outside Normals vis-à-vis clients. Few persons other than those offering resources (such as apartments, food, or jobs) or services (such as police) had reason to interact with the clients. Except for university students, state employees, and downtown shoppers, few Outside Normals shared the temporal-spatial arena around the Square. When community events were held in this space, events such as the annual summer art fair and the weekly farmer's market, the client population tended to withdraw, stating that they did not like the crowds and all the new people.

A Closer Look at the System

Careful scrutiny of this classification scheme reveals some interesting features. It is perhaps most important to note that, in nearly every dimension, normals, both insiders and outsiders, had more control than clients and other crazy people over those aspects of living that attest to independent, positive selfhood. Clients' resources, in particular, were subject to almost total control by normals. For example, a PACT client could not obtain SSI money without the cooperation of the PACT staff and the service chief in verifying the disability and its causes. SSI workers then controlled the disbursement of the money, determining whether and when the client would receive it. A financial guardian usually controlled the use of the money, and this control could, in turn, influence how a client utilized his time (i.e., the amount of money available for entertainment, school, and travel).

During treatment, PACT staff had almost complete control in each area. When there was exchange, it was not equivalent. Staff had access to information about clients which clients did not have in relation to staff. Clients were unable to exchange resources with staff, for they had few resources to offer. The list of inequalities was nearly endless.

Clients, and others like them, were equal in relation to each other. Most had virtually equivalent access to and control of resources, time, space, and information. Those on SSI received the same incomes. The quality, size, and location of their living spaces were similar and were shared symmetrically. Any restriction on such sharing was voluntarily negotiated. Clients entered each others' living spaces, spent time with each other almost at will, and made loans to and borrowed from each other. They did not have to make appointments to see each other, as they usually did with normals, and they could engage in activities with each other, such as drinking alcohol, smoking marijuana, and having sex, that they did not customarily engage in with normals, especially with Inside Normals. Clients could also exercise control of the information and knowledge passed between them. There were no medical records, staff meetings, and therapy sessions to be communicated. Clients could choose what information they shared with each other. They could also choose what they shared with staff, but such information, once shared with staff, was taken in a sense out of clients' control and put into a systematic communication network.

Such a system did not enable clients to prove themselves independent, competent, and adequate in the face of life tasks. Opportunities for experiencing or even testing independence were not in abundance within the confines of the system. But many clients demonstrated consistent inability or lack of desire to take responsibility for, or control of, these dimensions of their lives. Clients often viewed responsibility and decision-making as stressful, but they became more dependent, ineffective persons by attempting to alleviate this discomfort, that is, by seeking treatment as unequals in a system where the help-givers appeared adequate, independent, and in control. Inside Normals, who promoted independence and control for and among clients, were bound, because of the values and structure of the social and treatment system, to frustrate their own attempts. Within the existing system, not being hospitalized did not automatically remove the messages of weakness, powerlessness, and incompetence from clients' environments.

Most research on the difficulties encountered in reintegrating the chronic mentally disabled, during psychiatric treatment, into communities, has focused on the exclusionary role played by community members (e.g., Aviram and Segal 1973; Schwartz et al. 1974). Little attention has been paid to the role played by clients themselves in creating and perpetuating the circumstances. Instead of perhaps further demeaning clients by perceiving them as passive victims of discrimination, it is possible to accord them more dignity and autonomy by ascertaining whether they *want* to be "integrated" and whether their isolation or clustering might not represent reasonable strategies.

Given the prevalence and power of the asymmetry that clients experience in relation to normals, by interacting primarily with other clients, they may be availing themselves of more opportunities to experience autonomy, symmetry, and reciprocity than they would encounter in any other sphere. By staying within the client group, they may, consciously or unconsciously, be choosing to identify with others in terms of commonly held values, resources, and experiences. Relatively speaking, this may represent a "healthy" choice. The painful and real obstacles to interacting symmetrically with normals dictate that many clients will feel far more comfortable, as we all do, among others like themselves. Comer and Piliavin (1972; 1975) found that physically handicapped persons exhibited and experienced more discomfort with a physically normal interviewer than with a physically handicapped interviewer. The highlighting of differentness in relation to others, especially when that differentness is negatively valued, may be sufficiently stressful, to clients that they are innately wise to avoid such contacts.

In no way would I justify excluding these people from our lives or communities by saying "they want it this way." I would simply suggest that we view the processes of integration as being broadly interactive, that we acknowledge the client's capacity for choice, and that we not be ethnocentric, trying instead to understand the phenomenon from the insider's perspective. Most important, we should reexamine our own roles in perpetuating the asymmetries as we seek alternative means of relating to these people.

From a different perspective, Chamberlain (1978) suggests that one reason psychiatric patients ultimately concur with normals' evaluations of themselves as "sick" or "incompetent" is that they usually are not permitted or encouraged to help one another. This was true at PACT, but, as the CAS responses revealed, clients themselves perceived their friends as not giving help when it was needed. My ethnographic data are filled with clients' remarks about one anothers' craziness and incompetence. The empirical question should be raised as to whether these attitudes can be changed. Perhaps they are inevitably responsive to the messages that are explicit and implicit in the treatment system and our culture. We know very little about friendships among clients, their social and interpersonal networks, and the impact that these have on their lives and treatment.

In an excellent and extensive review of social networks and schizophrenia, Hammer et al. (1978) report that schizophrenic subjects tend to have smaller, more asymmetrical networks than non-schizophrenics. These networks are sparse, loosely interconnected, fluctuating, and often other-mediated. Such contacts are associated with rehospitalization, poor prognosis, and changes in levels of symptomatology. These researchers argue that the "reduced cultural predictability" of schizophrenics, as reflected in their speech and communication patterns, contributes to and is a part of what we call schizophrenia. This approach, which seems promising, focuses on cultural, value, and behavioral differences rather than on pathology.

Sokolovsky et al. (1978), investigating this subject in a Manhattan SRO hotel, confirmed that schizophrenic persons, impaired minimally to severely, had smaller networks than nonpsychotic residents. Relationships among the severely impaired schizophrenics tended to be dependent, loosely interconnected, and associated with higher rates of hospitalization. Relationships among the minimally impaired were more autonomous, goal-directed, and interconnected. These researchers point to the potential supportive and preventive features of friendships among schizophrenic outpatients, but they do not suggest modes of facilitation.

The usefulness of this classification scheme hinges upon what it tells us about the social and interpersonal relationships of clients. Inside Normals and Inside Crazies are the most powerful persons in the clients' everyday world, and these two groups provide the clients with the most paradoxically negative indications about themselves. It seems that the only persons with whom clients can have symmetrical, limitless relations are other crazies. In his relations with normals, the client encounters structures, codes, and regulations. These normals not only have more control of, and responsibility for, their own lives but often of the clients' lives as well. In addition, the normals who are most important in clients' lives (Inside Normals) usually stand in this relation *because* of the clients' psychiatric problems and consequent life difficulties. Thus, although these people are help-givers, they may also serve as potent daily reminders to clients of their own deficits and differentness in comparison with normals.

The real cultural craziness here is that not only do we describe these persons as pathologically dependent but we contribute to their dependencies. Not only do we view them as unintegrated within the community but we isolate them by constantly reminding them of their incompetencies and by introducing them to peers (in treatment programs like PACT) with whom they may be more comfortable. We provide professionals to help these persons, as a society seem to prefer to pay others to deal with them and thereby undermine any motivation that community members or other clients might have to participate in the caring and treatment process. We provide these networks and services even though hospital studies have shown that a steady diet of other clients and staff is detrimental to self-esteem and to "getting well." We negatively value these persons, collectively and as individuals, for their differentness and their dependencies, but we leave them little chance to give us anything except "getting better" (which means being more like us).

References

Aviram, U., and S. P. Segal. 1973. Exclusion of the mentally ill: Reflection of an old problem in a new context. *Archives of General Psychiatry* 29:126–131.

Chamberlain, J. 1978. *On our own: Patient controlled alternatives to the mental health system.* New York: McGraw-Hill.

Comer, R. J., and J. A. Piliavin. 1972. The effects of physical deviance upon face-to-face interaction: The other side. *Journal of Personality and Social Psychology* 23, 1:33–39.

Comer, R. J., and J. A. Piliavin. 1975. As others see us: Attitudes of physically handicapped and normals toward own and other groups. *Rehabilitation Literature* 36, 7:206–221.

Edgerton, R. B. 1967. *The cloak of competence: Stigma in the lives of the mentally retarded.* Berkeley: University of California Press.

Hammer, M., et al. 1978. Social networks and schizophrenia. *Schizophrenia Bulletin* 4(4):522–545.

Sokolovsky, J., et al. 1978. Personal networks of ex-mental patients in a Manhattan SRO hotel. *Human Organization* (Spring).

30

Strauss, J. S., Hafez, H., Lieberman, P., and Harding, C. (1985). The course of psychiatric disorder III: Longitudinal principles. *American Journal of Psychiatry, 142* (3), 289–296

Thirty or so years ago, schizophrenia was considered to be something akin to a death sentence—once you had it you had it, it was a devastating, life-altering disease, and if it changed at all over time it changed for the worse. John Strauss was one of a few American psychiatrists and other researchers during the 1970s and 1980s who, along with the World Health Organization studies of schizophrenia across cultures, conducted research that gave a different and more promising picture of the course of schizophrenia. This article reports on a study of the "illness course" among a small group of patients who were hospitalized for functional, that is, severe, psychiatric disorders. Data collected over the course of 2 years after hospital discharge revealed what the authors assessed as eight longitudinal principles for understanding the course of psychiatric disorder, grouped within the broad categories of longitudinal patterns and individual-environment interactions. These eight principles reflect identifiable phases of disorder and elements associated with a patient's remaining in one phase or moving on to a new one. The authors discuss the clinical and research implications of this perspective on the course of serious psychiatric disorders.

The Course of Psychiatric Disorder, III: Longitudinal Principles

The authors studied 28 patients hospitalized for functional psychiatric disorder in an attempt to explore systematically the course of psychiatric disorder. Data collected over the 2-year period following discharge suggested the existence of eight longitudinal principles for understanding the course of psychiatric disorder. These principles reflect identifiable phases and some of the factors involved in a patient's remaining in one phase or moving on to a new phase. The clinical and research implications of these principles are described.

(Am J Psychiatry 142:289–296, 1985)

Current views about the course of psychiatric disorder appear to be both incomplete and distorted. Two research practices have contributed to these shortcomings, which have limited the base of systematic inquiry underlying clinical practice. The first of these research strategies is the almost exclusive attention to outcome rather than course of disorder. The second is the tendency to look at course of disorder in a relative vacuum. This tendency leads to inadequate consideration of the disorder as taking place in a person evolving over time, a person who lives in an environmental context. In this report, we describe a study that attempted to reduce these shortcomings to provide a more complete perspective on the course of psychiatric disorder and the factors that influence it. It is our contention that until such a broad perspective is developed, an understanding of the nature of psychiatric disorder and the ability to provide optimum treatment will be severely limited.

Conceptualizations of the course of psychopathology fall into three groups: the natural history model, the diathesis-stress model, and the clinical model. The natural history model was brought to psychiatric thinking by Kraepelin, who focused on outcome of disorder (more than on the intervening course) as a way of identifying specific psychiatric diseases. Although noting its different courses, he defined dementia praecox essentially as a disease in which several different syndromes could be considered as representing a single disease because they all had a narrow range of outcomes.

The natural history model has been extremely important in the field of medicine generally and has contributed much to psychiatry. Although it has some validity, the validity is limited by certain problems. One of the most significant of these is that systematic data have recently become available indicating that even patients with the disorder for which the natural history model was established, schizophrenia (dementia praecox), do not all have the same outcome (1–3). Another problem for this model is that it does not have within it a structure for considering environmental impact. Recent research has shown that, even for schizophrenia, family environment (4) and perhaps life events (5), social supports (6), and psychosocial treatments (7) may have major effects on outcome.

A more recent model of the course of disorder, one more suitable for reflecting outcome heterogeneity and environmental impact, is the diathesis-stress model. This model, building on the natural history paradigm, suggests that although there is an underlying vulnerability for a disorder, its continued manifestation or recurrence is influenced by stress. This model provides a foundation for considering such factors as the impact of family environment and life events, but it too has certain shortcomings suggested by recent data. One major problem is the difficulty in defining diathesis and stress specifically. Events that could be predicted to be stressful, such as a death in the family, may for some people mobilize functioning and reduce symptoms rather than cause decompensation.

In addition to the problems with definition, the diathesis-stress model does not in itself provide a basis for thinking about the possibility that patients might play an active role in influencing the course of their disorder. And yet, even in psychotic disorders, it is highly likely that patients play a significant part in controlling their symptoms (8, 9). People also select their environments (which may be more or less stressful) and collaborate or "comply" with their treatment (or do not do so). The diathesis-stress model does not offer a basis for considering such patient contributions.

Finally, the diathesis-stress model does not emphasize possible shifts in vulnerability over time. If the patient becomes less likely to relapse under a given "stress" as time progresses, one must assume that there are changes in the patient that help to account for this shift in pathologic response.

Building on the natural history and diathesis-stress models to provide a structure that can define vulnerability and stress more specifically and account for change and the active role of the patient, we have described the Interactive Developmental Model (10). This model has two major principles: 1) The course of disorder is strongly affected by interactions between the individual and the environment. In these interactions, either the individual or the environment can be the initiator. 2) The individual develops over time. By develop we mean that the person's strengths and vulnerabilities change over time, frequently in the direction of human development more generally. This development, we hypothesize, influences the course of psychiatric disorder (11).

However, the Interactive Developmental Model was generated originally as a general and speculative statement to meet the data that were available. It is necessary next to construct this model in more detail and from an empirical base. Such a step requires an exploratory study to identify relevant variables and suggest longitudinal processes. In previous reports, we have outlined key variables (12) and discussed methodologic issues (13). In this report, we describe the longitudinal processes in the course of psychiatric disorder that have been suggested by our research. These processes are divided into two major types: 1) longitudinal patterns and 2) individual-environment interactions that contribute to these patterns.

Method

To explore systematically the course of psychiatric disorder, we carried out an intensive follow-along study of psychiatric patients. Twenty-eight patients hospitalized for functional psychiatric disorders were interviewed shortly after admission. Following discharge the subjects were interviewed at bimonthly intervals over the period of 1 year, and again at 2 years following discharge. The interviews focused on collecting data on symptoms and social functioning as they evolved across a variety of life "contexts" such as work, family,

Table 30.1. Characteristics of 28 Psychiatric Patients in a Study of Course of Disorder

Subject	Age (years)	Sex	Marital Status	Social Class[a]	Diagnosis[b]
1	31	F	Single	III	Schizoaffective disorder
2	26	M	Single	IV	Schizophrenia, paranoid type
3	24	M	Single	V	Schizophrenia, paranoid type
4	28	F	Single	III	Bipolar disorder, mixed type
5	37	F	Single	V	Schizophrenia, undifferentiated type
6	37	F	Divorced	II	Schizoaffective disorder
7	39	M	Divorced	II	Bipolar disorder, mixed type
8	26	F	Single	III	Bipolar disorder, manic type
9	43	F	Single	III	Schizoaffective disorder
10	34	F	Divorced	IV	Bipolar disorder
11	24	M	Separated	III	Schizoaffective disorder
12	37	M	Divorced	I	Major depression
13	26	F	Married	III	Major depression
14	39	F	Married	IV	Bipolar disorder, depressed type
15	26	F	Single	III	Major depression
16	23	F	Single	V	Major depression
17	20	M	Single	V	Bipolar disorder, manic type
18	38	M	Married	III	Atypical depression
19	28	F	Separated	V	Schizoaffective disorder
20	55	F	Married	III	Major depression
21	25	M	Single	IV	Major depression
22	22	F	Single	IV	Schizoaffective disorder
23	20	F	Single	IV	Schizoaffective disorder
24	28	M	Single	III	Bipolar disorder, manic type
25	29	M	Single	III	Schizophrenia, paranoid type
26	20	M	Single	V	Dysthymic disorder
27	24	F	Single	III	Schizophrenia, paranoid type
28	26	M	Single	III	Affective disorder, bipolar type

[a] Hollingshead-Redlich scale.
[b] According to *DSM-III*.

friendships, and treatment. Information was also collected on a range of environmental factors that might influence shifts or stabilities in these areas.

The interview schedules used in the study included open-ended and structured questions. After the interviews, ratings were made using several standard scales (1, 14, 15), and a narrative description of the previous 2 months' events and sequences was written.

Patients in the study were between the ages of 18 and 55 years, had a functional psychiatric disorder, and lacked any history of major problems with organic brain disorders or substance abuse. Because one focus of the study was the role of work following hospital discharge, another criterion for participation in the study was that the patient had worked at some time in the year before admission. Basic clinical and demographic characteristics of subjects in the sample are presented in Table 30.1.

Results

We have been able to find no published account of a similar research project that followed subjects and their environmental situations repeatedly over time. Regular observation of

Table 30.2. Longitudinal Principles in the Course of Disorder

A. Longitudinal patterns
   1. Nonlinearity of course
   2. Identifiable phases
      a. Moratoriums
      b. Change points
      c. Ceilings
   3. "Mountain climbing"
   4. Time decay of vulnerability
   5. Phases of environmental response
      a. Convalescence
      b. Backlash
B. Individual-environment interactions
   6. Identifiable sequences of individual-environment interaction
      a. Exaggerating feedback
      b. Corrective feedback
      c. Cumulative effect
   7. The active role of the patient
   8. The meaning of environmental events and personal behaviors

the evolution of our subjects and their disorders in relation to their environment allowed us to document the course, for example, of a subject who, when rehospitalized, recovered rapidly from one episode of a recurrent psychosis following her original discharge. She functioned well for 3 months, then, following a success at work, had an exacerbation involving increased symptoms and diminished ability to work. The subject took more medication, got assistance from family and co-workers, and improved somewhat. She stabilized over the next several months.

Our review of sequences such as these (which are so commonplace in clinical experience), using systematically collected data and follow-up, suggested a set of eight longitudinal principles. These principles are grouped into two categories: longitudinal patterns and individual-environment interactions (see Table 30.2).

Longitudinal Patterns

Principle 1: Nonlinearity of Course

Concepts of course of disorder drawn from previous research have sometimes been strange indeed. For example, a traditional 1-year outcome study of patient 14 in our sample would suggest the course shown in Figure 30.1. However, our bimonthly assessment of this patient produced the curve shown in Figure 30.2. The two points in Figure 30.1 are not incorrect, but assuming a straight line between them is inadequate and misleading when the goal is to understand longitudinal processes. In our subjects the course of disorder and recovery over the 2 years as measured by the Global Assessment Scale (14) and the Level of Function Scale (1) never followed a straight line.

Principle 2: Identifiable Phases

This principle states that particular kinds of differentiated phases can be identified within the nonlinear courses of disorder. One common pattern for subjects in our study is shown in Figure 30.3.

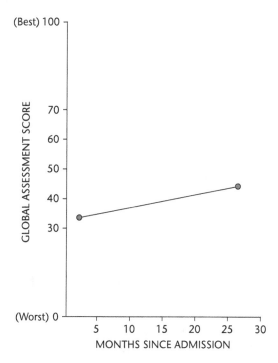

Figure 30.1. Traditional One-Year Outcome Study of Patient 14

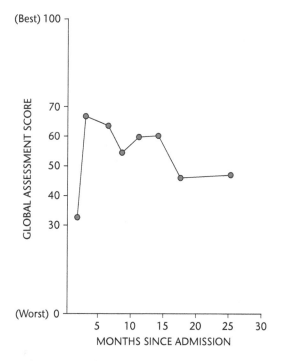

Figure 30.2. Bimonthly Assessment of Outcome of Patient 14

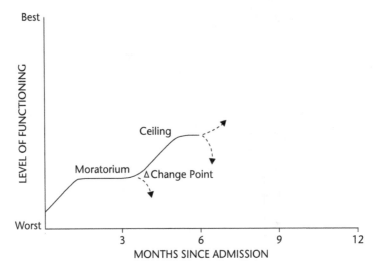

Figure 30.3. Common Pattern of the Course of Psychiatric Disorder in 28 Patients

Three commonly occurring phases can be discerned in such patterns. They are designated as moratoriums, change points, and ceilings.

Moratoriums. During certain periods, patients in our study experienced stability in symptoms and function. During such periods little measurable behavioral or symptom change was noted. We call these periods "moratoriums." Somewhat like the psychoanalytic concept of latency, the moratorium often appears to involve many important, although relatively hidden, changes. In such a case, patients often seemed to be reconstituting their identity, accumulating supports, or strengthening their skills in subtle ways. The following are three examples of moratoriums.

After her discharge, patient 1 went to work as a sales clerk in a store run like a large family. The job itself was well below the status of those she had achieved at her prehospitalization peak, but it felt "comfortable." The low demand of the job tasks and the warmth and support she received from several co-workers and from her boss contributed to this comfort.

Patient 22 stayed home with her parents and did very little socially or occupationally for 3 months following hospital discharge. After that period, she returned to work and increased her level of social and occupational function steadily over a 3-month period to a point well above the level she had lived at for several years before the onset of her psychiatric symptoms.

Patient 10, who may have been in a prolonged moratorium period, was rehospitalized because of an exacerbation of her longstanding anxiety and auditory hallucinations following an increase in her job responsibilities. After admission, these symptoms dropped rapidly to their usual level. Following 1 week at this plateau, she returned to her job, which had been adjusted to be less stressful. She was discharged from the hospital a few days later and remained without further incident at her pre-exacerbation moratorium level of functioning.

The existence of moratoriums following an episode of disorder appears to be universal, but their timing and duration vary widely. These variations may be related to the severity of illness and the number of previous episodes, among other things.

Change points. Change points involve considerable shifts in functioning or symptoms over a brief period.

Patient 1, who had been working as a sales clerk in the family-like store, decided she needed to move on to a job with more future and better pay. She found such a job, and as she planned to begin it she also started to consider using the increased money she would receive to move from her parents' house to an apartment where she could have more personal freedom to date, cook, and function more autonomously.

Change points can be stimulated by the patient's own desires for moving on or by family or other pressures. These points appear to follow the principles of crisis theory, which postulate that at such a time the patient can either improve markedly or decompensate. It is extremely difficult at this stage in our knowledge (since these points had not previously been identified and hence studied) to predict which direction the patient's course will take. Knowledge of the person's earlier patterns of response to stress, his or her other skills and needs, and the availability of social supports may help us anticipate the patient's future course, however.

Predicting the direction of change is especially difficult because symptoms frequently become worse at a change point, whether the person goes on to improvement or exacerbation. This phenomenon of temporary symptom exacerbation at such a point has also been noted by McCrory et al. (16).

An additional problem with change points emerges when the patient or clinician has to decide when symptom exacerbation is a prodromal sign of decompensation or simply a normal reaction to life's exigencies.

Patient 12, who had been diagnosed as having a major depression, started to become depressed 2 months after hospital discharge and wondered if he was becoming ill again. He had been considering a major career change that involved a lower-status but more lucrative job. When seen at follow-up 2 months later, he reported the symptoms to have disappeared and the job change to be well under way.

Ceilings. The ceiling is defined as the highest level of functioning reached in a given period of time. It is not an impenetrable level, but it is often particularly difficult for the person to surpass the ceiling without experiencing major decompensation and symptom exacerbation.

Patient 5 was a subject who would return rapidly to work following discharge from each of her several hospitalizations. She was very competent, but each time she was going to be promoted she would once again start to become psychotic.

Several subjects in the study experienced further progress beyond their ceiling after discharge, but also found such progress particularly stressful.

The irregular patterns in the course of disorder and the moratoriums, change points, and ceilings have several treatment implications. For example, patients, clinicians, and family members often become frustrated during moratoriums, seeming to expect that there should be a more or less straight line of progression and improvement. But excessive pressure for improvement during moratoriums might sometimes be deleterious, not allowing patients to gather their resources before approaching a change. In fact, patients may need all the moratorium time they can get because changes, when they do come, rarely come singly. If people get jobs, they have to deal with work settings, get used to a change in identity, shift roles with friends, perhaps take on new responsibilities in the family, and manage transportation.

Once the phases are noted, educational intervention by the clinician may be helpful, analogous to the interventions in family interactions described by Vaughn and Leff (4) and Liberman (17). Related adjustments to the quantity and quality of support, encouragement, and demand as well as possible shifts in medication and training using behavioral rehearsal may also be helpful.

Principle 3: "Mountain Climbing"

The course of disorder and its phases thus far have been described as a single process. In fact, as has been shown elsewhere (18), there are several different processes occurring simultaneously and operating as open-linked systems. Symptoms, social relations functioning, and occupational functioning are three such systems that are relatively independent of each other while also having some intercorrelation. In reviewing the evolution of disorder and recovery in our subjects, it appeared that these systems often reflected a pattern that we termed "mountain climbing." When a subject was well established in one context, such as social relations, perhaps following a period of moratorium he or she might attempt a change point in another context, such as work. This pattern of establishing a foothold in one area before attempting to make progress in another was relatively common.

Principle 4: Time Decay of Vulnerability

There appears to be a time decay phenomenon associated with vulnerability to various life events and situations during recovery from a symptomatic episode. The more recent the episode, the more vulnerable the person seems to be. This declining vulnerability may have an important biological analog. Post and Kopanda (19) have written about the possibility of a "kindling" phenomenon through which repeated exposure to certain chemicals may increase physiological reactivity to them rather than produce habituation. A time decay phenomenon might reflect the reversal of this process, an "unkindling," or reduced reactivity.

Principle 5: Phases of Environmental Response

Just as there are several longitudinal phases in the patient's disorder and functioning, there appear to be predictable phases of environmental responses as well.

Convalescence. Many patients reported that they are implicitly allowed a convalescence of about 2–4 months following discharge from the hospital. During this time demands are generally limited, and patients are given assistance and permission to reenter the stream of life gradually.

Backlash. When the implicit convalescent period ends, however, there often is a backlash during which family, friends, and clinicians appear to demand even more than they had before the exacerbation or onset of the illness. These demands often come as a surprise to patients who think that they have been doing well. The backlash phenomenon often causes considerable distress for all involved. An understanding of the patient's moratorium, change point, and ceiling phases during the postdischarge period would help those persons in the patient's environment titrate their own reactions and expectations more appropriately.

It is possible that as such environmental phases are clarified further, they may be found to include the same kind of moratoriums and change points seen in the individual. In fact, correspondences of certain individual and environmental phases may be crucial influences on the patient's improvement.

Individual-Environment Interactions

Principle 6: Identifiable Sequences of Individual-Environment Interaction

At a level more microscopic than the broad patterns described earlier, the subjects' experiences can be seen to reflect identifiable sequences in which they and their environments interact. Several types of cause-effect sequence appear to take place, including exaggerating and corrective feedback cycles and cumulative impacts.

Exaggerating feedback. In exaggerating feedback cycles ("positive feedback," in general systems terms), each event in the sequence exaggerates the situation further in a cyclic fashion. Feedback is used here to indicate the process by which a change in the person or the environment itself generates subsequent changes, which in turn influence the initial change.

> Patient 12 found that when he started to get depressed before a psychotic episode, he became preoccupied with astrology, paid less attention to work, performed more poorly, became more depressed, and became more preoccupied and progressively more disturbed.

Corrective feedback. In corrective feedback situations ("negative feedback," in the terms of general systems theory), a sequence of events occurs that returns a person to a previous, more modulated state.

> Patient 1, a young woman with schizoaffective disorder, noted that as she became more hyperactive on the job a co-worker would say things like, "Why don't you slow down? I'll help you with those customers." This intervention appeared to help the subject regain control of her activity level.

Cumulative effect. Cumulative impacts of more or less separate environment-individual interactions are common.

> Patient 11 moved, changed jobs, and separated from his family all within a few weeks. Then he was involved in an automobile accident (not through his fault) that left him without transportation for work or social contacts. This group of events was followed by a recurrence of symptoms.

Principle 7: The Active Role of the Patient

Many views of psychiatric disorder portray the patient as passive. Although such concepts of illness go back at least to Newton (Toulmin, 1982 unpublished paper), the principle described here suggests that the patient often has an active role in the process of decompensation and recovery.

Our subjects persistently described the role they took in affecting the course of their disorder both directly and through influencing their environment. This principle was noted, for example, in a patient's determination to function in spite of frightening symptoms, participation in a treatment regimen, attempts to undermine that regimen, or consumption of symptom-causing street drugs. The importance of the patient's active role is suggested by studies of patients' giving up on efforts to get better (20) and of their treatment participation (21). Besides giving up on improving and their participation in therapy, patients also have a major role in terms of their many ways of helping to control their symptoms, methods that appear to be most useful when symptoms are at low or moderate levels of intensity (8).

Principle 8: The Meaning of Environmental Events and Personal Behaviors

The implications to the person of the environmental event or situation will influence the course of the disorder (9, 22). For instance, a job failure may free the person to pursue a new line of work more compatible with certain basic needs.

Patient 6 was a very proud woman who quit her administrative job because she just couldn't take the pressures. Although job problems had previously been followed by a recurrence of her schizoaffective disorder, on this occasion her symptoms did not reappear. Rather, she found a job as a clerk in an office. In this job she pursued in comfort, and for the first time in her life, her interest in developing better relationships with co-workers.

Just as the meaning of the environmental situation affects the person's response, so the meaning of the person's behavior influences environmental responses.

When patient 6 was later laid off from her new job because of the deteriorating economy, her boyfriend threatened to break up with her because she was no longer contributing to the household.

These then are the longitudinal principles of the interactive developmental model. It should be noted that not all eight principles were identifiable in all subjects, but each principle was found often enough to warrant routine attention for clinical and research purposes. It also appears that there are interactions among the principles. For example, a moratorium may be most likely to end after time decay of vulnerability has reached a certain level.

An Illustrative Case

How do these various longitudinal principles operate together to influence the course of disorder for a particular patient?

Patient 14, mentioned earlier, was a 39-year-old married white woman with a 4-year history of bipolar disorder and three previous psychiatric hospitalizations. She was admitted to the hospital for the fourth time for a severe depressive episode when we first saw her as a research subject. In a schematic comparison of only her functioning level on admission and at 1-year follow-up, the line is straight, as shown in Figure 30.1. In fact, her course was far more complex, as shown in Figure 30.2.

When admitted to the hospital, the patient was extremely depressed. She said she was "no good" and was distanced from the people in her environment. She fended off practically all attempts to make contact with her.

In the course of treatment, both psychosocial and pharmacologic, she became less depressed, and her interactions with the environment increased. These changes made it possible for her to be discharged from the hospital. She returned to living with her family, which consisted of her husband and two children.

Because her job had been a very helpful part of her life, she returned to work immediately. Her supervisor and co-workers were supportive and were pleased to have her back, and they told her so. She in turn began joking with them again, completing an exaggerating feedback sequence moving her further away from her depressed state. She was very effective at her computer programming job, shouldered more than her share of the work, and even suggested effective procedural changes to help the group be more productive. If a moratorium occurred at all with this patient, it did so in the hospital and was of very brief duration. In fact, she returned very quickly to her pre-hospitalization ceiling of function.

During a plateau at this ceiling level (perhaps a second moratorium at a higher level), she did well for several months. In fact, she even pushed through her previous ceiling within the family context (mountain climbing). She lived in a very difficult family situation. Her children had minor but troublesome problems with the school authorities, and her husband had been diagnosed as having a major illness. With the support of her successes at work, the patient assumed a more active role in the family. She became more assertive than she had ever been and insisted that family members help with the housework. They responded well, and the situation improved. Thus, successes in the job and family contexts resulted in a positive cumulative impact on the patient.

At this time, however, the economy was on the decline and the regional office of the manufacturing company that employed the patient laid off many employees. She was lucky, however, or so it seemed. She did continue on the job, but in spite of the fact that her abilities were superior to those of several other workers, her hours were reduced and she was transferred to the evening shift.

The patient had a longstanding problem with not being very assertive. She had become more assertive at home, but she did not transfer her new advances at home to the work context. If she had taken a more active role in protesting the reduction of and change in hours, perhaps she would have avoided the shift in the job situation. Unfortunately, the job change had a major negative impact on her self-esteem and social contacts. There was only one co-worker, a rather dour and withdrawn woman, on the evening shift. There was no joking or praise for work well done. In addition, the cutback in hours reduced her salary and she felt less valuable for what she could contribute to the hard pressed family finances.

The patient became less assertive at home. While hoping for more praise and recognition from the family, she received more criticism instead. Before long, she was back in the hospital with a severe depression. The exaggerating feedback sequence (reduced work---->reduced money---->educed self-esteem---->reduced active role---->reduced self-esteem) appeared to have contributed to the recurrence.

This patient's situation illustrates how the course of decompensation and recovery in psychiatric disorder may be a complex evolving process. For her, a sequence involving positive changes in self-esteem, active role, and social contacts in the work setting led to increased ability to deal with another context, the family. But with the change of the economy, the role of her work in meeting, or at least not frustrating, certain needs was reduced. The snowball effect that apparently was set into motion had aroused more desperate coping mechanisms in the patient, perhaps the kind of conservation withdrawal described by Engel (unpublished 1972 paper). It is processes such as these that seem to influence the directions, timing, and structure of the moratoriums and change points, and the degree of vulnerability to decompensation.

Discussion

The need for a more adequate model to reflect the evolution of a psychiatric disorder is especially glaring now that increasing evidence has been generated showing that even people with the most severe and chronic mental illness may experience major changes, often with partial or full recovery. Furthermore, there is increasing evidence that these changes may be related to environmental factors such as family behavior and expectations, psychosocial treatment, social networks, and stressful life events. Thus, we know that a person with a psychiatric disorder may, over time, go from point A to a very different point B, and we know of some factors that may be involved in that change. But almost nothing is known about the processes by which the person gets to point B and the sequence of phenomena that may be involved.

Actually, the lack of information on the evolution, in contrast to the outcome, of psychiatric disorder is not so surprising: the problem of doing truly longitudinal research has been noted in developmental psychology, a field where there might have been an even more intensive focus in this direction (Elder, 1983 unpublished paper). Apparently the multiple cross-sectional model, with its assessment at no more than a few points in time and its ease of data collection and analysis, has been so seductive that the more complex understanding of the evolution of sequential processes has been all but ignored.

But the issues of sequence and patterns cannot be neglected indefinitely: they potentially hold answers for too many crucial questions. Are there critical periods in the recovery process when stressful life events may have an especially powerful impact? Is there a particular point in a chain of happenings during which a specific intervention, such as helping a patient return to work or starting intensive psychotherapy, may be especially helpful or noxious? Are there particular sequences of events in the evolution of disorder that in themselves lead to recurrence of the disorder? Although there are many clinical impressions regarding these essential questions, there has been almost no systematic research to help validate or correct the clinical impressions and to develop them further.

One of the major features inhibiting research on the evolution of disorder and recovery is the complexity involved. What characteristics should be studied? When should data be collected? To begin resolving these questions, it was essential to carry out exploratory research focused on identifying patterns and delineating key variables. Through such research, it is possible to begin to establish a truly longitudinal framework for understanding the processes of psychopathology. It is important in such an inquiry, as in any scientific effort, to be faithful to the phenomena being studied, even though this may lead to shifts in research method (13, 23, 24).

The Interactive Developmental Model of the course of psychiatric disorder has grown out of such efforts. With its longitudinal principles, it attempts to describe variables and processes to provide a structure for integrating and furthering what is known about the course of psychiatric disorder.

References

1. Strauss JS, Carpenter WT Jr: Characteristic symptoms and outcome in schizophrenia. Arch Gen Psychiatry 30:429–434, 1974
2. Ciompi L: The natural history of schizophrenia in the long term. Br J Psychiatry 136: 413–420, 1980
3. Harding CM, Strauss JS: The course of schizophrenia: an evolving concept, in Controversies in Schizophrenia. Edited by Alpert M. New York, Guilford Press (in press)
4. Vaughn CE, Leff JP: The influence of family and social factors on the course of psychiatric illness. Br J Psychiatry 129:125–137, 1976
5. Day R: Life events and schizophrenia: the "triggering" hypothesis. Acta Psychiatr Scand 64:97–122, 1981
6. Cohen C, Sokolovsky J: Schizophrenia and social networks: ex-patients in the inner city. Schizophr Bull 4:546–560, 1978
7. Maher L, Gunderson J: Group, family, milieu, and community support systems treatment for schizophrenia, in Disorders of the Schizophrenic Syndrome. Edited by Bellak L. New York, Basic Books, 1979
8. Breier A, Strauss JS: Self-control in psychiatric disorders. Arch Gen Psychiatry 40: 1141–1145, 1983
9. Lazarus RS: The stress and coping paradigm, in Models for Clinical Psychopathology. Edited by Eisdorfer C, Cohen D, Kleinman A, et al. New York, Spectrum Publications, 1981
10. Strauss JS, Carpenter WT Jr: Schizophrenia. New York, Plenum, 1981
11. Strauss JS, Kokes RF, Carpenter WT Jr, et al: The course of schizophrenia as a developmental process, in Nature of Schizophrenia: New Findings and Future Strategies. Edited by Wynne LC, Cromwell RL, Matthysse S. New York, John Wiley & Sons, 1978
12. Strauss JS, Loevsky L, Glazer W, et al: Organizing the complexities of schizophrenia. J Nerv Ment Dis 169:120–126, 1981
13. Strauss JS, Hafez H: Clinical questions and "real" research. Am J Psychiatry 138: 1592–1597, 1981

14. Endicott J, Spitzer RL, Fleiss JL, et al: The Global Assessment Scale: a procedure for measuring overall severity of psychiatric disturbance. Arch Gen Psychiatry 33:766–771, 1976

15. Overall J, Gorham D: The Brief Psychiatric Rating Scale. Psychol Rep 10:799–812, 1962

16. McCrory DJ, Connelly PS, Hanson-Mayer TP, et al: The rehabilitation crisis: the impact of growth. J Appl Rehabil Couns 11:136–139, 1980

17. Liberman RP: Social factors in schizophrenia, in Psychiatry 1982: The American Psychiatric Association Annual Review. Edited by Grinspoon L. Washington, DC, American Psychiatric Press, 1982

18. Strauss JS, Carpenter WT Jr: Prediction of outcome, III: five-year outcome and its predictors. Arch Gen Psychiatry 34:14–20, 1977

19. Post RM, Kopanda RT: Cocaine, kindling, and psychosis. Am J Psychiatry 133:627–634, 1976

20. Schmale AH: A genetic view of affects with special reference to the genesis of helplessness and hopelessness. Psychoanal Study Child 19:287–310, 1964

21. Van Putten T, May PRA: Subjective response as a predictor of outcome in pharmacotherapy: the consumer has a point. Arch Gen Psychiatry 35:477–480, 1978

22. Lieberman P, Strauss JS: Recurrence of mania: environmental factors and medical treatment. Am J Psychiatry 141:77–80, 1984

23. Bakan D: On Method: Toward a Reconstruction of Psychological Investigation. San Francisco, Jossey-Bass, 1973

24. Skinner BF: A case history in scientific method, in Cumulative Record, 3rd ed. New York, Appleton-Century-Crofts, 1972

31

Harding, C. M., Brooks, G. W., Ashikaga, T., Strauss, J. S., & Brier, A. (1987). The Vermont longitudinal study of persons with severe mental illness, II: Long-term outcome of subjects who retrospectively met DSM-III criteria for schizophrenia. *American Journal of Psychiatry,* 144, 727–735

Can people with serious mental illness who have been institutionalized from years of inpatient hospitalization not only be "managed" in the community but get better in the traditional sense of the term "recovery"? The Vermont Longitudinal Research Project is perhaps the most often cited and recognized study of the community psychiatry era in the United States in regard to confounding pessimistic expectations for persons with serious and persistent mental illnesses. Findings reported in this and a companion paper, also published in the *American Journal of Psychiatry*, were based on research conducted as part of a 32-year longitudinal study of 269 long-term state hospital patients who were discharged and placed in a community rehabilitation program during the 1950s. Part I covers 10-year follow-up data from first-stage research and 25-year follow-up interviews that the authors conducted. The data showed remarkable improvement in functioning and decreased symptoms, including remission, among the cohort. Part II, which we include here, involved a study of a subset of 118 patients who retrospectively met DSM-III criteria for schizophrenia. Patients showed similar improvement or recovery. The Vermont study provided strong support for the ability of persons with chronic mental illness to adjust to community living with appropriate supports and treatment.

The Vermont Longitudinal Study of Persons With Severe Mental Illness, II: Long-term Outcome of Subjects Who Retrospectively Met DSM-III Criteria for Schizophrenia

The authors present the findings from a long-term follow-up study of 118 patients from Vermont State Hospital who, when rediagnosed retrospectively, met DSM-III *criteria for schizophrenia at their index hospitalization in the mid-1950s. The patients were studied with structured, reliable, multivariate instrument batteries by raters who were blind to information in their records. The rediagnostic process is described, and results of the follow-up are presented. Outcome varied widely, but one-half to two-thirds of the sample had achieved considerable improvement or recovered, in contrast to statements in* DSM-III *that predict a poor outcome for schizophrenic patients.*

(Am J Psychiatry 1987; 144:727–735)

The third edition of the *Diagnostic and Statistical Manual of Mental Disorders (DSM-III)* of the American Psychiatric Association both reflects and shapes current American thinking about the course and outcome of schizophrenia. Heavily based on the Feighner criteria (1) and the Research Diagnostic Criteria (2), *DSM-III* pictures the schizophrenic patient as a person with increasing residual impairment.

A complete return to premorbid functioning is unusual—so rare, in fact, that some clinicians would question the diagnosis. However, there is always the *possibility* of full remission or recovery, although its frequency is unknown. The most common course is one of acute exacerbations with increasing residual impairment between episodes. *(DSM-III, p. 185)*

These impairments are said to include flattened affect, persisting delusions and hallucinations, and increasing inability to carry out everyday functions such as work, social relationships, or basic self-care. Such assumptions influence concepts of etiology (3) and course and outcome (4); in addition, they shape decisions about treatment (5), program implementation (6), economic planning (7), and social policy for mental health service delivery systems (8).

The advent of *DSM-III* has been seen by many clinicians and investigators as a major change in a field heretofore severely hampered in research and treatment relevant to schizophrenia by the lack of reliable definitions of diagnostic categories (9–11). With such a system in place (12), it is now possible to reaffirm or disconfirm the prevalent notions about the long-term course of schizophrenia.

This paper reports findings from the fifth very long-term follow-up study of schizophrenia conducted within the last decade (13–15) and the second such endeavor recently completed in the United States (16). It is the only study to date that has examined the long-term outcome of subjects rediagnosed as meeting the *DSM-III* criteria for schizophrenia.

The Vermont Longitudinal Research Project was a 32-year prospective follow-along study of a clinical research cohort (17–28). The prospectively gathered material has been combined with a systematic retrospective follow-back to document the lives of 97% (N=262) of the 269 original subjects.

In the mid-1950s, when they became subjects in the study, these patients were "middle-aged, poorly educated, lower-class individuals further impoverished by repeated and prolonged hospitalizations" (25, p. 29). Demographic, illness, and hospitalization characteristics of this cohort have been extensively described elsewhere (25–31).

The subjects were originally chosen for a rehabilitation program from the back wards of Vermont State Hospital because of their chronic disabilities and resistance to treatment. The chronicity criterion required subjects to have been disabled for 1 year before entry into the rehabilitation program. The term "disabled" was defined as inability to function in ordinary day to-day role capacities. Members of this cohort had been ill for an average of 16 years, totally disabled for an average of 10 years, and continuously hospitalized for 6 years. In addition, most patients had been given phenothiazines for 2 1/2 years without enough improvement to warrant discharge. They were provided with a comprehensive rehabilitation program and released to the community during the mid-to-late 1950s in a planned deinstitutionalization effort (17–25, 31).

In the follow-up data collection period (1980–1982), 97% of the original cohort was extensively studied in a structured and reliable manner (30–31). The catamnestic period for these patients ranged from 22 to 62 years. More detailed descriptions of the methodology, the study sample, and the overall status of the cohort at follow-up may be found in our companion paper in this issue.

Initial results for these subjects, whose original diagnoses had been made according to *DSM-I* criteria, indicated that from one-half to two-thirds of the cohort had significantly improved or recovered (28, 30). These findings were at odds with the prevailing assumptions about the long-term course of schizophrenia. It was possible, however, that this discrepancy had been generated by the use of the loosely formulated *DSM-I* diagnostic guidelines. Therefore, with the publication of *DSM-III* while we were in the midst of our study, we undertook the task of giving a retrospective rediagnosis from case records for each of the 269 patients in order to determine what their *DSM-III* status would have been at the time they were selected for the study.

The present paper examines the process of rediagnosis and assesses the long-term outcome achieved by the group who met the *DSM-III* criteria for schizophrenia at selection. The two hypotheses involved in this aspect of the study were statements of common conceptions about schizophrenia: 1) Members of this cohort diagnosed as having met the *DSM-III* criteria for schizophrenia at index hospitalization would still have signs and symptoms of schizophrenia at follow-up. 2) Members of this cohort diagnosed as having met the *DSM-III* criteria for schizophrenia at index hospitalization would have uniformly poor outcomes in critical areas of functioning such as work, social relations, and self-care at follow-up. Confirmation of these hypotheses would lend support to the validity of the statements about the long-term course and outcome of schizophrenia that are made in *DSM-III*.

Rediagnosis of Patients at Index Hospitalization

Originally, 213, or 79%, of the 269 subjects had been given a diagnosis of schizophrenia according to *DSM-I* guidelines. Table 31.1 presents a breakdown by age, sex, and diagnosis of the entire cohort at entry into the study in the mid-1950s.

We instituted several methods to achieve the retrospective rediagnosis. First, the two raters selected (J.S.S. and A.B.) were new to the project and blind to the outcome of each subject. The raters participated in two sets of interrater trials on 40 randomly selected cases (15% of the 269 subjects), which were independently assessed in a straight series without any discussion between raters. The case records and standardized record review abstracts from the time of the patient's entry into the study were stripped of all previous diagnostic assignments as well as any information about future episodes, hospitalizations, and other outcome information after index admission. (Index hospitalization was designated as the hospitalization during the 1950s during which transfer to the rehabilitation program occurred.) The *DSM-III* criteria were strictly applied.

The hospital records had been abstracted, as part of the overall goals of the larger project, in a structured and systematic manner by means of a battery of instruments known as the Hospital Record Review Form. This battery contained forms for extracting data about family and early life history, prodromal signs, and all hospital admissions. Interrater trials had revealed it to be a reliable instrument battery (31).

For a signs and symptoms checklist, we used Strauss's Case Record Rating Scale (32) and ratings from the World Health Organization's (WHO) Psychiatric and Personal History Schedule (33). This combination battery recorded behavioral descriptors and symptom dimensions noted by the clinician in recounting his or her impressions of the patient at the time of the original assessment. Case summaries and copies of the original chart

Table 31.1. DSM-I Diagnoses of 269 Chronic Psychiatric Patients at Entry Into the Vermont Study in the Mid-1950s

Diagnostic Category	Mean Age (years)	Subjects With Diagnosis (N=269)	
		N	%
Schizophrenia		213	79
Hebephrenic			
Men	36	13	
Women	41	9	
Catatonic			
Men	38	26	
Women	43	39	
Paranoid			
Men	43	48	
Women	45	59	
Undifferentiated			
Men	34	8	
Women	37	11	
Affective disorders		34	13
Men	39	16	
Women	38	18	
Organic disorders		22	8
Men	36	14	
Women	44	8	

information, such as admission and discharge summaries with ward notes but with all references to diagnosis deleted, were included in each diagnostic packet. Structured *DSM-III* diagnostic checklists from WHO and the Chestnut Lodge Follow-up Study (34) were used by those making the rediagnoses to systematically summarize all the evidence for each diagnosis to be assigned.

Concerns about the quality of the records might be raised, because throughout the United States records from most state hospitals are considered to be poor. Vermont State Hospital's records, however, were remarkably complete. Since most of our subjects had also been the subjects of early phenothiazine drug trials before their entry into the rehabilitation program, the records tended to be of good research quality both before and during the institution of the federally funded rehabilitation program in 1957. The records described the evolution of symptoms by using statements from the patients themselves and gave examples of behaviors to illustrate the presence of hallucinations, delusions, catatonic waxy flexibility, and other symptoms. Such clinical notes were entered often by psychiatrists, residents, and other members of the treatment team. There were also mental status reports, past medical histories, results of current physical examinations, medication charts, treatment plans, progress notes, and admission and discharge summaries. In addition, social workers had collected systematic family and personal histories.

We conducted two sets of interrater trials. Complete agreement was achieved on 57% of the first 21 cases. In an analysis of the cases about which there was disagreement, it was found that 56% of the time, the second diagnosis proposed by one rater agreed with the first diagnosis selected by the other rater. Each rater agreed with the eventual consensual diagnosis 71% of the time overall and 75% of the time for schizophrenia. In assessing the level of interrater agreement, after collapsing the data into four diagnostic categories (schizophrenia, schizoaffective disorder, affective disorders, and "other" disorders), we generated an overall kappa coefficient (35) for the first trial of .40 (p=.001) and a kappa of .40 (p=.02) for schizophrenia alone. In the second trial set of 19 cases, an overall kappa of .65 (p<.0001) was generated; the kappa for schizophrenia was .78 (p<.0007). Clearly, there was an improvement in levels of agreement after the raters had further experience with the records and the diagnostic system. On the basis of the variation in the observed statistic, we concluded that the kappa value fell within the range observed by Spitzer et al. (36).

After application of the *DSM-III* criteria to the entire set of cases, 118 subjects received a diagnosis of schizophrenia (see Table 31.2).

Fifty-four percent (114 of 213) of those who were diagnosed as having schizophrenia according to the *DSM-I* guidelines retained the same diagnosis with the *DSM-III* criteria. (An additional four members of the *DSM-III* schizophrenia group were shifted from the *DSM-I* affective disorders category.) The primary shift from the *DSM-I* category of schizophrenia occurred to the *DSM-III* categories of schizoaffective disorder and atypical psychosis, not to the affective disorders category as expected from the experience of previous investigators.

The process of rediagnosis provided subtype categories for this subsample. The paranoid subtype predominated in both the *DSM-I* (50%, or 107 of 213) and *DSM-III* (61%, or 50 of 82) classification systems. The remaining subtypes included undifferentiated (17%, or 14 of 82), catatonic (13%, or 11 of 82), and disorganized (9%, or seven of 82).

Method

Of the 118 subjects who met the *DSM-III* criteria for schizophrenia, at follow-up 70% (N=82) were alive and were interviewed, 24% (N=28) were deceased, 3% (N=4) refused

Table 31.2. Follow-up Status by *DSM-III* Category of 269 Chronic Psychiatric Patients in the Vermont Study Who Were Rediagnosed Retrospectively

| Subjects' Follow-up Status | Number of Subjects in Diagnostic Category | | | | | | Total | |
	Schizophrenia	Schizo-affective Disorder	Affective Disorder	Atypical Psychosis	Other	Organic Disorder	N	%
Alive and interviewed	82	25	29	13	19	10	178	66
Alive; refused participation	4	1	1	0	5	2	13	5
Could not be located	4	1	1	0	1	0	7	3
Deceased	28	4	16	5	7	10	70[a]	26
Total								
N	118	31	47	18	32	22	268[a]	
%	44	12	17	7	12	8		100

[a]For one patient there was not enough information to make adequate ratings.

to participate, and 3% were lost to follow-up. It should be noted that these figures are nearly identical to those reported for the larger cohort in our companion paper (see table 1 in that paper).

The present paper focuses on the long-term outcome of the 82 subjects who were alive and were interviewed 20–25 years after their entry into the project, because their data were the most reliable. The catamnestic period for these subjects ranged from 22 to 59 years.

Forty-five percent of the 82 subjects who met the *DSM-III* criteria for schizophrenia at index hospitalization had been hospitalized for more than 6 years before being transferred to the rehabilitation program in the 1950s. Twenty-four percent had been in the hospital from 2 to 6 years, and 31% had been hospitalized less than 2 years.

Demographic analysis of these 82 subjects produced the following information. The group was split evenly between the sexes (41 men and 41 women). Their ages (as of July 1,1981, which was the midpoint in the data collection period) ranged from 41 to 79 years. It should be noted that 91% (N=75) were above the age of 50; the average age for the group was 61 years. Fifty-five percent (N=45) of the subjects had not completed high school. Sixty-two percent (N=51) had never married, and only 10% (N=8) had remained married. Seventy-six, or 93%, were living in Vermont.

To carry out the follow-up study, our raters conducted two structured and reliable field interviews with each subject to ascertain current status and longitudinal patterns of community tenure. The raters were blind to previously recorded information about the subjects. Additional informants who knew each subject well were also interviewed, and ratings were verified. The six subjects who were not living in Vermont were interviewed with the same protocols. Another structured protocol (the Hospital Record Review Form, described at length elsewhere [31]) was used by a rater blind to all field information to abstract hospital and vocational rehabilitation records.

We used two structured interview batteries from the Vermont Community Questionnaire (30, 31), which included 15 standard scales and schedules, to assess the subjects' levels of functioning in a variety of areas at follow-up and to discern longitudinal shifts and patterns across the 20–25 years since the rehabilitation program began. All batteries were subjected to two sets of interrater trials 6 months apart and were found reliable (30, 31).

As part of the assessment, the two interviewers, who were new to the project and who had 5–8 years of clinical experience each, made ratings that provided a current clinical profile for each subject. The interviewers were blind to diagnostic record information when they made these symptom ratings, after the third hour of contact with each subject. The interviewers used the Research Diagnostic Criteria Screening Interview (36, 37), the Brief Psychiatric Rating Scale (38), and a reduced version of the Mini-Mental State examination (39) to make their assessments. This assessment package was designed to replace the Schedule for Affective Disorders and Schizophrenia (SADS) (40), proposed in our original design (27), because the extra time and costs required for the SADS interview were not funded.

In addition, the Global Assessment Scale (GAS) (41, 42) provided a single score (from 0 to 100) based on level of symptoms and social functioning. The scale's developers divided scores on the instrument into three categories (0–30 = poor, 31–60 = fair, 61–100 = good functioning). The interrater trials generated a Pearson coefficient of .85 (p < .0001) for the first set (N = 20) and .93 (p < .0001) for the second set (N = 20) on this scale alone.

The Strauss-Carpenter Levels of Function Scale (43) was used to identify some of the major components that constitute the overall level of functioning assessed by the GAS. Each of the nine items is scored from 0 (poorest) to 4 (best); they include hospitalizations, symptoms, amount and quality of friendships, amount and quality of work, ability to meet basic needs, fullness of life, and overall level of functioning. (We excluded quality of work because, unlike all the other assessments, it could not be cross-checked by separate informants. A visit to each subject's work site was not deemed to be in the best interests of our subjects, most of whose employers might have been unaware of their early history as state hospital patients.) The results of interrater trials on this instrument alone generated Pearson coefficients of .92 (p < .0001) on the first set (N = 21) and .92 (p < .0001) on the second set (N = 18).

Results

For one-half to two-thirds of these subjects who retrospectively met the *DSM-III* criteria for schizophrenia, long-term outcome was neither downward nor marginal but an evolution into various degrees of productivity, social involvement, wellness, and competent functioning. The more stringent *DSM-III* diagnostic criteria for schizophrenia failed to produce the expected uniformly poor outcome.

The combined data from the structured instrument battery described earlier, as well as all of the clinical observations obtained in the 3-hour interview sequence, indicated that 68% of the 82 subjects who met the *DSM-III* criteria for schizophrenia at index hospitalization did not display any further signs or symptoms (either positive or negative) of schizophrenia at follow-up. Forty-five percent of the sample displayed no psychiatric symptoms at all. For another 23%, symptoms had shifted to probable affective or organic disorders. One person was rated as a probable alcohol abuser (see Table 31.3).

Eighty-four percent of the 82 subjects had had psychotropic medications prescribed for them; 75% of these in a low to medium dose range (in chlorpromazine equivalents). Seventy-five percent of the subjects stated they were complying with their regimes, but field interviewers were eventually told, after hours of interview time had elapsed, that the

Table 31.3. Psychiatric Status at Follow-up of 82 Patients in the Vermont Study Originally Diagnosed as Schizophrenic and Rediagnosed According to the RDC

Diagnostic Category	Subjects With Diagnosis (N = 82)	
	N	%
No symptoms	37	45
Schizophrenia		
Positive symptoms		
Definite	1	1
Probable	7	9
Possible	0	0
Negavite symptoms		
Definite	7	9
Probable	7	9
Possible	0	0
Affective disorders		
Definite	1	1
Probable	8	10
Possible	0	0
Organic disorders		
Definite	1	0
Probable	9	11
Possible	0	0
Alcoholism		
Definite	0	0
Probable	1	1
Possible	0	0
Not enough information to rate	4	4

actual compliance pattern was closer to the following: about 25% of the subjects always took their medications, another 25% self-medicated when they had symptoms, and the remaining 34% used none of their medications. Adding the 34% who were noncompliers to the 16% who were currently not receiving any prescriptions for psychotropics means that 50% of the cohort was not using such medication.

A single score for psychological and social functioning was assigned each subject on the basis of the GAS. Figure 31.1 compares outcome scores of the subjects who met the *DSM-III* criteria for schizophrenia at index hospitalization with the scores of the subjects who met the *DSM-I* guidelines for schizophrenia at index hospitalization. Sixty percent or more of the subjects diagnosed as schizophrenic by both diagnostic systems scored over 61, designated by the developers of the scale as good functioning. No one scored in the poor functioning category (score of 30 or less). It should be noted that all but four subjects who met the *DSM-III* criteria for schizophrenia came from the pool of subjects diagnosed as meeting the *DSM-I* criteria for schizophrenia.

Figure 31.2 shows the GAS scores of the 82 subjects who met both *DSM-I* and *DSM-III* criteria for schizophrenia (including four subjects who were in other categories of *DSM-I* but who met *DSM-III* criteria for schizophrenia) and of the subjects who met *DSM-I* criteria but who were reclassified as fitting some category other than schizophrenia by *DSM-III* criteria (N = 71). A t test for the means of the two groups revealed no significant differences between them (t = -1.44, df = 149, n.s.).

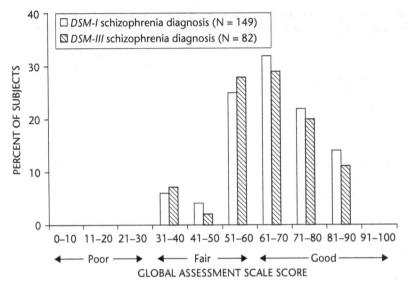

Figure 31.1. Global Assessment Scale Scores of Subjects in the Vermont Study Who Met *DSM-I* Criteria and Those Who Met *DSM-III* Criteria for Schizophrenia at Index Hospitalization

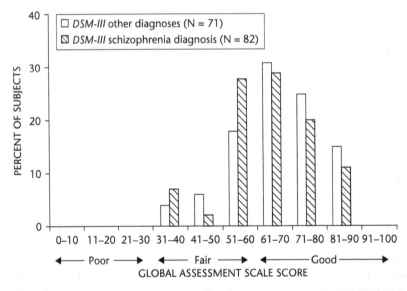

Figure 31.2. Global Assessment Scale Scores of Subjects in the Vermont Study Who Met Both *DSM-I* and *DSM-III* Criteria for Schizophrenia and Subjects Diagnosed as Schizophrenic by *DSM-I* Who Had Other Diagnoses According to *DSM-III*

Table 31.4 shows the findings from the Levels of Function Scale for living subjects originally diagnosed as meeting the *DSM-I* guidelines for schizophrenia, those for subjects who met the *DSM-III* criteria for schizophrenia, and those for subjects who met the *DSM-III* criteria for other categories. For most outcome variables in either diagnostic system, for any of the three groups, two-thirds to four-fifths of the subjects were found to be significantly improved.

Table 31.4. Results From the Strauss-Carpenter Levels of Function Scale at Follow-Up for Vermont Study Subjects Diagnosed as Schizophrenic by *DSM-I* and Rediagnosed by *DSM-III*

Area of Functioning	Patients With DSM-I Schizophrenia (N=149)		Patients With DSM-I and DSM-III Schizophrenia (N=82)[a]		Patients With DSM-I But Not DSM-III Schizophrenia (N=71)		$X^2(df=l)$[b]	P
	N	%	N	%	N	%		
Not in hospital in past year	125	84	67	82	61	86	0.23	.63
Met with friends every week or two	97	65	50	61	51	72	1.54	.21
Had one or more moderately to very close friends	113	76	56	68	61	86	5.62	.02
Employed in past year[c]	66	44	33	40	37	52	1.71	.19
Displayed slight or no symptoms	104	70	56	68	52	73	0.24	.62
Able to meet basic needs	119	80	66	81	57	80	0.00	1.00
Led moderate to very full life	113	76	60	73	57	80	0.71	.40

[a]Includes four subjects who were not schizophrenic according to *DSM-I* but who were given a *DSM-III* diagnosis of schizophrenia.
[b]Chi-square with Yates' correction for the comparison between the group diagnosed as schizophrenic by both *DSM-I* and *DSM-III* and the group with *DSM-I* schizophrenia only (now *DSM-III* other categories).
[c]Does not account for subjects who were widowed, retired, or elderly.

The only exception to the high levels of functioning across all diagnostic categories was the rating for employment, which was scored for one-half or fewer of the subjects. However, this rating did not take into account subjects who were retired or elderly.

The major difference between the subjects who met the *DSM-III* criteria for schizophrenia and those who met the *DSM-III* criteria for other diagnoses was fewer close friendships for the *DSM-III* schizophrenia sub-sample (68% versus 86%) ($\chi^2 = 4.89$, df=1, p=.03).

We compared these two groups by using a 2x2 chi-square test with Yates' correction. A small number of cases with missing values were included in the analysis category that reflected the least positive outcome. No significant differences in results were observed when we used this approach and when we used the standard method of excluding cases with missing values.

Discussion

Members of the Vermont cohort were once profoundly ill, back-ward, chronic patients who were provided with a comprehensive rehabilitation program and released to the community 20–25 years ago. The 5- to 10-year follow-up study found that two-thirds of these patients were out of the hospital but were expected to require continuous support by the mental health system in order to remain in the community (44). Further, the subsample of this group rediagnosed as having met the *DSM-III* criteria for schizophrenia at index hospitalization would be expected, according to that system's description of schizophrenia, to have a course with "increasing residual impairment between episodes" *(DSM-III,* p. 185), including continued symptoms, unemployment, social isolation, and inability to care for themselves.

Data from the present study demonstrated that these predictions were inadequate for the majority of subjects. Widely heterogeneous patterns of social, occupational, and psychological functioning evolved over time for these once schizophrenic patients. The more stringent diagnostic criteria of *DSM-III* failed to predict any better than the more loosely formulated *DSM-I* guidelines the true outcome for these schizophrenic patients.

Although these findings show some robustness, they come from a study that suffers from numerous flaws (see our companion paper in this issue). Although it was one of the more rigorously designed research studies of its type, the selection was biased toward the long-term institutionalized patient. The use of reliable, structured instrument batteries was a significant advance over many earlier studies, but the *DSM-III* diagnoses had to be made retrospectively. The updating of subjects' diagnoses to meet current diagnostic criteria is a problem common to all longitudinal studies. It is always a trade-off to try to second-guess the original clinician, who was able to see and interact with the patient. The original clinicians were apt to neglect noting signs and symptoms that were not present and to present data to substantiate their own diagnostic decisions. We were fortunate to have excellent records rich in descriptive passages of actual conversations and behaviors to aid in our own rediagnostic work, but we did not see the patients in person then.

The structured battery that determined the subjects' current functional status was solidly reliable. The two interviewers each had 5–8 years of clinical experience with caseloads of chronic patients before these investigations, and they spent several hours with each subject as well as with a variety of other informants (including other clinicians) who knew these clients or family members well.

Our findings of heterogeneity in functioning at outcome corroborate similar results from the four other long–term studies of schizophrenia that we have mentioned: the three European studies by Bleuler (15), Ciompi and Müller (13), and Huber et al. (14) and the Iowa 500 study (16). These studies have been extensively analyzed by us elsewhere (45). Diverse levels of functioning have been found also in shorter-term studies such as the WHO International Pilot Study of Schizophrenia (33, 46), the Rochester First Admission Study (47), the Boston State Hospital 12-Year Follow-Up Study (48), and the New York State Psychiatric Institute Diagnostic Study (49).

It has been argued that the more stringent the criteria, the better a sample will reflect "true" or "core" schizophrenia (50, 51), and that core schizophrenia has a uniformly poor outcome (5, 52–54). The rigorous inclusion/exclusion criteria of the *DSM-III* classification were designed to select for core schizophrenia, but since the findings of this study revealed outcome to be heterogeneous, the *DSM-III* criteria did not predict long-term outcome as well as expected. This finding was recently duplicated for prediction of very short-term outcome as well (49).

Hawk and associates (55) also found that narrowness of criteria did not predict homogeneous outcome functioning when they compared subjects rediagnosed according to four diagnostic systems, i.e., Langfeldt's criteria (51), Schneider's first-rank symptoms (56), *DSM-II,* and the Flexible System (57).

The focus on strictness of criteria evolved from the Kraepelinian notion that prognosis confirmed diagnosis (58). This theory stated that poor outcome reflected a unifying common denominator for clustering several differently expressed types of mental disorders under one umbrella, dementia praecox. If the patients recovered or improved, they had obviously been misdiagnosed, and another label was applied, such as reactive psychosis (59), schizophreniform states (51), or cycloid psychoses (60–61). In pursuing this argument further, Vaillant (62) cited 16 major attempts to reclassify "remitting schizophrenics" and concluded that most investigators were describing a blend known as Kasanin's schizoaffective disorder (63). Thus, there was no definitive system to describe schizophrenic patients who improved without recategorizing them as having another disorder.

A decade later, in 1975, Vaillant himself completed a 10- to 15-year follow-up of 51 patients who exhibited the classical profile of remitting schizophrenia, as cited from the literature by Stephens (64) and others. This profile included a positive family history of affective disorders, sudden onset with the patient reacting to a clear precipitant, bipolar-like symptoms, and remission within the first 2 years. Thirty-nine percent of the 51 study subjects developed a chronic course. Vaillant found no factors that could differentiate between the patients who would relapse and those who were later rediagnosed as having an affective disorder (65). He concluded that "diagnosis and prognosis should be treated as different dimensions of psychosis" (G.E. Vaillant, paper presented at the 128th annual meeting of the American Psychiatric Association, Anaheim, Calif., May 5–9, 1975).

In the current study, it should be noted that the 25 interviewed patients who were rediagnosed as schizoaffective, the three who had schizophreniform disorders, and the 13 who had atypical psychoses were all eliminated from the analyses that were done to determine the long-term outcome of "core" schizophrenia. These patients were considered to have a much better chance for a good long-term outcome. Despite this very stringent approach, there were still "core schizophrenics" who remitted—a finding that supports Vaillant's concept of the separate contributions of diagnosis and prognosis to long-term outcome (65, and the paper presented at the APA annual meeting).

In addition to incorporating the Kraepelinian idea that future course validates the original diagnosis, *DSM-III* was based on the Feighner, or St. Louis, criteria (1), which established the validity of a diagnosis by requiring deterioration from a previous level of functioning as well as a 6-month duration of illness with or without prodrome. Thus, in the *DSM-III* attempt to select out reactive, schizophreniform, and cycloid types, subjects are required to have been functioning poorly before they are entered into the classification and are expected to be functioning poorly at follow-up. Strauss and Carpenter (66) pointed out the tautology of such a scheme. They suggested that finding an outcome of chronic illness may be primarily related to the original selection of patients with a longstanding disorder as the entry criterion. However, the Vermont subjects were selected for their strong indications of chronicity (e.g., at selection these subjects had had an average of 6 years of continuous psychiatric hospitalization and 16 years of illness before entering the rehabilitation program). Despite this status, many of these very chronic patients appear to have recovered or improved considerably. This finding clearly supports those of the Bonn, Lausanne, Iowa, and Burghölzli studies, which found improvement or recovery two to three decades later (13–16).

One of the complications in analyzing data across earlier studies was the fact that those studies often used the criteria "recovered" or "improved" without defining either concept and commonly used only a single measure of outcome, such as "hospitalized" or "discharged" (see Shapiro and Shader [67] for a discussion). However, the work of Strauss and Carpenter (43, 68, 69) and many others has clearly demonstrated the partial independence in level of functioning at outcome in a variety of areas such as work, social relationships, symptoms, and hospitalization. In Strauss and Carpenter's "open-linked systems" approach (66) to analyzing the course of disorder, the best predictor of follow-up functioning was preepisode functioning in the same area (e.g., previous levels of work predicted current levels of work—a finding also supported by Brown et al. [70] and Monck [71]). Strauss and Carpenter pointed to the need for separate measurements of functioning in a wide variety of areas.

The Vermont Longitudinal Research Project found evidence to support this strategy. Within the middle range of outcome, there were subjects in the sample who were considered to be functioning well (e.g., working, with good family relationships and friends) but who still had delusions or hallucinations. Many subjects had learned either to devise ways of controlling their symptoms—an ability reported also by Breier and Strauss (72)—or had learned not to tell anyone about them anymore. Other subjects were working but were otherwise socially isolated. Some subjects had warm and extensive social networks but did not work. The picture was a complex and heterogeneous one.

Because narrowness of diagnostic criteria seems not to predict outcome, attention might be refocused on an analysis of this hidden underlying heterogeneity within samples (28, 73) in order to sort out other possible predictors of long-term outcome.

The implications of the findings from the Vermont cohort are many and varied. The present study provides strong evidence for the limited usefulness of the current diagnostic classification systems in predicting accurately the long-term outcome for people who meet the criteria for schizophrenia. Further, in each of the five major studies conducted in the past decade that assessed the long-term outcome of schizophrenia, one-half or more of the subjects had recovered or considerably improved in their functioning. Together, these findings offer an argument for a shift in our thinking about the proportions of schizophrenic patients who are able to achieve a better outcome than has heretofore been expected.

Acknowledgments

The following people contributed to this phase of the project: design and methodology: Brendan Maher, Ph.D.; the late Robert Shapiro, M.D.; Bonnie Spring, Ph.D.; Joseph L. Fleiss, Ph.D.; Jane Murphy, Ph.D.; Joseph M. Tobin, M.D.; Lee Robins, Ph.D.; Leona Bachrach, Ph.D.; Edward Zigler, Ph.D.; Stanley Herr, J.D.; and Jon Rolf, Ph.D.; additional aid with instrumentation: William Woodruff, M.D.; Alan Gelenberg, M.D.; Gerard Hogarty, M.S.W.; Paula Clayton, M.D.; Janet Mikkelsen, M.S.W.; and Thomas McGlashan, M.D.; data collection: Paul D. Landerl, M.S.W.; Carmine M. Consalvo, M.Ed.; Janet Wakefield, Ph.D.; William Deane, Ph.D.; Barbara Curtis, R.N.; and Robert Lagor, B.A.; data management: Susan Childers, A.C.S.W.; Lori Witham; Mary Ellen Fortini, Ph.D.; Sandi Tower; Andrea Pierce; Mary Noonan; Dorothy Myer; and Joanne Gobrecht; manuscript review: Luc Ciompi, Prof. Dr. Med.; Prof. John Cooper; Boris Astrachan, M.D.; Malcolm B. Bowers, Jr., M.D.; Richard Musty, Ph.D.; George Albee, Ph.D.; Thomas Achenbach, Ph.D.; Paul Carling, Ph.D.; Lawrence Gordon, Ph.D.; and Frederick Schmidt, Ph.D.; and manuscript preparation: Nancy L. Ryan.

References

1. Feighner JP, Robins E, Guze SB, et al: Diagnostic criteria for use in psychiatric research. Arch Gen Psychiatry 1972; 26:57–63
2. Spitzer RL, Endicott J, Robins E: Research Diagnostic Criteria: rationale and reliability. Arch Gen Psychiatry 1978; 35:773—782
3. Crow TJ: Schizophrenic deterioration. Br J Psychiatry 1983; 143:80–81.
4. Garmezy N: Process and reactive schizophrenia: some conceptions and issues, in The Role and Methodology of Classification in Psychiatry and Psychopathology: NIMH Public Health Service Publication 1584. Edited by Katz MM, Cole JD, Barton WE. Washington, DC, US Government Printing Office, 1965

5. Stephens JH, Astrup C: Treatment outcome in "process" and"non-process" schizophrenics treated by "A" and "B" types of therapists. J Nerv Ment Dis 1965; 140:449–456

6. Kirk SA, Therrien ME: Community mental health myths and the fate of former hospitalized patients. Psychiatry 1975; 38: 209–217

7. Lamb HR, Edelson MB: The carrot and the stick: inducing local programs to serve long-term patients. Community Ment Health J 1976; 12:137–144

8. Talbott JA (ed): The Chronic Mental Patient: Problems, Solutions, and Recommendations for a Public Policy. Washington, DC, American Psychiatric Association, 1979

9. Cooper JE, Kendell RE, Gurland BJ, et al: Psychiatric Diagnosis in New York and London: A Comparative Study of Mental Hospital Admissions. New York, Oxford University Press, 1972.

10. Fenton WS, Mosher LR, Matthews TM: Diagnosis of schizophrenia: a critical review of current diagnostic systems. Schizophr Bull 1981; 7:452–476

11. Romano J: On the nature of schizophrenia: changes in the observer as well as the observed (1932–1977). Schizophr Bull 1977: 3:532–559

12. Spitzer RL, Forman JBW, Nee J: *DSM-III* field trials, I: initial interrater diagnostic reliability. Am J Psychiatry 1979; 136: 815–817

13. Ciompi L, Müller C: Lebensweg und Alter der Schizophrenen: Eine katamnestische Lonzeitstudies bis ins senium. Berlin, Springer Verlag, 1976

14. Huber G, Gross G, Schüttler R: Schizophrenie: Verlaufs und sozialpsychiatrische Langzeituntersuchungen an den 1945 bis 1959 in Bonn hospitalisierten schizophrenen Kranken: Mono-graphien aus dem Gesamtgebiete der Psychiatrie. Bd 21. Berlin, Springer Verlag, 1979

15. Bleuler M: The Schizophrenic Disorders: Long-Term Patient and Family Studies. Translated by Clemens SM. New Haven, Yale University Press, 1978

16. Tsuang MT, Woolson RF, Fleming JA: Long-term outcome of major psychoses, I: schizophrenia and affective disorders compared with psychiatrically symptom-free surgical conditions. Arch Gen Psychiatry 1979; 36:1295–1301

17. Brooks GW: Opening a rehabilitation house, in Rehabilitation of the Mentally Ill. Edited by Greenblatt M, Simon B. Washington, DC, American Association for the Advancement of Science, 1959

18. Brooks GW: Rehabilitation of hospitalized chronic schizophrenic patients. In Chronic Schizophrenia. Edited by Appleby L, Scher J, Cumming J. Chicago, Free Press, 1960

19. Brooks GW: Motivation for work in psychiatric rehabilitation. Dis Nerv Syst 1961; 22:129–132

20. Brooks GW: Rural community influences and supports in a rehabilitation program for state hospital patients, in Mental Patients in Transition. Edited by Greenblatt M, Levinson DJ, Klerman GL. Springfield, Ill, Charles C Thomas, 1961

21. Brooks GW, Deane WN: Attitudes of released chronic schizophrenic patients concerning illness and recovery as revealed by a structured post-hospital interview. J Clin Psychol 1960; 16: 259–264

22. Brooks GW, Deane WN: The chronic mental patient in the community. Dis Nerv Syst 1965; 26:85–90

23. Brooks GW, Deane WN, Lagor RC, et al: Varieties of family participation in the rehabilitation of released chronic schizophrenic patients. J Nerv Ment Dis 1963; 136:432–444

24. Brooks GW, Deane WN, Laqueur HP: Fifteen years of work therapy. Dis Nerv Syst (Suppl) 1970; 31:161–165

25. Chittick RA, Brooks GW, Irons FS, et al: The Vermont Story. Burlington, Vt, Queen City Printers, 1961

26. Harding CM, Brooks GW: Longitudinal assessment for a cohort of chronic schizophrenics discharged twenty years ago. Psychiatr J Univ Ottawa 1980; 5:274–278

27. Harding CM, Brooks GW: Life assessment of a cohort of chronic schizophrenics discharged twenty years ago, in The Handbook of Longitudinal Research, vol II. Edited by Mednick S, Harway M, Finello K. New York, Praeger, 1984

28. Harding CM, Brooks GW, Ashikaga T, et al: Aging and social functioning in once-chronic schizophrenic patients 22–62 years after first admission: the Vermont story, in Schizophrenia, Paranoia, and Schizophreniform Disorders in Later Life. Edited by Hudgins G, Miller N. New York, Guilford Press (in press)

29. Harding CM, Strauss JS: The course of schizophrenia: an evolving concept, in Controversies in Schizophrenia: Changes and Constancies. Edited by Alpert M. New York, Guilford Press, 1985

30. Harding CM: Long-term outcome functioning of subjects re-diagnosed as meeting the DSM-III criteria for schizophrenia (doctoral dissertation). Burlington, University of Vermont, 1984

31. Harding CM, Brooks GW, Ashikaga T, et al: The Vermont longitudinal study of persons with severe mental illness, I: methodology, study sample, and overall status 32 years later. Am J Psychiatry 1987; 144:718–726

32. Strauss JS, Harder DW: The Case Record Rating Scale. Psychiatry Res 1981; 4:333–345

33. World Health Organization: Collaborative Project on Determinants of Outcome of Severe Mental Disorders (1977–1979): Research Protocols. Geneva, WHO, Aug 1978

34. McGlashan TH: The Chestnut Lodge follow-up study, I: follow-up methodology and study sample. Arch Gen Psychiatry 1984; 41:573–585

35. Fleiss J: Statistical Methods for Rates and Proportions. New York, John Wiley & Sons, 1973

36. Spitzer RL, Endicott J, Robins E: Research Diagnostic Criteria (RDC) for a Selected Group of Functional Disorders, 3rd ed. New York, New York State Psychiatric Institute, Biometrics Research, 1977

37. Research Diagnostic Criteria Screening Interview. New York, New York State Psychiatric Institute, Department of Psycho-physiology, 1976

38. Overall JE, Gorham DR: The Brief Psychiatric Rating Scale. Psychol Rep 1962; 10:799–812

39. Folstein MF, Folstein SE, McHugh PR: "Mini-Mental State": a practical method for grading the cognitive state of patients for the clinician. J Psychiatr Res 1975; 12:189–198

40. Endicott J, Spitzer RL: A diagnostic interview: the Schedule for Affective Disorders and Schizophrenia. Arch Gen Psychiatry 1978; 35:837–844

41. Spitzer RL, Gibbon M, Endicott J: The Global Assessment Scale (GAS). New York, New York State Psychiatric Institute, 1975

42. Endicott J, Spitzer RL, Fleiss JL, et al: The Global Assessment Scale: a procedure for measuring overall severity of psychiatric disturbance. Arch Gen Psychiatry 1976; 33:766–771

43. Strauss JS, Carpenter WT: Prediction of outcome in schizophrenia, III: five-year outcome and its predictors. Arch Gen Psychiatry 1977; 34:159–163

44. Deane WN, Brooks GW: Five-Year Follow-Up of Chronic Hospitalized Patients. Waterbury, Vermont State Hospital, Sept 1967

45. Harding CM, Zubin J, Strauss JS: Chronicity in schizophrenia: fact, partial fact, or artifact? Hosp Community Psychiatry (in press)

46. World Health Organization: The International Pilot Study of Schizophrenia. Geneva, WHO, 1973

47. Strauss JS, Kokes RF, Ritzler BA, et al: Patterns of disorder in first admission psychiatric patients. J Nerv Ment Dis 1978; 166: 611–625

48. Gardos G, Cole JO, LaBrie RA: A 12-year follow-up study of chronic schizophrenics. Hosp Community Psychiatry 1982; 33: 983–984

49. Endicott J, Nee J, Cohen JL, et al: Diagnosis of schizophrenia. Arch Gen Psychiatry 1986; 43:13–19

50. Langfeldt G: The Prognosis in Schizophrenia and the Factors Influencing the Course of the Disease. Acta Psychiatr Neurol Scand (Suppl) 1937; 13

51. Langfeldt G: Schizophreniform States. Copenhagen, E Munks-gaard, 1939

52. Achté KA: On Prognosis and Rehabilitation in Schizophrenia and Paranoid Psychoses. Acta Psychiatr Neurol Scand (Suppl) 1967; 196

53. Astrup C, Noreik K: Functional Psychoses: Diagnostic and Prognostic Models. Springfield, Ill, Charles C Thomas, 1966

54. Eitinger L, Laane CL, Langfeldt G: The prognostic value of the clinical picture and the therapeutic value of physical treatment in schizophrenia and the schizophreniform states. Acta Psychiatr Neurol Scand 1958; 33:33–53

55. Hawk AB, Carpenter WT Jr, Strauss JS: Diagnostic criteria and 5-year outcome in schizophrenia: a report from the International Pilot Study of Schizophrenia. Arch Gen Psychiatry 1975; 32:343–347

56. Schneider K: Clinical Psychopathology. Translated by Hamilton MW. New York, Grune & Stratton, 1959

57. Carpenter WT Jr, Strauss JS, Bartko JJ: A flexible system for the identification of schizophrenia: a report from the International Pilot Study of Schizophrenia. Science 1973; 182:1275–1278

58. Kraepelin E: Dementia praecox, in Clinical Psychiatry: A Textbook for Students and Physicians, 6th ed. Translated by Diefendorf AR. New York, Macmillan, 1902

59. Jaspers K: General Psychopathology. Edited and translated by Hamilton MW. Chicago, University of Chicago Press, 1963

60. Leonhard K: The question of prognosis in schizophrenia. Int J Psychiatry 1966; 2:633–635

61. Leonhard K: Cycloid psychoses: endogenous psychoses which are neither schizophrenic nor manic depressive. J Ment Sci 1961;107:633–648

62. Vaillant G: Prospective prediction of schizophrenic remission. Arch Gen Psychiatry 1964; 11:509–518

63. Kasanin J: The acute schizoaffective psychoses. Am J Psychiatry 1933; 90:97–126

64. Stephens JH: Long-term course and prognosis in schizophrenia. Semin Psychiatry 1970; 2:464–485

65. Vaillant GE: A 10-year follow-up of remitting schizophrenics. Schizophr Bull 1978; 4(II):78–85

66. Strauss JS, Carpenter WT: Characteristic symptoms and outcome in schizophrenia. Arch Gen Psychiatry 1974; 30:429—434

67. Shapiro R, Shader R: Selective review of results of previous follow-up studies of schizophrenia and other psychoses, in Schizophrenia: An International Follow-Up Study. By the World Health Organization. New York, John Wiley & Sons, 1979

68. Strauss JS, Carpenter WT: The prediction of outcome in schizophrenia, I: characteristics of outcome. Arch Gen Psychiatry 1972; 27:739–746

69. Strauss JS, Carpenter WT: The prediction of outcome in schizophrenia, II: relationships between predictor and outcome variables. Arch Gen Psychiatry 1974; 31:37–42

70. Brown GW, Bone M, Dalison B, et al: Schizophrenia and Social Care. London, Oxford University Press, 1966

71. Monck EM: Employment experience of 127 discharged schizophrenic men in London. Br J Preventive and Social Med 1963; 17:101–110

72. Breier A, Strauss JS: Self-control of psychotic disorders. Arch Gen Psychiatry 1983; 40:1141–1145

73. Hogarty GE: Treatment and the course of schizophrenia. Schizophr Bull 1977; 3:587–599

32

Lefley, H. P., & Bestman, E. W. (1991). Public-academic linkages for culturally sensitive community mental health. *Community Mental Health Journal, 27* (6), 473–488

This article combines two important themes in community psychiatry—culturally sensitive mental health care and public-academic linkages—that are even more relevant today than when it was published in 1991. Culturally sensitive care, also called cultural appropriate or culturally competent care, has received increasing attention in recent years. High percentages of African Americans, Latinos, and other racial-ethnic groups are served in community mental health centers and other community mental health settings, yet clinicians and other providers of care often are predominantly white and have not received training to increase their awareness of and sensitivity to the cultural traditions and preferences of their clients. Understanding of the special importance attached to family support for members of some ethnics groups, for example, is not a given for clinicians trained to provide individually oriented psychotherapy. In addition, as more and more emphasis is placed on evidence-based practice, there is concern that such practices, when applied to members of racial-ethnic groups not included among participants with whom the intervention was tested, may require modifications in order to provide the same benefits that others experience. Academic linkages to public mental health centers, the authors contend, can make available to clinicians, administrators, and others expertise in cultural competence theory, research, and training that can help to fill these gaps. Lefley and Bestman give a detailed description of the rationale for and development of culturally sensitive teams, treatment, training and staffing, based in part on their experience with the ethnically diverse client population of the University of Miami-Jackson Memorial Community Mental Health Center.

Public-Academic Linkages for Culturally Sensitive Community Mental Health

ABSTRACT: This paper traces the sixteen year history of a unique community mental health center which has combined academic and service provider roles in delivery of culturally appropriate care. Initially an arm of a department of psychiatry and derived from an anthropological research project, the center model was based on seven teams serving discrete ethnic communities, with subsequent development of a network of neighborhood-based "mini-clinics" as well as centralized aftercare facilities. The team staff-social scientists, clinicians, and paraprofessionals all of matching ethnicity to the populations served-became a core of "culture brokers" with a service, teaching, and research role at the interface of the university, medical center, and community. Subsequently the university was funded for a cross-cultural training institute for mental health professionals. Center staff extended training in culturally appropriate care to 174 mental health professionals from 97 facilities throughout the nation, as well as other spinoffs improving cultural expertise of staff in public sector agencies. Data on effectiveness of services and training are given and significant findings are discussed. The description includes the impact of historical shifts in funding, the effects of external events on community mental health center structure, and the current state of cross-cultural training and public-academic linkages in this particular program.

Public-academic linkages have always been desirable from both a service and training viewpoint. The need for well-trained practitioners in public service delivery, particularly in work with seriously mentally ill persons, is matched by the need of universities to provide educators who are well-versed in state-of-the-art theory, research, and practice. One of the best ways to accomplish this is for universities and public sector agencies to promote bridging positions for academicians in public sector service delivery.

Currently there is a multidisciplinary focus on training clinicians to serve seriously mentally ill persons (Cutler & Lefley, 1988; Faulkner et al., 1980; Lefley, Bernheim & Goldman, 1989). National Institute of Mental Health (NIMH) initiatives simultaneously emphasize serving minority populations, of whatever types or levels of psychopathology, in a "culturally sensitive" way. The extent to which various minority groups are represented in the seriously mentally ill population is variable and difficult to assess (Lefley, 1990; Snowden & Cheung, 1990). According to the latest national data base, American Indians and Blacks are admitted to all inpatient psychiatric services at rates over three times higher than those of Asians, about twice higher than Hispanics, and about one and one half times higher than Whites. In public sector state and county mental hospitals, American Indians and Blacks are admitted at rates four times greater than Asians, two to two and one-half times more than Hispanics, and two and one-quarter to two and two-thirds more than Whites. In all inpatient admissions, the order from highest to lowest is Blacks, American Indians, Whites, Hispanics, and Asians, although Hispanics are somewhat higher than Whites in state and county hospital admissions. Yet, in state and county mental hospitals, Asians, Hispanics, and Whites, in that order, have higher median inpatient stays than do Black or American Indian patients (Rosenstein, Milazzo-Sayre, MacAskill, & Manderscheid, 1987). Manderscheid (personal communication) indicates that by next year we should have a more precise count on ethnic distribution and other characteristics of persons with serious and persistent mental illnesses through the NIMH mental health supplement to the National Health Interview Survey.

Meanwhile, the variable picture shown in the above data suggests a range of possible differences in ethnic communities. These may include legitimate differences in prevalence and intensity of major types of psychopathology which require hospitalization. Alternatively, they may reflect variation in cultural belief systems, symptom thresholds, supportive networks, community stigma and tolerance levels, differential access to mental health systems and use of traditional healers, discrete patterns of stressors, and other socioeconomic and cultural variables affecting the developmental stage of presentation for services as well as precipitants of decompensation. Since there is now a large empirical literature on diagnostic and treatment deficits on the part of professionals working with culturally diverse patients, the data may also reflect practitioners' cultural ignorance or bias in evaluation, diagnosis, admissions practices, case disposition, and involuntary commitment decisions which are differentially applied to minority subgroups (Lefley, 1990; Snowden & Cheung, 1990).

Issues in Developing Culturally Sensitive Services

One of our first tasks, then, should be to develop a core group of mental health professionals who can apply and share expertise in their own cultures. The NIMH focus on supporting the training of minority group professionals is certainly a major step in this direction. Yet, we all recognize that it will be many years before we have an adequate representation of professionals from ethnic minority groups, or even of professionals from the mainstream culture who are trained in a trans-cultural perspective. Moreover, is provision of culturally-matched or culturally-trained clinicians within a traditional service framework sufficient to qualify as providing "culturally sensitive" services? Or, rather, do we need to reconceptualize the locus and mode of service delivery to meet requirements of cultural accessibility? Further, if a variable picture indeed exists with respect to major mental illnesses, which are increasingly viewed as equally distributed biogenetic disorders, should professionals try to identify and reduce those community stressors (including possible ecological variables) which may precipitate a differential pattern of decompensation? What is the role of professionals in secondary prevention of lesser emotional disorders—those which are not major psychotic conditions but are nevertheless distressful and disabling—in high risk communities? How do we differentiate that which is ethnocultural from the interacting variables of minority status, poverty, social discrimination, refugee status, migration, or the functional and emotional impact of culture loss and change?

In short, what comes under the rubric of "culturally sensitive services?" Rogler, Malgady, Costantino and Blumenthal (1987) attempted to answer this question for just one group by analyzing the literature on Hispanic mental health services for the past 15—20 years. Three broad approaches emerged. The first involved making traditional treatments more accessible to Hispanics by increasing the congruence between values of the professionals and indigenous Hispanic values, and also incorporating elements of the lay referral system to promote rather than impede service utilization. The second involved selecting available therapeutic modalities according to the perceived features of Hispanic culture—in most cases establishing a hierarchy of need, taking the cohesive extended family network into account, dealing with issues of culture change, and tailoring the therapeutic modality to the client's level of acculturation. The third approach involved "extracting elements from Hispanic culture to modify traditional treatments or use them as an innovative treatment tool" (p. 565). This typically has involved therapeutic content that mirrors the culture, but others have argued for bending or redirecting traditional cultural patterns (such as female subjugation) to facilitate individual therapeutic gains and ease adaptation to a new cultural system. Szapocznik et al. (1986) have argued for bicultural effectiveness training—the ability to negotiate both old and new cultural systems—as the desired goal for Hispanic-American youths and their families. For the most part, these cultural adaptations did not deal with aftercare or rehabilitative modalities needed for persons with serious mental illnesses.

A Culturally-Sensitive Community Mental Health Program

In March, 1974, when the University of Miami-Jackson Memorial Community Mental Health Center (CMHC) was first organized, many of these issues with respect to serving clients from minority cultures had already begun to appear in the literature. This CMHC, the first in Miami-Dade county, was funded to serve a catchment area in inner-city Miami rich in ethnic diversity, with almost 85% of the population of U.S. Black, Caribbean, Central or South American origin, and the balance composed primarily of Anglo elderly. The catchment area also had a median income of under $5000 and a multiplicity of social problems.

The grant was developed by faculty in the Department of Psychiatry at the University of Miami and awarded to its teaching hospital, Jackson Memorial, a large county facility and at that time the major public psychiatric resource for a metropolitan area of one and one half million people. The model evolved from a comprehensive three-year research effort, the Health Ecology Project, initiated and directed by Hazel H. Weidman, a social/medical anthropologist, and co-directed by departmental chairman James N. Sussex, a psychiatrist, and Janice Egeland, a medical sociologist who later went on to develop and direct the noted Amish Affective Disorders Study.

Funded by the Commonwealth Fund, the Health Ecology Project investigated health systems, beliefs, and behaviors of five ethnic groups: Bahamians, Cubans, Haitians, Puerto Ricans, and U.S. Blacks. These groups were the major constituents of the area designated for service by the CMHC. In this study of over 500 families (Weidman, 1978), preliminary findings indicated culturally-patterned differences in clustering of symptoms, culture bound syndromes with a large emotional component, unrecognized by orthodox medical or mental health professionals (Lefley, 1979b, Weidman, 1979); and differences in conceptions of bodily functioning (Scott, 1974). Alternative healing modalities were widely used for physical and emotional problems, often in conjunction with orthodox medical treatment. Orthodox mental health treatment, however, was almost never solicited, although interviews and daily health calendars maintained by the families indicated many stressors and a high degree of emotional distress.

Field data from the Health Ecology Project and elsewhere, on cultural variations in the distribution, manifestation, and conceptualization of mental health problems, together with emergent diagnostic and therapeutic problems among ethnic patients in the hospital system, strongly suggested that a community mental health center established along traditional lines would neither be maximally effective nor optimally utilized. Further, while all groups suffered from multiple socioeconomic and environmental stressors, the indications were that in many cases culturally specific therapeutic interventions might be required to deal with different ethnic groups living within the same poverty area.

The CMHC that was developed reflected the prevailing community mental health ideology of the day; the vistas of service were broad. To a greater extent than many other CMHCs, the program incorporated and served seriously and persistently mentally ill persons, if only because of their need and visibility in a poor inner-city area. But the mission focused on larger and more grandiose objectives: a) to provide fully accessible, culturally appropriate services that would encompass the full range of presenting complaints, including but in no way limited to major psychiatric disorders; and b) to alleviate environmental stressors by helping residents receive their fair share of adaptive resources. To this end, the CMHC developed six teams of indigenous mental health workers to serve the major demographic groups in the area: Anglo elderly, Bahamian, Cuban, Haitian, Puerto Rican, and U.S. Black. A seventh team primarily serving Black elderly was added. In each ethnic community the team had an advisory board which helped with needs assessment, staffing, and developing services. Combining research, community development, and clinical functions, each team was led by a social scientist, typically at the Ph.D. level, and each had a clinical social worker and part-time psychiatrist and psychologist, together with 3–5 trained paraprofessionals. Almost all staff, of all levels and disciplines, were of matching ethnicity to the populations served.

Team functions involved structured needs assessment, action-oriented research to bring needed resources into communities (day care programs, senior citizens programs), provision of social services, and consultation and education in accordance with how communities defined their needs. When the teams began to be viewed as a viable helping resource, a network of neighborhood "mini-clinics" was established in each of the ethnic communities. These functioned as aftercare clinics and outpatient units, as well as neighborhood centers for the local population. There was also an aftercare clinic, Community House, which offered a more structured medication and day treatment program than did the mini-clinics. These were the decentralized components of the CMHC. Crisis intervention, inpatient, and some partial hospitalization services were provided at Jackson Memorial Hospital, the centralized hospital system serving the entire county. Structurally, the CMHC consisted of the seven ethnic community teams, nine neighborhood clinics, administrative and research and evaluation sections; and affiliative relationships with special drug and alcohol services and primary health care clinics in the Black and Hispanic communities. Transitional housing was later added for aftercare clients.

In treatment of aftercare clients, two features of the teams and their mini-clinics are of particular interest. First, with their extensive community contacts, the paraprofessional neighborhood workers assigned to individual clients functioned as effective case managers long before the term had been coined. They obtained entitlement checks, medical care, housing, and other resources because they knew their own locales, were adept at networking, and had been trained to do community research. Secondly, some of the mini-clinics functioned as neighborhood centers, offering games and classes in macrame, art, guitar, exercises, health and the like, so that they attracted children, elders, and other community members. In this setting, aftercare clients had normalized roles. Former hospital patients received medication, counseling, and recreational activities alongside people from the surrounding community who had problems in living but no diagnosed mental disorder. Unfortunately, this situation did not remain constant for all teams, and the population of aftercare clients served in mini-clinics, hospital, or centralized aftercare clinic varied as a function of ethnic neighborhood and accessibility to resources. Hispanic and Haitian aftercare clients tended to be fewer in number and could be accommodated in the mini-clinics; whereas the larger caseload of young adult Anglo and Black clients with long-term mental illnesses required more centralized facilities. Increasingly, also, it was seen that the Bahamian team tended to serve Black-American clients (many of whom were of mixed Bahamian or West Indian descent), and ultimately the teams merged.

In addition to clinic-based services, teams were involved in home visits and in establishing a network of information, referral, and social service coordination for clients. Neighborhood outreach programs, needs assessment, casefinding and resource linkages were ongoing at the community level. Community-based consultation and education were balanced by case-centered consultation and direct services to individuals in the home, schools, churches, and boarding houses, including development of supportive networks for social isolates.

A new dimension in community mental health services, however, was provided by the selection of anthropologists and other social scientists for leadership positions. Programmatic research, in addition to needs assessment, included ethnographic and demographic profiles, and action-oriented research for community organization and development. The teams acted as initiators and coordinators of various projects to bring new resources into their communities or strengthen existing ones; conducted surveys to provide supportive data for community-requested programs; linked consumer groups with appropriate service agencies; and helped residents learn how to utilize these agencies for ameliorating specific neighborhood problems. And each of these efforts was oriented toward serving the needs of a specific ethnic community and conducted in its own cultural idiom. More specific examples of these projects may be found in Bestman, 1986 and Lefley and Bestman, 1.984.

"Culture-Brokers": the Academic-Public Bridging Role

Social scientists and clinicians on these teams were called "culture brokers"—a professional role in the health care delivery system first described by Weidman (1983), involving a bridging, interpretive, collaborative, and teaching function at the interface of the hospital and community and within the two systems. Culture brokers, as faculty in the Department of Psychiatry, had combined academic, applied social scientist, and service provider roles. Hospital linkages facilitated an exchange of transcultural clinical information with a wide range of medical staff as well as mental health practitioners.

In educating mental health and medical staff about culturally appropriate care, the culture broker focused on beliefs and practices that might impede or facilitate effective treatment, and also on adaptive strategies, strengths, and supports within the patient's cultural milieu. As a consultant and collaborator in specific cases, the culture broker played an interpretive and affiliative role in in-house treatment—sometimes functionally as a co-therapist—and an active role in aftercare. Examples of cultural interpretation might involve explaining a "rooted" patient to a crisis worker who was unable to diagnose the observed symptoms within traditional psychiatric nosology; or teaching a psychiatric resident how to differentiate legitimate paranoid ideation-i.e., ideas that are considered bizarre in the culture—from ideas of reference or persecution that would not be considered abnormal within the conceptual framework of the culture. In each of these examples, the condition might be interpreted by the patient as arising from a malevolent curse that requires ritualistic undoing, and chemotherapeutic or psychotherapeutic interventions will help only if the ritual is performed. On another level, cultural interpretation could involve the very mode of interviewing and eliciting cooperation from clients. In some cases the authority of the mental health professional conflicts with the authority relationships at home and the client is placed in a double bind. One example involved informing an intake worker that certain requests might be perfectly acceptable to a white middle-class client, such as asking a wife to bring her husband in for marital counseling, but would be so unacceptable in some traditional cultures (in this case Guatemalan immigrants) that this might explain why the wife did not return. In such cases, cooperation of a respected elder in the household or kinship network may be required in approaching the husband and insuring that the wife does not abandon therapy.

Concurrently, the culture broker facilitated understanding and utilization of services by the ethnic consumers within the context of their belief and value systems. In cases where diagnosis or treatment conflicted with cultural norms or expectations, the brokers sometimes took an active role in arranging appropriate interventions. In cases where it seemed advisable, they established linkages between the orthodox mental health care system and a traditional healer, even arranging an exorcism in intractable cases (see Lefley, 1984).

Program evaluation subsequently demonstrated the efficacy of these combined approaches. Empirical data on minority utilization, no-show rates, and dropout rates demonstrated that, when compared with normative or baseline data then available from other centers, the model had been successfully applied. For example, at a time when most community mental health centers were underutilized by minorities, our CMHC had a minority caseload of 80%. In addition to underutilization, cultural inaccessibility often results in minority members failing to keep appointments, with no-show rates ranging from 40% to 56% for Black and Hispanic patients (Herz & Stamps, 1977). In comparison, our CMHC had a mean no-show rate of 9.7 percent.

At that time, drop-out rates had been reported as high as 74% for Black clients and 75% for Mexican-Americans (Wolkon et al., 1974); and Sue (1977) assessing 14,000 CMHC clients reported the percentages of those who failed to return after one appointment as over 50% for Blacks, Asian Americans, and Native Americans and 42% for Chicanos, significantly higher than the 30% for whites. There is an admitted difficulty in comparing rates without controlling for baseline length of treatment. Long-term patients are less likely to drop out of treatment, and the Miami CMHC may have been overweighted for aftercare patients compared with the others. But the majority of the clientele were not in this category. Thus our mean dropout rate of 4%, with a high of 12%, appeared to be significantly lower than the norm. Other data on client satisfaction, and outcome measures based on goal-attainment scaling and recidivism rates, similarly demonstrated the effectiveness of this program model (see Lefley & Bestman, 1984). This program also demonstrated that interventions aimed at reducing environmental stressors—essentially case management such as helping the client obtain housing or medical care for a sick child—predicted therapeutic outcome in individual cases (Lefley, 1979a).

The Cross-Cultural Training Institute

In the course of treating our multi-ethnic clientele in the hospital and mini-clinics; in ongoing supportive contacts and home visits with families; and in consultation and interventions in the schools, criminal justice system, and other community agencies, a body of information emerged relevant to the application of culturally appropriate care. This information was shared in clinical case conferences, lectures, papers, articles, and books. Staff members were increasingly called on for consultation and continuing education workshops on minority and cross-cultural issues by local and state agencies, and later at the national level as well. Subsequently NIMH funded a three-year Cross-Cultural Training Institute for Mental Health Professionals (CCTI). The CCTI was a highly intensive eight-day training experience that ultimately trained 174 practicing mental health professionals representing 97 institutions and agencies throughout the United States.

Because this was a funded research and demonstration project, rather than an educational workshop alone, we were able to be selective in choosing applicants so that we could accomplish two missions. The first was to orient the training toward structural as well as content changes in service delivery to minority groups. The second was to require trainees' participation in a comprehensive evaluation of process and outcome. This was essentially a research project on the transfer of training to practice.

In selecting trainees, preference was given to candidates from agencies which (a) served catchment areas with sizeable numbers of Black, Hispanic, or other minority populations, and (b) were willing to release at least two participants at the same time, preferably an administrator as well as direct service staff. Knowing the resistance which one lone change agent is likely to incur, we wanted to train persons in a position to provide administrative as well as professional support for knowledge sharing, spinoff cross-cultural training efforts, and agency-wide changes. We also wanted to insure as many minority participants as possible, to share their own cultural expertise, learn about the cultures of other ethnic minorities, and function as motivators and catalysts to get new programs off the ground in their own agencies. The ethnic breakdown was 52% non-minority white, 48% minority; and 65% of the mental health agencies sent at least one administrator over the course of the training.

Training included didactic materials, cultural immersion (community experiences) experiential role-playing and simulations, and action plan development and implementation, with on-site technical assistance provided after the CCTI ended. The training was accompanied by a comprehensive evaluation component. Short-term evaluation utilized participant feedback in rating the workshops, and objective measures looked at changes in knowledge and skill levels, reductions in cognitive, social, and attitudinal distance, understanding of values, and behaviorally demonstrated (videotaped) therapeutic effectiveness. Long-range evaluation looked at effects on clinical and administrative practice, agency changes and spinoff effects, and impact on cultural accessibility for clients in terms of minority utilization and dropout rates. A cost-effectiveness study determined the savings obtained by reducing clients' failure to keep scheduled appointments. And a follow-up was obtained of the long-range impact of the training on the participant's own work, self-concept, analytic perceptions of his/her own professional education, and views of good mental health care. (More detailed curriculum and evaluation materials may be found in Lefley & Pedersen, 1986),

Significant rises in learning occurred on all cognitive measures, and significant changes in social distance which varied as a function of the ethnicity of the trainee. With training, trainees' perceptions of the values and world view of a contrast culture moved closer to those of persons representing that culture. Videotaped vignettes of interviewing skills with a client from a different cultural background, rated blind by over 1000 community viewers of Black, Hispanic, and Anglo backgrounds, indicated a significant increase in therapist skills and sensitivity after training, with controls for practice effects. Reports of the long-range subjective impact, 6 to 18 months after CCTI training, indicated changes in participants' work, self-concept as mental health professionals, cultural self-awareness, assessments of deficits in their own professional education, and views of good mental health care.

In long-range evaluation of action plans submitted by 61% of the agencies, more than half fulfilled goals formulated by the trainees, including ethnic needs assessments, community liaison and outreach, affirmative action plans, ethnic representation on boards, continuing education, special services, and quality assurance. Confirming the wisdom of the selection process, the scores of action plans developed by agencies that sent at least one administrator were significantly higher ($p < .01$) than those of agencies whose trainees were primarily clinical. There were multiple spinoff effects, ranging from total restructuring and decentralization of an urban CMHC to improve its services to ethnic minorities, to replications of cross-cultural training at the home site.

Perhaps the most significant findings, however, were those which suggested the impact of training on clients. It was hypothesized that increased cultural awareness in clinicians and administrators would be reflected in an observed decrease in clients' drop-out rates, both in clinicians' personal caseloads, and in overall agency rates due to culturally sensitive procedures initiated by administrator-participants. Comparison of rates six months before and six months after CCTI attendance, using the prior period for baseline percentages, indicated the following: 1) there was an increase in minority utilization, both in clinician and agency caseloads; 2) there was a significant reduction in agency dropout rates, overall ($p < .001$) and for specific ethnic groups; 3) for individual clinicians, there was a significant reduction in the dropout rates of Hispanic clients. This could not be attributed to the passage of time alone. Normative data from the NIMH Annual Biometry Inventory on all federally funded CMHCs indicated remarkable stability in dropout rates, with less than .02% deviation over a two year period (see Lefley, 1986).

Finally, a cost-benefit analysis suggested a projected mean annual savings of $152,930 based on only one output unit—the last scheduled appointment. The cost-benefit to individual clients and their families in terms of productivity, improved role functioning, improved interpersonal relations, and subjective wellbeing cannot be assessed here, but they also must be considered in the analysis. So, too, must the cultural sensitivity and skills that will later be extended to other clients.

Following the success of the CCTI, specialized cultural training was developed for paraprofessionals working with children, families, and chronic patients. The culture brokers became consultants to the local school system, helped develop curriculum for its desegregation center, and became involved in training major police departments and protective services on cultural beliefs and practices of the populations they served. The CMHC was awarded a contract to provide cross-cultural training for five Deinstitutionalization Projects throughout Florida. The CMHC was funded for a Mental Health Human Services Training Center to train paraprofessional staff to increase their effectiveness in providing services to Cuban and Haitian entrants (Bestman, 1986). The CCTI continued to provide technical assistance and to provide cross-cultural training workshops oriented toward the growing population of deinstitutionalized patients with serious and persistent mental illnesses.

Changing Trends and Future Directions

As is well known, replication of successful research and demonstration projects is contingent on favorable events in the external environment—fiscal, sociological, and ideological. Modes of delivering mental health services and training practitioners are interrelated with events in the larger society. These include the characteristics, numbers, and needs of consumers; governmental changes in administrative infrastructure and the distribution of funding; restrictions of third-party payments that affect locus, mode, and duration of treatment; and changes in social and professional thought regarding the parameters and priorities of mental health services (Lefley, 1988a). Like all federally funded CMHCs, the University of Miami-Jackson Memorial CMHC ultimately became free standing. Its name was changed to New Horizons CMHC. With changes in federal administration, the major funding source shifted to block grants to the states.

In contrast to many other centers, New Horizons had had a good track record in serving the seriously and persistently mentally ill population. This underserved group now became the first priority for states wishing to reduce their hospital beds. In line with this trend, New Horizons now began to focus on tertiary prevention. This involved efforts to prevent rehospitalization through building up community support services. With diminished funding, the CMHC's prior focus on community organization for primary prevention of sociologically-based stress disorders could no longer be sustained. Because we are now increasingly aware of the need for conceptual distinctions among sociogenic, psychogenic and biogenic disorders, it is important to state that community mental health centers cannot and should not claim a capability of primary or secondary prevention of biologically-based mental illnesses. However, poverty and racism continue to be issues that affect not only the mental health of populations, but the adjustment of the seriously mentally ill (Lefley, 1990). Secondary prevention efforts continue to be maintained with groups at risk for emotional disorders such as AIDS patients, conduct-disordered children, refugees, homeless persons, assault victims, etc. And tertiary prevention of decompensation and relapse in persons with serious and persistent mental illnesses is continuously emphasized in terms of intensive case management and a range of other community-based services.

At New Horizons, the ethnic community teams and mini-clinics are now gone, and the center has developed a more traditional structure based on service categories rather than ethnicity. The ethnic team model has changed to a multi-ethnic staff, although there is insufficient funding to hire enough Spanish and Creole-speaking individuals. Today, the idea of cultural sensitivity embedded in cultural pluralism persists primarily in specialized programs. There is a 12-bed Haitian residential program and an 18-bed Hispanic (primarily Cuban) residential program. These are primarily for entrants but also serve to house homeless clients and others referred from these cultures for residential services. Day treatment has culturally specific therapy groups: a Spanish-speaking group and a Creole-speaking Haitian group. There are also special issues groups, e.g., a group on special problems of Black males, as well as individual counseling. The center has expanded its services in other areas. In addition to outpatient services, case management, and day treatment, New Horizons now has its own 20-bed crisis stabilization unit and crisis intervention services; a substance abuse program; child and adolescent services; a 30-bed Adult Residential Treatment Services (ARTS) program with an array of services for persons who would otherwise be hospitalized; geriatric services; a homeless program, with a 15-bed emergency residential facility and a 20-bed short-term (six months) residence for the homeless mentally ill.

New Horizons continues to be the major provider of mental health services to the Afro-American and Afro-Caribbean populations of Miami. At this writing the CMHC is reviving its Haitian services for work with Haitian children and parents referred from the juvenile justice system. Three staff members and a substance abuse specialist also do consultation and education in the schools with Haitian children. In response to the needs of seriously mentally ill patients, a 70-member family group has been organized and a core group meets regularly. An affiliate of the National Alliance for the Mentally Ill and of Florida AMI, New Horizons AMI is composed primarily of Afro-American families, with a few Hispanic and Haitian members as well. In addition to its support group function, the focus now is principally on education and advocacy in minority communities.

In terms of public-academic liaison, the initial faculty of cultural specialists is still available and often engages in cross-cultural training as a team, despite the departure of some from the New Horizons staff. All remain on the faculty, or adjunct faculty, of the University of Miami, and all teach in other schools as well: Barry University School of Social Work, Miami-Dade Community College, and others. The past few years have seen a great deal of cross-fertilization and cooperative ventures. Lectures on Cuban, Afro-American, Haitian, and other Afro-Caribbean cultures are periodically given to health and mental health personnel, criminal justice system, and other public service staff. Barry University School of Social Work and the Department of Psychiatry at the University of Miami have collaborated in setting up three new courses which interweave cultural perspectives and working with the seriously mentally ill. Under contract with the state, Barry's social work professors train New Horizons staff in crisis intervention and case management, and work closely with the University of Miami and New Horizons in developing new training initiatives for transcultural work with chronic patients and their families. New Horizons works with the University of Miami AIDS project, handling referrals from the research component for mental health counseling. Their staff work with AIDS mothers and pregnant women with AIDS, as well as handling other referrals from the various projects at the medical center. University of Miami faculty continue to provide training, consultation, and research assistance to New Horizons staff.

In other linkage projects, University of Miami faculty lecture and work closely with staff at the South Florida State Hospital as part of the legislatively funded Task Force on Public Psychiatry. A psychiatry professor, head of an inpatient unit, regularly does consultation at the state hospital with residents in training. Psychiatric residents at the University of Miami are involved as rotating resource persons for family support groups developed by CAMI (the major local AMI group), in public lectures sponsored by CAMI, and in learning from families and some patients the phenomenological experience of serious mental illness (Lefley, 1988b). Currently, we have psychiatric residents in a rotation at Fellowship House, the local Psychosocial Rehabilitation Center.

Meanwhile, at the University of Miami-Jackson Memorial Medical Center, training in cultural sensitivity continues at various levels. In previous years, cross-cultural materials in a crammed curriculum were often viewed as exotica that were peripheral to one's "real" education. Currently we are trying to interweave both culture-specific insights and a transcultural perspective with regular training rather than focusing on specialized lectures. Thus, cultural perspectives are introduced as much as possible into clinical case conferences in both adult and child psychiatry, and are a component of training psychiatric residents to work with families of persons with chronic mental illnesses (Lefley, 1988b). It is hoped that instilling a transcultural perspective, a fulfillment of Weidman's (1983) original dream, will enable practitioners to attain not only the skills for working with particular cultures, but a sensitivity that will enable them to listen, understand, and heed the implicit conceptual framework of all persons with whom they work. This, after all, is the essence of the good clinician.

References

Bestman, E.W. (1986). Intervention techniques in the Black community. In H.P. Lefley & P.B. Pedersen (eds.), *Cross-cultural training for mental health professionals* (pp. 213–224). Springfield, IL: Charles C. Thomas.

Cutler, D.L. & Lefley, H.P. (Eds.) (1988). Training professionals to work with the chronically mentally ill. *Community Mental Health Journal,* 24(4), whole issue.

Faulkner, L.R., Cutler, D.L., Krohn, D.D., Factor, R.M., Goldfinger, S.M., Goldman, C.R. et al. (1989). A basic residency curriculum concerning the chronically mentally ill. American Journal of Psychiatry, 146, 1323–1327.

Hertz, P. & Stamps, P.L. (1977). Appointment-keeping behavior re-evaluated, *American Journal of Public Health,* 67, 1033–1036.

Lefley, H.P. (1979a). Environmental interventions and therapeutic outcome. *Hospital & Community Psychiatry,* 30, 341–344 (a).

Lefley, H.P. (1979b). Prevalence of potential falling-out cases among the Black, Latin, and non-Latin White populations of the city of Miami. *Social Science and Medicine,* 13B, 113–114.

Lefley, H.P. (1984). Delivering mental health services across cultures. In P. Pedersen, N. Sartorius, & A. Marsella (Eds.), *Mental health services: The cross-cultural context.* New York: Sage.

Lefley, H.P. (1986). Evaluating the effects of cross-cultural training: Some research results. In H.P. Lefley & P.B. Pedersen (Eds.), *Cross-cultural training for mental health professionals* (pp. 265–307). Springfield, IL: Charles C. Thomas.

Lefley, H.P. (1988a). Linked changes in mental health service delivery and psychiatric education. *Psychiatric Quarterly,* 59 (2), 121–139.

Lefley, H.P. (1988b). Training professionals to work with families of chronic patients. *Community Mental Health Journal,* 24, 338–357.

Lefley, H.P. (1990). Culture and chronic mental illness. *Hospital & Community Psychiatry,* 41, 277–286.

Lefley, H.P., Bernheim, K.F., & Goldman, C.R. (1989). National forum addresses need to enhance training in treating the seriously mentally ill. *Hospital & Community Psychiatry,* 40, 460–362, 470.

Lefley, H.P. & Bestman, E.W. (1984). Community mental health and minorities: A multi-ethnic approach. In S. Sue & T. Moore (Eds.), *The pluralistic society: A community mental health perspective* (Chap, 4, pp. 116–148). New York: Human Sciences.

Lefley, H.P. & Pedersen, P.B. (1986). Cross-cultural training for mental health professionals. Springfield, IL: Charles C. Thomas.

Rogler, L.H., Malgady, R.G., Costantino, G., & Blumenthal, R. (1987). What do culturally sensitive mental health services mean? The case of Hispanics. *American Psychologist,* 42, 565–570.

Rosenstein, M.J., Milazzo-Sayre, L.J., MacAskill, R.L., & Manderscheid, R.W. (1987). Use of inpatient psychiatric services by special populations. In R.W. Manderscheid & S.A. Barrett (Eds.), *Mental health, United States, 1987* (DHHS Publication No. ADM 87–1518, Chap. 3, Tables 3.1, 3.5). Washington, DC: U.S. Government Printing Office.

Scott, C.S. (1974). Health and healing practices among five ethnic groups in Miami, Florida. *Public Health Reports,* 89, 523–532.

Snowden, L.R. & Cheung, F.K. (1990). Use of inpatient mental health services by members of ethnic minority groups. *American Psychologist,* 45, 347–355.

Sue, S. (1977). Community mental health services to minority groups. *American Psychologist,* 32, 616–624.

Szapocznik, J., Rio, A., Perez-Vidal, A., Kurtines, W., Hervis, O., & Santisteban, D. (1986). Bicultural effectiveness training (BET): An experimental test of an intervention modality for families experiencing intergenerational/intercultural conflict. *Hispanic Journal of Behavioral Sciences,* 8, 303–330.

Weidman, H.H. (1978). *Miami Health Ecology Project Report: A statement on ethnicity and health.* Volume I. Unpublished report. Miami, FL: University of Miami School of Medicine.

Weidman, H.H. (1979). Falling-out: A diagnostic and treatment problem viewed from a transcultural perspective. *Social Science and Medicine,* 13B, 95–112.

Weidman, H.H. (1983). Research, science, and training aspects of clinical anthropology: An institutional overview. In D. Shimkin and P. Golde (Eds.), *Anthropology and health services in American society.* Washington, DC: University Press of America.

Wolkon, G.W., Moriwaki, S., Mandel, D., Archuleta, J., Bunje, P., & Zimmerman, S. (1974). Ethnicity and social class in the delivery of services. *American Journal of Public Health,* 64, 709–712.

33

Davidson, L., Hoge, M. A., Merrill, M. E., Rakfeldt, J., & Griffith, E. E. H. (1995). The experience of long-stay inpatients returning to the community. *Psychiatry, 58,* 122–132

Davidson and colleagues' article, based on in-depth qualitative interviews the authors conducted, is noteworthy for the rare glimpse it gives of the experiences of persons with serious mental illnesses living in their home communities after long stays in state psychiatric hospitalizations. The authors report the apparently contradictory finding that the people they interviewed lived "stark, empty, lonely" lives in the community [p. 125], yet preferred those lives to the ones they had in state hospitals, which offered more activities and, in some ways, more of a sense of community than they had found in their new neighborhoods and communities. Freedom is the key ingredient that explains this preference, according to the authors. This finding, they argue, points to the need for greater emphasis on consumer choice and partnership with treatment providers in community mental health treatment, along with greater attention to social and recreational activities. Such changes must be implemented in concert with an understanding of and appreciation for the lives of people with mental illness outside of their lives as patients of mental health centers and systems, in order to help these persons become participating members of their communities. These themes and elements would loom larger over the course of this decade and up to the present.

The Experiences of Long-Stay Inpatients Returning to the Community

[W]hen I look back at you, Patricia, as I watch you smoking and staring, when I see the way you are suffering and are alone, somehow, despite all they have said about you, I see you and a tenderness fills my heart. You are precious and good. You are not trash to be discarded or a broken object that must be fixed. You are not insane. You do not belong in institutions for the rest of your life ... .

P. E. Deegan (1993: 11)

Many states are presently engaged in another round of deinstitutionalization. With the majority of state hospital beds having been emptied in earlier downsizing efforts, the current round is focused on long-stay inpatients who either have been hospitalized continuously for extended periods or have been unable to adapt to community living during multiple previous attempts. While understanding that the move to community-based treatment is inspired by both humanitarian and economic considerations, those of us who are administrators charged with receiving these long-stay patients upon discharge, as well as the staff who work with them in community settings, have become concerned about the wisdom of this policy directive. Reasons for concern include the severity of illness and multiple needs experienced by these profoundly disabled patients, and the level of risk to which they are exposed in the community, particularly in the urban areas to which many patients return upon discharge. Such concerns are reflected in ongoing discussions about whether there is an abiding need of asylum and sanctuary for the seriously disabled (Hall and Brockington 1991; Lamb and Peele 1984; Wasow 1993; Wing 1990), with the related sentiment that it may now be time to declare a "moratorium" on deinstitutionalization (Lamb 1992).

Rather than trying to resolve the deinstitutionalization debate on a national level, Bachrach (1993) has recently suggested that decisions about the wisdom of continued hospital downsizing are perhaps best made on the local level. Given the wide variability of community characteristics, patient needs, and service system resources, it may make more sense to ask for whom, when, and where deinstitutionalization will be effective in enhancing clinical outcomes and quality of life. Grounded in a concern for patients' day-to-day lives, this principle of emphasizing the local context may be preferable to assuming that deinstitutionalization will always be the best policy regardless of the community and service system to which a particular person will be discharged (cf. also Hoge et al. 1994).

In moving toward a refraining of deinstitutionalization as a local question to be considered within the context of patients' lives, it has become apparent that an important dimension of this issue has been largely overlooked. Little mention has been made thus far in the debates on deinstitutionalization of the experiences and preferences of those people affected most directly by the fate of this policy direction: the patients themselves (Herman and Smith 1989; Lord et al. 1987; Thornicroft and Bebbington 1989). In other

441

domains, such as housing (Levstek and Bond 1993; Tanzman 1993) and clinical care (Bene-Kociemba et al. 1982; Lebow 1982; Massey and Wu 1993), surveys of consumer opinions are becoming commonplace and have assumed an important role in shaping programs. However, policy debates about deinstitutionalization have yet to appeal to this body of first-person experience, either by incorporating the findings of existing surveys or by requesting that such studies be conducted.

We were able to identify only seven studies that have inquired about the experiences and preferences of long-stay inpatients (Dickey et al. 1981; Herman and Smith 1989; Jones et al. 1986; Lord et al. 1987; MacGilp 1991; Okin and Pearsall 1993; Solomon 1992). Conducted in the United States, the United Kingdom, and Canada, these studies have focused primarily on the quality of life and clinical status of approximately 400 people with severe mental illness living in the community after extended periods of inpatient care. These participants expressed considerable dissatisfaction with community living in areas such as unemployment, inadequate housing, and a lack of basic living skills and support, yet the vast majority preferred life in the community to life in the hospital. However, most of these studies did not explicitly ask participants to describe the impact of being discharged on their quality of life, nor did they ask participants to compare their level of dissatisfaction in the community with that experienced in the hospital. While these studies suggest that most patients have a strong preference for the community despite its several serious drawbacks, we do not yet know why, nor do we know if and how they perceive their lives as actually having changed as a result of returning to the community following extended inpatient care.

In this report, we present the findings of a study that asked long-stay inpatients about their experiences of returning to the community following discharge from a state hospital. To introduce these patients' voices into our ongoing local policy debate about the wisdom of continued downsizing, we adopted an action research strategy that allowed us to assess if and how they perceived their lives to have changed as a result of returning to New Haven following extended periods of inpatient care. To answer the questions raised by previous studies, we chose to conduct in-depth interviews concerning patients' lives both in and out of the hospital and the reasons for their preferences for hospital or community living. Such interviews belong in the tradition of qualitative research methods that have been attracting attention in clinical and community psychiatry (Barham and Hayward 1991; Davidson and Strauss 1995; Lovell 1990; Strauss 1989), having produced many important insights into both the beneficial and deleterious effects of treatment settings during the era of extended inpatient care (Edelson 1970; Goffman 1961; Stanton and Schwartz 1954). Since Estroff's (1981) introduction of this methodology into community settings, it has proven most useful in affording investigators access to the entirety of the person's day-to-day life both in and outside of treatment (Lewis 1990), offering a person–centered approach to complement existing service-centered, outcome-oriented, quantitative studies (Jones et al. 1986). As the opening passage from Patricia Deegan (1993), a leader of the mental health consumer movement, attests, concerns arising from a patient's own experiences may differ from those derived from a provider or policy maker's point of view. It is primarily with the patient's perspective, with the experiences of those whose lives have been impacted most directly by deinstitutionalization, that we are concerned in the following.

Method

All long-stay patients discharged from the regional state hospital to New Haven from July 1992 to June 1993 were invited to be interviewed for the study. Patients were considered to be eligible for the study if discharged as part of a community-based initiative targeting

Table 33.1. Subject Characteristics

N = 12		Total duration of hospitalizations	
		Mean	10 years
		Range	3–35 years
Gender		*Age*	
Female	8	Mean	42 years old
Male	4	Range	22–56 years old
Number of hospitalizations		*Race*	
Mean	12	Caucasian	7
Range	5–60+	African-American	4
		Hispanic	1
		Diagnosis	
Schizophrenia	6	Major affective disorder	3
Schizoaffective disorder	3	Co-existing drug or alcohol abuse	5

individuals who either had been hospitalized for over 2 years or had more than 5 previous hospitalizations. Of the 16 patients who met these criteria, 3 declined to participate and 1 died before she could be interviewed. Demographic characteristics, diagnosis, and hospitalization history for the remaining 12 patients who make up the sample for the study are summarized in Table 33.1. From these data it is clear that the sample chosen for the study, with a mean of 12 hospitalizations and a mean cumulative duration of 10 years spent in the hospital, may be accurately described as patients with an extended period of inpatient care prior to their most recent return to the community.

Participants were interviewed between 6 and 9 months after discharge. Two semi-structured interviews were developed for the study. The first interview schedule was used with the patients themselves, focusing on what their lives were like in the community, a retrospective account of life in the hospital, and how they experienced the transition from hospital to community. The second interview schedule was used with mental health providers to obtain additional information about each patient's transition to the community and how the staff viewed his/her adjustment and quality of life following discharge. Interview schedules began with open-ended questions in order to minimize the impact of interviewer bias and to elicit a spontaneous narrative of life in and out of the hospital. It was also important to begin with a spontaneous description from each participant because we did not know a priori what the most relevant categories would be in assessing each person's satisfaction with life during and after hospitalization. Focused prompts followed open-ended questions to facilitate elaboration of details for those participants who required a more structured inquiry and to ensure that a set of core areas were explored with each participant. Examples of specific prompts include questions about sexual and religious activity; about participation in social activities and groups; and about the resumption of family or community activities that the person had enjoyed prior to the onset of illness, such as participation in holiday celebrations and partaking of favorite ethnic foods.

All interviews were audiotaped and transcribed to facilitate data analysis. At the completion of each set of patient and provider interviews, the investigator conducting the interviews composed a narrative summary of the events and experiences described by the participant and his/ her caregivers. Following completion of data collection, each of the 5 investigators independently reviewed all 12 sets of transcripts and narrative summaries to identify the salient themes in each patient's experiences. The research team then met to reach consensus on themes that could be identified across multiple participants, and then reviewed the transcripts again for confirmatory and disconfirmatory evidence of the presence or absence of each theme in each set of interview data. A final review was then conducted to distill patients' descriptions of each theme; these first-person accounts are included in the presentation of findings that follows.

Findings

We have focused our presentation of findings on the three central themes that emerged most clearly from the interviews with both patients and their mental health providers: (1) similarities between hospital and community, (2) strong preference for life in the community, and (3) disadvantages and dangers in community living.

Similarities Between Hospital and Community

The most striking finding that was consistent across all interviews was the stark, empty, lonely, and tragic nature of the participants' lives regardless of setting. Plagued by such long periods of unremitting mental illness, their daily lives both in and out of the hospital largely consisted of sleeping, smoking cigarettes, drinking soda and coffee, and watching television or listening to the radio for hours at a time. Productive activity of any sort was virtually nonexistent, as were true friendships or romantic involvements. Living spaces were sparsely furnished and frequently unclean, and participants complained of insufficient financial resources. They mentioned, as the few bright spots in an otherwise monotonous and dreary existence, the van trips and recreational activities that were organized for them by staff. It seemed insignificant if these trips were organized by state hospital staff to take patients off hospital grounds or by community-based staff to bring otherwise isolated individuals together for an activity in New Haven. Similarly, the minimal socializing that occurred happened either at the state hospital canteen or at equally impersonal venues in the community, such as McDonalds or Dunkin Donuts restaurants. The following passages from two different participants-the first describing life in the hospital and the second, life after discharge–captured these stark similarities:

> Well, [I'm] at the canteen every day. My mother sent money, [so I'd] buy cigarettes, buy candy, buy coffee, buy gum, buy soda, buy tea, buy soup, saltines and cheese and ham and bagels, and you know, buy food, and listen to the music.
>
> I just sit at my table and drink soda or water and smoke and listen to the radio and get a few memories by listening to the music. Or occasionally, I'll turn on the TV and watch a pretty good movie. And we get together and sometimes we go out [to] McDonald's and have a little bite to eat.

In addition to feeling that their lives were presently impoverished, few of the people we interviewed had any sense that the future might hold promise for improvements. Of those who did, their hopes seemed so unrealistic—a college education, full-time employment, marriage, and children—that we were left with the impression that these hopes served as defenses against recognition of the impact and limitations that mental illness had imposed on their lives. The words of a 55-year-old man who had been hospitalized on and off since age 29, and who had since given up all hope for a better future, expressed the sense of quiet desperation that characterized the group:

> Well, there's nothing really out here for me ... . I'll say a prayer, say God help me or heal me or take [me]. But it hasn't worked so far ... . It's hard for me to concentrate, and sometimes

when someone says something I may get a reminder of the past, I live in the past. Every day is the present, but it holds nothing for me. As far as the future, I have no future worth mentioning, … I know I'm going to die mentally ill. I don't know what else I'll die from physically, but as far as hopes, I don't see any hope … I fear that I'll get sicker and linger on and suffer more than I'm suffering now.

Strong Preference for Life in the Community

While we were struck first by the tragic nature of these people's lives, whether in the hospital or in the community, we were equally impressed with the resounding preference they expressed for life in the community. Despite the remarkable and unfortunate similarities described above between life in and out of the hospital, all of those interviewed found community living to be significantly more satisfying. Even though they were experiencing considerable stress and symptomatology in the community, antihospital sentiments were even more pronounced. The comments of a 53-year-old woman who had had over 60 hospitalizations since age 16 illustrated this sentiment well:

I had enough of [the state hospital], 35 years [there] is too much for me … . I'm not institutionalized … I would rather be home any day than be in [the state hospital] … I wouldn't go back [there] again. I'd commit suicide … I'd kill myself … hang myself with a sheet. I'm sick of [the state hospital]. I [have] been there long enough.

While less graphic in their descriptions, other participants were equally adamant in stating this preference. One younger woman who had been most recently hospitalized for 2 years claimed: "I didn't have to be locked up … for two years. Two years is a long time for somebody. It's like they don't see it. The doctors and workers don't want to admit that. But it is, it's a long time." Another woman whose most recent hospitalization had lasted 4 years agreed; "Four years are a hell of a lot of years, and a hell of a lot of rotten Christmases and rotten Easters."

Given the apparent commonalities between life in and out of the hospital, the question remains as to why there was such a strong preference for community living. We were able to identify five factors that contributed to this preference.

First and foremost, participants talked about the importance of having their "freedom." They described at length their loss of freedom in the state hospital: being locked on a unit or restrained as if in jail; being unable to make simple decisions about where to go, what to do, and when to go to sleep, wake up, or eat because these decisions were being made by staff; and having to cater to staff in order to get passes, smokes, or other favors. These stories conveyed the loss of control that is experienced upon entry into the hospital. Participants were equally vivid in their description of the freedom they were able to regain upon discharge—freedoms so mundane and taken for granted by those of us who do not live in institutions that we may never have thought to ask about them. As the man who had earlier stated that there was "nothing out here" for him described:

[It's] just the idea of being on the outside where I can walk down the street if I want to. I don't have to be back at a certain time … I have more hours to myself where I'm not waiting for something … . You can come and go as you please, and if you've got to smoke, you smoke.

Regaining basic freedom and control over one's own life, even if one then chooses to be relatively inactive, appeared to be the principal reason for the participants' preference of community life.

A second element in this preference stemmed from a perceived lack of safety in the hospital. Participants feared both the clinical and whimsical actions of hospital staff and viewed fellow patients as dangerous and unpredictable. Ironically, although they were now living in an urban environment marked by poverty, drugs, violence, and criminal victimization, they viewed the community as safer than the hospital. They thought it possible to minimize risk in the community by staying off the streets at night, retreating to their apartments or rooms, and locking their doors. The state hospital, by contrast, involved constant exposure and vulnerability to the actions of others, with no personal or protected space for a safe retreat. Far from viewing the hospital as providing sanctuary or asylum, when asked if they felt safe there, participants' more typical responses were as follows:

> Not really, 'cause you never knew who was going to hit you or if you'd wind up in restraints.
> I was afraid that if I made one wrong move someone would knock me down.

On a related theme, the ability to achieve privacy was a third reason given by participants for their community preference. Retreating to a private living space appeared to serve as a vehicle for minimizing stress and achieving distance from the constant challenges of daily living. Having a place to retreat to and having control over the decision to retreat were both highly valued, as was having the key to one's own bedroom or apartment door.

Proximity to family was a fourth factor in the preference for the community. Contact with family during hospitalization was hampered by the distant location of the state hospital. While returning to New Haven made contact with family more feasible, these relationships often appeared to the interviewers and the participants' mental health providers as full of conflict. Nonetheless, a sense of family membership was described as important, even if contacts were brief or chaotic.

Finally, as a fifth reason for preferring life outside of the hospital, participants expressed the importance of being in their home communities. Familiarity with people and places, and having skills in negotiating the local area were offered as the reasons for this attachment. Clearly for some participants, attachment to a home community, even if plagued by drugs and violence, holds a value comparable to the importance placed on being close to one's family of origin. As a 27-year-old woman with a history of 16 hospitalizations remarked:

> I like New Haven. It's my home. I was born and raised here. I know people, and people know me. I always liked New Haven. I always will, you know … [In New Haven] I know what to do if I *want* to do it. I know when to do it. I know how to do it.

Disadvantages and Dangers in Community Living

Despite this young woman's comments about knowing people and having access to activities in New Haven, participants reported minimal use of social and recreational resources in the community. They identified as significant drawbacks to community living the loneliness and lack of any sense of group membership or belonging that came from living alone in one's own apartment with little to do during the day, evenings, or weekends. Despite their loneliness, participants seldom took advantage of the structured social and recreational activities available to them through the local psychosocial rehabilitation program. Outside of their trips to McDonalds or the local convenience store, they ventured out of their apartments only for treatment appointments and informal events organized by their residential providers such as pizza parties in a staff apartment or weekend bowling trips. As mentioned earlier, descriptions of these community-based activities shared with fellow patients did not differ from descriptions of field trips and other events organized by hospital staff on and off the state hospital campus.

In contrast to this extreme social isolation, participants reported having some sense of group membership while in the hospital. Fellow patients and select staff were all that participants reported missing about the hospital after discharge. While they talked about having friends in the hospital, it should be noted that these relationships were seldom close and seemed to be based on the shared experience of living together in a closed setting. For example, one woman stated that she had many friends in the hospital; but when asked to describe these friendships, she paused and then said sadly, "We were just confined together, I guess." Said another: "I had nothing in common with the other patients except that I was another nut with them, you know." It was nevertheless within this context of forced togetherness that participants reported taking part in such regular social activities as attending the hospital chapel for Sunday services and trading stories and smokes while hanging out at the hospital canteen.

While group membership emerged in the hospital out of forced togetherness, no such force existed in the community. Given the range of options available to them outside a closed milieu, participants chose largely to distance themselves both from formal treatment settings—even that of a consumer-oriented social club—and from fellow patients, perhaps hoping to shed the identity of being mentally ill. We would be tempted to view such distancing as a move toward health and a nonpatient identity if it were not for the fact that the participants remained acutely uncomfortable in the larger community as well. Some of those interviewed were direct and eloquent in talking about stigma and their lack of acceptance by the community, about how people laughed or screamed at them and made them feel generally unwelcome. When asked if he went to any parties in the community, for example, one man replied simply: "I wouldn't fit in because I'm bipolar." Others, like the young woman who stopped attending church services after discharge, expressed her discomfort more indirectly:

"I don't own a dress," she responded when asked if she went to church.
"If you had a dress, would you go?" asked the interviewer.
"No. Churches are crowded these days, and I wouldn't want to just go and try to mingle around them, you know. All I['d] have to do is listen to the radio to the word of God if I wanted to hear it".

While the lack of affiliation and group membership was the primary disadvantage to community living identified by the participants themselves, their mental health providers were mostly concerned with the decreases in clinical stability and increases in high-risk behaviors they witnessed following discharge. Many of the participants in this sample have required hospitalizations at the local community mental health center, and for some these hospitalizations have been repeated and at times lengthy. Symptom levels and substance use appear to have increased, leading to conflicts with peers, staff, family, and landlords. High-risk behaviors have also increased, including prostitution, unsafe sexual practices, and poor social judgments that have led to victimization. In addition, several participants have experienced exacerbations of serious medical illnesses, such as diabetes and HIV infection. One young woman whom we intended to interview died suddenly of a systemic infection of unknown origin. Optimal medical care has not been received by all individuals because of the fragmented and office-based nature of general medical practice and participants' decisions not to follow prescribed self-care regimens. While participants showed some awareness of these increases in instability and risk experienced in the community, it was undoubtedly their treaters and the interview team who were most concerned about these dangers attendant upon discharge.

Discussion

All of the participants in this study painted a picture of life in the community as lonely, empty, and isolated; filled with many hours of solitary distraction by television and radio; with little money and only occasional trips to nearby fast-food restaurants and convenience stores for limited, impersonal, social interactions. Returning to the community has also meant added difficulties for these patients in terms of increased clinical instability, risk of victimization, and difficulties meeting complicated medical needs. These factors, combined with the unemployment, inadequate housing, and lack of basic living skills and support identified by participants in earlier studies, help to account for why questions continue to be raised about the wisdom of downsizing and closing our state hospitals (e.g., Lamb and Shaner 1993).

Yet all of the participants interviewed also held a strong preference for life in the community. Along with the majority of patients surveyed in previous studies, they supported continued deinstitutionalization by agreeing that they should have been discharged from the hospital. What the participants in this study were able to describe were the reasons why they continued to find community living significantly more satisfying despite its serious drawbacks, Through the in-depth interviews they were able to convey quite poignantly what is perhaps the subtle and difficult to appreciate nature of the reasons for this preference. Freedom to come and go as one pleases and not to be told what to do every hour of the day, protection from constant exposure to insult and assault, and a place for personal retreat and privacy came across in these interviews as the primary reasons for wanting to be outside of the hospital. While basic to our sense of human dignity, these reasons get overlooked to the extent that most of us living outside of oppressive contexts take them for granted as part and parcel of our daily lives. But for patients for whom these needs have been sacrificed in the pursuit of structure and containment of symptomatology, it may be precisely their fundamental dignity and autonomy as human beings that is at stake in debates about deinstitutionalization. This sentiment is reflected in the passage from Patricia Deegan (1993) that opened this paper. It was also embodied in the emphatic statements made by participants in this study as they described their preferences for what remains a fairly empty life in the community—but one they feel is at least full in regard to the possibility for them to be free and in control of their own destinies.

As we listened to participants stress the centrality of their desire for dignity and autonomy in determining their preference for community living, we began to wonder if the importance of these concerns for patients is being adequately addressed in existing mental health policy and programming. At this point we are left with a series of unanswered questions regarding how to balance our patients' needs for safety, structure, and a sense of belonging and identity with their desires for freedom, autonomy, choice, privacy, and access to family and community.

A first question is how to balance our participants' desires for choice and autonomy with an acknowledgment of what Geller and his colleagues (1990) have described as the "hazards of freedom." What participants liked most about life outside the hospital was that no one was telling them what to do when, no one else had the keys, and they could come and go, smoke or not smoke, when and as they pleased. Yet what came across in interviews as most concerning about life in the community were some of the ways in which they were exercising this freedom: abuse of drugs and alcohol, poor social judgment that placed them at risk of victimization, unsafe sexual practices, and a dangerous lack of adherence to medical regimens and care. While there is always a risk that freedom will be misused, as it often is by individuals who are not psychiatrically disabled, this issue becomes more complicated in the case of individuals whose judgment may be compromised by the very illnesses we are responsible for treating.

How can we ensure safety without transferring the rigid and authoritarian relationships established in the state hospital to the community along with these patients? Can we develop collaborative treatment relationships in the community that provide needed structure, but that also allow for what Deegan (1992) has called "the dignity of risk and the right to failure"? In other words, can we develop models of treatment that support patient choice and prompt patients' growth into self-responsible and self-determining adults? How to do this while cognizant of the serious dangers described above provides an important opportunity for discussion between clinicians, consumers, administrators, and family members (e.g., *Innovations and Research* 1993).

A second question is how to go beyond simplistic notions of normalization and community integration. Community-based treatment and rehabilitation programs as well as hospitals highlight an individual's unwanted identity as a mental patient and prolong unwanted associations with other patients. On the other hand, attempts at mainstreaming inject patients into communities where they are unwanted and subject them to the repeated microtrauma of stigma and rejection. Our participants evoked the image of immigrants who have fled a familiar environment due to unacceptable conditions but find themselves in a new environment and culture where they now stand out as different and are generally unwelcome. Like other minorities faced with the dilemma of assimilating into the majority group, people with psychiatric disabilities remain a marginalized group within the larger community. The plight of these patients is even more difficult, however, for they are ambivalent about using a primary coping strategy of immigrants and minority groups, which is to search out those of the same cultural identity in order to find support and solace.

How can we help these discharged patients to feel less isolated and alienated in the community? We can agree that for them to be sequestered in their own apartments is not an acceptable outcome; nor was it the hope of deinstitutionalization. While we had recognized by the mid-1970s (e.g., Reich and Siegel 1973; Smith and Hart 1975) that such a state of affairs had become the unwitting result of early attempts at deinstitutionalization, community-based programs developed since that time promised to meet many of the basic needs of discharged patients and to enhance their quality of life in the community (Stroul 1988). And certainly these programs have succeeded to some extent (Parrish 1989). But for most people with severe psychiatric disabilities, community placement has not yet been translated into community integration. Patients may have returned to the community, but they have not yet found a home there.

In order to promote more effective community integration, we need to recognize that the process of assimilation is exceedingly complex, and we must search for innovative ways of helping people to find a home within the general community. When that is not yet possible, we need to turn our attention to helping patients build connections and a sense of belonging and positive identity within their community of peers. Our local service system embodies some of the advances in service delivery of the last decade by bringing clinical services out of the office, providing assertive outreach, and making intensive efforts to transition patients to the community though a social club over a several month period of time. Yet these efforts have been focused primarily on the individual (Hoge et al. 1992; Toro 1990) and have only just begun to target the cultivation of supportive social networks in the community (e.g., Bebout et al. 1993). In addition to network development, intensive community treatment may need to put more of an emphasis on individualized support for normalizing social and recreational activities for patients who would not participate in such activities on their own at first, much as we are currently doing in the residential and vocational areas in supported independent living, supported employment, and supported education.

While we find that these implications challenge our own thinking about programmatic and policy issues in mental health service delivery, these questions do not represent the most important outcome of this study. The most valuable aspect of this project has been the access it has afforded us to the lives and voices of the patients to whom we are responsible in both our daily clinical work and our program and policy development. On this score, we have found this research process and its results to be both persuasive and disconcerting. Participating in these interviews has lent a clarity and commitment to the hospital down-sizing efforts in our own service system, as we have become convinced by these patients of the real advantages to the freedom, privacy, and access to family and community afforded by their return. We have also found it useful to share these findings with our staff in foster-ing in them an appreciation of the value of their own efforts in helping severely disabled patients to achieve the benefits of living outside of hospital settings. On the other hand, we have been troubled by the tragic nature of these peoples' lives even as they have been glad to return from the hospital to the community. In bearing witness to their suffering, we feel compelled to redouble our efforts to help them feel more at ease and at home within our community, ever mindful of the limits imposed by their disabilities and by the consider-able stigma that continues to permeate their attempts at having a normal life.

Following Bachrach's (1993) principle of emphasizing the local context in discussions of mental health service delivery, we recognize that these findings may not necessarily be generalizable to other patients in other service systems. We offer the research strategy described in this paper as one that may be useful in these other communities, however, as a method for assessing the needs of severely disabled patients in both hospital and commu-nity settings, and for injecting the desires and preferences of these patients into local policy debates regarding hospital downsizing, the future of deinstitutionalization, and optimal forms of mental health service delivery.

References

Bachrach, L. L. *The biopsychosociallegacy of de-institutionalization.* Presentation delivered at the First Annual Conference of the Center for Mental Health Policy, Services and Clinical Research of the Connecticut Mental Health Center, New Haven, CT, October 1993.

Barham, P., and Hayward, R. *From the Mental Patient to the Person.* Routledge, 1991.

Bebout, R. R., Harris, M., Swayze, F. V., et al. *The Community Connections Social Support Network Intervention Model.* National Institute on Alcohol Abuse and Alcoholism, 1993.

Bene-Kociemba, A., Cotton, P. G., and Fort-Gang, R. C. Assessing patient satisfaction with state hospital and aftercare services. *American Journal of Psychiatry* (1982) 139:660–62.

Davidson, L., and Strauss, J. S. Beyond the bio-psychosocial model: Integrating disorder, health and recovery. *Psychiatry,* (1995) 58:44–55.

Deegan, P. E. The Independent Living Movement and people with psychiatric disabilities: Taking back control over our own lives. *Psychosocial Rehabilitation Journal* (1992) 15:3–19.

Deegan, P. E. Recovering our sense of value after being labeled mentally ill. *Journal of Psychosocial Nursing* (1993) 31:7–11.

Dickey. B., Gudeman. J. E., Hellman. S., et al. A follow-up of deinstitutionalized chronic patients four years after discharge. *Hospital and Community Psychiatry* (1981) 32:326–30.

Edelson, M. *Sociotherapy and Psychotherapy.* University of Chicago Press, 1970.

Estroff, S. E. *Making It Crazy: An Ethnography of Psychiatric Clients in an American Community.* University of California Press, 1981.

Geller, J. L., Fisher, W. H., Simon, L. J., et al. Second-generation deinstitutionalization. II. The impact of *Brewster v. Dukakis* on correlates of community and hospital utilization. *American Journal of Psychiatry* (1990) 147:988–93.

Goffman, E. *Asylums: Essays on the Social Situation of Mental Patients and Other Inmates.* Doubleday, 1961.

Hall, P., and Brockington, I. F. *The Closure of Mental Hospitals,* Gaskell, 1991.

Herman, N. J., and Smith, C. M. Mental hospital depopulation in Canada: Patient perspectives. *Canadian Journal of Psychiatry* (1989) 34:386–91.

Hoge, M. A., Davidson, L., Hill, W. L, et al The promise of partial hospitalization: A reassessment. *Hospital and Community Psychiatry* (1992) 43:345–54.

Hoge, M. A., Davidson, L., Griffith, E. E. H., et al. *Managed care in public sector psychiatry.* Hospital and Community Psychiatry (1994) 45; 1085–9.

Jones, K., Robinson, M., and Golightley, M. Long-term psychiatric patients in the community. *British Journal of Psychiatry* (1986) 149:537–40.

Lamb, H. R. Is it time for a moratorium on deinstitutionalization? *Hospital and Community Psychiatry* (1992) 43:669.

Lamb, H. R., and Peele, R. The need for continuing asylum and sanctuary. *Hospital and Community Psychiatry* (1984) 38:798–802.

Lamb, H. R., and Shaner, R. When there are almost no state hospital beds left. *Hospital and Community Psychiatry* (1993) 44:973–76.

Lebow, J. Consumer satisfaction with mental health. *Psychological Bulletin* (1982) 91:241–69.

Levstek, D. A., and Bond, G. R. Housing cost, quality, and satisfaction among formerly homeless persons with serious mental illness in two cities. *Innovations and Research* (1993) 2:1–8.

Lewis, D. A. From programs to lives: A comment. *American Journal of Community Psychology* (1990) 18:923–26.

Lord, J., Schnarr, A., and Hutchison, P. The voice of the people: Qualitative research and the needs of consumers. *Canadian Journal of Community Mental Health* (1987) 6:25–36.

Lovell, A. M. Managed cases, drop-ins, drop-outs, and other by-products of mental health care. *American Journal of Community Psychology* (1990) 18:917–21.

Lovell, A. M. Seizing the moment: Power, contingency, and temporality in street life. In Rutz, H. J., ed., *The Politics of Time* (pp. 86–107). American Anthropological Association, 1992.

MacGilp, D. A quality of life study of discharged long-term psychiatric patients. *Journal of Advanced Nursing* (1991) 16:1206–15.

Massey, O. T., and Wu, L. Service delivery and community housing: Perspectives of consumers, family members, and case managers. *Innovations and Research* (1993) 2:9–15.

Okin, R. L., and Pearsall, D. Patients' perceptions of their quality of life 11 years after discharge from a state hospital. *Hospital* and *Community Psychiatry* (1993) 44:236–40.

Parrish, J. The long journey home: Accomplishing the mission of the Community Support Movement. *Psychosocial Rehabilitation Journal* (1989) 12:107–24.

Reich, R., and Siegel, L. Psychiatry under siege: The chronically mentally ill shuffle to oblivion. *Psychiatric Annals* (1973) 3.

Smith, W. G., and Hart, D. W. Community mental health: A noble failure? *Hospital and Community Psychiatry* (1975) 26:581–83.

Solomon, P. The closing of a state hospital: What is the quality of patients' lives one year post-release? *Psychiatric Quarterly* (1992) 63:279–96.

Stanton, A., and Schwartz. M. *The Mental Hospital: A Study of Institutional Participation in Psychiatric Illness and Treatment.* Basic Books, 1954.

Strauss, J. S. Subjective experiences in schizophrenia: Toward a new dynamic psychiatry II. *Schizophrenia Bulletin* (1989) 15:179–88.

Stroul, B. A. *Community Support Systems for Persons with Long-Term Mental Illness: Questions and Answers.* National Institute of Mental Health, 1988.

Tanzman, B. An overview of surveys of mental health consumers' preferences for housing and support services. *Hospital and Community Psychiatry* (1993) 44:450–55.

Thornicroft, G., and Bebbington, P. Deinstitutionalization: From hospital closure to service development. *British Journal of Psychiatry* (1989) 155:739–53.

Toro, P. A. Evaluating professionally operated and self-help programs for the serious mentally ill. *American Journal of Community Psychology* (1990) 18:903–7.

Wasow, M. The need for asylum revisited. *Hospital and Community Psychiatry* (1993) 44:207–8.

Wing, J. K. The functions of asylum. *British Journal of Psychiatry* (1990) 157:822–27.

34

Hopper, K., Jost, J., Hay, T., Welber, S., & Haugland, G. (1997). Homelessness, severe mental illness, and the institutional circuit. *Psychiatric Services, 48* (4), 659–665

Hopper and colleagues article hearkens back to both Jacqueline Wiseman's *Stations of the Lost*, in which she described the stations of jail, detoxification services, and life on the Skid Rows of American cities for alcoholic men during the 1960s and 1970s, and to the "revolving door" syndrome of deinstitutionalization during the 1970s and 1980s. The authors, who studied a group of persons with diagnoses of severe mental illness who were admitted to a shelter in Westchester County in 1995, found that an "institutional circuit" of jail, shelter, psychiatric hospitals, and other mental health custodial institutions constituted an alternative to stable community living for these persons. The institutional circuit is dual, involving both the institutions of which individuals are on the looping circuit *and* the institutional responses that have replaced the asylums of another era, as opposed to long-term permanent housing in the community with supports. A corollary to the authors' main argument is that the emergency response to homelessness, and particularly to homelessness and mental illness, which began out of the best humanitarian impulses, has become a business with a self-perpetuating cycle of customers and companies to serve them. Alternatives to the institutional circuit, the authors argue, in addition to mental health services such as critical time intervention and assertive outreach, must include the availability of permanent affordable housing for persons with serious mental illnesses.

Homelessness, Severe Mental Illness, and the Institutional Circuit

Objective: Research on homelessness among persons with severe mental illness tends to focus on aspects of demand, such as risk factors or structural and economic forces. The authors address the complementary role of supply factors, arguing that "solutions" to residential instability—typically, a series of institutional placements alternating with shelter stays—effectively perpetuate homelessness among some persons with severe mental illness. *Methods:* Thirty-six consecutive applicants for shelter in Westchester County, New York, in the first half of 1995 who were judged to be severely mentally ill by intake workers were interviewed using a modified life chart format. Detailed narrative histories were constructed and reviewed with the subjects. *Results:* Twenty of the 36 subjects had spent a mean of 59 percent of the last five years in institutions and shelters. Analysis of the residential histories of the 36 subjects revealed that shelters functioned in four distinctive ways in their lives: as part of a more extended institutional circuit, as a temporary source of transitional housing, as a surrogate for exhausted support from kin, and as a haphazard resource in essentially nomadic lives. The first pattern dominated in this group. *Conclusions:* Shelters and other custodial institutions have acquired hybrid functions that effectively substitute for more stable and appropriate housing for some persons with severe mental illness. *(Psychiatric Services* 48:659–665, 1997)

Inquiry into the nexus of homelessness and severe mental illness has moved away from the concerns of the early and mid-1980s—how many and how bad—to closer examinations of "what went wrong" and "how it might be fixed." Depictions of the longitudinal course of homelessness aside, much of the descriptive task has been accomplished. Meta-analyses have narrowed the range of estimates of prevalence of severe mental illness among homeless people, drawn useful distinctions among subpopulations of that group, and recognized that, despite methodological caveats, different contexts are likely to produce different rates of disorder (1,2).

Ethnographic studies have yielded fine-grained descriptions of street and shelter life (3,4), supplemented by comparative inventories of victimization and hardship (5,6). To be sure, "base rates" research on homelessness and mental illness continues in circumscribed pockets of inquiry—among veterans, prisoners, and forensic patients (7–10); in less heavily urbanized areas (11); and as they relate to risk of HIV infection (12). But the bulk of the research effort has shifted to more sophisticated analyses of the causes of (or pathways to) homelessness for persons with severe mental illness, and to careful evaluations of programs and housing models designed to arrest and prevent the recurrence of homelessness among them (13–15).

This paper takes a different approach. It argues that de facto "solutions" to precarious housing—shelters and custodial facilities linked in haphazard chains of time-limited occupancy—should be considered among the inertial forces that sustain homelessness among persons with severe mental illness.

Causal analyses of homelessness have become progressively more refined. Nonetheless, the tendency is still for explanations to migrate, at least in relative emphasis, toward polar extremes—one stressing vulnerability and pathology, and the other stressing underlying social structure (16). The first of these is best exemplified by the burgeoning of "risk factor" analyses in studies of homeless individuals and, to a lesser extent, homeless families. Diagnostic assessments, life history interviews, and inventories of recent stressful events have all been used to identify factors disproportionately found among homeless populations that are likely to be causally related to the occurrence of homeless "episodes."

Statistical techniques (multivariate analyses, regression models, and survival analysis), along with computations of relative risk and odds ratios, are then used to take the measure of the factors' differential contributions to such episodes. Male gender, African-American ethnicity, longstanding psychiatric disorder (especially when coupled with substance abuse), childhood out-of-home placements, and disruptive life events have all been shown to increase the risk of homelessness among single adults (17,18).

Structural analyses, undertaken in part as a corrective to the focus on individual disability, shift the focus to "fundamental causes," understood as the unequal distribution of resources (material and social) that limit one's exposure to risks and enhance one's ability to deal with misfortunes (19). Inventories typically include persistent poverty, dearth of affordable housing, injurious social and economic policies, and depleted social networks (20,21). Lately, attempts have been made to synthesize the two approaches (22,23).

These approaches to the "etiology" of homelessness share the epidemiological premise that homelessness is a condition akin to a disease or disorder. They further assume that methods for mapping the distribution and determinants of affliction in human populations can be usefully applied to instances of "social pathology" as well. Accordingly, even those with a structural bent tend to ignore the institutional mechanics of shelters, what might be called the supply side of relief, except insofar as such places provide convenient sampling sites. To extend the disease analogy, homelessness is what shelters "treat"; there is little reason to inquire into the intentions or routines of deliberating agents, whether clients or keepers.

Etiologic analyses seek to disentangle the bundles of early trauma, rigged life chances, bad habits, threadbare supports, co-existing ailments, and external forces that propel persons with severe mental illness into homelessness, sometimes repeatedly. No one disputes the productivity of such analyses, but their limits concern us. By ignoring the actions of shelter users and street-level bureaucrats (24), they miss ingredients that may be central to "making it crazy" (25) on the margins today.

This paper argues that, in addition to personal "risk factors" and structural "root causes," homeless service systems should be viewed as independent agents shaping the course of homelessness. It offers provisional evidence that these and allied systems may have the perverse institutional effect of perpetuating rather than arresting the "residential instability" that is the underlying dynamic of recurring literal homelessness (26) and that so often harries the lives of persons with severe mental illness. It concludes that any attempt to "unravel" the causes of homelessness and its association with mental illness (27) must seek not only to plumb the backgrounds of shelter users and street dwellers but also to take account of the institutions that serve them.

Methods

Setting

Narrative histories for this project were collected as part of a feasibility study of methods for tracking homeless individuals over time. Interviews were conducted in the first half of 1995 at the shelter adjoining the Single Homeless Assessment Center, the central intake site for single adults seeking shelter in Westchester County, New York. The intake process includes a clinical assessment of psychiatric history and current diagnoses. For this study, shelter applicants were considered severely mentally ill if they were already receiving Supplemental Security Income (SSI) for psychiatric reasons or if intake workers referred them for SSI evaluation. That is, for purposes of tracking the fate of homeless people thought to be severely mentally ill, we accepted the classification itself as ethnographic fact.

The original intent was to compile histories of residential instability that would refine the risk profile of the cohort to be followed. A close reading of these histories, however, has enabled us to describe how shelters and allied facilities have functioned over time in managing the basic needs of a population no single system seems prepared to claim.

Procedure

Sixty-two consecutive applicants for shelter who were also considered mentally ill were approached for participation in the study; 36 consented to participate. Refusers did not differ significantly from consenters in demographic characteristics; consenters were younger and had more foster care history than comparable subjects recruited from the same site a year earlier (28).

Subjects' whereabouts and support for the preceding five years were mapped using a version of the life chart pioneered by Harding and colleagues (29), as modified by World Health Organization researchers in a long-term study of schizophrenia (30). The three fieldworkers who conducted the interviews were college graduates recruited for the study. One was enrolled in a doctoral research program. They were trained in field methods and interview technique by the first author. Twelve pilot interviews using the life chart schedule were conducted before the study began.

Subjects were guided through a reconstruction of places of residence, treatment experiences, family relations, and sources of income for the past five years, beginning with the circumstances leading them to request shelter. Anchor points—incidents clearly fixed in the subject's memory—were used to prompt and order other recollections. Special attention was paid to reasons for changes in residence. Inconsistencies were flagged and resolved later in the interview.

The process could be painstaking. Each interview lasted from 45 minutes to two and a half hours. A second fieldworker was on hand to take notes during the process. The raw data of the life chart were reviewed by both workers, assembled the same night into coherent narratives, and then read by the first author. Gaps or contradictions in the account were highlighted. The next day, the interviewer reviewed the narrative with the subject, making emendations as needed. In several cases, further corrections were made as new material surfaced in the course of follow-up interviews. These narratives, data from a brief structured interview, and the official intake record of the Single Homeless Assessment Center formed the basis for the analysis.

Analysis

Narratives were independently reviewed by the fieldworkers and by the first author to identify and measure periods of past homelessness, institutional stays, and other placements.

In this way, a complete inventory of residence was compiled for each subject. Time the subject was literally homeless was computed, both for the entire five years and for the noninstitutionalized portions of those years—the time effectively at risk of homelessness. For purposes of this analysis, persons were considered to be institutionalized, and thus not substantially at risk of becoming homeless, while residing in jails or prisons, hospitals, detoxification and rehabilitation facilities, and segregated housing located on the grounds of psychiatric hospitals.

The narratives were detailed enough with respect to the circumstances leading to past episodes of homelessness to enable us to identify a provisional list of functions played by shelters in these lives. Armed with that list, investigators rereviewed the narratives, amended the list of functions, and classified each five-year history by the dominant pattern of shelter use exemplified. These patterns were then compared with the officially recorded reason for homelessness in the intake record.

Results

As Table 34.1 indicates, the 36 subjects did not differ markedly from cohorts in other studies of single homeless adults with severe mental illness. They were predominantly young, of minority status, not well educated, and with substantial foster care experience. As Table 34.2 shows, their residential histories reveal that women were more successful in negotiating doubled-up arrangements (staying with kin whether rent was contributed or not; staying with nonkin, or with someone not a romantic partner, for less than one week without making a rent contribution). However, the histories are chiefly notable for the amount of time spent literally homeless; on average, subjects spent 20 percent of the past five years on the street or in shelters and 29 percent of the time at risk—that is, not in

Table 34.1. Characteristics of 36 Homeless Adults Eligible for Supplemental Security Income Who Sought Shelter at the Single Homeless Assessment Center in Westchester County, New York

Characteristic	Total (N = 36)		Males (N = 26)		Females (N = 10)	
	N	%	N	%	N	%
Age						
17 to 29 years	15	42	12	46	3	30
30 to 39 years	10	28	7	27	3	30
40 to 49 years	7	19	5	19	2	20
50 years or older	4	11	2	8	2	20
Ethnicity						
Black	23	64	15	58	8	80
White	11	31	9	35	2	20
Hispanic	2	6	2	8	0	0
Education						
Less than high school	16	44	13	50	3	30
High school or general equivalency diploma	9	25	5	19	4	40
Some college	11	31	8	31	3	30
Psychiatric history						
Previously hospitalized	36	100	26	100	10	100
Taking psychiatric medications	34	94	24	92	10	100
Foster care	8	22	7	27	1	10

Table 34.2. Five-Year Residential Histories of 36 Homeless Adults, by Months in Various Settings and Percentage of the Five Years in Each Setting[1]

Group	Own or Shared Housing[2]		Doubled Up[3]		Institutionalized[4]		Literally Homeless[5]		
	Mean months	% of five years	Mean months	% of five years	Mean months	% of five years	Mean months	% of five years	% of five years at risk[6]
Total sample (N=36)	19.7	33	6.9	11	17.1	29	12.0	20	29
Male (N=26)	20.5	34	5.5	9	16.8	28	12.6	21	29
Female (N=10)	17.6	29	9.7	16	17.7	29	12.8	21	30
First time homeless (N=5)	18.7	31	17.0	28	15.2	25	0	0	0

[1] Not included in the total were community mental health housing and time spent in the Job Corps, foster care, a state-affiliated group home, or residential school. Periods when subjects could not recall their housing status were not counted.

[2] Making a rent contribution to obtain regular access to housing; staying for one week or more with a partner in a "romantic relationship" whether rent was contributed or not; or staying overnight in a motel paid out of pocket (when not accounted for on a shelter or mental health housing roster)

[3] Staying with kin whether rent was contributed or not; staying with nonkin or with someone not a romantic partner for less than one week without making a rent contribution

[4] Psychiatric hospitalization, prison or jail, detoxification facility, rehabilitation, or mental health housing on the grounds of state psychiatric facilities

[5] A shelter, motel, or drop-in center; living on the street; or living in a nomadic manner

[6] Time literally homeless/(60 months-time institutionalized)

Table 34.3. Official Reasons for Homelessness Noted in the Intake Records of 36 Homeless Adults

Reason	Total Subjects	
	N	%
Evicted		
By landlord for nonpayment of rent	2	6
By landlord for behavior problems	2	6
Because dwelling was a fire hazard or conditions were untenable	3	8
By family for behavior problems	3	8
Institutional discharge		
From prison or jail	7	19
From a psychiatric hospital	3	8
Other		
Lost job or was relocated	2	6
Unspecified	14	39

institutions. (These figures rise to 23 percent and 33 percent, respectively, if five persons who had never been previously homeless are excluded.)

Table 34.3 shows the reasons for the subject's current homelessness. Subjects' intake records either resorted to using the category of "other" or identified eviction (formal or informal) and institutional discharge as the chief reasons for homelessness. Strikingly, nearly a third (32 percent) of the 22 shelter seekers for whom a reason was listed had come directly from jail or prison.

Table 34.4. Four Patterns of Shelter Function Among 36 Homeless Adults Who Were Interviewed About Their Five-Year Residential Histories

Pattern of Function	Mean Months in Institutions	% of Five Years in Institutions	Mean Months Literally Homeless	% of Five Years Literally Homeless	Mean Months in Shelters	% of Five Years in Shelters	Excerpts From Narrative of Interview
Institutional circuit (N=20)	24.2	40.4	14.0	23.3	11.2	18.7	Has lived virtually an institutionalized life Institutionalized since age eight; jailed after flare-up at residential work program Succession of residences: jail, parents' home, own place, retreat for alcoholics, shelter, rehabilitation facility, hospital Has never lived in a place of his own Used the hospitals as an alternative to the shelter system but also would occasionally stay at shelters when he was between treatment facilities
Surrogate for informal assistance (N=5)	7.6	12.6	1.8	2.8	.6	1.0	Long-standing structure of support (kin and friends) collapsed after subject's injury and convalescence After lengthy prison term, moved with daughter to mother and aunt's apartment; wore out welcome and moved on, leaving daughter behind Long psychiatric history; sister intervened recently to prevent subject from moving back with his elderly father After long absence, moved back to New York City, but funds gave out, as well as support from friends and kin (sister recovering from surgery)
Crisis and temporary housing (N=6)	15.3	25.6	6.3	10.4	6.0	10.0	Usually on own in marginal housing, but evicted from unsuitable dwelling Usually in shared housing, but after brief jail term came to shelter Burned out of apartment with wife and later separated after she was hospitalized Moved a lot in last five years, occasionally resorting to shelters when out of work and without income
Nomadic (N=5)	5.6	9.3	25.8	42.9	9.7	16.1	Wandering for a long time; homeless most of the time since 1970 Haphazard ill-planned bus trip to New York City area, footloose (mostly in California) Confirmed nomad, with stays at monasteries, retreats, missions, on the road, in a tent, and in abandoned houses; even worked for a time as a nanny

Table 34.4 presents four patterns of how shelters have functioned in the lives of these individuals—patterns that reveal further institutional linkages. For many subjects, shelters repeatedly provided the bridgework from confinement to community, and back again. At first glance the shelters seem to be functioning as discharge planning units for people who are otherwise difficult to place. However, for 20 subjects, shelter stays appeared to be part of a more durable pattern, of a life lived on the "institutional circuit" with occasional breaks for temporary housing on their own. Persons in this group had spent on average of 40 percent of the last five years in institutions; shelters accounted for an additional 19 percent of those years. Thus, if we ignore time spent in a place of one's own (alone or shared), as well as time doubled-up with others, in specialized community-based housing, and on the street, we can still account for 59 percent of the last five years in these persons' lives.

"Release from institution" cited as a reason for homelessness often simply marked a transition from one institution to another. For some young adults in this group, the latest shelter stay coincided with a bid for independence as they negotiated the transition from foster care or emergency housing placements with their parents.

Other shelter functions were also apparent in the subjects' histories. For some, the shelter functioned as a time-limited resource, a way station en route to another habitat of often tenuous stability. For others, it served as a surrogate for informal (usually kin-based) assistance that had either been exhausted or for other reasons was no longer available. For still others, it provided fleeting refuge for nomadic souls who nowhere put down roots, let alone engaged in rehabilitation or treatment.

The cases of those who had never before been homeless offer telling counterpoints to the institutional circuit pattern. Two of the five were young men who had only recently left foster care settings; the other three were middle-aged men and women whose kin-based sources of assistance had, for the first time, failed them. For the younger group, the shelter system both extended the institutional apparatus that had largely defined their life to date and broke with it at a crucial transitional point, the passage to adulthood. For the middle-aged individuals, it substituted for informal supports.

In all these cases, shelter proved a transitory resource; the stays of all five were relatively brief, and once they left, they did not return in the next year. Three found independent housing on their own, one was placed in supportive housing for persons with mental illness, and one returned home to Alabama.

Discussion

An alternative approach to the causation (or, better, the perpetuation) of homelessness takes its lead from historical accounts of the manifold "uses of charity" (31) and looks at how institutional resources are actually deployed. It observes, for example, that the function of confinement for disabled persons is not fixed but variable, subject to the needs and capacities of households, demands of seasonal labor, and exigencies of wartime (32–34). Problem-oriented, suspicious of bureaucratic boundaries, and careful not to confuse site of custody with category of need met, this approach asks how dilemmas of subsistence and housing (compounded by individual disability) are solved in everyday practice over time.

The old notion of the "latent" function of institutions (35,36) resurfaces, now put to the mundane task of accounting for the whereabouts of those formerly housed in special-purpose quarters. For example, Rochefort and Mechanic (37) remarked on the variety of "nontraditional institutions" that were pressed into service as functional equivalents of asylum in the wake of widespread deinstitutionalization, itself a hodgepodge of what they termed "design and inadvertence." Dear and Wolch (38) decried the growth of "service-dependent ghettoes" where legions of the formerly hospitalized were exiled. This fresh (and often short-lived) profusion of reclaimed rooming houses, board-and-care facilities, and single-room-occupancy hotels, in turn, represented the rediscovery of the value of cheap marginal housing for the unstable or misfit (39,40). But when the capacity of such alternatives is exhausted, or access to them is foreclosed, other arrangements must be made.

Sosin and Grossman (41) found that homeless clients of residential treatment facilities and shelters were distinguished from their housed, poor, and mentally ill counterparts chiefly by the latter's access to such "tangible resources" as a steady income. (Members of both groups made frequent use of soup kitchens.) That is, shelters and treatment beds served as in-kind surrogates for a commodity others could afford to purchase. Obviously, persons with severe mental illness are not the only group to suffer income shortages, but they may find it more difficult to arrange informal makeshifts, especially when psychiatric problems are compounded with substance use (42).

In implicit recognition of their multipurpose nature, contemporary shelters have been compared not to the missions or flophouses of skid row but to 19th century police station lodgings and almshouses (43,44), to total institutions (45,46), to refugee camps for the American poor (47), and, pointedly, to "open asylums" (48). Four decades after the first stirrings of deinstitutionalization, attempts to locate the enduring but reconfigured functions of "custody and asylum" (49) must, it seems, take public shelters into account.

This argument rests on a simple logic of displacement: if persons with severe mental illness are moved from hospitals, and kin-based alternatives prove unavailable or unequal to the task, they must be relocated somewhere, no matter what the classification or official provenance of that place is. As certain institutional resources dry up, others—market-based, informal, or bureaucratic—are cobbled together to provide some semblance of the ordered subsistence that encompassing institutions like asylums once ensured. Especially when disreputable populations are involved—for example, the indigent chronic inebriate at the turn of the century (34), resistance may be expected from institutional quarters unused to catering to such a clientele and eager to dispose of them elsewhere ("not in my back ward"). In other cases, bureaucratic niceties of design and classification grudgingly give way in the face of the de facto "hybridization" of institutional function (50,51).

Unplanned, accidental, or haphazard as such accretions of function may be, they not uncommonly acquire inertial forces of their own. Over time, accommodating "inappropriate referrals" can become routinized, even accepted practice. Consider the designation of shelters as legitimate "housing placements" in some hospital discharge plans. Neither the utilities nor the clientele of facilities serving as the functional equivalents of hospitals or halfway houses is adequately captured by the conventional names for such places.

Studies explicitly located in this tradition first reframe the immediate issue of sheltering the homeless, mentally ill or not, as part of the more durable problem of holding surplus and potentially troublesome populations in "abeyance" (52). They then attempt to describe how contemporary shelters actually work in this respect (43,53,54). Homelessness is treated less as social pathology than as a variable state that is defined by degrees of "regular access to a conventional dwelling" (55).

Just as labor economists have learned to examine alternative employments in military service, prisons, hospitals, and the informal economy in accounting for the officially unemployed, so students of abeyance are learning to seek out alternative residences for erstwhile (and would-be) patients who in times past would have been hospitalized. Just as alternative sources of work can lure and harbor people who are ill suited for conventional jobs, or barred for various reasons from attaining them, so alternative dwellings can work to keep difficult people out of conventional housing.

This report reflects that tradition. Prudence dictates caution in interpreting these results; the numbers are not large, "heavy users" may be over-represented, and other uncontrolled sources of bias may have gone undetected. Nevertheless, the continuing dominance of institutional stays in the lives of the 36 subjects is impressive. Solomon (56) has written about the imitative couplings that increasingly join clinical and criminal justice systems in the handling of difficult patients, such that the jobs of case managers and parole officers begin to resemble one another. Less formal modes of institutional articulation are apparent here. The couplings at work in these histories are not extended versions of coercive surveillance, but largely haphazard and uncoordinated transfers across institutional domains.

In this respect, today's homeless poor people with psychiatric disabilities strongly resemble their skid-row counterparts of the 1960s. That kinship was apparent to some early analysts (57,58), but with few exceptions (39,40) it has been ignored or denied since. Marginal lives spent on the institutional circuit today are not much different from those played out on "the loop" (jails, detoxification facilities, missions, and flophouses) in the skid rows of the 1960s (59); nor, indeed, are they much different from the shuttle round of saloons, fleabag hotels, missions, jails, almshouses, hospitals, and asylums that turn-of-the-century homeless drunks navigated (60).

Not that there aren't "good reasons" for any one facility refusing the long-term view. Displacement of problems and the timeworn desire to run an establishment unencumbered by the demands of people whose needs do not fit neatly into prescribed niches and whose eagerness to get with the program is suspect no doubt explain much of the mobility of the subjects in this study. Whether such reasons justify the hidden costs of disheveled systems is another question.

Public mental health care in the U.S. may have once represented, in Dowdall's words (61), "an unusually clear example of a highly institutionalized organizational field," but only irony salvages that characterization for the population studied here. When the locus of extended care was disaggregated, traditional lines of bureaucratic responsibility were disrupted. Recreating them outside the hospitals through networks of coordinated care has proven difficult, in part because the relevant agencies tend to have parochial ideas about their proper domains of work. Community-based systems of care were supposed to counter and correct for that tendency, but have manifestly fallen short of that goal. When sufficient resources are dedicated, the premise of flexible, coordinated care has proven sound, even for homeless persons with severe mental illnesses (13).

Thus one solution to the disarray depicted in this report would be to establish a special-purpose "alternative system" for this population. But the costs of such a parallel system are likely to be prohibitive. More feasible options, such as mobile relocation and stabilization units designed for "critical time intervention" (62) or modified assertive community treatment teams (14), also recommend themselves as interim measures.

However, in the face of a severe shortage of affordable housing for income-constrained households in Westchester County that shows no sign of lifting soon (63), stepped-up efforts to serve the needs of a relative few amount to little more than queue-jumping. Service providers have little choice but to advocate for the special needs of their clients, but that ought not to be mistaken for a solution to homelessness.

References

1. Fischer PJ: Alcohol, Drug, and Mental Health Problems Among Homeless Persons: A Review of the Literature, 1980–1990. Washington, DC, US Department of Health and Human Services, 1991
2. Lehman AF, Cordray DS: Prevalence of alcohol, drug, and mental disorders among the homeless: one more time. Contemporary Drug Problems 20:355–384, 1993
3. Koegel P: Through a different lens: an anthropological perspective on the homeless mentally ill. Culture, Medicine, and Psychiatry 16:1–22, 1992
4. Liebow E: Tell Them Who I Am. New York, Free Press, 1993
5. Fischer PJ: Criminal behavior and victimization among homeless people, in Homelessness: A Prevention-Oriented Approach. Edited by Jahiel RI. Baltimore, Johns Hopkins University Press, 1992
6. Lehman AF, Kernan E, DeForge BR, et al: Effects of homelessness on the quality of life of persons with severe mental illness. Psychiatric Services 46:922–926, 1995
7. Rosenheck RA, Leda C, Gallup P, et al: Initial assessment data from a 43-site program for homeless chronically mentally ill veterans. Hospital and Community Psychiatry 40:937–942, 1989
8. Solomon PL, Draine JN, Marcenko MO, et al: Homelessness in a mentally ill urban jail population. Hospital and Community Psychiatry 43:169–171, 1992
9. Michaels D, Zoloth SR, Alcabes P, et al: Homelessness and indicators of mental illness among inmates in New York City's correctional system. Hospital and Community Psychiatry 43:150–155, 1992
10. Martell DA, Rosner R, Harmon RB: Base-rate estimates of criminal behavior by homeless mentally ill persons in New York City. Psychiatric Services 46:595–601, 1995
11. Kales JP, Marone MA, Bixler EO, et al: Mental illness and substance use among sheltered homeless persons in lower-density populations areas. Psychiatric Services 46:592–595, 1995
12. Susser E, Valencia E, Miller M, et al: Sexual behavior of homeless mentally ill men at risk for HIV. American Journal of Psychiatry 152:583–587, 1995
13. Making a Difference: Interim Status Report of the McKinney Research Demonstration Program for Homeless Adults With Serious Mental Illness. Rockville, Md, Center for Mental Health Services, 1994
14. Dixon LB, Krauss N, Kernan E, et al: Modifying the PACT model to serve homeless persons with severe mental illness. Psychiatric Services 46:684–688, 1995
15. Pion GM, Cordray DS: Meeting the needs of homeless persons with multiple diagnoses through supportive housing and services. Paper presented at Health and Human Services and Housing and Urban Development Advisory Group meeting, Washington, DC, Aug 14, 1996
16. Shinn M: Homelessness: what is a psychologist to do? American Journal of Community Psychology 20:1–24, 1992
17. Susser E, Lin S, Conover S: Risk factors for homelessness among aftercare patients of an urban state hospital. American Journal of Psychiatry 148:1025–1030, 1991
18. Koegel P, Melamid E, Burnam MA: Childhood risk factors for homelessness among homeless adults. American Journal of Public Health 85:1642–1649, 1995
19. Link BG, Phelan J: Social conditions as fundamental causes of disease. Journal of Health and Social Behavior 36(extra issue):80–94, 1995
20. Cohen CI, Thompson KS: Homeless mentally ill or mentally ill homeless? American Journal of Psychiatry 149:816–823. 1992
21. Rossi PH, Wright JD: The urban homeless: a portrait of urban dislocation. Annals of the American Academy of Political and Social Science 501:132–142, 1989
22. Susser E, Moore R, Link B: Risk factors for homelessness. Epidemiological Reviews 15: 546–556, 1993
23. Koegel P, Burnam MA, Baumohl J: The causes of homelessness, in Homelessness in America. Edited by Baumohl J. Phoenix, Ariz, Oryx, 1996
24. Lipsky M: Street-Level Bureaucracy. New York, Russell Sage, 1980
25. Estroff SE: Making It Crazy. Berkeley, University of California Press, 1980

26. Sosin M, Piliavin I.. Westerfelt .H: Toward a longitudinal analysis of homelessness. Journal of Social Issues 46:157–174, 1991
27. Susser E., Lovell A. Conover S: Unravelling the causes of homelessness and of its association with mental illness, in Epidemiology and Prevention of Mental Disorders. Edited by Cooper B, Helgasson T. London, Routledge, 1989
28. Haugland G, Siegel C, Hopper K, et al: Mental illness among homeless individuals in a suburban county. Psychiatric Services 48:504–509, 1997
29. Harding CM, Brooks GW, Ashikaga T, et al: The Vermont longitudinal study of persons with severe mental illness: 1. methodology, study sample, and overall status 32 years later. American Journal of Psychiatry 144:718–726, 1987
30. The Life-Chart Schedule. Geneva, World Health Organization, 1992
31. Mandler P (ed): The Uses of Charity. Philadelphia, University of Pennsylvania Press, 1990
32. Brown P: Peasant survival strategies in late imperial Russia: the social uses of the mental hospital. Social Problems 34:311–329, 1987
33. Warner R: Recovery From Schizophrenia. Boston, Routledge & Kegan Paul, 1985
34. Baumohl J, Tracy S: Building systems to manage inebriates: the divergent paths of California and Massachusetts, 1891–1920. Contemporary Drug Problems 21:557–591, 1994
35. Merton RK: Social Theory and Social Structure, rev ed. Glencoe, Ill, Free Press, 1957
36. Bachrach LL: Managed care: II. some "latent functions." Psychiatric Services 47: 243–244, 253, 1996
37. Rochefort DA, Mechanic D: Deinstitutionalization: practice and promise, in From Poorhouses to Homelessness. Edited by Rochefort DA. Westport, Conn, Auburn House, 1993
38. Dear M, Wolch J: Landscapes of Despair: From Deinstitutionalization to Homelessness. Princeton, NJ, Princeton University Press, 1987
39. Hoch C, Slayton RA: New Homeless and Old: Community and the Skid Row Hotel. Philadelphia, Temple University Press, 1989
40. Groth P: Living Downtown. Berkeley, University of California Press, 1994
41. Sosin MR, Grossman S: The mental health system and the etiology of homelessness. Journal of Community Psychology 19:337–350, 1991
42. Segal S, Baumohl J: Engaging the disengaged: proposals on madness and vagrancy. Social Work 28:319–323, 1980
43. Hopper K, Baumohl J: Held in abeyance: rethinking homelessness and advocacy. American Behavioral Scientist 37:522–525, 1994
44. Culhane D: The quandaries of shelter reform. Social Service Review 66:428–440, 1992
45. Stark LB. The shelter as "total institution" American Behavioral Scientist 37:553–562, 1994
46. Dordick GA: More than refuge: the social world of a homeless shelter. Journal of Contemporary Ethnography 24:373–404, 1996
47. Kozol J: Rachel and Her Children. New York, Crown, 1988
48. Walsh J: Are shelters becoming open asylums? In These Times 9(9):3, 22
49. Bachrach LL: Deinstitutionalization: An Analytical Review and Sociological Perspective. Rockville, Md, National Institute of Mental Health, 1976
50. Rice SA: The failure of the municipal lodging house. National Municipal Review 11:358–362, 1922
51. Hopper K: Public shelter as a "hybrid institution": homeless men in historical perspective. Journal of Social Issues 46:13–29, 1991
52. Mizruchi E: Regulating Society, rev ed. Chicago, University of Chicago Press, 1987
53. Hopper K, Baumohl J: Redefining the cursed word: a historical interpretation of American homelessness, in Homelessness in America. Edited by Baumohl J. Phoenix, Ariz, Oryx, 1996
54. Bogard CJ, McConnell JJ, Gerstel N, et al: Surplus mothers: assessing family shelters as gendered abeyance structures, Paper presented at the annual meeting of the Eastern Sociological Association, Philadelphia, March 30–31, 1995
55. Rossi PH: Down and Out in America. Chicago, University of Chicago Press, 1989

56. Solomon P: Research on the coercion of persons with severe mental illnesses, in Coercion and Aggressive Community Treatment. Edited by Dennis DL, Monahan J. New York, Plenum, 1996

57. Rooney JF: Societal forces and the unattached male: an historical review, in Disaffiliated Man. Edited by Bahr HM. Toronto, University of Toronto Press, 1970

58. Baumohl J, Miller H: Down and out in Berkeley. Report prepared for the City of Berkeley-University of California Community Affairs Committee, May 1974

59. Wiseman JP: Stations of the Lost: The Treatment of Skid Row Alcoholics. Englewood Cliffs, NJ, Prentice-Hall, 1970

60. Baumohl J: Editor's introduction: alcohol, homelessness, and public policy. Contemporary Drug Problems 16:281–300, 1989

61. Dowdall GW: The Eclipse of the State Mental Hospital. Albany, State University of New York Press, 1996

62. Susser E, Valencia E, Conover S, et al: Prevention of homelessness among mentally ill men: a randomized clinical trial of a critical time intervention. American Journal of Public Health 87:256–262, 1997

63. Housing in Westchester County. New Brunswick. NJ, Rutgers University, Center for Urban Policy Research, 1991

IV

The Recovery Era (1998–Present)

Martha Staeheli Lawless and Michael Rowe

> Mere reforms to the existing mental health system are insufficient … transformation is not accomplished through change on the margins but, instead, through profound changes in kind and in degree. Applied to the task at hand, transformation represents a bold vision to change the very form and function of the mental health service delivery system to better meet the needs of the individuals and families it is designed to serve … Transformation … implies profound change—not at the margins of a system, but at its very core. In transformation, new sources of power emerge and new competencies develop.
>
> *Transforming Mental Health Care in America. The Federal Action Agenda: First Steps*[1, p.1]

By the end of the 1990s, a movement toward recovery-oriented interventions and approaches had gained ascendancy at policy and, to a lesser degree, practice levels in public mental health services. Pharmacological interventions continued to be prominent, but studies began to show that second-generation antipsychotic medications, introduced with much fanfare in the preceding decade, did not produce fewer side effects and were not more effective than their predecessors, as was first thought. While these new medications did not carry the *same* side effects as first-generation antipsychotics, they instead produced a range of metabolic side effects resulting in increased rates of comorbid conditions such as obesity, diabetes, and heart disease.[2] These side effects were particularly problematic for people with complex pharmacological profiles or with multiple prescribers who are not working in coordination with each other. Also of concern was the growing influence of the pharmaceutical industry on the prescribing practices of mental health professionals, leading to several high-profile investigations of pharmacology investigators and experts who failed to disclose the contributions they had received from the pharmaceutical industry, resulting in allegations of conflict of interest.[3]

Consumer movements and the call for nonmedical interventions have a long history in mental health,[4–6] but these efforts began to coalesce in the early 1990s with the development of consumer-run and peer-delivered services and the increased involvement of consumers and family members in service system design and evaluation. Mental health systems of care, responding in part to such pressures and to advances in the field, began to give greater attention to psychosocial and rehabilitative interventions. Some of these, such as assertive community treatment (ACT), had been in place for decades in some mental health systems but were now beginning to be disseminated more broadly. Others, such as the employment of people in recovery as mental health staff, were early in their development. Taken together, these services and supports helped to begin to shift in discussion from a sole focus on reducing psychiatric hospitalizations and supporting people's stable lives in the community, toward an additional focus on their full involvement and membership in those communities. Rehabilitative approaches of supported housing and supported employment offer practical illustrations of efforts directed toward or consistent with this goal. The supported housing approach, for example, reversed a longtime incremental approach to housing in which people with mental illness who have been hospitalized or not fared well in independing housing in the past are prepared, incrementally, for independent living by slowly advancing through group home to halfway house to eventual placement in independent housing. In its place, supported housing proponents and theorists argued that people are always "ready for housing," although they may need, and should be able to choose from among, a variety of social supports to help them maintain their housing.[7]

It is beyond the scope of this chapter to provide an in-depth analysis of the recovery movement, but a brief review will help to establish the context in which our contemporary classics have been written. A number of definitions of recovery have been offered. Generally these fall into one of two categories. The first is remission or elimination of the symptoms and effects of the illness or disease in the traditional medical sense of the term, as with, say, recovery from pneumonia with no, or few, remaining symptoms or limitations on normal activities. The second, and more common meaning, in contemporary community mental health, involves winning back one's life as a whole person, including one's capacity for self-determination, friendship, meaningful activities, and valued roles, *even if* and *even when* the symptoms and functional constraints of mental illness persist. In the latter form of recovery, psychiatric disability comprises one element of a person's life, rather than subsuming his or her identity.[8]

The person lives a life "in recovery" in the second sense of the term, but mental health services can support the person's recovery by being "recovery-oriented." "Person-centered care," for example, privileges the client's choice of the treatment she wants and the clinician, while bringing his clinical skills and training to the treatment endeavor, helps her work through her options to develop and maintain, or change, that plan over time. [9–11] Culturally competent care, which is consistent with and informs person-centered care, highlights the importance of culture, race, religion, sexual orientation, gender, and other social elements of both the person with the mental illness and the practitioner or treatment milieu, with the implicit, or explicit, message that a singular vision of mental health treatment is no longer sufficient for much of America's population.[12,13] The recovery vision and principles suggest that the supports needed to facilitate and promote recovery can be found not only in formal treatment interventions but also in churches, schools, clubs, neighborhoods, and cafés. Indeed, such psychosocial practices and programs, and informal, naturally occurring arrangements had been in place for years in the community mental health era, with an upsurge in consumer-run organizations beginning in the early 1990s.[14,15] People in recovery became an ever more important source of information about recovery processes and were increasingly being looked to as guides for others navigating their own "recovery journeys."[16]

If recovery has been the preeminent philosophy in community mental health during our present era (and perhaps for a few years before the date we have given for its start), the notion of "evidence-based treatment" has been the most influential in terms of specific treatment models. Let us use the example of a successful treatment model—motivational interviewing—to try to clarify the relationship between the two in the case of mental health treatment. Motivational interviewing describes people as, at any given point, being at a certain stage along a continuum of motivation, rather than as "having" or "not having" motivation. The clinician assesses the client's location on the motivational continuum and seeks to intervene clinically in a manner appropriate for the client at that point. Intervene at the wrong place on the continuum, and you may thwart the client's progress by "asking" too little or too much of her.[17,18] Motivational interviewing, although it appears to be consistent with the recovery philosophy, and certainly does not contradict it, could be practiced by or taught to individual clinicians in a way that is more or less recovery oriented.

The introduction of evidence-based practice (EBP) in psychiatry began to take root in the late 1990s.[19,20] In increasingly complicated and expensive managed and public health care systems, EBP became a way of prioritizing funding for interventions with proved effectiveness. A 1998 conference convened by the Robert Wood Johnson Foundation identified six models of psychiatric treatment—illness management and recovery, family psychoeducation, standardized (algorithmic) pharmacological treatment, supported employment, and integrated treatment for co-occurring disorders—as being evidence-based as a result of positive findings for each from randomized clinical trials.[20]

The New Hampshire–Dartmouth Psychiatric Research Center received funding from the federal Substance Abuse and Mental Health Services Administration to develop toolkits with the input of multiple stakeholders, including persons with mental illnesses and practitioners, for each designated practice.[21–23] Toolkits, which include instructional guides, videos, and fidelity scales, are disseminated through state mental health authorities and local mental health authorities to clinicians, administrators, and consumers of mental health services and their families. The toolkits were evaluated beginning in 2002 to determine how well they accomplished their goals of educating mental health professionals and people in recovery, and starting in 2005 have been refined based on these evaluations.[20] The EBP roster has also been expanded to include supported housing and consumer-operated services and programs for older adults and adolescents.

The introduction of EBPs did not come without controversy. Some criticize the use of tools developed for general medicine for mental health treatment. Others argue that manualization neglects both the "art" and individualized nature of clinical care. Others point out that many of the clinical trials from which EBPs derived their designation were tested on homogeneous groups that do not reflect the racial, ethnic, and cultural makeup of the client population of many public mental health systems. Finally, questions of the feasibility, cost, and time required for training of clinicians in EBPs have been raised, given that many clinicians have been trained in different approaches to practice, and that many mental health workers lack professional training, are not required to obtain continuing education or practice according to a governing body's standards, or do not have access to technology that would make knowledge dissemination more feasible.[20,24]

Funding for mental health services followed a similar state-of-the-art and science approach. The Medicaid Rehabilitative Services Option (MRO), added by many states, was designed so that the country's largest source of mental health funding—the Centers for Medicare and Medicaid Services—could provide people with serious mental illness more flexible recovery supports beyond those offered in a purely clinical model.[25,26] Services reimbursed under the MRO vary by state but include ACT, peer services, rehabilitative coordination, and recreational activities that occur in the community or at home as aids to the client's ability to function independently. As of this writing, Georgia and South Carolina have added peer services to their MROs, and other states have added rehabilitative coordination and integrated dual diagnosis treatment. Although states' use of the MRO mechanism for funding mental health and psychosocial services is likely to increase, the option has been slow, overall, to take hold in the field.

A notable state effort to create more flexible funding pathways is New Mexico's effort to redesign its mental health care system in 2004 with the designation of ValueOptions New Mexico, a privately owned and managed behavioral health care entity, as the state's sole provider of mental health services. Under this system, several federal funding streams are to be leveraged by one company so that reimbursement for services is simplified and patients receive seamless and comprehensive services. ValueOptions, the company that oversees every aspect of the behavioral health care system from credentialing to billing, cites prevention of mental illness, recovery, and resiliency as the foundational principles of their service provision. Evaluation of this system has not been done as of this writing.[27]

At the federal policy level, an important impetus for mental health reform was the work of Second Lady Tipper Gore, named the White House Mental Health Advisor under the Clinton Administration for her previous advocacy of mental and physical health coverage parity and reduction of stigma related to mental illness and mental health care.[28] Ms. Gore announced in 1999 that her mother had been hospitalized several times for it during Ms. Gore's childhood, and that she, too, had personal experience with depression., In the same year, Ms. Gore chaired the first-ever White House Conference on Mental Health, in which people with mental illness were invited to talk about their experiences, and She also encouraged President Clinton to support the Mental Health Equitable Treatment Act, which unsuccessfully sought federal parity for mental and physical health coverage.

The U.S. Surgeon General, Dr. David Satcher, worked with the National Institute of Mental Health to commission a series of papers for a report on the nature of mental health disorders and the state of current treatment practices. The 1999 report, *Mental Health: A Report of the Surgeon General,* was groundbreaking in its scope and its emphasis on recovery from mental illness. The report, which reviews the theorized causes and symptoms of mental illness and cites public health statistics regarding the ubiquity (one in four adults) of mental health problems in the United States, argues that mental and physical health are inextricably linked and that mental health is fundamental to good general health. It also called for new efforts to dispel stigma surrounding mental illness that discourages many from seeking treatment, and called for parity with general health care coverage for mental health treatment. Mental illness is normal, the report argued, and treatment is effective when it is readily available and accessible. Access, however, is complicated by significant disparities due to poverty, social class, geography, and cultural competence, especially in minority populations.[8]

Rather than addressing cultural and racial health disparities in a separate section, the committee members chose to weave the current state of knowledge about nonwhite populations into the general text of the report.[29,30] Many in the field thought that the report did not address adequately the mental health needs and experiences of populations of color. A supplement, published in 2001, outlined ways in which cultural mores affect mental health treatment for African Americans, Asians, Hispanic/Latinos, and Native American/Pacific Islanders, and noted that access to, and the success of, treatment is affected significantly by the cultural background of patients and their clinicians. People in minority populations are more often diagnosed with serious mental illness and less likely to seek and receive services. The services they do receive are generally of poorer quality than those for whites, and minority groups are severely underrepresented in mental health services research. Because of these disparities, the mental illness imposes an even greater burden on nonwhite groups. The report advocated the development of culturally responsive treatment and related services to address the mental health needs of each of these populations.[31]

Although Surgeon General reports are not federal policy documents per se, they represent the policy orientation of the sponsoring administration, the Substance Abuse and Mental Health Services Administration. With the end of the Clinton Administration in 2000 and rejection of the Mental Health Eqitable Treatment Act, the Surgeon General's 1999 and 2001 reports provided, at a minimum, national policy-related reference points for advocates' efforts as President Bush took office.

In 2001, the Bush Administration launched the New Freedom Initiative with the stated purpose of promoting access to life "in the community for everyone." It would do this, in part, by building on the 1999 *Olmstead v. L.C.* Supreme Court decision and the Americans with Disabilities Act, both of which, in different ways, mandated the full inclusion of people with psychiatric disabilities in their communities. *Achieving the Promise,* the New Freedom Commission's 2004 report, argued that the U.S. mental health system delivered fragmented services that did not support and promote recovery from mental illness. The report called for a transformed system of care in which (1) the importance of mental health to general health would be recognized and addressed in health care systems, (2) care would be driven by the needs of the individuals and families who receive it, (3) disparities in care would be eliminated, (4) early screening for mental illness would be conducted and early referral to treatment would occur, (5) care would be driven by research findings, and (6) technology would be employed as a tool for gaining access to information on mental health and other relevant services.[32]

The New Freedom Commission Report called for recovery-focused mental health care driven by the needs and desires of people with psychiatric disabilities and their families and offering meaningful choices among services types and approaches. It emphasized the need to offer services that are evidence based, collaborative in nature, and community based, with the goal of increasing peoples' abilities and opportunities to live in the communities of their choosing and participate as citizens with full, productive lives. The report was seminal but unfortunately did not come with funding to back its recommendations.

Following publication of *Achieving the Promise*, the Department of Health and Human Services invited six other federal departments—Education, Justice, Labor, Housing and Urban Development, Veterans' Affairs, and the Social Security Administration—to collaborate in a study process that led to publication in 2005 of *The Federal Mental Health Action Agenda.* This report pledged collaboration among agencies to develop inventories of current policy and programs that address the goals set forth by the New Freedom Commission Report and to propose methods for achieving them. As with its predecessors, its chief goal was to promote the message that mental illness is treatable and recovery is possible. In addition, the report and the proposed continuing agency collaboration set goals of increasing access to effective mental health and reducing suicide by helping states develop mental health infrastructures to promote recovery; increasing the capabilities and cultural competence of the mental health workforce; improving mental health care in primary care settings; promoting early intervention for children, increasing translation of knowledge from research to practice; supporting employment opportunities for people with psychiatric disabilities; and developing electronic health records. While federal agencies would provide support for this work, the onus of transformation would fall to individual states.

The federal government has begun to issue policy and provide limited funding for states and municipalities—from Transformation State Incentive Grants[33] to Medicaid reimbursement for peer-specialists[34,35]—to refashion their services to better address the needs of people with psychiatric disabilities. Recovery-oriented services appear to be on the rise and to have some momentum at state and federal levels. With increasing emphasis on cultural competence, self-determination, and person-centered care, the person in recovery may be poised to take greater control over his or her own treatment. As this trend progresses, the question of its relationship to academic psychiatry's focus on the neurobiology and pharmacology of mental illness will become more pressing. Another pressing issue, to which we've hardly done justice in this chapter, is the fact that, fifty-plus years after the cense of state psychiatric hospitals began their long decline and the idea of a life in the community for people with mental illnesses began to take root, institutionalization of people with mental illness, in the sense of segregation from society, occurs more often today, and at very high rates, via incarceration rather than psychiatric hospitalization.[36,37] The recovery movement, and EBPs, have had little impact on this fact to date, and their role will be limited without changes in policy such as those we are beginning to see in federal and state attempts to develop new programs for released offenders returning to their communities.[38]

Since we began work on this chapter, a new president has taken office and health care reform has been enacted. In a sense, then, we are already in a new future, one of which we can see only the hazy outline at present. The continuation of our current era, or its own new one, could result in expanded mental health coverage. What mental health care will look like in a redesigned health care system in the United States, however, remains to be seen as that new system, should it survive challenges to it, is rolled out over the next few years.

References

1. Substance and Mental Health Services Administration. (2005). *Transforming mental health care in America: The federal action agenda: First steps.* Rockville, MD: Author.
2. U.S. Medical Directors Council of the National Association of State Mental Health Program Directors. (2006). *Morbidity and mortality in people with serious mental illness.* Alexandria, VA: Author.
3. Safer, D. J. (2002) Design and reporting modifications in industry sponsored comparative psychopharmacology trials. *Journal of Nervous and Mental Disease, 90,* 583–592.
4. Deegan, P. E. (1996). Recovery as a journey of the heart. *Psychiatric Rehabilitation Journal, 19,* 91–97.
5. Jacobson, N., Greenley, D. (2001). What is recovery: A conceptual model and explication. *Psychiatric Services, 52*(4), 482–485.
6. Roberts, G., Wolfson, P. (2004). The rediscovery of recovery: Open to all. *Advances in Psychiatric Treatment, 10,* 37–49.
7. Culhane, D. P., Stephen M., Trevor R. Hadley (2002). The Impact of Supportive Housing for Homeless People with Severe Mental Illness on the Utilization of the Public Health, Corrections, and Emergency Shelter Systems: The New York-New York Initiative. *Housing Policy Debate 13.1,* 107–163.
8. (1999). *Mental health: A report of the surgeon general.* Rockville, MD.: Department of Health and Human Services, Substance Abuse and Mental Health Services Administration: National Institutes of Health.
9. O'Brien, C., O'Brien, J. (2000). *The origins of person-centered planning: A community of practice perspective.* Syracuse, NY: Responsive Systems Associates, Inc.
10. Tondora, J., Pocklington, S., Gorges, A., Osher, D., Davidson, L. (2005). *Implementation of person-centered care and planning. From policy to practice to evaluation.* Washington D.C.: Substance Abuse and Mental Health Services Administration.
11. Adams. N., Grieder, D. (2005). *Treatment planning for person-centered care: The road to mental health and addiction recovery.* San Diego, CA: Elsevier Academic Press.
12. Delphin, M., Rowe, M. (2008). Continuing education in cultural competence for community mental health practitioners. *Professional Psychology: Research and Practice, 39*(2), 182–191.
13. National Alliance of Multi-Ethnic Behavioral Health Associations. (2008). Blueprint for the National Network to Eliminate Disparities in Behavioral Health. Washington, D.C.
14. Davidson, L., et al. (1999). Peer support among individuals with severe mental illness: A review of the evidence. *Clinical Psychology Science & Practice, 6*(2), 165–187.
15. Mead, S.,Copeland, M. E. (2000). What recovery means to us: Consumers' perspectives. *Community Mental Health Journal, 36*(3), 315–328.
16. Miller, W. R., Rollnick, S. (eds.) (1991). *Motivational interviewing: Preparing people to change addictive behavior.* New York: Guilford Press.
17. Rollnick, S., Miller, W. R. (1995). What is motivational interviewing? *Behaviour Cogn Psychother, 23,* 325–334.

18. Davidson, L., et al. (2005). Peer support among individuals with severe mental illness: A review of the evidence. In Davidson, L., Harding, C., Spaniol, L., editors. *Recovery from severe mental illnesses: Research evidence and implications for practice, Vol 1* (pp. 412–450). Boston: Center for Psychiatric Rehabilitation.

19. Goodman, K. (2003). *Ethics and evidence-based medicine: Fallibility and responsibility in clinical science.* Cambridge: Cambridge University Press.

20. Bond, G. R., Becker, D. R., Drake, R. E., Rapp, C. A., Meisler, N., Lehman, A. F., et al. (2001a). Implementing supported employment as an evidence-based practice. *Psychiatric Services, 52,* 313–322.

21. Bond, G. R., Drake, R. E., Mueser, K. T., Latimer, E. (2001b). Assertive community treatment for people with severe mental illness. *Disease Management and Health Outcomes, 9,* 141–159.

22. Drake, R. E., Merrens, M. R., Lynde, D. W. (2005). *Evidence-based mental health practice: A textbook.* New York: W. W. Norton.

23. Drake, R. E., Goldman, H. H., Leff, H., et al. (2001). Implementing evidence-based practices in routine mental health service settings. *Psychiatric Services, 52,* 179–182.

24. O'Brien Danm Ford Laurie, Malloy, JoAnne (2005). Person-centered planning: Using vouchers and personal budget to support recovery and employment for people with psychiatric disabilities. *Journal of Vocational Rehabilitation 23*(2), 71–79.

25. Turner, T. P. *Ten Models for Transforming State Mental Health Systems.* Washington, D.C.: National Association of State Mental Health Program Directors. http://www.nasmhpd. org/general_files/meeting_presentations/TF%20nonT%20TTI%20conf/h%20Non%20 T-SIG%20States%20intro%20FINAL.pdf. Accessed September 7, 2010.

26. Dixon, L., Goldman, H. H. (2004). Forty years of progress in community mental health: The role of evidence-based practices. *Administration and Policy in Mental Health, 31*(5), 381–392.

27. Hill, B. B. (2008). New Mexico and ValueOptions use braided funding to transform the state's behavioral health services. http://www.valueoptions.com/company/Coverage/A_New_ System_for_NewMexico.htm. Accessed January 28, 2008.

28. Short, J., Shogan, C., Owings, N. (2005). The influence of first ladies on mental health policy. *White House Studies, 5*(1), 65–76.

29. Chang, D. (2003). An introduction to the politics of science: Culture, race, ethnicity, and the Supplement to the Surgeon General's Report on Mental Health. *Culture, Medicine and Psychiatry, 27,* 373–383.

30. Goldman, H. H. (2003). Commentary: Making culture count in mental health reports from the surgeon general. *Culture, Medicine and Psychiatry, 27,* 387–389.

31. National Institutes of Health. (2001). *Mental health: Race, culture, and ethnicity.* Rockville, MD: Department of Health and Human Services, Substance Abuse and Mental Health Services Administration.

32. The President' New Freedom Commission on Mental Health. (2003). *Achieving the promise: Transforming mental health care in America. Final report.* Rockville, MD: Department of Health and Human Services.

33. Mental Health Transformation State Incentive Grants RFA. Rockville, MD. Substance Abuse and Mental Health Services Administration, Center for Mental Health Services. http://www. samhsa.gov/grants/2005/nofa/sm05009_mht_sig.aspx. Accessed September 7, 2010.

34. Sabin James, E., Daniels, N. (2003). Managed Care: Strengthening the Consumer Voice in Managed Care: VII. The Georgia Peer Specialist Program. *Psychiatric Services, 54,* 497–498.

35. Peebles, S. A., Mabe, P. A., Davidson, L., Fricks, L., Buckley, P.F., Fenley, G. (2007). Recovery and systems transformation for schizophrenia. *Psychiatric Clinics of North America, 30,* 567–583.

36. Belcher, J. (1988). Are jails replacing the mental health system for the homeless mentally ill? *Community Mental Health Journal, 24*(3), 185–195.

37. Draine J., Salzer M. S., Culhane, D. P, Hadley, T. R. (2002). Role of social disadvantage in crime, joblessness, and homelessness among persons with serious mental illness <http://www.ps.psychiatryonline.org/cgi/content/abstract/53/5/565>. *Psychiatric Services, 53*, 565–573.
38. Second Chance Act Prisoner Reentry Initiative FY. (2009) Competitive Grant Announcement. Washington, D.C.: U.S. Department of Justice, Office of Justice Programs' Bureau of Justice Assistance. http://www.ojp.usdoj.gov/BJA/grant/09SecondChanceReentrySol.pdf. Accessed September 7, 2010

Government, Legislative, and Policy Classics

35

Talbott, J. A., & Lamb,
H. R. Introduction and
recommendations. In
H. Richard Lamb, ed. (1984).
The homeless mentally
ill: A task force report of
the American Psychiatric
Association. Washington,
D.C.: American Psychiatric
Association, 1–10

The "new homelessness" in the United States began in the late 1970s and became a national issue in the late 1970s and early 1980s, as the single adult males of the Skid Row era of homelessness were joined by younger single men and women (and by new homeless families and youth, as well) who were poorer, more likely to be African American, had a higher incidence of mental illness than their Skid Row predecessors and compatriots, and were more visible than the latter on the downtown streets of American cities. There would be a robust debate during the 1980s and beyond about whether homelessness was a problem of persons with mental illness or drug addictions, or a socioeconomic problem caused by lack of low income housing and a lack of jobs and income supports, with the most vulnerable persons, including those with behavioral health disorders, falling "over the edge," in Martha Burt's phrase, into homelessness. Richard Lamb's edited volume takes up the issues of identification of mentally ill persons among those who are homeless, development of better service delivery systems, medical and legal issues, and the politics of homelessness, among other topics. Lamb and colleagues make an argument for a vigorous, coordinated national response led locally by community mental health systems. (Sue Estroff's "Medicalizing the Margins," in this volume, uses a critique of this volume as its starting point.) The excerpt here is Talbott's and Lamb's introduction to the volume, including a series of recommendations for a targeted response to homelessness and mental illness in America.

Summary and Recommendations

A large number of difficult and often seemingly overwhelming social issues, most of which elude easy solutions, confront us today. Principal among them is the widespread, serious, and increasing phenomenon of homelessness in America, many of whose victims are seriously and/or chronically mentally ill. To address this problem, the American Psychiatric Association appointed a Task Force on the Homeless Mentally Ill in 1983, realizing that while all citizens have a responsibility for the welfare of the homeless, psychiatrists have an additional responsibility for the mentally ill among them.

The recommendations in this report reflect that general obligation as citizens to address the problems of this heterogeneous population as well as our specific obligation as psychiatrists to help the large number of homeless mentally ill. Recommendations for additional action on the part of the American Psychiatric Association and American psychiatrists will be contained in a joint position paper formulated by the Association's Task Force on the Homeless Mentally Ill, its Committee on the Chronically Mentally Ill, and its Council on Psychiatric Services.To provide a basis for the recommendations below, we will begin by summarizing the major points of this study of the homeless mentally ill in America. Both here and in the recommendations, the reader is referred to individual Chapters for more detailed information. It should be noted, however, that most of the points are discussed in more than one Chapter.

Summary

Homelessness is not a new phenomenon. Large urban centers have always attracted vagabonds, derelicts, and hoboes, but until recently these unfortunate individuals tended to cluster in certain areas, often called skid rows. Today, however, we are experiencing a new phenomenon—one of unprecedented magnitude and complexity—and hardly a section of the country, urban or rural, has escaped the ubiquitous presence of ragged, ill, and hallucinating human beings, wandering through our city streets, huddled in alleyways, or sleeping over vents.

This rapidly growing problem of homelessness has emerged as a major societal tragedy and has recently commanded increasing attention from all segments of society, including the government, the media, and the public at large. The individuals affected are now regarded as an eyesore at best and the victims of a moral scandal at worst.

It now is apparent that a substantial portion of the homeless are chronically and severely mentally ill men and women who in years past would have been long-term residents of state hospitals. They now have no place to live because of efforts to depopulate public hospitals coupled with the unavailability of suitable housing and supervised living arrangements in "the community," inadequate continuing medical-psychiatric care and other supportive services, and poorly thought-out changes in the laws governing involuntary treatment.

Homelessness has historically reflected the interaction between the most vulnerable of our population and the scarcity or plenty of our resources. Those members of society least able to care for themselves have always been at greatest risk for loss of residence and affiliation—for example, the never-institutionalized alcoholic, the unemployed, and the migrant and the refugee. Today their ranks are swelled by the addition of thousands of people suffering from severe and chronic mental disorders, including major psychotic disorders, alcoholism, drug abuse, and severe personality disorders, who have been discharged or diverted from institutions.

The causes of homelessness are many and complex, and the homeless comprise different populations with different needs. Some of the homeless are undomiciled because they have lost their jobs, others because of the gentrification of urban areas without a concomitant replacement of inexpensive housing. Still others suffer from substance abuse or severe and chronic mental disorder and disability. Thus each person's needs can be identified only by knowing which subset of the homeless population he or she belongs to.

The concept of deinstitutionalization per se was not bad. The idea that many, if not most, of the severely and chronically mentally ill suffering from serious illnesses such as schizophrenia and manic-depression could be cared for as well in community programs as in institutions, if not better, was in itself not a bad idea. It was clinically sound and economically feasible.

However, the way deinstitutionalization was originally carried out, through the poorly planned discharge of thousands of mentally ill residents of state hospitals into inadequately prepared or programmatically deficient communities, was another thing altogether. In addition, as a result of the states' admission diversion policies, increasing numbers of "new" chronically mentally ill individuals have never been institutionalized, and have further expanded the homeless mentally ill population.

Vital resources for both groups have been lacking. They include adequate and integrated community programs for these individuals; an adequate number and range of community residential settings, with varying degrees of supervision and structure; a system of follow-up, monitoring, and responsibility for ensuring that services are provided to those unable to obtain them; and easy access to short-term and long-term inpatient care when indicated. The consequences of these gaps in essential resources have been disastrous (see Chapters 2 and 3).

An emphasis on homelessness per se deflects attention from the basic, underlying problem of the lack of a comprehensive support system for the severely and chronically mentally ill. As was noted above, it was not the concept of deinstitutionalization, but its implementation, that was flawed. All services available to patients while they resided in state facilities, including the function of asylum, were not available when they returned to community settings (see Chapter 3). In addition, in hospitals such services are provided under one roof, and no such umbrella existed in the community.

While temporary housing such as shelters may be an important stopgap measure for many of the homeless mentally ill, increasing the number of shelters merely postpones the day of reckoning when we will have to try to provide all the services needed as well as a system to glue them together. Such a support system can be familial or institutional (that is, provided by mental health programs), or a combination of both, but society must ensure that the system exists and is adequate.

Society's ambivalence about wanting the mentally ill kept out of sight, while at the same time opposing involuntary incarceration, must be better resolved. When deinstitutionalization occurred, society reacted vehemently to the presence on our cities' streets of the most seriously and chronically ill patients. Yet society has increasingly rejected the idea of involuntarily committing such patients to state hospitals for long periods of time. Currently few states have commitment laws that give family members or those responsible for treatment easy access to prompt treatment for persons whose mental illness has worsened or whose condition has deteriorated severely. Society cannot continue to have it both ways.

These major points of the Task Force report lead to three general statements that relate to proposed solutions to the problems of the homeless mentally ill.

First, there is no single, simple solution to the problems of homelessness. Because of the different subpopulations of the homeless, the different causes of and reasons for homelessness, and the different needs of the various subgroups, no one solution will meet all the needs of the homeless. Moreover, while temporary housing, such as shelters, is a necessary step, it is only a short-term solution.

Second, solutions must be targeted to the differing populations. Obviously such diverse groups as the unemployed, those displaced by gentrification, alcoholics and drug abusers, and the severely and chronically mentally ill have very different needs. The solutions for those who are unemployed include job assessment, placement, and retraining; for those displaced by gentrification, an ambitious new program of low-cost housing; for those suffering primarily from substance abuse and alcoholism, outreach services, detoxification facilities, medical treatment, and a host of specialized programs; and for those suffering from severe and chronic mental illnesses, supervised housing, medical and psychiatric care, aggressive case management and follow-up, and a multiplicity of other services.

Lastly, the recommendations that follow will deal only with the mentally ill homeless, the group with which this report deals, not with the homeless in general. To come to grips, with the problems of the homeless mentally ill, we must address both short- and long-term issues simultaneously; thus the recommendations suggest both immediate and long-range actions. While other advocates and agencies will address the problems of other groups of homeless Americans, and some of their proposals will apply to the entire population of the homeless, we will confine our recommendations specifically to the homeless mentally ill.

The recommendations that follow are proposed as optimal solutions that all concerned segments of society should work to carry out. Clearly their implementation, however, will depend on society's willingness to reallocate resources to meet this pressing problem.

Recommendations of the Task Force

Major Recommendation

To address the problems of the homeless mentally ill in America, a comprehensive and integrated system of care for this vulnerable population of the mentally ill, with designated responsibility, with accountability, and with adequate fiscal resources, must be established.

Derivative Recommendations

1) *Any attempt to address the problems of the homeless mentally ill must begin with provisions for meeting their basic needs: food, shelter, and clothing.* The chronically mentally ill have a *right,* equal to that of other groups, to these needs being met.

2) *An adequate number and ample range of graded, step-wise, supervised community housing settings must be established.* (See Chapter 6.) While many of the homeless may benefit from temporary housing such as shelters, and some small portion of the severely and chronically mentally ill can graduate to independent living, for the vast majority neither shelters nor mainstream low-cost housing are appropriate. Most housing settings that require people to manage by themselves are beyond the capabilities of the chronically mentally ill. Instead, there must be settings offering different levels of supervision, both more and less intensive, including quarterway and halfway houses, lodges and camps, board-and-care homes, satellite housing, foster or family care, and crisis or temporary hostels.

3) *Adequate, comprehensive, and accessible psychiatric and rehabilitative services must be available, and must be assertively provided through outreach services when necessary.* (See Chapters 5, 8, and 9.) First, there must be an adequate number of direct psychiatric services, both on the streets and in the shelters when appropriate, that provide (a) outreach contact with the mentally ill in the community, (b) psychiatric assessment and evaluation, (c) crisis intervention, including hospitalization, (d) individualized treatment plans, (e) psychotropic medication and other somatic therapies, and (f) psychosocial treatment. Second, there must be an adequate number of rehabilitative services, providing socialization experiences, training in the skills of everyday living, and social rehabilitation. Third, both treatment and rehabilitative services must be provided assertively—for instance, by going out to patients' living settings if they do not or cannot come to a centralized program. And fourth, the difficulty of working with some of these patients must not be under-estimated (see Chapters 7, 9, and 11).

4) *General medical assessment and care must be available.* (See Chapter11.) Since we know that the chronically mentally ill have three times the morbidity and mortality of their counterparts of the same age in the general population, and the homeless even higher rates, the ready availability of general medical care is essential and critical.

5) *Crisis services must be available and accessible to both the chronically mentally ill homeless and the chronically mentally ill in general.* Too often, the homeless mentally ill who are in crisis are ignored because they are presumed, as part of the larger homeless population, to reject all conventional forms of help. Even more inappropriately, they may be put into inpatient hospital units when rapid, specific interventions such as medication or crisis housing would be more effective and less costly. Others, in need of acute hospitalization, are denied it because of restrictive admission criteria or commitment laws. In any case, it will be difficult to provide adequate crisis services to the homeless mentally ill until they are conceptualized and treated separately from the large numbers of other homeless persons.

6) *A system of responsibility for the chronically mentally ill living in the community must be established, with the goal of ensuring that ultimately each patient has one person responsible for his or her care.* Clearly the shift of psychiatric care from institutional to community settings does not in any way eliminate the need to continue the provision of comprehensive services to mentally ill persons. As a result, society must declare a public policy of responsibility for the mentally ill who are unable to meet their own needs; governments must designate programs in each region or locale as core agencies responsible and accountable for the care of the chronically mentally ill living there; and the staff of these agencies must be assigned individual patients for whom they are responsible. The ultimate goal must be to ensure that each chronically mentally ill person in this country has one

person—such as a case manager or resource manager—who is responsible for his or her treatment and care.

For the more than 50 percent of the chronically ill population living at home or for those with positive ongoing relationships with their families, programs and respite care must be provided to enhance the family's ability to provide a support system. Where the use of family systems is not feasible, the patient must be linked up with a formal community support system. In any case, the entire burden of deinstitutionalization must not be allowed to fall upon families (see Chapter 13).

7) *Basic changes must be made in legal and administrative procedures to ensure continuing community care for the chronically mentally ill.* (See Chapter 12.) In the 1960s and 1970s more stringent commitment laws and patients' rights advocacy remedied some egregious abuses in public hospital care, but at the same time these changes neglected patients' right to high-quality comprehensive outpatient care as well as the rights of families and society. New laws and procedures must be developed to ensure provision of psychiatric care in the community—that is, to guarantee a right to treatment in the community.

It must become easier to obtain conservatorship status for outpatients who are so gravely disabled and/or have such impaired judgment that they cannot care for themselves in the community without legally sanctioned supervision. Involuntary commitment laws must be made more humane to permit prompt return to active inpatient treatment for patients when acute exacerbations of their illnesses make their lives in the community chaotic and unbearable. Involuntary treatment laws should be revised to allow the option of outpatient civil commitment; in states that already have provisions for such treatment, that mechanism should be more widely used. Finally, advocacy efforts should be focused on the availability of competent care in the community.

8) *A system of coordination among funding sources and implementation agencies must be established.* (See Chapters 2, 5, and 8.) Because the problems of the mentally ill homeless must be addressed by multiple public and private authorities, coordination, so lacking in the deinstitutionalization process, must become a primary goal. The ultimate objective must be a true system of care rather than a loose network of services, and an ease of communication among different types of agencies (for example, psychiatric, social, vocational, and housing) as well as up and down the governmental ladder, from local through federal. One characteristic of a genuine system is the ability to flexibly alter roles, responsibilities, and programs as specific service needs change, and this ultimate end must be striven for.

9) *An adequate number of professionals and paraprofessionals must be trained for community care of the chronically ill.* Among the additional specially trained workers needed, four groups are particularly important for this population: (a) psychiatrists who are skilled in, and interested in, working with the chronically mentally ill; (b) outreach workers who can engage the homeless mentally ill on the streets; (c) case managers, preferably with sufficient training to provide therapeutic interventions themselves; and (d) conservators, to act for patients too disabled to make clinically and economically sound decisions.

10) *General social services must be provided.* Besides the need for specialized social services such as socialization experiences and training in the skills of everyday living (referred to in Recommendation 3), there is also a pressing need for generic social services. Such services include escort services to agencies and potential residential placements, help with applications to entitlement programs, and assistance in mobilizing the resources of the family.

11) *Ongoing asylum and sanctuary should be available for that small proportion of the chronically mentally ill who do not respond to current methods of treatment and rehabilitation.* (See Chapter 3.) Some patients, even with high-quality treatment and rehabilitation efforts, remain dangerous or gravely disabled. For these patients, there is a pressing need for ongoing asylum in long-term settings, whether in hospitals or in facilities such as California's locked skilled nursing facilities that have special programs for the mentally ill.

12) *Research into the causes and treatment of both chronic mental illness and homelessness needs to be expanded.* While our knowledge has greatly advanced in recent years (see Chapters 4 and 10), it is still limited. Treatment of chronic mental illness remains largely palliative, and definitive treatment will occur only with an adequate understanding of etiologic processes. In addition, our understanding of differential therapeutics—that is, what treatment works for which patients in what settings—is in its infancy and requires increased resources and attention.

13) *More accurate epidemiological data need to be gathered and analyzed.* Currently the research findings of incidence of mental illness among homeless groups are highly variable, ranging up to 91 percent; these differences depend largely on such methodological issues as where the sample is taken, whether standardized scales or comparable criteria of illness are used, and theoretical biases (see Chapters 4 and 14). Better data, using recognized diagnostic criteria, need to be acquired.

14) *Finally, additional monies must be expended for longer-term solution for the homeless mentally ill.* Although health and mental health costs and funding in this country have recently increased, the homeless mentally ill have not been beneficiaries of this increase. Therefore adequate new monies must be found to finance the system of care we envision, which incorporates supervised living arrangements, assertive case management, and an array of other services. In addition, financial support from existing entitlement programs such as Supplemental Security Income and Medicaid must be ensured.

In summary, the solutions to the problems of the mentally ill homeless are as manifold as the problems they seek to remedy. However, only with comprehensive short- and long-term solutions will the plight of this most neglected population in America be addressed.

36

National Association of State Mental Health Program Directors. (2006). *Morbidity and mortality in people with serious mental illness.* Alexandria, VA: NASMHPD

The news that people with serious mental illnesses die, on an average, more than two decades earlier than those among the general population in the United States shocked even those who had known for years of the poor health and health care of persons with mental illness and of the gaps in coordination between mental health and primary care. That part of the increased risk for morbidity and mortality among this population is due to "second-generation" antipsychotics, which replaced first-generation drugs because they produced fewer neurologic side effects but are associated with other health risks such weight gain and diabetes, is a sobering finding regarding the potential for pharmaceutical fixes to mental illness and their facilitation of "a life in the community." Like a 1999 Institute of Medicine report, *To Err Is Human,* on medical error in U.S. hospitals, the 2006 report of the National Association of State Mental Health Program Directors reports on research that was published elsewhere, but the organization's visibility and resulting capacity to publicize its work in the home states of its members contributed to making the theme of early mortality perhaps the most widely discussed topic in public mental health of the past several years. Time will tell the degree to which these findings prod public health efforts to address morbidity and mortality among people with mental illnesses who also carry the health risks of poverty, lack of access to health care in general, and others, or end in another instance of, in Sue Estroff's term, "medicalizing the margins" of people whose mental illness is embedded in their poverty and social exclusion from mainstream life. The excerpt here is the Executive Summary of the NASHMPD report.

I. Foreword

It has been known for several years that persons with serious mental illness die younger than the general population. However, recent evidence reveals that the rate of serious morbidity (illness) and mortality (death) in this population has accelerated. *In fact, persons with serious mental illness (SMI) are now dying 25 years earlier than the general population.*

Their increased morbidity and mortality are largely due to treatable medical conditions that are caused by modifiable risk factors such as smoking, obesity, substance abuse, and inadequate access to medical care.

This report reviews the causes of excess morbidity and mortality in this population and makes recommendations to improve their care. It presents a roadmap for strategic approaches to reduce excess illness and premature death among the persons served by State Mental Health Authorities.

State Mental Health Authority (SMHA) stakeholders need to embrace two guiding principles:

1. Overall health is essential to mental health.
2. Recovery includes <u>*wellness.*</u>

This is the thirteenth technical report developed by the National Association of State Mental Health Program Directors (NASMHPD) Medical Directors Council. It is based on a relevant literature review, a series of work-group conference calls, and a two-day meeting of medical directors, commissioners, researchers, and other technical experts. This report provides the overarching context for two previous reports, *Polypharmacy* and *Integrating Primary Care with Behavioral Health* and our forthcoming report on *Smoking Policies and Practices.* We must all work together to fight this epidemic of premature death and its contributing causes.

Joe Parks, MD
Chair, Medical Directors Council

II. Executive Summary

A. Overview—The Problem

People with serious mental illness (SMI) die, on average, 25 years earlier than the general population. State studies document recent increases in death rates over those previously reported. This is a serious public health problem for the people served by our state mental health systems. While suicide and injury account for about 30–40% of excess mortality, *60% of premature deaths in persons with schizophrenia are due to medical conditions such as cardiovascular, pulmonary and infectious diseases.*

People with serious mental illness also suffer from a high prevalence of modifiable risk factors, in particular obesity and tobacco use. Compounding this problem, people with serious mental illness have poorer access to established monitoring and treatment guidelines for physical health conditions.

B. Increased Mortality and Morbidity are Largely Due to Preventable Conditions

Among persons with SMI, the "natural causes" of death include:

Cardiovascular Disease (CVD) Risk Factors

Modifiable Risk Factors	Estimated Prevalence and Relative Risk (RR)	
	Schizophrenia	*Bipolar Disorder*
Obesity	45–55%, 1.5–2X RR[1]	26%[5]
Smoking	50–80% 2–3X RR[2]	55%[6]
Diabetes	10–14% 2X RR[3]	10%[7]
Hypertension	> 18%[4]	15%[8]
Dyslipidemia	Upto 5X RR[4]	

1. Davidson S, et al. *Aust N Z J Psychiatry.* 2001;35:196–202. 2. Allison DB, et al. *J Clin Psychiatry.* 1999; 60:215–220. 3. Dixon L, et al. *J Nerv Ment Dis.* 1999;187:496–502. 4. Herran A, et al. *Schizophr Res.* 2000;41:373–381. 5. MeElroy SL, et al. *J Clin Psychiatry.* 2002;63:207–213. 6. Ucok A, et al. Psychiatry Clin Neurosci. 2004;58:434–437. 7. Cassidy F, et al. *Am J Psychiatry.* 1999;156:1417–1420. 8. Allebeck. Schizophr Bull. 1999;15(1)81–89

- Cardiovascular disease
- Diabetes (including related conditions such as kidney failure)
- Respiratory disease (including pneumonia, influenza)
- Infectious disease (including HIV/AIDS)

The rates of mortality from these diseases for the SMI population are several times those of the general population.

There are a number of other factors that place people with SMI at higher risk of morbidity and mortality, including:

- **Higher rates of modifiable risk factors**
  - Smoking
  - Alcohol consumption
  - Poor nutrition/obesity
  - Lack of exercise
  - "Unsafe" sexual behavior
  - IV drug use
  - Residence in group care facilities and homeless shelters (exposure to tuberculosis and other infectious diseases as well as less opportunity to modify individual nutritional practices)

- **Vulnerability due to higher rates of**
  - Homelessness
  - Victimization/trauma
  - Unemployment
  - Poverty
  - Incarceration
  - Social isolation

- **Impact of symptoms associated with SMI**
  - Example: paranoid ideation causing fear of accessing care
  - Example: disorganized thinking causing difficulty in following medical recommendations
- *Symptoms can mask symptoms of medical/somatic illnesses*
- *Psychotropic medications may mask symptoms of medical illness and contribute to symptoms of medical illness and cause metabolic syndrome*
- *Polypharmacy*
- *Lack of access to appropriate health care and lack of coordination between mental health and general health care providers*

C. The Impact of Medications

Modifiable Risk Factors Affected by Psychotropics
Overweight/obesity
Insulin resistance
Diabetes/hyperglycemia
Dyslipidemia

Beginning with the introduction of clozapine in 1991, and the subsequent introduction of five newer generation antipsychotics over the next decade or so, antipsychotic prescribing in the US has moved to the use of these second generation antipsychotics. This has occurred despite their significantly greater cost, largely due to a decrease in neurologic side effects and the perception that people using them may experience better outcomes, especially improvement in negative symptoms. However, with time and experience *the second generation antipsychotic medications have become more highly associated with weight gain, diabetes, dyslipidemia, insulin resistance and the metabolic syndrome* and the superiority of clinical response (except for clozapine) has been questioned. Other psychotropic medications that are associated with weight gain may also be of concern.

D. Access to Health Care

Druss[ii] suggests that having SMI may be a risk factor and lead to problems in access to health care because of:

- Patient factors: Amotivation, fearfulness, social instability
- Provider factors: Competing demands, stigma
- System factors: Fragmentation

He also provides us with examples from his research and that of colleagues regarding Overuse, Underuse, and Misuse *(Three Types of Poor Quality,* Chassin 1998) of services related to the population with SMI:

Overuse

- Persons with SMI have high use of somatic emergency services (Salisberry et al 2005, Hackman et al 2006)

Underuse

- Fewer routine preventive services (Druss 2002)
- Lower rates of cardiovascular procedures (Druss 2000)
- Worse diabetes care (Desai 2002, Frayne 2006)

Misuse

- During medical hospitalization, persons with Schizophrenia are about twice as likely to have infections due to medical care postoperative deep venous thrombosis and postoperative sepsis (Daumit 2006)

E. What Should Be Done? Recommendations and Solutions

These proposed recommendations and solutions are organized at four levels of action: national; state; provider agencies and clinicians; and, persons served, families and their communities. We have identified several major actions necessary to address the issues described in this report.

1. *Prioritization of the public health problem of morbidity and mortality and designation of the population with SMI as a priority health disparities population.*
2. *Tracking and monitoring of morbidity and mortality in populations served by our public mental health systems (surveillance).*
3. *Implementation of established standards of care for prevention, screening, assessment, and treatment.*
4. *Improved access and integration with physical health care services.*

National Level

1. Designate the Population with SMI as a Health Disparities Population

a. Federal designation of people with SMI as a distinct at-risk health disparities population is a key first step, followed by development and adaptation of materials and methods for prevention in this population as well as inclusion in morbidity and mortality surveillance demographics.

2. Adopt Ongoing Surveillance Methods

a. Establish a committee at the federal level to recommend changes to national surveillance activities that will incorporate information about health status in the population with SMI.

b. Engage at the national and state levels, per the IOM report, in developing the National Health Information Infrastructure (NHII) to assure that EHR and PHR templates include the data elements needed to manage and coordinate general health care and mental health care.

3. Support Education and Advocacy

a. Share information widely about physical health risks in persons with SMI to encourage awareness and advocacy. Educate the health care community. Encourage persons served and family members to advocate for wellness approaches as part of recovery.

b. Build on the development of SAMHSA evidence-based practices by creating a toolkit that is focused on health status and healthy lifestyles.

c. Promote adoption of recommendations in the NASMHPD Technical Reports on Polypharmacy and Smoking to implement policies and programs addressing these risk factors.

State Level

1. Prioritize the Public Health Problem of Morbidity And Mortality and Designate the Population with SMI as a Priority Health Disparities Population.

a. Collect surveillance data on morbidity and mortality in the population with SMI.

b. Apply a public health approach and population based interventions.

2. Improve Access to Physical Health Care

a. Require, regulate, and lead the public behavioral health care system to ensure prevention, screening, and treatment of general health care issues.

b. Build adequate capacity to serve the physical health care needs of the SMI population.

3. Promote Coordinated and Integrated Mental Health and Physical Health Care for Persons with SMI

a. Utilize the system transformation recommendations from the New Freedom Commission, Institute of Medicine and SAMHSA to achieve a more person-centered mental health system. Specifically, implement the following selected recommendations, as identified in the IOM report, and modified to address the morbidity and mortality issues.

- *Create high-level mechanisms to improve collaboration and coordination across agencies*
- *Promote integration of general healthcare and mental health records*
- *Revise laws and other policies to support communication between providers*

b. Implement the recommendations found in the 11th NASMHPD Technical Paper: Integrating Behavioral Health and Primary Care Services.

4. Support Education and Advocacy
a. Develop and implement toolkits and guidelines to help providers, self-help/peer support groups and families understand how to facilitate healthy choices while promoting personal responsibility.
b. Establish training capacity. A key component of this plan will be training and technical assistance for the mental health workforce on the importance of the issues.
c. Involve academic and association partners in planning and conducting training.
d. Address stigma/discrimination.

5. Address Funding
a. Assure financing methods for service improvements. Include reimbursement for coordination activities, case management, transportation and other supports to ensure access to physical health care services.
b. As a health care purchaser, Medicaid should:

- *Provide coverage for health education and prevention services (primary prevention) that will reduce or slow the impact of disease for people with SMI.*
- *Establish rates adequate to assure access to primary care by persons with SMI.*
- *Cover smoking cessation and weight reduction treatments.*
- *Use community case management to improve engagement with and access to preventive and primary care.*

6. Develop a Quality Improvement (QI) Process that Supports Increased Access to Physical Health care and Ensures Appropriate Prevention, Screening and Treatment Services.
a. Establish a system goal for quality health care with the same priority as employment, housing or keeping people out of the criminal justice system.
b. Join with the Medicaid and Public Health agencies at the state level to develop a quality improvement (QI) plan to support appropriate screening, treatment and access to health care for people being served by the public mental health system, whether Medicaid or uninsured.
c. Assure that all initiatives to address morbidity and mortality have concrete goals, timeframes and specific steps. Gather performance measurement data and use to manage overall system performance.
d. Use regulatory, policy and other programming opportunities to promote personal responsibility for making healthy choices by changing the locus of control from external (program rules, regulations, staff) to the individuals we serve (self-control and management).
e. Continue to promote adoption of recommendations in the NASMHPD Technical Reports on Polypharmacy and Smoking to implement policies and programs addressing these risk factors.

Provider Agencies/Clinicians

1. Adopt as Policy that Mental Health and Physical Healthcare Should Be Integrated.
2. Help Individuals to Understand the Hopeful Message of Recovery, Enabling their Engagement as Equal Partners in Care and Treatment.

3. Support Wellness and Empowerment of Persons Served, to Improve Mental and Physical Well-Being

a. Support personal empowerment and individual responsibility, enabling individuals to make healthy choices for recovery to promote their individual recovery efforts; this means engaging people with SMI in their health care in new ways.

4. Ensure the Provision of Quality, Evidence-Based Physical and Mental Health Care by Provider Agencies and Clinicians.

a. Utilize the system transformation recommendations from the New Freedom Commission, Institute of Medicine and SAMHSA to achieve a more person-centered mental health system.

b. Implement standards of care for prevention, screening and treatment in the context of better access to health care.

c. Improve comprehensive health care evaluations.

d. Assure that all initiatives to address morbidity and mortality have concrete goals, timeframes and specific steps. Gather performance measurement data and use to manage overall system performance.

5. Implement Care Coordination Models.

a. Assure that there is a specific practitioner in the MH system who is identified as the responsible party for each person's medical health care needs being addressed and who assures coordination all services.

Persons Served/Families/Communities

1. Encourage the Persons We Serve, Families and Communities to Develop a Vision of Integrated Care.

a. Share information so that the mental health community and others become more aware of the co-morbid physical health risks and integrated care approaches.

2. Encourage Advocacy, Education and Successful Partnerships to Achieve Integrated Physical and Behavioral Health Care.

a. Encourage integrated physical and behavioral health care as a high priority similar to employment, housing and staying out of the criminal justice system.

3. Pursue Individualized Person Centered Care that is Recovery and Wellness Focused.

a. Support individualized partnerships, between the person served and the care provider, for integrated behavioral and physical health care.

First Person and Literary Classics

First Person and Literary
Classics

37

McDiarmid, J. S. (2005).
Scrambled eggs for brains.
Psychiatric Services, 56 (1), 34

This one was a find, recent as it is. With a title like "Scrambled eggs for brains" under the "Personal Accounts" section of the journal *Psychiatric Services*, one might guess at any number of tones that Joy S. McDiarmid's essay was likely to adopt or reflect. Dark humor, self-pity, outrage, a Yankee Doodle–like owning of the stigmatized label as a response to those who paste it on the so-labeled person, are a few. None of these qualities apply, quite, to this piece or prepare the reader for the richness of life and language the author manages to achieve in the space of a few hundred words. But enough said. Let the author speak for herself of her life, her experience of mental illness, and the electroconvulsive treatment—"a stupefying zap, a brain fry, an invasion at the core of my being" [p. 34]—that she received in the 1960s and writes of 40 years later.

Scrambled Eggs for Brains

I am 63 years old and have never married. I have lived alone, except for the 13 years I lived with a business partner and the past six years, when I have lived with a companion-caregiver. She, by happenstance, is the daughter of my first psychiatrist.

I graduated from a girls' school and went directly to university, destined to take undergraduate studies to enter medicine. That was not to be—I couldn't handle "the stress," but I did graduate with a bachelor of arts in psychiatry and English. Then I took the traditional trip to Europe while contemplating postgraduate studies.

The year was shortened as a result of my having to see a psychiatrist in London. The psychiatrist suggested I fly home and gave me pills to do so. Thus began what I refer to as my "stolen years"—a ten-year gap in my life during which I had three years of electroconvulsive therapy (ECT) followed by seven years of recovery, rediscovery, and thoughts about "what to do" next.

This was the decade during which my friends fell in love, married, had babies, and went to graduate school, while I sat in a room (either in hospital or out) staring through a window—if there was one!—at nothing, a blank slate for life. You could say, "Oh, she's just feeling sorry for herself." And you'd be right. However, I think a dash of self-pity is normal—in the end, it is a fine motivator to get off one's butt.

For me, ECT in the 1960s was a stupefying zap, a brain fry, an invasion of the core of my being, the personal center of my universe. And I never said, "You have my permission to take this from me." I hasten to add that I am not alone in that thought. I do understand that those who administered the procedure, who performed ECT research in the early 1960s, were caught between a rock and a hard place. Sometimes ECT was all that could be offered to a patient like me, because drug therapy was in its infancy—and the medications available had failed. For me, however, ECT was a barbaric abuse of a human being.

The Process

In the waiting room, I sit in terror. I wear a hideous striped blue dressing gown that covers only parts of my body. New slippers, though. Who gave me those? No hood to hide behind. I feel as though I'm on my way to the executioner. My body stinks of the familiar nervous sweat I used to love in my locker room days. Other people, dressed the same as I, are all around, waiting for the same event, the only thing we have in common.

I do not look, and neither do they. We are soldiers in a camp, each person selfishly protecting his or her small space of being: a very old and torn vinyl chair. I sneak a peek. Across the room, an older lady. Around the room, people older than I, more women than men. All keep their heads bowed. Me too. I am ashamed. I hate being here. I am so scared. My heart races. I can't hold my knees together in a ladylike way, as I was taught. Who cares? This is definitely not a tea party! I was not invited here: I did not come willingly. I am a captive in a locked ward who trudged down to the bowels of this freaky cold hospital in lockstep with the others, shepherded by a nurse who had a silly old-style white cap on her head and a man in white who looked big and strong and who kept us marching.

I follow the others, who also look glassy eyed and terrified. I don't belong here, I scream inside. What did I do? Why am I here?

I don't know what is to happen to me; I haven't been told a thing. How long will I be gone in that room across the hall? What happens afterward and, worse still, where will I be taken? No one is here to protect and love me, to be with me. I don't understand why anyone would make me do this.

My name is called. Obediently I rise and follow the nurse. My head starts spinning. I don't want to see the equipment; I call it the black box (although it is in fact brown), because it is dark and evil.

I see the big, busy, uneven eyebrows of Dr. A, and his very dark, brown, beady eyes. I feel sick to my stomach, and I feel like I am either peeing or pooping myself. I don't care. I see the eyes of another doctor—Dr. A's son—who is seven years older than me. This is embarrassing. I climb on the table. People take hold of me. I can smell the room. I know an anesthetic is coming. I hate the mask. I hate white, especially men in white coats—doctors, and nurses too, for that matter. White means pain. My pulse races. The jelly that goes on my temples messes my hair, squiggles around. I feel the sodium pentothal injection prick the skin. I taste it, and then comes a weird shudder inside my head. I go into oblivion, sur-rendering the care of my brain, of myself, to strangers, people I do not trust.

I cannot tell you what they did to me, only what I learned in dribs and drabs much later in life. (Funny, I was never curious enough to ask.) I know that bilateral electrodes were placed on top of the jelly on my temples and that someone flipped a switch, after which my self-worth and memories of my early years (birth to the age of about 15 years) were gone, stolen in a flash of electricity. The first thing I remember in that recovery room was the taste of cotton batten.

I survived! No saliva. A metallic mouth. Nice nurse. Achy legs, neck. Weak. I had a froggy voice, so I couldn't even talk to myself. Soft words. Blotto. If I was living in a hospital, I'd wake up, sometime, in my bed near the window. I went to occupational therapy in a dungeon. All these people, fried like me, doing silly things. I was supposed to knit. Ha! The afghan grew, from a scarf into a jagged rug and then went to the junk heap, I guess.

Unending trooping to the ECT room. Feelings of horror, a zombie. One night a young man in white came to my room. He touched me in all the places one shouldn't. Then he climbed on top of me and mumbled something, as his hand went over my mouth—something like, "This should make you feel better." What was this? Another experiment? Couldn't be! I tell Dr. A, and he looks like he is going to explode. Did I do something wrong? I blot it from my mind. Already I have done so many bad things.

More treatments, more waiting for someone to come and say, "There, there, dear, it'll be over soon." But no one did. The nights were dark, shadows on the walls, people with big rings of jangly keys. But I never went anywhere. Just bed 2 on the psycho ward. Locked in, no one to talk to. Brusque nurses. Did I eat? I don't remember, except for medications, apple juice (which I hate to this day) and Coca-Cola (which I never drank again).

And then one day my father came and took me away, home. I kept looking out the win-dow, crying. What for? The terrible thing is, I had to go back to "that room." I "graduated" to outpatient, and one time I was with my aunt, waiting for the white coats in that room.

Who took me home afterward? Did someone pick up my aunt? Or did we go by cab? When did it all end? The spring of 1963, I think.

Reflections on Ect

I had some 60—count 'em, 60—ECT treatments. I should say that I never felt like a victim of ECT. It was all that was available to "help." I know and accept that. "They knew not what they did." I refer to my parents. My mother's father was manic-depressive, his youngest daughter too. The other side of the family had mental illness. Fear gripped them all, and the best way to get rid of fear is to act, put us out of sight. I never did forgive my father for signing the consent form without telling me (asking me?) something—anything. Where were the explanations to help with my fear?

Obviously ECT stole years from me, leaving me with memory loss and gaps in my life. The experience of ECT is as clear to me right now and— pardon the pun—as electrifying as when it first happened in the dark during the winter of 1960. ECT leaves a searing imprint on my brain. The smells and disorientation. My memories of childhood come from a scrapbook I have that shows my mother's early life and a glimpse of mine—a dozen photos, maybe.

I also believe that ECT breeds and fuels self-absorption, even in a "normal" person. But for those with bipolar traits, it can get you into trouble. One cannot help but focus on self— and yet the real job is to turn that focus elsewhere. But who teaches one these "tricks" that can fill a toolkit of recovery and remotivation for a new life post-ECT? It's a revolting merry-go-round of learning, ECT, memory gaps, relearning, readjusting, and reengaging with life and friends but keeping your "secret." My stories stayed with me, and only recently have I divulged even smidgeons to two trusted friends. My stories and scary thoughts were owned by me alone for nearly 40 years.

I still doubt that adequate descriptions of the process and side effects are provided to ECT patients. But I urge health care professionals to fully explain the procedure, the feelings, the emotions, and the recovery of memory so that we have more informed patients and families, so there are fewer "surprises" that can affect a lifetime. Then there is less erasure of self. This is one outcome I missed.

My Years After Ect

In the years post-ECT, I did pull myself up by my bootstraps. I grabbed some grit, left Dr. A. and psychiatry behind. It was a brave new world for me. I got into graduate school on a scholarship, specializing in communications. I passed, got a career as a librarian, and then switched directions because I had a passion for writing. I craved the freedom of the no-rules life of the late 1960s.

As the decade changed to the 1970s and new psychotropic medications became available, my experiences could be characterized in one phrase: some good days, some bad days, but it was all that could be done. I passed through a very ugly time when my parents died, my mother of tongue cancer and my father of lung cancer, followed by the death of my beautiful grandmother shortly thereafter. These serial deaths sent me down to the depths of utter despair, and I had a huge "break"—mania, depression, psychosis, obsessive-compulsive behavior, horrible hallucinations, dreadful delusions, identity crisis. Quite frankly, I was crazy, but I hid it—or thought I did. I traveled, worked, and freaked people out, until one night, in another city while on business, I admitted myself to emergency psychiatry and the staff called a new psychiatrist for me, one who coached me home on the aircraft and into whose office I walked the next morning. He told me, softly, gently, and firmly, that I had a dissociative disorder and that life would be difficult, for the rest of my life.

Never did I seriously consider suicide. I was desperate, yes. Disarrayed, cluttered, isolated, failing exhaustive drug therapy, avoiding interaction with friends, threatened by more mental illness. Every little aspect of my life was overwhelmingly failing. And, once again, I was not a traveler in life. Furthermore, I was financially broke.

For several months, my psychiatrist treated me with the older type of drugs, powerful ones. I sat and observed life as it went by, too stoned to know much of what was going on. Then, slowly, I began to sort out the puzzle, again, and pull myself up by my bootstraps, again. Life opened a crack and moments of joy flooded in, enough to convince me I had the energy for another "go" on the train.

Would I submit to ECT now if drug therapy failed me? Truthfully, I don't know. I'd likely try lithium first. God willing, I hope I can escape further ECT. But if I had to submit in order to get another chance to go on living, then I would need a mitt full of information to fully understand the current procedures, risks, and benefits of ECT. Once times 60 is enough.

38

Weiner, S. (2007). A Socialist youth: An adult needing the welfare state. *The Suspicious Humanist,* 2/10/07

Stephen Weiner attended Stanford University in the late 1960s and had a series of mental health problems that, as he says, have made him "an adult needing the welfare state." This need has not kept him from making a contribution to the welfare state he acknowledges the need for, and to his fellow citizens. Weiner is the self-publisher and lead writer of *The Suspicious Humanist: A Journal of the Arts & Opinion*, which he started years ago with his late father. In Weiner's essays, there is little talk of recovery and much talk of struggle and the devastating impact of mental illness in his life, yet his work could be said to represent one face of the recovery movement. He writes about current affairs, the Communist era and its very personal meaning to him growing up with parents who were socialists and sometime Communists, and his experience of mental illness. But, as with Ms. McDiarmid, let's have Mr. Weiner tell a little bit of his own story. This excerpt from *The Suspicious Humanist* touches on all the themes noted above.

A Socialist Youth; An Adult Needing the Welfare State

My parents, as I have often written in these spaces, were members of the Communist Party USA before and after I was born in 1951. So I grew up hearing about FBI agents coming to the door to harass them, and getting my father fired from several jobs. I am named after Steve Nelson, the commander of the Abraham Lincoln Brigade of mostly Communist volunteer soldiers in the Spanish Civil War against the fascist uprising against the legally-elected Republic led by General Francisco Franco, who was promptly aided by Hitler and Mussolini while American, Britain and France stupidly and shamefully remained neutral. As I wrote here a few months ago, my father was wounded in Spain and again in the South Pacific in World War Two. I grew up seeing my father's very visible wounds and feeling awe, love and gratitude towards him for risking his life to try, essentially, to prevent the Holocaust and the whole world war. As I also wrote, my mother, from a traditionally absolute pacifist long-time Quaker background, decided that Hitler could not be defeated nonviolently, and worked as one of a multitude of women in war industry, a "Rosie the Riveter."

I grew up as a good reader, loving it since the age of four, when my mother said I taught myself to read. That meant reading left-wing books my parents had, mostly published by the Communist-controlled International Publishers and the Communist magazine Masses and Mainstream. I read Steve Nelson's book about his sedition conviction under a Pennsylvania law in his home town of Pittsburgh, a conviction that I believe was later overturned by either the Pennsylvania or U.S. supreme courts because the law was a violation of free speech conditions. Not until many years later, when I was at least a teenager or maybe a young adult, did I learn that I was named after him. But here's the point: I was almost a classic "red diaper baby," the Left's term for us children of the Left, and I was heavily influenced by these books, which also included material on poverty in the U.S. and other capitalist countries. We, strangely enough, lived in Orinda, a heavily right-wing suburb of Berkeley, and the New Left was making a lot of news in Berkeley. My father hung out on weekends at the Cafe Mediterraneum on Telegraph Avenue in Berkeley, holding many adult conversations, and I was fascinated. I wanted to be a socialist, though not a communist, as soon as possible

Well, I've made it plain that I was exposed to Communist ideas; what I need to make clear also is that from a very early age I rejected Soviet and Chinese style communism. I did this partly because my father was breaking with it and constantly pointing out the atrocities of those governments, especially under Stalin (whom both my parents had previously supported) and because I was of course taught about the undemocratic, evil nature of Communism in public school, In addition, I followed the political news on my own from a very young age, and was horrified and disgusted by the Berlin Wall, which the

East Germans/Soviets built in August 1961, I believe, when I was nine years old. I hated school myself (I was labelled a "hyperactive underachiever") and felt so imprisoned by it that I related to all the East Germans who tried to get past the Wall and were shot to death by Communist police and soldiers. The Communists had turned an entire country into a prison.

So I could never be a Communist, but I was disgusted by the politics of the Right picked up by my friends and most of my fellow students from their parents. A great deal of it had to do with attacking welfare programs, particularly among black people in Oakland. Even from a fairly young age, it disgusted me that these children of privilege,—we all were living in one of the most affluent towns in the Bay Area—would attack poor people so viciously. This brings me to the central theme of this article, my instinctive gut level support from the beginning for the welfare state, as it was frequently termed in Britain, the Scandinavian countries, and other places like New Zealand. I knew that individuals and families were frequently overwhelmed financially (mine was because my father had to leave his first career, soil science, due to what he told me later was sexual harassment by his male boss, and the businesses he started, like publishing calligraphy books, were financial failures), and I believed that governments had a right and duty to help them. My parents at some point left the Communist Party, but neither of them ever abandoned the liberal ideals of Franklin D. Roosevelt's New Deal.

So I entered my older childhood and my teens determined to be a democratic socialist, not a communist. All sorts of groups and tendencies had a presence in Berkeley. I started by giving the American Civil Liberties Union and the Congress of Racial Equality contributions when I was 11 years old. When I was 13, in the summer of 1965, I discovered *Liberation Magazine,* published in New York by the War Resisters League as I recall, and *Freedom,* an anarchist magazine published in London. But I really increased my involvement in the fall of 1965, when I was a high school freshman, and I heard that the prominent and now-legendary group Students for a Democratic Society was holding weekend meetings in Berkeley. My parents agreed to give me rides to and from the meetings (after all, wasn't I a red diaper baby and wasn't it therefore predictable I'd get involved with the New Left?), but they refused to let me formally join, fearing government harassment for my membership, the kind of harassment they had had to endure. So I didn't formally join then, which was ok with me because SDS was such a loose, almost anarchic organization that many people who were involved were not formal members. At that point, SDS was totally nonviolent, which was to change within three years. The quick march of SDS from the democratic Left to a violently pro-communist group impelled me, in 1968, to join the Socialist Party-Young Peoples Socialist League run by the followers of Max Shachtman, an older leader who had gone from orthodox communism in the 1920s to Trotskyism (followers of the Russian revolutionary Leon Trotsky who lost out in a power struggle with ultra-dictator Joseph Stalin for leadership of the Soviet Union and the world Communist movement) to democratic socialism, the belief in an egalitarian society with much state control of the economy but with democratic freedoms intact.

That's who I was politically as a young kid. I would have to face the Vietnam draft when I turned 18 in 1969, which made politics very personal to me, but I was also motivated by concern over poverty and racism. I never really challenged the need for government economic-assistance programs, though I read plenty of arguments against them by reading literature of the Right, like William F. Buckley's magazine *National Review.* I was always willing to listen to and read the conservative viewpoint, and I agreed with them mostly on the evils of Communism, but they never shook my faith in the need for the welfare state.

But now I must start to change the subject somewhat, for I need to write about the development of my lifelong diagnosed (many times) mental illness, which began on August 28,

1965 when I was 13 and has long since become the reason that I've accepted help from government programs and reached the point I am today, when I live mostly on Social Security Disability (SSDI) money, receive food stamps, and live in a HUD-subsidized apartment building for people with "serious and persistent mental illness." It is what turned my theoretical advocacy of the welfare state to a desperate need for it.

I am going, here, to need to discuss some of the mental issues, some of the things I felt and thought over many decades and in many ways, thoughts and feelings that, when I told them to psychiatrists and other mental health professionals, got me diagnosed with a variety of mental illnesses for the 42 years from 8/28/65 until now. Early on, in my early teens, some things occurred to me that were extremely distressing: I started worrying that I was "queer," homosexual, even though I'd had a long childhood history of having crushes on girls; I started worrying that some malevolent force was going to suddenly change me into a girl (I don't think that's because I was sexist and regarded female as inferior, I think it's because anyone of either sex would be horrified to suddenly have their sex switched on them without warning or their control) and I had to check continually that I was still a boy by putting a hand in my pocket and subtly checking my testicles; and worst of all, everything and everybody seemed literally, physically, ultimately unreal to me, which was intensely lonely because it meant I was the only sentient being in the universe, completely without companionship. A year or so later, I developed an intense fear of my mother's menstrual blood, and had the strong feeling/thought that if I saw any in the house, even a tiny drop, it would render the universe unreal (of course, a huge part of me already felt/thought the universe was unreal anyway, including my mother). I basically did not report these feelings to anyone, even psychiatrists I asked my parents to let me see, because I felt that by doing so I would be rendering the psychiatrist unreal. I was a tortured mess.

Over the months, years and decades different feeling/thoughts rose up out of me to keep me a tortured mess: I started fearing that I would cause an earthquake when I was with my father in the San Francisco Bay Area; I moved from Berkeley to Philadelphia where my mother lived to escape from the earthquake. Later, in Philadelphia, I developed a terror that I would hear on the news that there would be a huge California earthquake and that would be my fault, and also a signal to pick up nearby knives and stab my mother to death. At that point I became absolutely terrified and admitted myself to a mental hospital, with the aid of a good psychiatrist. I've had four psychiatric hospitalizations to date. All of them have involved my suicidality (my sister was a suicide and a bad but seductive example), or my fear that I've been inadvertently evil by murdering people in my sleep, or my continuing feelings/thoughts of derealization, of physical unreality.

What was I doing for work during all these decades, and why did I decide I was unable to work enough to support myself financially, not to mention my daughter, who is 34 now? Well, in high school, I finally learned how to get good grades, how to study, how not to disrupt class (fortunately, one's late high school grades are about all the colleges care about). I started high school in Orinda, but moved across the country in the middle of my sophomore year when my mother moved to Connecticut to escape my father's harassment after she divorced him. New England was a rude shock to me after an all-California childhood, I can tell you that. But, precisely because my family life was such a mess and, as I have said, I was a tortured mess inside, I threw myself into my studies for the first time and was no longer a "hyperactive underachiever." As a result, I was admitted to Carleton College in Minnesota, a very good liberal arts college but relatively unknown outside the Midwest. I chose the Midwest because it was in between my parents, and I had had to choose between them for my home before a judge in a custody battle instigated irresponsibly by my father. I was hypersensitive about choosing either the East Coast or the West Coast for that reason.

Also, Bob Dylan was from Minnesota and had dropped out of the University of Minnesota after a year. At that time, believe me, I wanted to be Bob Dylan.

What I did instead was go back to California, to Stanford University in Palo Alto 60 miles south of where my father then lived in Sausalito. He had finally become the bohemian poet he was always meant to be, and was organizing poetry readings and trying to sell his calligraphy books and calligraphy posters. He was interesting and loving, but I was wary of his weird moods and deep anxieties. The truth is, I became an excellent student in a way I was never an excellent worker in the decades to come. Nearly all my course work involved a lot of reading, and I liked nothing better than to read.

I also at that time had a girlfriend, D, whom I had originally met and been nonsexual friends with since high school. We got together on a camping trip in New Brunswick Canada when she initiated sexual contact with me in the tent we were sharing. Well, I was willing enough. But here came one of the biggest ongoing disasters of my life: sex, instead of making or helping me feel united with her or even close to her, made me feel even more alone in the universe. And we had a lot of sex, at least at the beginning before my torture during it led to my aversion to the whole thing and the total collapse of our marriage. By that time we had a baby daughter and by the time D and I divorced in 1974, I was very attached to her. But we were separated from each other when she was a little younger than three and D went to graduate school in Seattle and I moved to Philadelphia.

The truth is, that in conventional terms, I was never a success again, or even close. I applied for many jobs in journalism and publishing (I'd been first a religion major then a communication major and had idealized reporters since I was a little boy) and got hardly any of them. Most times I never got past the interview stage and many times not even that. I'm sure my inner agitation and disorganization showed up in the interviews. I did during those years work at a couple of interesting jobs, at the Solar Energy Research Institute, a federal laboratory in Golden Colorado (when I lived in Denver) where I wrote abstracts of scholarly articles on alternative energy but never believed the evidence of my own eyes that I had written the right words down, and thus did a very slow job, and another job when I moved back to California after Denver, at the private legal publishing firm Commerce Clearing House, where I abstracted occupational safety and health cases for lawyers' newsletters, but there I simply could not concentrate on the complex material and went on company disability and then state disability and then social security. I have not worked for pay since then, fall 1987. I knew I was, in their language, completely and permanently disabled.

All this time I was active in various democratic socialist groups, led by Michael Harrington, the left-wing intellectual who had written *The Other America,* about poverty, and had inspired Presidents Kennedy and Johnson to start their anti-poverty programs. Harrington had been/was a long-time Shachtmanite (Shachtman himself died in 1972, but not before inspiring future groups of both Marxists and neoconservatives). Harrington was my hero; I stayed in his faction of the old Socialist Party, which had splintered, mostly over Vietnam. I guess it should be obvious that my socialism made it even easier to make the decision to leave the regular workforce and live on disability.

Clinical and Systems Theory, Conceptual, and Historical Texts

39

Rosenheck, R. (2000). The delivery of mental health services in the 21st century: Bringing the community back in. *Community Mental Health Journal, 36* (1), 107–124

It does not take much first-era digging into the linked movements of deinstitutionalization and community psychiatry to find broad concerns with social justice and human and civil rights. Correspondingly, it takes little digging to find these values in today's recovery and community integration movements. In this article, Robert Rosenheck writes that the Community Mental Health Center movement of the 1960s and beyond failed to meet its goals even with strong public support, while today's goals of community-based care for persons with mental illness are threatened with failure due to the lack of that support. In the first case, public support for community-based care could not overcome lack of practitioner knowledge of, and orientation toward, community care. In the second case, lack of public support could undermine community-based care even with the advantages of a vastly improved knowledge base and effective treatments that have been developed over the past 40 years. Rosenheck argues that advocates and planners should eschew efforts to broaden the scope of public mental health care to incorporate social and community changes that, theoretically, could enhance the goal of community integration persons with mental illnesses. Instead, they should focus on providing the effective, but not inexpensive, community-based services they can offer now. They should also educate and persuade the public and legislators to support this narrower but critical agenda targeted to persons with the most serious mental illnesses, the group that has been least well served by mental health reform movements of the past. It will be interesting to take another look at this article a few years from now to see (or to see if we can see) how health care reform has responded to the issues Dr. Rosenheck addresses here.

The Delivery of Mental Health Services in the 21st Century: Bringing the Community Back In

ABSTRACT: The community mental health movement of the 1960s enjoyed widespread public support but poorly served its intended target population of seriously mentally ill individuals because: (1) its professional values and technology were, at least initially, not well-oriented toward serving people with severe mental illness; (2) organizational structures linking Community Mental Health Centers with State Mental Health Agencies, State Hospitals, and other relevant service agencies were lacking; (3) ideologically driven aspirations diverted energies and resources into diffuse goals related to the achievement of social justice; and (4) performance objectives were not operationally defined or monitored. Since that time professional technologies and organizational linkages have substantially improved, but there has been a loss of public support for safety net services for the least well off, in part due to a general ascendence of individualist market values, declining civic engagement and reduced support for specialized services for the disadvantaged. A new community mental health movement would be less oriented towards stimulating broad community change, and more narrowly focused on building support among decision makers and the public at large to expand the availability of costly but effective and improved services for people with severe and persistent mental illness.

Thirty years ago the community mental health movement was a source of direction and hope for an entire generation of mental health professionals. As we confront sharp budgets cuts and the growing influence of hard-edged industrial management styles, it is hard to remember the expansive days when the federal government was going to blanket the country with over 2,000 Community Mental Health Centers (CMHCs) to provide a comprehensive range of services to all who needed them. Changes in our society and in the world over the past 30 years, along with new developments in the academic fields of political science and sociology, make this an auspicious moment to review the relationship between mental health service delivery and the community in which it is embedded.

Community mental health is no longer at the center of mainstream psychiatric circles these days, but elsewhere in our society major questions are being raised about the loss of community, the growing dominance of an amoral market-oriented culture, the widespread loss of faith in established institutions, and the need to reassert collective values and expectations. This national dialogue, from which our field has been largely absent, is likely to be of importance for the continued development of mental health service systems in the future, especially those for the least well off. We need to get our bearings in this new framework.

506

A Glance Backward

The community mental health movement of the 1950s and 1960s was a creature of its time. At its base were: (1) the social optimism of the years following victory in World War II; (2) the faith that scientific medicine, including psychiatry, had immense potential to improve our lives; and (3) the expectation that the federal government would play an important role in bringing the benefits of psychiatric treatment to the public (Grob, 1991; Rochfort, 1993).

Implementation: From Idea to Practice

The fight against mental illness would not, however, have a D-day-like triumph, because reality would not live up to ambitious aspirations that were based more on theory than on data. Five factors may help account for this missed success.

Professional Disinterest

First, although promoted to the Congress as a necessity for the humane treatment of the institutionalized mentally ill, one of the major and by now, well-known, failings of the CMHC movement, was that the treatment and care of severely disabled patients received limited emphasis (Grob, 1991; Chu and Trotter, 1972). It would be years before the basic needs of severely mentally ill people—needs for practical assistance in housing, income supports and structured activities—featured prominently on the radar screens of mainstream mental health professionals (Goldman and Morrissey, 1985).

Disconnection from State Agencies

Second, in addition to the mismatch of professional interest and the core obligation to the least well off, only weak organizational ties linked CMHCs to state mental hospitals, where most severely mentally ill patients still remained. State mental health agencies were only peripherally involved in CMHC planning, and the federal government provided CMHC funds directly to local agencies (Grob, 1991).

Social Activism

Third, by the time the centers actually began operation, in the mid- to late 1960s, the civil rights movement had captured the imagination of much of liberal America and many in the mental health field began to see in Community Mental Health, an opportunity to contribute to a movement of historic importance.

Lack of Accountability

Fourth, although evaluation was identified as one of the core tasks of the CMHCs, operational goals were rarely articulated and accountability was minimal. Oversight of the program within the federal government was assigned to the NIMH, but that agency lacked experience providing administrative oversight at the national level and had no capacity to evaluate the performance of hundreds of programs across the country.

In spite of these important shortcomings, crucial foundations were laid during this period and much good was accomplished. The establishment of institutions devoted to providing mental health services in urban population centers was a major accomplishment in itself, and a necessary prerequisite for any further developments.

Corrective Refocusing and Maturation

During the later 1970s and 1980s, the CMHCs, like institutions in many other sectors of society, became less focused on ideology and more committed to measurable performance. As goals narrowed, many of the impediments described above were identified and corrected, and others faded with time.

For better and for worse, the idealism associated with community mental health ideology ran its course and dissipated with the urban riots of the late 1960s and the furor over the war in Vietnam and Watergate (Nye and Zelikow, 1997). By the mid 1970s the failure of CMHCs to address the needs of their primary target population had been highlighted (Chu and Trotter, 1974) and corrective efforts were initiated. New professional models of community support were developed and tested (Turner and TenHoor, 1978; Stein and Test, 1980), and efforts to encourage their dissemination were initiated.

In the 1980s, the Reagan Administration converted federal funding for mental health to a block grant program and responsibility for the CMHCs devolved from the Federal Government back to the states. As a result CMHCs were organizationally integrated with the same State Mental Health agencies that were responsible for the State Hospitals (Rochfort, 1993; Hogan, 1996; Goldman, Morrissey, Ridgely, Frank, Newman, and Kennedy, 1992). As the mission of the CMHCs became more clearly focused on care of the severely mentally ill, that target population was operationally defined and given explicit priority. Accountability increased, although systematic assessment of performance and outcomes have yet to be implemented on a large scale.

Community psychiatry thus matured from its beginnings as a relatively untested ideological vision to become a mature professional sub-specialty with clear goals, specific treatment technologies, and potentially measurable outcomes. Conventional biomedical approaches to diagnosis, pharmacotherapeutic treatment, and psychosocial rehabilitation were shown to be effective. Improved systems of service delivery were tested (Goldman et al., 1992) and public policy initiatives were proposed, and in many cases successfully promoted, to address needs for housing, income support, and employment.

Consumer movements also emerged that involved both families of people with severe mental illness and "consumer-survivors" themselves (Lefley, 1996). While 8 of 11 (72%) national mental health professional groups were founded before 1960 (Rickards, 1992), 8 of 9 (89%) public interest advocacy groups focusing on mental health were established after 1960, and 4 (55%) were established after 1980 (Havel, 1992). These organizations became important advocates for expanded and improved services and spurred development of empowering self-help programs and consumer operated services. Unfortunately, in spite of efforts at coalition building (Ross, 1992), these groups have not been mutually supportive of one another and, in the extreme, some consumer groups, deny the existence of mental illness altogether, regarding both diagnosis and treatment as advocated by professionals and family organizations, as oppressive. Thus while the movement of mental health treatment from closed state-run institutions to communities stimulated the development of grass roots advocacy groups, divisive ideological differences emerged that weakened their effectiveness (Ross, 1992).

Resources for Mental Health Services

The impact of new technologies and skilled management approaches is ultimately limited by the availability of resources to support them. At first glance resources for mental health services seem to have expanded during these years. From 1972 to 1992 staffing of mental health organizations increased by 56%; expenditures increased by 353%; and outpatient admissions

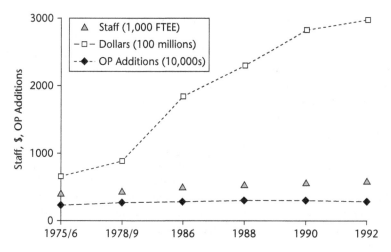

Figure 39.1 Mental Health Service Resources: 1969/72–1992

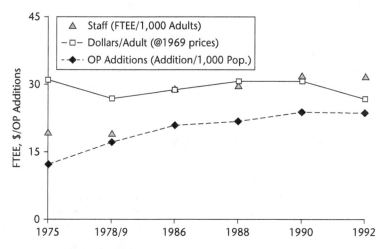

Figure 39.2 Mental Health Resources, 1969/72–1992: Adjusted for Inflation and Adult Population

increased by 26%—suggesting substantial improvement in both resources and access to care (Figure 39.1) (Redick et al., 1996). However, inflation increased medical prices during these years and thus reduced the actual value of health care dollars by 300%, while the adult population of the nation grew by 44%, increasing the aggregate demand for services (US Department of Commerce, 1996). When one takes these changes into account, inflation adjusted mental health expenditures per adult per year actually *declined* slightly—by 12.5% overall, or 0.5% per year—from 1969–1992, as did new outpatient mental health additions per adult in the general population—by 2.8% overall or 0.05% per year (Figure 39.2). Thus resources for mental health declined or, at best, remained roughly constant through this 20-year period.

Changing Needs and Deteriorating Communities

The adequacy of health resources must be judged in relationship to the need for those services. During the 1980s this need was anything but stable. With the decline in the availability of public hospital beds and shortened lengths of stay, sicker and sicker patients were placed in the community. The growing epidemic of drug and alcohol addiction created havoc in the lives of increasing numbers of people with serious mental illness, people who were far more exposed to such hazards as hospital use declined (Drake and Wallach, 1989). Data from the VA system, for example, show that during the 1980s the proportion of dually diagnosed inpatients doubled from 20% to 40% (Rosenheck, Massari, Astrachan and Suchinsky, 1991).

In the early 1980s, large numbers of homeless people began to appear in public spaces in urban centers—many of the most visible displaying manifest symptoms of severe mental illness. Commentators initially suggested that the rise in homelessness was attributable to the closing of state hospitals, the weakening of civil commitment laws, and the general failure of the community mental health movement. Additional research, however, pointed more clearly to broad structural changes in American society that adversely affected many low income people, especially those with special disadvantages such as severe mental illness (Burt, 1992).

The ready availability of crack cocaine, distinguished by its especially low cost, in major cities after 1985 also contributed directly to homelessness and to the deterioration of urban communities, bringing additional crime, gang warfare and social breakdown (Jencks, 1994). Ironically the urban ghettos of the 1950s and 1960s that were targeted for intervention by early community mental health practitioners, were described by observers of the urban world of 1980s and 1990s as relatively benign environments—wholesome communities in which poverty could be harsh, but in which positive community institutions maintained an intact fabric of social life (Wilson, 1987, 1996; Massey and Denton; 1993).

Thus, while resources remained constant or declined, needs increased.

A "Mean Season" for the Least Well Off

The generous if naive liberalism of the 1960s was also supplanted by a skepticism about services for the poor and disabled. Conservative critics maintained that welfare made the poor worse off by sapping their incentives to work (Murray, 1984) and both professionals (Satel, 1994; Shaner, Eckman, Roberts, Wilkins, Tucker, Tsuang, and Mintz, 1995) and journalists (Haner and O'Donnel, 1995) suggested that many people on disability programs like SSI were using their benefits to support their addiction to alcohol and drugs. Even though mental health resources, as we have seen, were held nearly constant relative to population and inflation, massive cuts occurred in general social welfare programs such as the Social Services Block grant (Title XX of the Social Security Act) (Smith and Lipsky, 1993); Supplemental Security Income (SSI); and Aid to Families with Dependent Children (Bane, 1988). These reductions added strain to the disabled mentally ill and on the low income communities in which they lived (Wolch and Dear, 1987).

Privatization and Managed Care

After the defeat of President Clinton's 1993 proposal for a comprehensive national health care system, privatization of health care accelerated and various forms of managed care, diverse payors' cost-saving initiatives, swept the country and proved to be effective at reducing service utilization and cost. Mental health services have been especially affected by this development. Resource reductions of 30%–40% have been observed in association with the advent of managed care in several settings (Ma and McGuire, 1998; Goldman, McCulloch and Sturm, 1998;

Rosenheck, Druss, Stolar, Leslie and Sledge, under review; Leslie and Rosenheck, in press) and have been shown to affect severely mentally ill people no less than those with milder disorders. Evidence of adverse clinical impacts has also been observed in some studies (Popkin, Lurie, Manning, Harman, Callies, Gray, and Christianson, 1998; Mechanic 1998).

It is, thus, ironic that as concepts and methods for fostering the community survival of people with severe mental illness became more focused and effective, other changes in society worked against realizing their potential benefit: (1) mental health resource levels stagnated; (2) the community and environmental circumstances in which seriously mentally ill people lived deteriorated; and (3) political support for addressing the needs of the poor and disabled weakened. The humanitarian idealism of the 1960s had successfully generated political support in an era of limited technical service capability. In contrast, by the far less generous 1990s, health care technologies and management strategies had improved and the aggregate need for services had increased sharply; but resources to support these improved services were in short and diminishing supply.

Cultural Impact of the Demise of Communism

In the late 1980s, the demise of the command and control economies of the Soviet block gave western societies, and especially the United States, a bloodless social, cultural, and economic triumph (Yergin and Stanislaw, 1998). The sweetness of the Western victory was attenuated, however, by uncertainty about what it was that actually had triumphed. In one view the triumph was attributed to the workings of market economies unfettered by intrusive government management. A second camp, however, pointed out that the truly unregulated markets of the type that had existed in America in the later 19th century had produced one of the great crises of American society in which monied interests almost superseded the democratic process. It had been government regulation, in this view, that had made free market economies compatible with democracy (Kuttner, 1997).

A third perspective, however, gave credit to neither pure markets nor regulating governments. This middle view accepted the role of both markets and governments in the coordination of modern economic and social life, but claimed that the crucial element in effective societies was something the reformers of Eastern Europe had celebrated as civil society—a space between private life and government in which citizens band together spontaneously and effectively for common purpose. In this third zone, in which neither market self-interest nor governmental authority predominated, larger personal aspirations for the good life and a fair society could hold sway.

In a seminal tract entitled *To Empower People,* Peter Berger and John Neuhaus (1977) argued that civil society is the key to the success of democratic society and is characterized by informal organizations, neither public nor private, that arise when people take issues into their own hands, making an active investment to influence both government and the electorate on the issues of the day.

In an influential empirical study of government reform in Italy during the 1970s, Robert Putnam showed that the same basic governmental reform had strikingly different impacts in different regions of the country. Using a combination of survey data and indices of government performance, Putnam showed that the crucial determinant of the effectiveness of government was the existence of strong civic culture—a local pattern of social activism characterized by: (1) high levels of interpersonal trust; (2) active participation in public and community affairs (as manifested by voting, reading the newspapers, and joining both political and recreational associations); and (3) mutual cooperation even in the context of competition (Putnam, 1993).

This new communitarianism, it has been suggested, with its focus on empowerment, civil society, and citizen participation, might offer a new path for linking citizens and government; for generating public support for the public good; and for providing critical input, oversight and support for public institutions (Dionne, 1998). Thus unlike the professional activism of the 1960s in which experts sought to lead or heal communities, the civic mobilization of the 1990s would seek to facilitate the shaping and pursuit of a common agenda by consumers, family, government and professional advocates, together.

Declining Civic Engagement in the US

When Robert Putnam turned his empirical lens from Italy to the United States he found evidence of steadily *declining* civic engagement from 1945 to 1990. Each year, fewer Americans voted and fewer were active in civic institutions from political parties to PTAs. The central symbol in his provocative study of social relationships in the US, entitled "Bowling Alone," was the fact that while Americans have been bowling more frequently in recent years, they are more likely to bowl alone rather than in groups or leagues (Putnam, 1995). Between 1965 and 1985 informal socializing declined by one quarter, and time devoted to clubs and organizations declined by half (Putnam, 1996). The core institutions of the civil society that won the cold war, it appeared, were in decline. Although still subject to debate, Putnam's thesis is strikingly consistent with a large body of data showing declining trust in government, in corporate leaders, in, doctors, and other societal authorities (Blendon, Benson, Morin, Altman, Brodie, Brossard and James, 1998).

Civic Culture and Health Care: Loss of Faith in Authority

For those of us in the health care world, it is notable that these studies collectively suggest that eroding confidence in physicians and negative attitudes towards managed care may not be specifically attributed to changes in the organization of health care service delivery. Since these changes occurred simultaneously with the development of more general negative attitudes toward societal authorities and institutions they may not be specific to health care institutions, at all. In 1993, even before the recent explosion in managed care, 83% of the public thought that waste, greed, and profiteering were the main reasons for high health care costs and confidence in medicine was at its lowest level in 27 years (Blendon et al., 1993). The major decline in confidence in medicine occurred between 1966 and 1982, long before the explosion in managed care (Blendon et al, 1998).

Civic Culture, Health and Mental Health

What implications, if any, does this emerging view of the crisis in American community life have for the delivery of mental health services? Five questions deserve consideration. (1) Does civic culture have any direct relationship to the epidemiology of mental illness? (2) Is a strong civic culture associated with the delivery of superior mental health services or with more integrated delivery of diverse of health care and social services to those with multiple complex needs? (3) Does the emergence of managed care reflect the decline in civic culture and the abandonment of yet another institution of community life to corporate dominance? (4) Does the mental health community have any role to play in restoring civic culture in American society? (5) What implications do new conceptualizations of community and society have for building coalitions to promote services for people with severe mental illness?

We have few answers to these questions at present. The main reason for raising them, at this stage, is to suggest a new research agenda for community mental health. However some data are available and are worthy of review.

(1) Does Civic Culture Have Any Direct Relationship to the Epidemiology of Mental Illness?

Direct evidence of the relationship of civic culture and mental health is extremely limited. Epidemiologic studies have suggested that higher mortality rates are found in association with lower levels of civic culture (Kawachi, Kennedy, Lochner, Prothrow-Stith, 1997) as well as with greater residential segregation on the basis of income (also presumed to be an indicator of low levels of civic unity) (Waitzman and Smith, 1998).

Of more direct relevance to mental health, the National Co-Morbidity Study (NCS), the only nationally representative study of mental illness ever undertaken, found that people living in rural areas, in which civic culture is stringer, have lower levels of psychiatric co-morbidity than those in urban areas (Kessler, McGonagle, Zhao, Nelson, Farmer Regier, 1994). In addition, the NCS clearly suggests that there has been a general increase in the prevalence of mental illness in recent years, a finding which also corresponds to the decline in civic culture in America, and which may reflect the impact of eroding social ties and deteriorating community life. Although little studied, civic culture is a potentially important factor in the epidemiology of mental illness and deserves further examination.

(2) Is a Strong Civic Culture Associated with Delivery of Superior Mental Health Services or with More Integrated Delivery of Diverse Health Care and Social Services to Those with Multiple Needs?

While Putnam found superior delivery of social services and greater satisfaction in regions of Italy with high levels of civic culture (Putnam, 1993), there have been virtually no published empirical studies of regional differences in the quality or effectiveness of mental health services in the US.

Several studies, however, have attempted to evaluate the relationship of service system integration, the degree of cooperativeness among agencies to outcomes of treatment for people with serious mental illness (Goldman et al., 1992). The largest and most recent of these is the Access to Community Care and Effective Services and Supports (ACCESS) program which is examining the relationship of service system integration, service delivery, and client outcomes among homeless people with mental illness at 18 sites in 9 states (Rosenheck, Morrissey, Lam, Calloway, Johnsen, Goldman, Calsyn, Teague, Randolph, Blasinsky, and Fontana, 1998). Recent analysis using measures of civic culture provided by Robert Putnam reveal significant relationships between civic culture, service system integration, service use, and housing outcomes (Rosenheck, Morrissey, Lam, Calloway, Stolar, Johnsen, Randolph, Blasinsky, and Goldman, under review). These data are the first to show a relationship between measures of civic culture and service system performance in the United States. The ACCESS program will ultimately evaluate the impact of strategies for improving service system integration, but the findings cited here, suggest considerable potential relevance of social integration to the performance of mental systems. They may also suggest that, if as Putnam and others indicate, social capital is declining in the US, establishing well functioning community-based service systems may be increasingly difficult.

(3) Does the Emergence of Managed Care Reflect the Decline in Civic Culture and the Abandonment of Yet Another Institution of Community Life to Corporate Dominance?

The future of mental health services under managed care is, at present, deeply uncertain, especially as it applies to services for people with severe mental illness. There is widespread concern among patients, their families, and providers, that economic incentives will impair service delivery to severely ill patients (Hall and Beinecke, 1998). Some studies of Medicaid managed care for the disabled mentally ill have shown modest savings with no evidence of adverse effect on outcomes (Hausman et al., 1998; Dickey et al., 1998). Others, however, have found deterioration in both service delivery and outcomes (Popkin et al., 1998). In Tennessee, to take an extreme case, the mismanagement of the program led to a serious and potentially enduring erosion of treatment capacity in the public mental health system (Chang et al., 1998).

Although corporate consolidation has dramatically reduced the number of managed behavioral health care companies and, presumably both increased the power of those that remain and reduced their investment in community health (Schlesinger and Gray, 1998b), professional and mental health advocacy groups have been critical of the narrow range of services they provide (Hall, Edgar and Flynn, 1997). The impact of these criticisms is, as yet, unclear and may ultimately represent a conflict of representative voluntary organizations, and immense corporations with little attachment to local communities. The presumed erosion of civic engagement in US communities would sharply reduce the possibility of mounting counter pressure to strengthen support for such services. Whatever the eventual outcome, the civic culture perspective throws important new light on the nature of challenge that lies ahead into sharp relief.

(4) Does the Mental Health Community Have any Role to Play in Restoring Civic Culture in American Society?

It is here that the new community psychiatry most diverges from that of the 1960s. Refocused on an important but specialized clinical mission, it is hard to find either mental health professionals or advocates who are arguing for the application of mental health technologies beyond the realm of alleviating the distress and dysfunction associated with psychiatric and substance abuse disorders. While strengthening social support and enhancing empowerment among individual clients has become an important theme in the treatment of individuals, mental health intervention at the level of entire communities seems to have been abandoned, and, most likely, appropriately so.

(5) What Implications Do New Conceptualizations of Community and Society Have for Building Coalitions to Promote Concern for the Mentally Ill?

We come, now to the last and most challenging of our five questions: how to support the empowerment of localities while assuring due attention to the needs of people with severe mental illness. If we take seriously the disaffection of the American public from an activist government—a disaffection whose persistence is revealed by the fact that every presidential candidate since Lyndon Johnson has campaigned against Washington and for community-centered government—we must allow issues of mental health policy and mental health service priorities to devolve to States and localities. Such a position, however, is perilous because advocates for small stigmatized minorities like the seriously mentally ill are generally unlikely to be able to marshal sufficient resources to influence policy at the local, or even state, level.

Theda Skocpol (1988) and others have suggested that a general principle in crafting social policy is that programs are most likely to receive sustained support if they offer benefits to both the least well off and better off or middle class, constituencies. In the community mental health movement of the 1960s and 1970s services to better off clients in many ways displaced priority from the least well off and diverted CMHCs from their primary tasks. Now that progress has been made in providing services to the severely mentally ill, it may be possible to expand the mission of community mental health providers to address the needs of a larger segment of the population without jeopardizing care of the least well off. The artificial divisions between services for people with psychiatric illness and for those with addictive disorders have been divisive and weakening in this respect. Given the importance of providing integrated services to those with both disorders, the dually diagnosed, such a division is both clinically inappropriate as well as politically ill-advised.

What is required, in effect, is a reversal of roles. In the old community mental health model, mental health professionals, authorities by virtue of their special technical expertise, operating in the tradition of progressive reformers, took on the role of social engineers. They aspired to address the problems of people with serious mental illness and the wider social pathologies of the communities in which they lived, with both legislators and community advisory boards supporting their efforts.

The public seems now to reject that model. No less respectful of technical expertise, the public expects health care professionals to demonstrate the value of the services they provide to primary consumers, clients and their families, and to join with them in advocating the case for services to the larger community. This remains a process of political advocacy rather than of market sales, but in either case it imposes new demands on professionals and implies a different position for them as partners with consumers and families in a joint effort to achieve public recognition and support.

Conclusion

The situation faced by community mental health advocates on the eve of the 21st century was thrown into sharp relief recently when the Mayor of New York announced a plan to eliminate methadone maintenance because the treatment itself fosters drug dependence, even though it is clearly effective in treating heroin addiction (Massing, 1998). The proposal was greeted with universal scorn by professional experts and researchers, but was only withdrawn, after sustained criticism in the media and presumably by the concerted efforts of community advocates.

The original community mental health movement, while short on output, received broad support because its approach was consonant with the values current during the long progressive era of federal expansion. The community mental health movement of the 21st century, in contrast, although armed with superior medical and managerial technologies, will operate in the context of federal devolution and the new localism. This context will impose greater challenges than previous eras, but holds the possibility of generating a renewed societal commitment to improving the welfare of people with severe mental illness.

References

Bane M.J. (1988). Politics & Policies of the Feminization of Poverty in Weir M., Orloff A.S. & Skocpol T. (Eds.) *The Politics of Social Policy in the United States.* Princeton, New Jersey: Princeton University Press.

Barber B.R. (1998). *A Place for Us: How to Make Society Civil and Democracy Strong.* New York, NY: Hill and Wang.

Berger P.L. & Neuhaus J. (1996). *To Empower People: From State to Civil Society.* Washington, DC. AEI Press.

Blendon R.J., Benson J.M., Morin R., Altman D., Brodie M., Brossard M. & James M. (1997). Changing Attitudes in America in Nye JS, Zelikow PD & King DC (Eds.) *Why People Don't Trust Government.* Cambridge, MA: Harvard University Press.

Blendon R.J., Hyams T.S. & Benson J.M. (1993). Bridging the gap between expert and public views on health care reform. *JAMA, 269*(19), 2573–2578.

Burt M.A. (1992). *Over the Edge: The Growth of Homelessness in the 1980s.* New York and Washington. The Russell Sage Foundation and the Urban Institute Press.

Chang C.F., Kiser L.J., Bailey J.E., Martins M., Gibson W.C., Schaberg K.A., Mirvis D.M. & Applegate W.B. (1998). Tenessee's failed managed care program for mental health and substance abuse services: JAMA, 279(11), 864–869.

Chu F.D. & Trotter S. (1974). *The Madness Establishment: Ralph Nader's Study Group Report on the NIMH.* New York, NY: Grossman.

Dear M. & Wolch J. (1987). *Landscapes of despair: From deinstitutionalization to homelessness.* Princeton, New Jersey: Princeton University Press.

Dickey B., Norton E., Norman S.L., Azeni H., Fisher W.H. (1998). Managed Mental Health Experience in Massachusetts in Mechanic D (Ed.) *Managed Behavioral Health Care: Current Realities and Future Potential.* San Francisco, CA: Jossey-Bass.

Dionne E.J. (1998). *Community Works: The Revival of Civil Society in America.* Washington, DC: Brookings.

Drake RE, Wallach MA. (1989). Substance abuse among the chronically mentally ill. *Hosp and Community Psychiatry 40,* 1041–1045.

Goldman H.H. & Morrissey J.P. (1985). The Alchemy of Mental health policy: Homelessness and the fourth cycle of reform. *American Journal of Public Health, 75,* 727—731,

Goldman H.H., Morrissey J.P., Ridgely M.S., Frank R.G., Newman S.J. & Kennedy C. (1992). Lessons from the Program on Chronic Mental Illness. *Health Affairs 11* (3), 51–68.

Goldman W., McCulloch J. & Sturm R. (1998). Costs and Use of Mental Health Services Before and After Managed Care. *Health Affairs, 17* (2), 40–52.

Grob G. (1991). *From Asylum to Community: Mental Health Policy in Modern America.* Princeton, NJ: Princeton University Press.

Hall L.L. & Beinecke R. (1998). Consumer and family views of managed care in Mechanic D (Ed.) *Managed Behavioral Health Care: Current Realities and Future Potential.* San Francisco, CA: Jossey-Bass.

Hall L.L., Edgar E.R. & Flynn L.M. (1997). *Stand and Deliver; Action Call to a Failing Industry. The NAMI Managed Care Report Card.* Arlington, VA: National Alliance for the Mentally Ill.

Haner J. & O'Donnell J.B. (1995). "America's Most Wanted Welfare Program," *Baltimore Sun,* January 23, p. 1.

Hausman J.W., Wallace N., Bloom J.R. (1998). Managed Mental Health Experience in Colorado in Mechanic D (Ed.) *Managed Behavioral Health Care: Current Realities and Future Potential.* San Francisco, CA: Jossey-Bass.

Havel J.T. (1992). Association and public interest groups as advocates. *Administration and Policy in Mental Health, 20*(1) 27–44.

Hogan M.F. (1996). State Mental Health Systems: Their Evolution and Use of Economic Tools in Moscarelli M, Rupp A, & Sartorius N. *Handbook of Mental Health Economics and Health Policy, Volume 1: Schizophrenia.* Chichester, UK: John Wiley & Sons (p. 515–524).

Jencks C. (1994). *The Homeless.* Cambridge, MA: Harvard University Press.

Kawachi I., Kennedy B.P., Lochner K., Prothrow-Stith D. (1997). Social Capital, Income Inequality and Mortality. *American Journal of Public Health, 87,* 1491–1498.

Kessler R.C., McGonagle K.A., Zhao S., Nelson C.B., Farmer M.E., Regier D.A. (1997). Lifetime and 12-month prevalence of DSM-III-R psychiatric disorders among persons aged 15–54 in the United States: Results from the National Co-Morbidity Study. *Archives of General Psychiatry, 51,* 8–19.

Koyonagi C & Goldman HH. (1991). The quite success of the national plan for the chronically mentally ill. *Psychiatric Services,* 42(9): 899–905.

Kuttner R. (1997). *Everything for Sale: The Virtues and Limits of Markets,* New York, NY: Knopf.

Lefley H. (1996). Impact of Consumer and Family Advocacy Movements on Mental Health Services in Levin B.L. & Petrila J. (Eds.) *Mental Health Services: A Public Health Perspective.* New York, NY: Oxford.

Leslie D.L. & Rosenheck R.A. (in press). Shifting from Inpatient to Outpatient Care? Mental Health Utilization and Costs in a Privately Insured Population. *American Journal of Psychiatry.*

Ma C. & McGuire T.G. (1998). Costs and incentives in a behavioral health care-out. *Health Affairs, 17* (2), 53–69.

Massey D.S. & Denton N.A. (1993). *American Apartheid: Segregation and the Making of the Underclass.* Cambridge, MA: Harvard University Press.

Massing M. (1998, September 6). Winning the Drug War Isn't So Hard After All. *New York Times Magazine.*

Mechanic D., Ed. (1998). *Managed Behavioral Health Care: Current Realities and Future Potential.* San Francisco, CA: Jossey-Bass.

Murray C. (1984). *Losing Ground: American Social Policy 1950–1980.* New York, NY: Basic Books.

Nye J.S., Zelikow P.D. (1997). Conclusion: Reflections, Conjectures, and Puzzles, in Nye JS, Zelikow PD & King DC, Eds. *Why People Don't Trust Government.* Cambridge, MA: Harvard University Press.

Orfield G. (1988). Race and the Liberal Agenda: The Loss of the Integrationist Dream, 1965–1974, in Weir M, Orloff A.S. & Skocpol T. (Eds.) *The Politics of Social Policy in the United States.* Princeton, New Jersey: Princeton University Press. Popkin M.K., Lurie N., Manning W., Harman J., Callies A., Gray D. & Christianson J. (1998). Changes in process of care for Medicaid patients with schizophrenia in Utah's prepaid mental health plan. *Psychiatric Services, 49(4),* 518–523.

Putnam R.D. (Winter, 1996). The Strange Disappearance of Civic America. *The American Prospect,* pp. 34–48.

Putnam R.D. (January, 1995). Bowling Alone: America's Declining Social Capital. *Journal of Democracy, 6,* 65–78.

Putnam R.D. (1993). *Making Democracy Work: Civic Traditions in Modern Italy,* Princeton, New Jersey: Princeton University Press.

Redick R.W., Witkin M.J., Atay J.E., & Manderscheid R.W. (1996). Highlights of Organized Mental Health Services in 1992 and Major National and State Trends, in Manderscheid R.W. & Sonnenschein M.A., *Mental Health, United States, 1996,* Rockville, MD, US Department of Health and Human Services.

Rickards L.D. (1992). Professional and organized provider associations. *Administration and Policy in Mental Health 1992; 20(1),* 11–25.

Rochfort D.A. (1993). *From Poorhouses to Homelessness.* Westport, CT: Auburn House.

R.A. Rosenheck, B. Druss, M. Stolar, D. Leslie & W. Sledge (under review). Effect of Declining Mental Health Service Use on Employees of a Large Self-Insured Private Corporation,

Rosenheck R.A., Massari L.M., Astrachan B.M. & Suchinsky R. (1991). Mentally Ill Chemical Abusers Discharged from VA Inpatient Treatment: 1976–1988. *Psychiatric Quarterly 61,* 237–249.

Rosenheck R. & Horvath T. (1998). Impact of VA Reorganization on Patterns of Mental Health Care. *Psychiatric Services, 49(1),* 56.

Rosenheck R.A., Morrissey J., Lam J., Calloway M., Johnsen M., Goldman H.H., Calsyn R., Teague G., Randolph F., Blasinsky M. & Fontana A. (1998). Service System Integration, Access to Services and Housing Outcomes in a Program for Homeless Persons with Severe Mental Illness. *American Journal of Public Health, 88(11),* 1610–1615.

Rosenheck R.A., Morrissey J., Lam J., Calloway M., Stolar M., Johnsen M., Randolph F., Blasinsky M., & Goldman H. (under review). Service Delivery and Community: Social Capital, Service Systems Integration, and Outcomes Among Homeless Persons with Severe Mental Illness.

Ross E.C. (1992). Success and failure of advocacy groups: A legislative perspective. *Administration and Policy in Mental health, 20(1),* 57–66.

Satel S. (1994). Hooked. It's time to get addicts off welfare, *New Republic, 210(4),* 18–20.

Schlesinger M. & Gray B. (1998). A Broader Vision for Managed Care, Part 1: Measuring the Benefit to communities. *Health Affairs, 17* (3), 152–168.

Skocpol T. The Limits of the New Deal System and the Roots of Contemporary Welfare Dilemmas in Weir M., Orloff A.S., Skocpol T., Eds. (1988). *The Politics of Social Policy in the United States.* Princeton, NJ: Princeton University Press.

Shaner A., Eckman T.A., Roberts L.J., Wilkins J.N., Tucker D.E., Tsuang J.W., Mintz J. (1995). Disability Income, Cocaine Use and Repeated Hospitalization Among Schizophrenic Cocaine Abusers. *New England Journal of Medicine,* 333(9), 777–783.

Smith S.R., & Lipsky M. (1993). *Nonprofits for Hire: The Welfare State in the Age of Contracting.* Cambridge, MA: Harvard University Press.

Stein L.I., Test M.A. (1980). Alternative to mental hospital treatment: I. Conceptual model, treatment program, and clinical evaluation. *Archives of General Psychiatry, 37,* 392–397.

Turner J.C. & TenHoor W.J. The NIMH Community Support Program: Pilot approaches to a needed social reform. *Schizophrenia Bulletin* 4(3), 319–349.

US Department of Commerce. (1996). *Statistical Abstracts of the United States 1996.* Washington, DC.

Waitzman N.J. & Smith K.R. (1998). Separate but lethal: The effects of economic segregation on mortality in metropolitan America. *The Milback Quarterly, 76*(3), 341–373.

Wilson W.J. (1987). *The truly disadvantaged: The inner city, the underclass, and public policy.* Chicago, IL: University of Chicago Press.

Wilson W.J. (1996). *When Work Disappears: The World of the New Urban Poor.* New York, NY: Knopf.

40

Thornicroft, G. & Tansella, M. (2004). Components of a modern mental health service: A pragmatic balance of community and hospital care. *British Journal of Psychiatry, 185, 283–290*

Graham Thornicroft and Michele Tansela, U.K. psychiatrists, return to an issue that many have thought resolved in modern community psychiatry—that of the proper balance between hospital- and community-based services. It may be that if recovery-based approaches to public mental health care carry the day, paradoxically psychiatric hospitalization, in the right circumstances and with the right coordination of care for transition back to the community, can be divested of some of its historical trappings as places of imprisonment and institutionalization, and provide the functions of emergency care, brief respite, and recuperation for episodes of acute psychiatric illness that are consistent with support for the self-determination of persons with mental illnesses. Thornicroft and Tansela propose a stepped model of care for countries and regions with low, medium, and high levels of resources. In low-resource regions, primary care will receive the lion's share of resources. Specialized mental health services and a wider range of acute inpatient and long-term outpatient clinical and residential services will come into play increasingly in higher-resource countries, but all areas should have a combination of inpatient and outpatient services. While the authors agree that there is no scientific evidence to support the sole use of hospital services, there is, they contend, no proof that community services alone can bear the weight of a comprehensive system of care, either. Their article is noteworthy for its "ideally realistic" or "realistically idealistic" approach to systemic mental health care: Starting from the reality of varied resource limitations or abundance in given countries or regions, what are appropriate standards of care for public mental health systems?

Components of a Modern Mental Health Service: A Pragmatic Balance of Community and Hospital Care

Background There is controversy about whether mental health services should be provided in community or hospital settings. There is no worldwide consensus on which mental health service models are appropriate in low-, medium- and high-resource areas.

Aims To provide an evidence base for this debate, and present a stepped care model.

Method Cochrane systematic reviews and other reviews were summarised.

Results The evidence supports a balanced approach, including both community and hospital services. Areas with low levels of resources may focus on improving primary care, with specialist back-up. Areas with medium resources may additionally provide out-patient clinics, community mental health teams (CMHTs), acute in-patient care, community residential care and forms of employment and occupation. High-resource areas may provide all the above, together with more specialised services such as specialised outpatient clinics and CMHTs, assertive community treatment teams, early intervention teams, alternatives to acute in-patient care, alternative types of community residential care and alternative occupation and rehabilitation.

Conclusions Both community and hospital services are necessary in all areas regardless of their level of resources, according to the additive and sequential stepped care model described here.

Declaration of interest None.

The public health impact of mental disorders is profound (Murray & Lopez, 1996; World Health Organization, 2001a). The estimated disability-adjusted life-years in 2000 attributable to mental disorders represents 11.6% of total disability in the world—more than double the level of disability caused by all forms of cancer (5.3%) and higher than the level of disability due to cardiovascular disease (10.3%).

Historically, the response of the mental health services can be seen in three periods: the rise of the asylum, the decline of the asylum and the reform of mental health services (Wing & Brown, 1970; Grob, 1991; Desjarlais *et al*, 1995; Thornicroft & Tansella, 1999). In the third period, community-based and hospital-based services commonly aim to provide treatment and care that are close to home, including acute hospital-care and long-term residential facilities in the community; respond to disabilities as well as to symptoms; are able to offer treatment and care specific to the diagnosis and needs of each individual; are consistent with international conventions on human rights; are related to the priorities of service users themselves; are coordinated between mental health professions and agencies;

and are mobile rather than static. We have described this as the 'balanced care' approach (Thornicroft & Tansella, 2002).

This paper summarises and extends a review prepared for the Health Evidence Network of the World Health Organization European Regional Office (WHO-EURO) (Thornicroft & Tansella, 2003). The Health Evidence Network is an information service initiated and coordinated by WHO-EURO which provides the best evidence available in the field of public health (http://www.who.dk/hen). Working with over 30 partner organisations, it aims to deliver timely information to health care decision-makers in the WHO European Region by providing summaries from a wide range of existing sources, including websites, databases, documents, national and international organisations and institutions. It comprises two services: answers to questions to support the decision-making process, and ready access to sources of evidence such as databases, documents and networks of experts.

Method

This paper focuses upon the following key questions: (a) How far should mental health services be provided in community and/or hospital settings? (b) What service components are necessary and which are optional? (c) What are the differing service development priorities for areas (countries and regions) with low, medium and high levels of resources?

The recent growth of mental health services research has provided substantial evidence in relation to these questions, but few attempts have been made to review these results as a whole and to put them in a resource context so that they are usable for the planning and provision of services at national and regional levels. The aim of this review is therefore to summarise such evidence, and to propose a stepped care model that contextualises the relevance of this evidence to areas at different stages of economic development. It refers to mental health services for adults of working age, and does not directly address other important groups, such as children, older people or those whose primary problem is drug or alcohol misuse. We appreciate, however, that for regions with fewer resources, where the majority of service provision is at the primary care level, these distinctions may be less relevant.

The procedure used was that first we searched Medline for the period 1980 to April 2003, using the search terms MENTAL *and* COMMUNITY *and* HOSPITAL (3177 records were extracted). Only English-language articles were examined to include those relevant journals with higher impact factors (1810 records); of these 141 were review articles, which were considered in preparing this paper. In addition, the authors searched the Cochrane Library and included other relevant systematic reviews. This procedure allowed us to summarise the evidence for distinct service components, and to recommend three particular blends of these components as suitable for areas with low, medium and high level of resources, as a contribution to the debate about resource-appropriate models of care.

Results

The results of this review are organised in relation to the level of resources available, as proposed by the WHO World Health Report (World Health Organization, 2001*a*: pp. 112–115). Table 40.1 indicates that areas with a low level of resources are likely to need to provide most or all of their mental health care in primary health care settings, delivered by primary care staff, with specialist back-up to provide training, consultation for complex cases, and in-patient assessment and treatment of cases that cannot be managed in primary care (Mubbashar, 1999; Saxena & Maulik, 2003). Some low-resource countries may in fact be in a pre-asylum stage (Njenga, 2002) in which apparent community care in fact represents widespread neglect of mentally ill people. Where asylums do exist, policy makers face choices about whether to upgrade the quality of care offered (Njenga, 2002) or to use the resources of the larger hospitals to establish decentralised services instead (Alem, 2002).

Differences in mental health services between low-resource and high-resource countries are vast. In Europe, for example, there are 5.5–20.0 psychiatrists per 100000 population, whereas the figure is 0.05 per 100 000 in African countries (Njenga, 2002); the average number of psychiatric beds is 8.70 in the European region and 0.34 in Africa (Alem, 2002). About 5–10% of the total health budget is spent on mental health in Europe (Becker & Vázquez-Barquero, 2001), whereas in the African continent 80% of countries spend less than 1% of their limited total health budget on mental health. These and other relevant comparative data are available from the WHO Project Atlas website (World Health Organization, 2001b) and from the World Bank (2002). For example, although health spending represents some 7.9% of global gross domestic product, with an average expenditure expressed in international dollars (based on purchasing power parities) of I$523 on health services, this average varies significantly across countries and regions, ranging from I$82 per person in Africa to I$2078 in the Organization for Economic Cooperation and Development (OECD) countries (Poullier et al, 2002). Further, for both Europe and Africa there are also considerable and often growing variations both between countries and between regions within countries, not only in health expenditure but also in social care. As a consequence the forms of service provision relevant to low-resource areas will be very different from those relevant to medium- and high-resource areas.

Areas (countries or regions) with a medium level of resources may first establish the service components shown in column 2 of Table 40.1, and later, as resources allow, choose to add some of the wider range of more differentiated services indicated in column 3. The choice of which of these more specialised services to develop first depends upon local factors, including service traditions and specific circumstances; consumer, carer and staff preferences; existing service strengths and weaknesses; and the way in which evidence is interpreted and used. This stepped care model also indicates that the forms of care relevant and affordable in areas with a high level of resources will include elements from column 3, in addition to the components in columns 1 and 2 which will usually already be present. The model is therefore both additive and sequential, in that new resources allow extra levels of service to be provided over time, in terms of mixtures of the components within each step, when the provision of the components in the previous step is complete.

Decisions on the planning and investment of funds to improve mental health will need to include a wide range of stakeholders, often bringing divergent or even conflicting perspectives to this task. It is now increasingly common in many countries for service users and family members or carers to participate routinely in such decision-making.

Step A: Primary care mental health with specialist back-up

Well-defined psychological problems are common in general health care and primary health care settings in every country, and cause disability which is usually in proportion to the number of symptoms present (Ormel et al, 1994). In areas with a low level of resources (Table 40.1, column 1), the large majority of cases of mental disorder should be recognised and treated within primary health care (Desjarlais et al, 1995). The WHO has shown that the integration of essential mental health treatments within primary health care in these countries is feasible (World Health Organization, 2001a).

Table 40.1. Mental Health Service Components Relevant for Countries and Regions with Low, Medium and High Levels of Resources

Low Level of Resources	Medium Level of Resources	High Level of Resources
Step A	**Step A + step B**	**Step A + step B + step C**
Step *A: Primary care with specialist back-up*	Step B: *Mainstream mental health care*	Step C: *Specialised/ differentiated mental health services*
Screening and assessment by primary care staff	Out-patient/ ambulatory clinics	Specialised clinics for specific disorders or patient groups, including:
Talking treatments, including counselling and advice Pharmacological treatment Liaison and training with mental health		• eating disorders • dual diagnosis • treatment-resistant affective disorders • adolescent services
specialist staff, when available Limited specialist back-up available for:	Community mental health teams	Specialised community mental health teams, including:
• training • consultation for complex cases		• early intervention teams • assertive community treatment
• in-patient assessment and treatment for cases that cannot be managed in primary care, for example in general hospitals	Acute in-patient care	Alternatives to acute hospital admission, including:
		• home treatment/crisis resolution teams • crisis/respite houses • acute day hospital
	Long-term community-based residential care	Alternative types of long-stay community residential care, including:
		• intensive 24 h staffed residential provision • less intensively staffed accommodation • independent accommodation
	Employment and occupation	Alternative forms of occupation and vocational rehabilitation:
		• sheltered workshops • supervised work placements • cooperative work schemes • self-help and user groups • club houses/transitional employment programmes • vocational rehabilitation • individual placement and support service

Step B: Mainstream mental health care

Mainstream mental health care refers to a range of service components, which may be necessary in areas that can afford more than a primary care-based system with specialist back-up. However, the recognition and treatment of the majority of people with mental illnesses, especially depression and anxiety-related disorders, remains a task that falls mostly to primary care. Von Korff & Goldberg (2001) reviewed 12 different randomised controlled trials of enhanced care for major depression in primary care settings. They found that interventions directed solely towards training and supporting general practitioners have not been shown to be effective. They argued that interventions should focus on low-cost case management, coupled with flexible and accessible working relationships between the case manager, the primary care doctor and the mental health specialist. In other words, the whole process of care needs to be enhanced and reorganised to include the following key elements: active follow-up by the case manager, monitoring treatment adherence and patient outcomes, adjustment of treatment plan if patients do not improve, and referral to a specialist when necessary (Von Korff & Goldberg, 2001). This could be seen as a major reversal of what is considered by many to be the conventional approach: enhancing the training of family doctors. Rather, the evidence now strongly suggests that improving outcomes of chronic diseases such as depression does appear to require more than changing the skills of one profession alone: namely, the combination of several concurrent active ingredients.

Mainstream mental health care can be considered to be an amalgam of the core components described below.

Out-patient and ambulatory clinics

Out-patient and ambulatory clinics vary according to:

(a) whether patients can self-refer, or need to be referred by other agencies such as primary care;
(b) there are fixed appointment times or open access assessments;
(c) doctors alone or other disciplines also provide clinical contact;
(d) whether direct or indirect payment is made;
(e) methods used to enhance attendance rates;
(f) how the clinic responds to nonattenders;
(g) the frequency and duration of clinical contacts.

There is surprisingly little evidence on any of these key characteristics of outpatient care (Becker, 2001), but there is a strong clinical consensus in many countries that such clinics are a relatively efficient way of organising the provision of assessment and treatment, provided that the clinic sites are accessible to local populations. Nevertheless, these clinics are simply methods of arranging clinical contact between staff and patients, and so the key issue is the content of the clinical interventions: namely, to deliver treatments that are known to be evidence-based (Roth & Fonagy, 1996; Nathan & Gorman, 2002; BMJ Publishing Group, 2003).

Community Mental Health Teams (CMHTs)

Community mental health teams are the basic building block for community mental health services. The simplest model of provision of community care is for generic (non-specialised) teams to provide the full range of interventions (including the contributions of psychiatrists, community psychiatric nurses, social workers, psychologists and occupational therapists), prioritising adults with severe mental illness, for a local defined geographical catchment area (Thornicroft et al, 1999; Department of Health, 2002). A series of studies and systematic reviews, comparing community mental health teams with a variety of local usual services, suggests that there are clear benefits to the introduction of generic, community-based multidisciplinary teams: they can improve engagement with services, increase user satisfaction, increase met needs and improve adherence to treatment, although they do not improve symptoms or social function (Tyrer *et al*, 1995, 1998, 2003; Thornicroft *et al*, 1998; Burns, 2001; Simmonds *et al*, 2001). In addition, continuity of care and service flexibility have been shown to be more developed where a community mental health team model is in place (Sytema *et al*, 1997).

Case management. Within community mental health teams, case management is a method of delivering care, rather than being a clinical intervention in its own right, and at this stage the evidence suggests that it can most usefully be implemented within the context of the community mental health team (Holloway & Carson, 2001). It is a style of working that has been described as the 'coordination, integration and allocation of individualised care within limited resources' (Thornicroft, 1991). There is now a considerable literature to show that this style of working can be moderately effective in improving continuity of care, quality of life and patient satisfaction, but there is conflicting evidence as to whether it has any impact on the use of in-patient services (Saarento *et al*, 1996; Hansson *et al*, 1998; Mueser *et al*, 1998; Ziguras & Stuart, 2000; Ziguras *et al*, 2002). Case management needs to be carefully distinguished from the much more specific and more intensive assertive community treatment (see below).

Acute In-patient Care

There is no evidence that a balanced system of mental health care can be provided without acute beds. Some services (such as home treatment teams, crisis houses and acute day hospital care, see below) may be able to offer realistic alternative care for some voluntary patients. Nevertheless, people who need urgent medical assessment, or those with severe and comorbid medical and psychiatric conditions, or those experiencing severe psychiatric relapse and behavioural disturbance, or those with high levels of suicidality or assaultativeness, or with an acute neuropsychiatric condition, or elderly patients with concomitant severe physical disorders, will usually require high-intensity immediate support in acute in-patient hospital units.

There is a relatively weak evidence base on many aspects of in-patient care, and most studies are descriptive accounts (Szmukler & Holloway, 2001). There are few systematic reviews in this field, one of which found no difference in outcomes between routine admissions and planned short hospital stays (Johnstone & Zolese, 1999). More generally, although there is a consensus that acute in-patient services are necessary, the number of beds required is highly contingent upon what other services exist locally and upon local social and cultural characteristics (Thornicroft & Tansella, 1999). Acute in-patient care commonly absorbs most of the mental health budget (Knapp *et al*, 1997). Therefore, minimising the number of bed-days used, for example by reducing the average length of stay, may be an important goal, if the resources released in this way can be used for other service components. A related policy issue concerns how to provide acute beds in a humane and less institutionalised way that is acceptable to patients, for example in general hospital units (Quirk & Lelliott, 2001; Tomov, 2001).

Long-term community-based residential care

It is important to know whether patients with severe and long-term disabilities should be cared for in larger, traditional institutions, or be transferred to long-term community-based residential care. The evidence here, for areas with medium and high resource levels, is clear. When deinstitutionalisation is done carefully for those who had previously received long-term in-patient care for many years, the outcomes are more favourable for most patients who are discharged to community care (Tansella, 1986; Thornicroft & Bebbington, ,1989; Shepherd & Murray, 2001). The Team for the Assessment of Psychiatric

Services study in London (Leff, 1997), for example, completed a 5-year follow-up of over 95% of 670 people without dementia discharged from long-stay residential care and found that:

(a) two-thirds of the patients were still living in their new residence;
(b) there was no increase in the death rate or the suicide rate;
(c) very few patients became homeless, and none was lost to follow-up from a staffed home;
(d) over a third were briefly readmitted, and at follow-up 10% of the sample were in hospital;
(e) patients' quality of life was greatly improved by the move to the community;
(f) there was little difference between total hospital and community costs, and overall community care was more cost-effective than long-stay hospital care.

However, there is less evidence available on the treatment and care needs of the never-institutionalised group of long-term patients (Holloway et al, 1999), and so careful local assessment of the needs of this population will be especially important. The range and capacity of community residential long-term care that will be needed in any particular area is also highly dependent upon which other services are available locally, and upon social and cultural factors, such as the amount of family care that is provided (van Wijngaarden et al, 2003).

Employment and Occupation

Rates of unemployment among people with mental disorders are usually much higher than in the general population (Warr, 1987; Warner, 1994). Traditional methods of occupation and day care have been provided by day centres or a variety of psychiatric rehabilitation centres (Shepherd, 1990; Rosen & Barfoot, 2001). There has been little scientific research into these traditional forms of day care, and a review of over 300 papers found no relevant randomised controlled trial (Marshall et al, 2001). Non-randomised studies have given conflicting results, and for areas with medium levels of resources it is reasonable at this stage to make pragmatic decisions about the provision of rehabilitation and day care services if the more differentiated and evidence-based options discussed below are not affordable (Marshall et al, 2001; Catty et al, 2003).

Step C: Specialised and Differentiated Mental Health Services

The stepped care model suggests that areas with a high level of resources may already provide all or most of the service components in steps A and B, and are then able to offer additional components from the following options (step C; Table 40.1).

Specialised Out-patient and Ambulatory Clinics

Specialised out-patient facilities for specific disorders or patient groups are common in many high-resource areas and may include services dedicated, for example, to those with eating disorders; patients with dual diagnosis (psychotic disorder and substance misuse); people with treatment-resistant affective or psychotic disorders; those requiring specialised forms of psychotherapy; mentally disordered offenders; mentally ill women with babies; and those with other specific disorder groups (such as post-traumatic stress disorder). Local decisions about whether to establish such specialist clinics will depend upon several factors, including their relative priority in relation to the other specialist services described below, identified services gaps and the financial opportunities available.

Specialised community mental health teams

Specialised community mental health teams are by far the most researched of all the components of balanced care, and most recent randomised controlled trials and systematic reviews in this field refer to such teams (Mueser *et al*, 1998). Two types of specialised community mental health team have been particularly well developed as adjuncts to generic teams: assertive community treatment teams and early intervention teams.

Assertive community treatment teams. Assertive community treatment teams provide a form of specialised mobile outreach treatment for people with more disabling mental disorders, and have been clearly characterised (Deci *et al*, 1995; Teague *et al*, 1998; Scott & Lehman, 2001). There is now strong evidence that assertive community treatment can produce the following advantages in areas with high levels of resources:

(a) reduced admissions to hospital and use of acute beds;
(b) improved accommodation status and occupation;
(c) increased service user satisfaction.

Assertive community treatment has not been shown to produce improvements in mental state or social behaviour. It can reduce the cost of in-patient services, but does not change the overall costs of care (Latimer, 1999; Phillips *et al*, 2001; Marshall & Lockwood, 2003). Nevertheless, it is not known how far this approach is cross-culturally relevant and indeed there is evidence that it may be less effective where usual services already offer high levels of continuity of care, for example in the UK, than in settings where the 'treatment as usual' control condition may offer little to patients with severe mental illness (Burns *et al*, 1999, 2001; Fiander *et al*, 2003).

Early intervention teams. There has been considerable interest in recent years in the prompt identification and treatment of first- or early-episode cases of psychosis. Much of this research has focused upon the time between the first clear onset of symptoms and the beginning of treatment, referred to as the 'duration of untreated psychosis'; other studies have placed more emphasis upon providing family interventions when a young person's psychosis is first identified (Addington *et al*, 2003; Raune *et al*, 2004). There is now emerging evidence that longer duration of untreated psychosis is a predictor of worse outcome for the disorder; in other words, if patients wait a long time after developing a psychotic condition before they receive treatment, then they may take longer to recover and have a less favourable long-term prognosis. Few controlled trials of such interventions have been published, and a recent Cochrane systematic review (Marshall & Lockwood, 2004) has concluded that there are 'insufficient trials to draw any definitive conclusions, ... the substantial international interest in early intervention offers an opportunity to make major positive changes in psychiatric practice, but this opportunity may be missed without a concerted international programme of research to address key unanswered questions'. It is therefore currently premature to judge whether specialised early intervention teams should be seen as a priority (Larsen *et al*, 2001; McGorry & Killackey, 2002; McGorry *et al*, 2002; Warner & McGorry, 2002; Friis *et al*, 2003; Harrigan *et al*, 2003).

Alternatives to Acute In-patient Care

In recent years three main alternatives to acute in patient care have been developed: acute day hospitals, crisis houses and home treatment/crisis resolution teams.

Acute day hospitals. Acute day hospitals offer programmes of day treatment for those with acute and severe psychiatric problems, as an alternative to admission to in-patient units. A recent systematic review of nine randomised controlled trials has established that acute day hospital care is suitable for about 30% of people who would otherwise be admitted to hospital, and offers advantages in terms of faster improvement and lower cost. It is reasonable to conclude that acute day hospital care is an effective option when demand for in-patient beds is high (Wiersma *et al*, 1995; Marshall *et al*, 2001).

Crisis houses. Crisis houses are houses in community settings which are staffed by trained mental health professionals and offer admission for some patients who would otherwise be admitted to hospital. A wide variety of respite houses, havens and refuges have been developed, but the term 'crisis house' is used here to mean facilities that are alternatives to non-compulsory hospital admission. The little available research evidence suggests that they are very acceptable to their residents (Davies *et al*, 1994; Sledge *et al*, 1996*a, b*; Szmukler & Holloway, 2001), may be able to offer an alternative to hospital admission for about a quarter of those who would otherwise be admitted, and may be more cost-effective than hospital admission (Sledge *et al*, 1996*a,b*; Mosher, 1999). Nevertheless, there is emerging evidence that female patients in particular prefer non-hospital alternatives (such as crisis houses) to acute in-patient treatment, and this may reflect the lack of perceived safety in hospital (Killaspy *et al*, 2000).

Home treatment and crisis resolution teams. Home treatment and crisis resolution teams are mobile community mental health teams offering assessment for patients in psychiatric crises and providing intensive treatment and care at home. A Cochrane systematic review (Catty *et al*, 2002) found that most of the research evidence comes from the USA and the UK, and concluded that home treatment teams reduce days spent in hospital, especially if the teams make regular home visits and have responsibility for both health and social care (Joy *et al*, 2002).

Alternative Types of Long-Stay Community Residential Care

These are usually replacements for long-stay wards in psychiatric institutions (Shepherd *et al*, *1996;* Trieman *et al*, 1998; Shepherd & Murray, 2001). Three categories of such residential care can be identified:

(a) 24 h staffed residential care (high staffed hostels, residential care homes or nursing homes, depending on whether the staff have professional qualifications);

(b) day-staffed residential places (hostels or residential homes which are staffed during the day);

(c) lower supported accommodation (minimally supported hostels or residential homes with visiting staff).

There is limited evidence as to the cost-effectiveness of these types of residential care, and no completed systematic review (Chilvers *et al*, 2003). It is therefore reasonable for policy makers to decide upon the need for such services with local stakeholders (Hafner, 1987; Nordentoft *et al*, 1992; Rosen & Barfoot, 2001; Thornicroft, 2001).

Alternative Forms of Employment and Occupation

Although vocational rehabilitation has been offered in various forms to people with severe mental illness for over a century, its role has weakened because of discouraging results, financial disincentives to work and pessimism about outcomes for these patients (Lehman *et al*, 1995; Polak & Warner, 1996; Wiersma *et al*, 1997). However, recent alternative forms of occupation and vocational rehabilitation have again raised employment as an outcome priority. Consumer and carer advocacy groups have set work and occupation as one of their highest priorities, to enhance both functional status and quality of life (Becker *et al*, 1996; Thornicroft *et al*, 2002). There are recent indications that it is possible to improve vocational and psychosocial outcomes with supported employment models, which emphasise rapid placement in competitive jobs and support from employment specialists (Drake *et al*, 1999). This individual placement and support model emphasises competitive employment in integrated work settings with follow-up support (Priebe *et al*, 1998); studies of such programmes have been encouraging in terms of increased rates of competitive employment (Marshall *et al*, 2001; Lehman *et al*, 2002).

Discussion

This review makes clear that there is no compelling argument and no scientific evidence favouring the use of hospital services alone. On the other hand, there is also no evidence that community services alone can provide satisfactory and comprehensive care. Both the evidence available so far, and accumulated clinical experience, therefore support a balanced approach, incorporating elements of both hospital and community care (Thornicroft & Tansella, 2002).

The material resources available will severely constrain how this approach is applied in practice. In low-resource areas it may be unrealistic to invest in any of the components described here as mainstream mental health care (step B), and the focus will need to be upon primary mental health care, where the main role for the relatively few specialist mental health staff is to support primary care staff (step A, column 1, Table 40.1). Areas that can afford a more differentiated model of care may first consolidate their mainstream mental health care (step B), with the capacity of each service component decided as a balance between the known local needs (Thornicroft, 2001), the resources available and the priorities of local stakeholders. In general, as mental health systems develop away from an asylum-based model, the proportion of the total budget spent on the large asylums gradually decreases. In other words, new services outside hospital can only be provided by using extra resources (which is uncommon) or by using the resources that are transferred from the hospital sites and staff (which is the more usual case). Interestingly, the evidence from cost-effectiveness studies of deinstitutionalisation and the provision of community mental health teams is that the quality of care is closely related to the expenditure upon services, and overall community-based models of care are largely equivalent in cost to the services that they replace.

Over time, and as resources allow, each of the components of the mainstream model can be complemented by additional and differentiated options, described here as specialised differentiated mental health services (step C). Notably, the evidence base for these more recent and innovative forms of care is stronger than for any of the service components in steps A or B, described above in relation to lower resource countries. Indeed, few high-quality scientific studies have been carried out in low-income countries (Patel & Sumathipala, 2001; Isaakidis *et al*, 2002). Consequently, the relevance of most published research in this field to less economically developed countries may be low. This schema therefore places the evidence of effective services within the appropriate resource context; 'resource' here refers not only to the monetary investments made, but also to the available numbers of staff, their levels of experience and expertise, their therapeutic orientation and the contributions available from the wider social and family networks (Desjarlais *et al*, 1995).

Two important implications arise from this approach. First, the stepped care model suggests that there should be a degree of coordination between service components, in particular between the provision of primary and specialist care. We recognise that such planning mechanisms may be weak in some areas. Second, this model implies that the training of mental health staff should be fit for purpose according to the service stage reached (A, B or C) and the level of resources in the area of practice (high, medium or low). In practice it is likely that in any particular area some but not all of the service components described here will be present, and that such identified gaps may inform local planning for service developments.

In recent years there has been a debate between those who are in favour of the provision of mental health treatment and care in hospitals, and those who prefer to use primarily or even exclusively community settings, in which the two forms of care are often seen as incompatible. This false dichotomy can now be replaced by an approach that balances both community services and modern hospital care. However, since this framework cannot be applied in the same way in settings with different resources, the stepped care model presented in this paper suggests a sequential view of how to develop a balance of services in any specific context, moving over time from the left column to the right column in Table 40.1. In this way, implementing the components of a modern mental health service can be seen as a pragmatic exercise undertaken by all those with an interest in improving care.

Acknowledgement

This review is based upon an evidence synthesis prepared for the WHO Regional Office for Europe's Health Evidence Network (http://www.euro.who.int/document/hen/mental-health.pdf).

Clinical Implications

- Countries with low levels of resources should focus on (a) establishing and improving services in primary care settings, along with (b) the provision of specialist back-up.
- Medium-resource countries, in addition to (a) and (b), may then develop 'mainstream' mental health care with the following components: (i) out-patient/ambulatory clinics; (ii) community mental health teams; (iii) acute in-patient care; (iv) long-term community-based residential care; and (v) employment and occupation.
- High-resource countries may include (a) and (b), and then develop evidence-based specialised/differentiated care for each of (i)-(v).

Limitations

- Within countries there may be wide variations between regions, so that different resource levels apply when planning services.
- The model proposed is most directly applicable to health systems that have a high degree of coordinated planning and commissioning of services.

- There remain many areas of mental health services, most notably in-patient care and out-patient/ambulatory services, where relatively little research on effectiveness or cost-effectiveness has been conducted.

References

Addington, J., Coldham, E. L , Jones, B., et al (2003) The first episode of psychosis: the experience of relatives. *Acta Psychiatrica Scandinavica,* 108, 285–289.

Alem, A. (2002) Community-based vs. hospital-based mental health care: the case of Africa. *World Psychiatry,* I, 99–100.

Becker, T. (2001) Out-patient psychiatric services. In *Textbook of Community Psychiatry* (eds G. Thornicroft & G. Szmukler). pp. 277–282. Oxford: Oxford University Press.

Becker, T. & Vázquez-Barquero, J. L. (2001) The European perspective of psychiatric reform. *Acta Psychiatrica Scandinavica Supplementum,* 8–14.

Becker, D. R., Drake, R. E., Farabaugh, A., et al (1996) Job preferences of clients with severe psychiatric disorders participating in supported employment programs. *Psychiatric Services,* 47, 1223–1226.

BMJ Publishing Group (2003) *Clinical Evidence.* London: BMJ Books.

Burns, T. (2001) Generic versus specialist mental health teams, In *Textbook of Community Psychiatry* (eds G, Thornicroft & G. Szmukler), pp, 231–241. Oxford: Oxford University Press.

Burns, T, Creed, F., Fahy, T, et al (1999) Intensive versus standard case management for severe psychotic illness: a randomised trial. UK 700 Group. *Lancet,* 353, 2185–2189.

Burns. T., Fioritti, A., Holloway, F, et al (2001) Case management and assertive community treatment in Europe. *Psychiatric Services,* 52, 631–636.

Catty, J., Burns, T., Knapp, M., et al (2002) Home treatment for mental health problems: a systematic review. *Psychological Medicine,* 32, 383–401.

Catty, J., Burns, T. & Comas, A. (2003) *Day centres for severe mental illness* (Cochrane Review). *Cochrane Library,* issue I. Oxford: Update Software.

Chilvers, R., Macdonald, G. & Hayes, A. (2003) *Supported Housing for People With Severe Mental Disorders* (Cochrane Review). Oxford: Update Software.

Davies, S., Presilla, B., Strathdee, G., et al (1994) Community beds: the future for mental health care? *Social Psychiatry and Psychiatric Epidemiology,* 29, 241–243.

Deci, P. A., Santos, A. B., Hiott, D.W., et al (1995) Dissemination of assertive community treatment programs. *Psychiatric Services,* 46. 676–678.

Department of Health (2002) Community *Mental Health Teams. Mental Health Policy Implementation Guide.* London: Department of Health.

Desjarlais, R., Eisenberg, L., Good, B., et al (1995) *World Mental Health. Problems and Priorities in Low Income Countries.* Oxford: University Press.

Drake, R. E., Mc Hugo, G. J., Bebout, R. R., et al (1999) A randomized clinical trial of supported employment for inner-city patients with severe mental disorders. *Archives of General Psychiatry,* 56, 627–633.

Fiander, M., Burns, T., McHugo, G. J., et al (2003) Assertive community treatment across the Atlantic: comparison of model fidelity in the UK and USA. *British Journal of Psychiatry,* 182, 248–254.

Friis, S., Larsen.T. K., Melle, I., et al (2003) Methodological pitfalls in early detection studies: the NAPE Lecture 2002. Nordic Association for Psychiatric Epidemiology. *Acta Psychiatrica Scandinavica,* 107, 3–9,

Grob, G. (1991) From Asylum to *Community. Mental Health Policy in Modern America.* Princeton, NJ: Princeton University Press.

Hafner, H. (1987) Do we still need beds for psychiatric patients? An analysis of changing patterns of mental health care. *Acta Psychiatrica Scandinavica,* 75, 113–126.

Hansson, L., Muus, S.,Vinding, H. R., *et al* (1998) The Nordic Comparative Study on Sectorized Psychiatry: contact rates and use of services for patients with a functional psychosis, *Acta Psychiatrica Scandinavica,* 97, 315–320.

Harrigan, S. M., McGorry, P. D. & Krstev, H. (2003) Does treatment delay in first-episode psychosis really matter? *Psychological Medicine,* 33, 97–110.

Holloway, F., & Carson, J. (2001) Case management: an update. *International Journal of Social Psychiatry,* 47, 21–31.

Holloway, F., Wykes, T, Petch, E., *et al* (1999) The new long stay in an inner city service: a tale of two cohorts. *International Journal of Social Psychiatry,* 45, 93–103.

Isaakidis, P., Swingler, G. H., Pienaar, E., *et al* (2002) Relation between burden of disease and randomised evidence in sub-Saharan Africa: survey of research. *BMJ,* 324,702.

Johnstone; P., & Zolese, G. (1999) Systematic review of the effectiveness of planned short hospital stays for mental health care. *BMJ,* 318, 1387–1390.

Joy, C., Adams, C., & Rice, K. (2002) Crisis intervention for people with severe mental illness. *Cochrane Library,* issue 2, Oxford: Update Software.

Killaspy, H., Dalton, J., McNicholas, S., *et al* (2000) Drayton Park, an alternative to hospital admission for women in acute mental health crisis. *Psychiatric Bulletin,* 24, 101–104.

Knapp, M., Chisholm, D., Astin, J., *et al* (1997) The cost consequences of changing the hospital-community balance: the mental health residential care study. *Psychological Medicine,* 27, 681–692.

Larsen.T. K., Friis, S., Haahr, U., *et al* (2001) Early detection and intervention in first-episode schizophreniacritical review. *Acta Psychiatrica Scandinavica,* 103, 323–334.

Latimer, E. A. (1999) Economic impacts of assertive community treatment: a review of the literature. *Canadian journal of Psychiatry,* 44, 443–454.

Leff, J. (1997) Care *in the Community. Illusion or Reality?* London: Wiley.

Lehman, A. F., Carpenter, W.T., Goldman, H. H., *et al* (1995) Treatment outcomes in schizophrenia: implications for practice, policy, and research. *Schizophrenia Bulletin,* 21, 669–675.

Lehman, A. F., Goldberg, R., Dixon, L. B., *et al* (2002) Improving employment outcomes for persons with severe mental illnesses. *Archives of General Psychiatry,* 59,165–172.

Marshall, M., & Lockwood, A. (2003) Assertive community treatment for people with severe mental disorders (Cochrane Review). *Cochrane Library,* issue I. Oxford: Update Software.

Marshall., M., & Lockwood, A. (2004) Early intervention for psychosis (Cochrane Review). *Cochrane Library,* issue 2. Chichester: John Wiley.

Marshall, M., Crowther, R., Almaraz-Serrano, A., *et al* (2001) Systematic reviews of the effectiveness of day care for people with severe mental disorders: (I) acute day hospital versus admission; (2) vocational rehabilitation; (3) day hospital versus outpatient care. *Health Technology Assessment* 2, 1–75.

McGorry, P. D., & Killackey, E. J. (2002) Early intervention in psychosis: a new evidence based paradigm. *Epidemiologia e Psychiatria Sociale,* II, 237–247.

McGorry, P. D., Yung, A. R., Phillips, L. J., *et al* (2002) Randomized controlled trial of interventions designed to reduce the risk of progression to first-episode psychosis in a clinical sample with subthreshold symptoms. *Archives of General Psychiatry,* 59, 921 -928.

Mosher, L. R. (1999) Soteria and other alternatives to acute psychiatric hospitalization: a personal and professional review. *Journal of Nervous and Mental Disease,* 187, 142–149.

Mubbashar, M., (1999) Mental health services in rural Pakistan. In *Common Mental Disorders in Primary Care* (eds M. Tansella & G. Thornicroft), pp. 67–80, London: Routledge.

Mueser, K.T., Bond, G. R., Drake, R. E., *et al* (1998) Models of community care for severe mental illness: a review of research on case management. *Schizophrenia Bulletin,* 24, 37–74.

Murray, C., & Lopez, A. (1996) The *Global Burden of Disease, Vol. I. A Comprehensive Assessment of Mortality and Disability From Diseases, Injuries and Risk Factors in 1990, and Projected to 2020.* Cambridge, MA: Harvard University Press.

Nathan, P., & Gorman, J. (2002) *A Guide* to *Treatments That Work.* Oxford: Oxford University Press.

Njenga, F. (2002) Challenges of balanced care in Africa. *World Psychiatry,* I, 96–98.

Nordentoft, M., Knudsen, H. C., & Schulsinger, F. (1992) Housing conditions and residential needs of psychiatric patients in Copenhagen. *Acta Psychiatrica Scandinavica,* 85, 385–389,

Ormel, J., Von Korff, M., Ustun, B., *et al* (1994) Common mental disorders and disability across cultures. Results from the WHO Collaborative Study on Psychological Problems in General Health Care. *JAMA,* 272, 1741–1748.

Patel, V., & Sumathipala, A. (2001) International representation in psychiatric literature: surveys of six leading journals. *British Journal of Psychiatry,* 178, 406–409.

Phillips, S. D., Burns, B. J., Edgar, E. R., *et al* (2001) Moving assertive community treatment into standard practice. *Psychiatric* Services, 52, 771–779.

Polak, P., & Warner, R. (1996) The economic life of seriously mentally ill people in the community. *Psychiatric Services,* 47, 270–274.

Poullier, J.-P., Hernandez, P., Kawabata, K., *et al* (2002) *Patterns of Global Health Expenditures: Results for 191 Countries.* World Health Organization Discussion Paper No. 51. Geneva: WHO.

Priebe, S., Warner, R., Hubschmid, T., *et al* (1998) Employment, attitudes toward work, and quality of life among people with schizophrenia in three countries. *Schizophrenia Bulletin,* 24, 469–477.

Quirk, A., & Lelliott, P. (2001) What do we know about life on acute psychiatric wards in the UK? A review of the research evidence. *Social Science and Medicine,* 53, 1565–1574.

Raune, D., Kuipers, E., & Bebbington, P. E. (2004) Expressed emotion at first-episode psychosis: investigating a career appraisal model. *British Journal of Psychiatry,* 184, 321–326.

Rosen, A., & Barfoot, K. (2001) Day care and occupation: structured rehabilitation and recovery programmes and work. In *Textbook of Community Psychiatry* (eds G. Thornicroft & G. Szmukler), pp. 296–308. Oxford: Oxford University Press.

Roth, A., & Fonagy, P. (1996) *What Works for Whom? A Critical Review of Psychotherapy Research.* New York: Guilford Press.

Saarento, O., Hansson, L., Sandlund, M., *et al* (1996) The Nordic comparative study on sectorized psychiatry. Utilization of psychiatric hospital care related to amount and allocation of resources to psychiatric services. *Social Psychiatry and Psychiatric Epidemiology,* 31, 327–335.

Saxena, S., & Maulik, P. (2003) Mental health services in low and middle income countries: an overview. *Current Opinion in Psychiatry,* 16, 437–442.

Scott, J., & Lehman, A. (2001) Case management and assertive community treatment. In *Textbook of Community Psychiatry* (eds G. Thornicroft & G. Szmukler), pp. 253–264. Oxford: Oxford University Press.

Shepherd, G. (1990) *Theory and Practice of Psychiatric Rehabilitation.* Chichester: John Wiley.

Shepherd, G., & Murray, A. (2001) Residential care. In *Textbook of Community Psychiatry* (eds G. Thornicroft & G. Szmukler), pp. 309–320. Oxford: Oxford University Press.

Shepherd, G., Muijen, M., Dean, R., *et al* (1996) Residential care in hospital and in the community: quality of care and quality of life. *British Journal of Psychiatry,* 168, 448–456.

Simmonds, S., Coid, J., Joseph, P., *et al* (2001) Community mental health team management in severe mental illness: a systematic review. *British Journal of Psychiatry,* 178, 497–502.

Sledge, W. H., Tebes, J., Rakfeldt, J., *et al* (1996a) Day hospital/crisis respite care versus inpatient care. Part I: Clinical outcomes. *American Journal of Psychiatry,* 153, 1065–1073.

Sledge, W. H., Tebes, J., Wolff, N., *et al* (1996b) Day hospital/crisis respite care versus inpatient care, Part II: Service utilization and costs. *American Journal of Psychiatry,* 153, 1074–1083.

Sytema, S., Micciolo, R., & Tansella, M. (1997) Continuity of care for patients with schizophrenia and related disorders: a comparative south-Verona and Groningen case-register study. *Psychological Medicine,* 27, 1355–1362.

Szmukler, G., & Holloway, F. (2001) In-patient treatment. In *Textbook of Community Psychiatry* (eds G. Thornicroft & G. Szmukler), pp. 321–337. Oxford: Oxford University Press.

Tansella, M. (1986) Community psychiatry without mental hospitals: the Italian experience: a review. *Journal of the Royal Society of Medicine,* 79, 664–669.

Teague, G. B., Bond, G. R. & Drake, R. E. (1998) Program fidelity in assertive community treatment: development and use of a measure. *American Journal of Orthopsychiatry,* 68, 216–232.

Thornicroft, G. (1991) The concept of case management for long-term mental illness. *International Review of Psychiatry,* 3, 125–132.

Thornicroft, G. (2001) *Measuring Mental Health Needs* (2nd edn). London: Gaskell.

Thornicroft, G., & Bebbington, P. (1989) Deinstitutionalisation: from hospital closure to service development. *British Journal of Psychiatry,* 155, 739–753.

Thornicroft, G., & Tansella, M. (1999) *The Mental Health Matrix: A Manual to Improve Services.* Cambridge: Cambridge University Press.

Thornicroft, G., & Tansella, M. (2002) Balancing community-based and hospital-based mental health care. *World Psychiatry,* 1, 84–90.

Thornicroft, G., & Tansella, M. (2003) *What Are the Arguments for Community-Based Mental Health Care?* Copenhagen: World Health Organization (European Region) Health Evidence Network.

Thornicroft, G., Wykes,T., Holloway, F., *et al* (1998) From efficacy to effectiveness in community mental health services. PRiSM Psychosis Study 10. *British Journal of Psychiatry,* 173, 423–427.

Thornicroft, G., Becker,T., Holloway, F., *et al* (1999) Community mental health teams: evidence or belief? *British Journal of Psychiatry,* 175, 508–513.

Thornicroft, G., Rose, D., Huxley, P., *et al* (2002) What are the research priorities of mental health service users? *Journal of Mental Health,* II, 1–5.

Tomov, T. (2001) Central and Eastern European Countries, In *The Mental Health Matrix: A Manual to Improve Services* (eds G. Thornicroft & M. Tansella), pp. 216–227. Cambridge: Cambridge University Press.

Trieman, N., Smith, H. E., Kendal, R., *et al* (1998) The TAPS Project 41: homes for life? Residential stability five years after hospital discharge. Team for the Assessment of Psychiatric Services. *Community Mental Health Journal,* 34, 407–417.

Tyrer, P., Morgan, J., Van Horn, E., *et al* (1995) A randomised controlled study of close monitoring of vulnerable psychiatric patients. *Lancet,* 345, 756–759.

Tyrer, P., Evans, K., Gandhi, N., *et al* (1998) Randomised controlled trial of two models of care for discharged psychiatric patients. *BMJ,* 316, 106–109.

Tyrer, P., Coid, J., Simmonds, S., *et al* (2003) Community mental health teams (CMHTs) for people with severe mental illnesses and disordered personality (Cochrane Review). *Cochrane Library,* issue 2, Oxford: Update Software.

Van Wijngaarden, G. K., Schene, A., Koeter, M., *et al* (2003) People with schizophrenia in five countries: conceptual similarities and intercultural differences in family caregiving. *Schizophrenia Bulletin,* 29, 573–586.

Von Korff, M., & Goldberg, D. (2001) Improving outcomes in depression. The whole process of care needs to be enhanced. *BMJ,* 323, 948–949.

Warner, R. (1994) *Recovery from Schizophrenia* (2nd edn). London: Routledge.

Warner, R., & McGorry, P. D. (2002) Early intervention in schizophrenia: points of agreement. *Epidemiologia e Psichiatria Sociale,* II, 256–257.

Warr, P. (1987) *Work, Unemployment and Mental Health.* Oxford: Oxford University Press.

Wiersma, D., Kluiter, H., Nienhuis, F. J., *et al* (1995) Costs and benefits of hospital and day treatment with community care of affective and schizophrenic disorders. British Journal *of Psychiatry,* 167 (suppl. 27), 552–559.

Wiersma, D., Nienhuis, F. J., Slooff, C. J., *et al* (1997) Assessment of needs for care among patients with schizophrenic disorders 15 and 17 years after first onset of psychosis. *Epidemiologia e Psichiatria Sociale,* 6, 21 -28.

Wing, J. K., & Brown, G. (1970) *Institutionalism and Schizophrenia.* Cambridge: Cambridge University Press.

World Bank (2002) *World Development Report 2002. Building Institutions for Markets.* Washington, DC: World Bank.

World Health Organization (2001*a*) *World Health Report 2001. Mental Health: New Understanding, New Hope.* Geneva: WHO. http://www.who.int/whr2001/2001/main/en/

World Health Organization (2001*b*) *Atlas: Mental Health Resources in the World 2001.* Geneva: WHO. http://www.who.int/mental _ health/media/en/244.pdf

Ziguras, S. J., & Stuart, G. W. (2000) A meta-analysis of the effectiveness of mental health case management over 20 years. *Psychiatric* Services, 51, 1410–1421.

Ziguras, S. J., Stuart, G. W., & Jackson, A. C. (2002) Assessing the evidence on case management. *British Journal of Psychiatry,* 181, 17–21.

41

Frank, R. B., & Glied, S. A. (2006). *Better but not well: Mental health policy in the United States since 1950.* Baltimore: Johns Hopkins University Press

Frank and Glied employ an economic approach to the history of mental health policy in the United States during the last half of the twentieth century. Their book gives a mainly positive scorecard to mental health services, systems, and resources today compared to 1950, but a more pessimistic view of policy and resources as they affect persons with serious and persistent mental illness. This group, the authors claim, received benefits from mental health exceptionalism in traditional state-fueled policies and programs, and again requires special attention to come to parity with other recipients of mental health care. The authors propose the creation of a new federal agency, reporting to the president, which will coordinate and enhance the availability of federal resources now scattered in a number of programs. Their book raises provocative questions about the relative balance between the benefits of mainstreaming services to people with mental illness versus setting aside targeted services (mental health exceptionalim) to address their special needs and vulnerabilities. The excerpts here are from Chapter 4, discussing the changes in financing and delivery of mental health care from 1950 to 2000, and Chapter 6, which analyzes the transition from policy directed by state mental health program directors and organized psychiatry, to mainstream policy makers, due in good part to the watershed events of the passage of federal Medicaid, Medicare, and Supplemental Security Income (SSI) legislation as part of the Great Society initiatives.

Chapter 4: Health Care Financing and Income Support

Between 1950 and 2000 the financing and delivery of mental health care underwent structural changes as dramatic as those in the Eastern European nations after the Soviet Union's disintegration. In a matter of twenty years, starting in the mid-1960s, mental health care moved largely from a centrally planned, state-owned and operated enterprise to a system dominated by market forces, though it still retained a large amount of public financing. These primary financing changes—not technological breakthroughs or demographic shifts—have transformed the lives of people with mental illness.

In the early 1960s choices about which services to provide and how much to spend on these services were made by state legislators. Legislators allocated a yearly budget for their state's centrally organized mental health system, whose focal point was the state mental hospital. People with a serious mental illness had few, if any, real choices about their care.

Today mentally ill individuals have become consumers, choosing their care—and allocating the financial resources associated with that care—from a broad array of institutions and services. They can usually weigh for themselves whether to enter a psychiatric hospital, a general hospital, a partial hospital (an institutional setting offering services similar to those of a hospital, without the overnight stay), a clinic, or a private office—each with its own assortment of services, providers, and intensities of care. Providers of care now compete for consumers on the basis of price, quality, and convenience—the very ingredients with which any business, whether a grocery store or an electronics outlet, vies for consumers. Health care markets differ from others, and the mental health care market has its own unique imperfections. Nonetheless, today there are markets for insurance and mental health care services where none existed before.[1]

The emergence of insurance and markets in mental health care turned individuals into consumers and thrust providers into the role of suppliers, with many of the commercial connotations of those labels. In the 1950s and early 1960s severely ill patients were cared for in what the sociologist Erving Goffman labeled "total institutions," which took pervasive control over all aspects of life. Outside institutional walls, less severely ill people sought counseling from a few public dispensaries or from office-based psychiatrists, for which they paid out of pocket. Today in the United States 86 percent of adults—and 80 percent of mentally ill adults—have some form of public or private insurance that confers varying degrees of protection against the high cost of care.[2]

Financing policies have been the principal driver of system change, as they have engineered the disintegration of the centralized mental health system. With its disintegration came the erosion of what we call mental health exceptionalism.

Financing Mental Health Care, 1950–2000

The first health economist to focus on mental health care financing was Rashi Fein. In *Economics of Mental Illness* (1958) he furnished an estimate of at least $1.14 billion for nominal spending in 1956. Fein estimated that state governments accounted for the lion's share of this funding. They were responsible for 59 percent of overall mental health care spending, while the federal government spent 25 percent. The remaining 16 percent came from other sources such as out-of-pocket payments and private insurance. Fein could not obtain data on private insurance. He did, however, estimate spending on private psychiatrists and private psychiatric hospitals on the basis of available information, and some of these costs may have been paid by private insurance.

Table 41.1 provides a summary of the level and composition of mental health service spending over the last five decades. Using data collected from a wide range of public and private sources, the table reports spending in current dollars. Spending grew more than seventyfold, from $1.14 billion in 1956 to $85.4 billion in 2001, faster than overall health care spending, with all the excess growth taking place in the 1956–71 period. Even after taking account of economy-wide inflation, mental health care spending grew dramatically over this period.

These changes occurred because of specific policy and market developments. First, Medicaid was established in 1965. Just six years later, in 1971, it already accounted for roughly 16 percent of all mental health spending. Medicaid contributed to a drastic reduction in states' share of direct spending on mental health services. In Fein's study states were responsible for 59 percent of overall spending in 1956. By 1971 the share of direct state spending dropped precipitously to about 23 percent, roughly the share today.

Table 41.1. Level and Share of Spending for Mental Health Services, by Payer (in Current Dollars)

	1956	*1971*[a]	*1987*[b]	*1997*[b]	*2001*[c]
Medicare	—	2.6%	8.3%	12.8%	7.3%
Medicaid	—	14.2%	16.0%	20.4%	27.4%
Private insurance	—	12.3%	22.2%	23.9%	21.9%
Out of pocket	16.0%	35.6%	19.2%	16.9%	12.8%
State	59.0%	30.4%	25.3%	20.0%	23.4%
Other direct federal mental health spending[d]	25.0%	3.5%	6.1%	4.1%	5.0%
Miscellaneous	—	1.4%	2.9%	1.9%	2.2%
Total spending	$1.14 bn	$8.96 bn	$35.7 bn	$70.8 bn	$85.4 bn

[a]Levine and Levine (1975). To make the 1971 estimates comparable to the more recent estimates, we used estimates of the percentage of nursing home, hospital, and outpatient spending that was attributable to senile dementia, mental retardation, and related disorders not covered by the National Health Accounts approach. Using figures from Mark et al. (2005), we estimated that about 86% of nursing home spending was attributable to dementia. We allocated this spending according to aggregate shares by payers, largely Medicaid (60%), out-of-pocket spending (30%), and other payers. We then used data from U.S. PCMH (1978b, app. Table 10) to categorize the diagnostic mix by major types of treatment settings. We identified diagnoses that cover senile dementia and related conditions. These accounted for between 2% (outpatient) and 5% (state mental hospitals) of spending by setting. We subtracted these numbers from the total and allocated the amount subtracted to payer categories on the basis of the composition of spending in 1971.
[b]Coffey et al. (2000).
[c]Mark et al. (2005).
[d]These include expenditures such as the Veterans Administration and the Alcohol, Drug Abuse, and Mental Health block grant.

In fact, state spending share did not so much evaporate as shift. Since 1965 states have been required by federal law to make matching contributions to federal Medicaid spending. If states' Medicaid matching contributions are added to their direct outlays, total state spending was roughly 36 percent in 1971, 33 percent in 1987, 28 percent in 1997, and 35 percent in 2001. State funds shifted dramatically away from direct spending on services toward Medicaid matching.

The expansion of public and private insurance arrangements over the latter half of the century led to a marked decline in out-of-pocket spending, from nearly 36 percent in 1971 to about 13 percent in 2001. Millions of people who are not seriously mentally ill now have greater protection against financial losses associated with mental illness. Finally, the federal government's role in paying for mental health care has grown as a result of the 1965 passage of Medicaid and Medicare, two different forms of public health insurance. This, too, represented a shift in the form of funding, as the federal government began spending most of its mental health dollars through insurance mechanisms.

The changes in overall spending patterns are clear. Between 1956 and 1971 the state share of spending dropped by nearly half. Since 1971 there has been significant growth in the federal and private insurance shares, greater protection for consumers against financial losses, and stability in state spending.

The Delivery of Mental Health Services, 1950–2000

The locus and nature of mental health services delivered to patients also changed greatly in the postwar period. The magnitude of the shifts in care can be seen in data on treatment episodes: in 1955, 77 percent of treatment episodes took place in inpatient settings (state mental hospitals and other hospitals), whereas by 1975 only 28 percent were in inpatient facilities (U.S. President's Commission on Mental Health, 1978b, app. Table 2). The absolute number of outpatient episodes is even more telling: the 379,000 outpatient treatment episodes in 1955 mushroomed thirteen years later to almost 2 million (Grob, 2001).

The shift away from state mental hospitals has been called *deinstitutionalization,* but the reality was that patients were often discharged to other types of institution—general hospitals or nursing homes—particularly after Medicaid was created in 1965. Indeed, instead of the term *deinstitutionalization,* many prefer to call the shift *transhospitalization* (Geller, 2000). Over the decade of the 1960s the nursing home population swelled from about 470,000 to almost 928,000, a nearly twofold growth (Grob, 2001).

The shift in care can be seen in Table 41.2, which depicts trends from 1971 to 2001 in the composition of mental health services. The table highlights the diminished role of state mental hospitals, whose share of overall spending fell by more than two-thirds. At the same time, the use of general hospital psychiatric units grew as a portion of total spending on mental health care, from 9.7 percent in 1971 to 16 percent in 2001.

Reorienting the mental health system toward community-based treatment became the stated goal of national policy when President Kennedy created in 1963 the Community Mental Health Centers (CMHCs) program. Table 41.2 shows that by 1971 CMHCs and outpatient psychiatric clinics accounted for nearly 8 percent of specialty mental health spending. In terms of treatment episodes, CMHCs supplied 15.4 percent of all such episodes in the United States in 1971. That share rose to 24.7 percent by 1975 (U.S. President's Commission on Mental Health, 1978b, app. Table 2).

The shift in emphasis away from public hospitals and toward community-based treatment was accompanied by growth in the mental health professions, especially psychotherapists. Markets for psychotherapy have grown quickly since the 1960s, and Table 41.2

Table 41.2. Share of Spending for Specialty Mental Health Services

	1971[a]	1987[b]	1997[b]	2001[c]
State mental hospitals	23.0%	23.9%	13.3%	7.0%
Private psychiatric hospitals	3.0	7.0	7.2	14.0
General hospitals	9.7	16.6	16.3	16.0
Nursing homes	28.0	12.0	6.2	7.0
CMHCs/OP clinics	7.9	10.6	15.1	18.0
Psychiatrists	8.7	7.7	9.7	8.7
Psychologists/social worker	1.0	10.3	13.4	8.0
Drugs	5.6	7.5	12.3	21.0

Note: Percentages do not add to 100 because some services are not shown.
[a]Levine and Levine (1975).
[b]Coffey et al. (2000).
[c]State and private psychiatric estimates are based on Mark et al. (2005) and expenditure shares from U.S. DHHS CMHS, 2004, Table 8a.

shows astonishing growth (thirteenfold) in the share of treatment resources spent on psychologists and social workers. The share of spending on psychotherapy appears to have declined between 1997 and 2001.

Innovations in pharmacology, along with expanded insurance coverage for prescription drugs, propelled spending on drugs. The spending share for drugs grew from about 5.6 percent in 1971 to 12.3 percent in 1997. The growth was even more rapid from 1987 to 2001, a time of substantial innovation in psychopharmacology, when the annual growth rate in spending on prescription drugs ranged from about 9 to 22 percent (Coffey et al., 2000; Mark et al., 2005).

To some extent, the shift in the pattern of care toward community-based services reflects changing attitudes and beliefs. The immediate post-World War II period ushered in a period of optimism about the potential for community-based treatment (Grob, 1994, 2001). During the war the military had successfully pioneered treatment of soldiers' stress disorders near their base, rather than transporting them back to military hospitals. Many military psychiatrists, once they returned to civilian life, tried to adapt these techniques of bringing care closer to home. They were also influenced by the Freudian emphasis on social and environmental factors in shaping mental health. Some hoped that early intervention in the community would prevent hospitalization.

This positive vision of the benefits of community-based treatment occurred in parallel with growing concern about the benefits and costs of institutional care.Reports about the quality of care in mental hospitals outraged the public, particularly in a climate that placed growing importance on respecting the rights of psychiatric patients. But the shift in care owes much more to the profound changes in the financing of care over this period than to these changing perceptions.

NOTES

1. It should be noted that the availability of meaningful choice of ambulatory care for people with severe mental illnesses is complicated and frequently quite limited.

2. For recent data on this issue, see McAlpine and Mechanic (2000) and Sturm and Wells (2000).

Chapter 6: Policy Making in Metal Health—Integration, Mainstreaming, and Shifting Institutions

In the 1950s and 1960s mental health policy making was the domain of governors and their state mental health program directors. Organized psychiatry wielded great influence and was deeply involved in consequential debates about the future of mental health care in the United States. Today, by contrast, state Medicaid directors, the Social Security commissioner, the administrator of the Centers for Medicare and Medicaid Services (CMS), and human resource directors in U.S. corporations are the voices with the greatest influence on the direction of mental health policy. These policy makers have little direct connection with the specialty mental health sector. Many of their offices did not even exist in 1950. They are mainstream policy makers. The decline of mental health exceptionalism in public policy has been accompanied by a parallel decline in exceptionalism in policy making.

Mental Health Policy Making at Midcentury

In the 1950s mental health policy was primarily the responsibility of the states, who also paid for most care (Fein, 1958). Most of this funding was allocated to the activities of the public mental hospital, and these hospitals were managed by psychiatrists. The people most directly associated with the direction and management of mental health care were in state government, closely linked to the profession of psychiatry.

In the aftermath of World War II, a sizable number of psychiatrists developed the belief that the mental hospital should no longer be the central institution of the mental health care system. This increasingly popular view of mental health delivery began to weaken the links among state government, the state hospital, and the profession of psychiatry. Organized psychiatry debated the direction of mental health delivery throughout the 1950s. Community-based psychiatry gained the upper hand through the leadership of psychiatrists such as Robert Rappaport, Harry Solomon, and Walter Barton.

The initial reforms that began to reorient mental health care in the United States emanated from the states and from state organizations such as the Governors Conference and the Council of State Governments (Grob, 2001). Individual states such as New York, California, and Massachusetts were among the first to adopt policies that began to shift resources in the direction of community-based mental health services. These states created grant programs with incentives for the development and expansion of community-based mental health clinics, albeit with modest funding. Other states followed suit, and during the 1950s there was a dramatic expansion in the number of outpatient mental health clinics, the majority of which were funded by state government. This growth in community clinics was driven in part by a belief in community-based treatment and by the hope that such care would reduce reliance on expensive state mental hospitals.

State officials and their ideas were also central to efforts aimed at identifying mental health care as a nationwide problem that had to be addressed in consistent policy terms. For example, when the Joint Commission on Mental Illness and Health (JCMIH) was created in the 1950s by a set of private interest groups and philanthropic organizations, the director of the commission was Jack Ewalt, the mental health commissioner in Massachusetts. The 1950s and early 1960s were a time when mental health became a matter for national policy. The creation of the National Institute of Mental Health in the late 1940s gave mental health policy a voice in the federal government. Technical specialists, such as the NIMH director Robert Felix, influenced the emerging federal interest in mental illness from the perspective of the specialty mental health sector. The policy statements that resulted from this initial effort of developing a national approach to mental health policy were based on ideas emerging from the professions and the states.[1] The JCMIH pointed to a two-pronged strategy for improving mental health care. One prong involved improving the conditions and the treatment capacity of public mental hospitals; the other worked at developing a community-based system of care primarily aimed at people with severe mental disorders.

Federal mental health policy until 1963 was limited to establishing a bully pulpit that helped activate a variety of interests to work on altering the directions of mental health care in the United States. The federal government's expanding role in social insurance and in civil rights contributed to a view that it might work in concert with localities to fix mental health care and avoid the political clout associated with interests linked to state mental hospitals. At this point, state interests and proponents of community mental health care began to part company on matters of federal policy. The shape of the new Community Mental Health Centers (CMHCs) legislation emphasized new institutions that bypassed states by forming federal-local partnerships based on financing arrangements that mimicked the Hill-Burton hospital expansion program (the 1946 federal initiative that funded the expansion of hospital beds in the United States).[2] The NIMH was given responsibility for managing the new CMHC program. Yet, while a shift was taking place regarding what shape the mental health system would take, the debate stayed primarily within the mental health community.

This growing federal interest was not accompanied by a massive injection of funds. States remained the main funders of mental health services. State officials such as Ewalt, Milton Greenblatt, and others continued to have great influence on the shape of mental health delivery.

Watershed Events in Mental Health Policy: Medicaid, Medicare, and SSI

The launch of President Johnson's Great Society initiative in 1964 unleashed forces that would fundamentally change mental health care financing and delivery in the United States—and the political institutions that had shaped mental health policy. The passage of Medicaid, Medicare, and later the Supplemental Security Income (SSI) program greatly expanded the resources available to treat mental illness. These programs made the federal government a much more significant payer and regulator of mental health care. At the same time, they began to take mental health policy making out of the hands of the mental health sector.

The debate over coverage of mental health care under Medicare offered the first indication that powerful new institutions were being created that would exert great influence over the care of people with mental illness, yet the mental health community would have only a modest say over what would emerge. Before the implementation of Medicare, organized psychiatry engaged in a series of attempts to influence the new program's design. During the debate in 1965, the modern argument over parity in insurance benefits for mental health care first surfaced. The mental health community called on Congress to abandon the practices of the private health insurance sector and offer comprehensive and comparable insurance benefits for mental health care and other medical care under the Medicare program. The arguments for equal treatment of mental health care were based on fairness—that it is wrong to discriminate against people with mental disorders. The arguments against equal coverage took aim at the difficulties in defining mental illness, the lack of evidence of effective treatments, the high costs of covering mental health services, and the uncertainty in making actuarial cost estimates (Frank, 2000). Congress chose to follow the private health insurance market as a model for choosing nearly all features of the benefit design under Medicare, including mental health. Concerns with the program's budget, disruption of existing health care arrangements, and program administration won the day.

The American Psychiatric Association's preparation for the implementation of the Medicare program also illustrated the new political and organizational context within which psychiatry (and mental health groups generally) had to operate in order to affect mental health policy. The specialty mental health concerns in policy were increasingly focused on preserving benefits in the context of a larger policy-making apparatus whose agenda reached far beyond issues of mental health care. The enactment of Medicare was accompanied by a new set of regulatory standards. Accreditation by the Joint Commission on Accreditation of Hospitals (JCAH, known today as JCAHO) was a central feature of quality assurance in Medicare. At the time, even though the JCAH had adopted APA standards for accreditation of psychiatric facilities, 33 percent of general hospitals and 66 percent of psychiatric hospitals were not accredited. The APA also proposed that a psychiatrist be appointed to the health insurance and medical review advisory councils for the Medicare program.

The ambulatory mental health benefit in Medicare carried high levels of cost sharing and strict limits on service utilization, so its immediate impact was muted. Mental health in Medicare remained a small share of Medicare spending for decades after its enactment. The late 1980s saw some expansion in Medicare coverage of care for mental disorders. Limits on psychotherapy were relaxed, the range of providers that could independently treat mental disorders was expanded to include psychologists and social workers, and a partial-hospital benefit was added. These changes resulted in expanded use of services and spending for mental health care (Rosenbach and Ammering, 1997).

Medicaid was similar to Medicare in terms of the role of the mental health community in policy making, but it had very different effects on mental health delivery. The program's focus on the poor and disabled and on the provision of long-term care for elderly persons meant that it included substantial numbers of people with mental illnesses who had previously relied on state mental health agencies for their care. The poor elderly mentally ill population was dramatically affected by the enactment of Medicaid. In 1963 there were 148,842 residents of state mental hospitals aged sixty-five or older, who accounted for 41 percent of all residents. By 1969, four years after the enactment of Medicaid, the number of these residents had declined to 111,420, or 22.7 percent of all residents (Kramer, 1977). During this same period the population of nursing homes nearly doubled. Following the enactment of Medicaid states faced a choice between hospitalizing indigent elderly people with dementia—and paying 100 percent of the costs in state mental hospitals—and placing them in nursing homes—and paying 17 percent to 50 percent of the costs (nursing homes also had lower per diem rates).

For poor and disabled people (after 1972) under age sixty-five, Medicaid also provided a form of health insurance for treatment of mental disorders, which was paid for under Medicaid's basic benefit. Again the costs to states of providing mental health services in the context of Medicaid were low. This presented strong inducements to mental health directors attempting to meet the mental health needs of their states under tight budgets to expand services by shifting priorities toward Medicaid-eligible populations and services covered by Medicaid. Of course, this strategy required that state mental health spending be applied to the state Medicaid match. As Medicaid grew to become the nation's largest mental health care payer, an increasingly large share of state mental health funds was being directly linked to Medicaid dollars.

Although Medicaid quickly became a central source of mental health funding, mental health concerns did not strongly influence Medicaid policy making. This lack of influence was noted in recommendations made by President Carter's Commission on Mental Health. The first recommendation of the Panel on Cost and Financing noted, "Stronger Federal leadership is needed with regard to the Medicaid mental health programs. This includes: Providing States with technical assistance in developing comprehensive mental health plans" (U.S. PCMH, 1978b). The largest payer for mental health care in the United States was simply not attuned to mental health issues, in part because state mental health agencies were generally not a central part of the Medicaid policy-making process.

During the 1980s and 1990s state mental health agencies showed great creativity in developing ways of capturing more federal funds to pay for mental health care. Each new success added more funds to the public mental health care budget while state mental health policy makers surrendered ever more discretion over who would be served and with what services (Frank et al., 2003). The result was that state mental health agencies could exercise less and less stewardship over mental health care for the poor and disadvantaged in their states.

Beginning in the 1960s, the period of introduction of Medicare and Medicaid, the federal government also introduced and expanded federal social insurance programs—Supplemental Security Income (SSI) and Social Security Disability Insurance (SSDI) offer income supports for disabled populations.

The introduction of these programs complemented Medicaid's effects in facilitating the shift of people with mental illness to the community. But state welfare agencies administer SSI, following federal rules. The federal Social Security Administration has authority over SSDI, and the federal Center for Medicare and Medicaid Services (formerly the Health Care Financing Administration) administers Medicare. Thus, the shift toward these programs also led to the creation of a new set of bureaucracies that were lifelines for people with mental illness but had little understanding of the unique aspects of creating community-based care and support of people with severe mental illnesses. Overall, mental health policy associated with Medicare, Medicaid, SSI, and SSDI was largely the by-product of policy aimed at health and disability insurance generally.

The federal block grant to state mental health agencies is the only remaining federal source of discretionary funds to these agencies. The Substance Abuse and Mental Health Services Administration (SAMHSA) controls the block grant. SAMHSA's staff is made up of experts in mental health care and substance abuse treatment delivery. The advisory councils are populated by people representing specialty providers, state mental health agencies, the mental health professions (e.g., psychiatry, social work, and psychology), managed behavioral health care industry representatives, and academics with specialized expertise in mental health. It has expertise—but few resources.

NOTES

1. The statement in 1961 by the JCMIH offered a conclusion that has become a modern refrain: the therapeutic possibilities in mental health are far better than the outcomes actually realized. The failure of the mental health system to achieve its potential stems from barriers to accessing treatment and the inappropriate care of many who enter treatment (JCMIH, 1961; US DHHS, CMHS, 1999).
2. The CMHC grant mechanism was modified to pay for operating expenses for a limited time and for training of mental health workers.

References

Coffey, R. M., T. Mark, E. King, et al. 2000. *National Expenditures for Mental Health and Substance Abuse Treatment*, 1997. SAMHSA Publication SMA-00–3499. Rockville, Md.: Substance Abuse and Mental Health Services Administration.

Fein, R. 1958. *Economics of Mental Illness.* New York: Basic Books.

Frank, R. G., H. H. Goldman, and M. Hogan. 2003. Medicaid and mental health: Be careful what you ask for. *Health Affairs* 22(1):101–13.

Geller, J. L. 2000. The last half-century of psychiatric services as reflected in psychiatric services. *Psychiatric Services* 51(1):41–67.

Grob, G. 1994. *The Mad among Us: A History of the Care of America's Mentally Ill.* Cambridge: Harvard University Press.

Grob, G. 2001. Mental health policy in twentieth-century America. In U.S. Department of Health and Human Services, Center for Mental Health Services, *Mental Health, United States, 2000*, ed. R. W. Manderscheid and M. J. Henderson. DHHS Publication (SMA) 01–3537. Rockville, Md.: Substance Abuse and Mental Health Services Administration, Center for Mental Health Services, 3–14.

Kramer, M. 1977. *Psychiatric Services and the Changing Institutional Scene*, 1950–1985. DHEW Publication (ADM) 77–483. Rockville, Md.: Alcohol, Drug Abuse and Mental Health Administration.

Mark, T. R., R. Coffey, R. Vandivort-Warren, et al. 2005. U.S. spending for mental health and substance abuse treatment, 1991–2001. *Health Affairs* (Web exclusive) W5:133–42.

Rosenbach, M. L., and C. J. Ammering. 1997. Trends in part B mental health utilization and expenditures, 1987–1992. *HCFA Review* 19(3):19–42.

U.S. President's Commission on Mental Health. 1978b. *Task Panel Reports*, vol. 2. Washington, D.C.: U.S. Government Printing Office.

42

Hopper, K. (2007). Rethinking social recovery in schizophrenia: What a capabilities approach might offer. *Social Science and Medicine*, 65(5), 868–879

Kim Hopper's article begins with a sympathetic but sober assessment of the recovery movement: strong on rhetoric with its message of hope and weak on evidence of its impact on the lives of persons with serious mental illnesses. He then takes up the question of whether recovery can serve both rhetorical and practical functions. Advocates and researchers have looked outside the confines of public mental health in the past—to the disability and civil rights movements, for example—for inspirations and models. Hopper looks to economics and Amartya Sen's capabilities theory. "[I]nstead of satisfaction or utility or some package of 'primary goods,' Sen proposes that we consider *not* resources but rather *the valued things people are able to do or to be* as a result of having them—the *capabilities* they command." (874) Training in hydroelectric engineering, for example, is a capability only if there are hydroelectric plants around and a shortage of people to run them. Capabilities theory goes beyond matching skills to local needs, however, to include the development of choices and capacities that may be exercised by persons—poor, marginalized, or otherwise spoken *for*—to influence local choices about how commitments that affect them and resources they need are made and allocated, respectively. The capabilities approach, Hopper argues, may be applied to the substantive unfreedoms of persons with mental illness who are not thriving in, or integrated as full members of, their communities, and may be a tool for enhancing the impact of the recovery movement. "Like poverty," he writes, "disability can be recast as capabilities deprivation because it interferes with a person's ability to make valued choices and participate fully in society." (874) If the person's impairment is his or her mental illness, then disability is its "social reception and consequence," (874) and mental health reform must address both. Dr. Hopper has written a brief piece for this volume, preceding his article, to elucidate further some aspects of capabilities theory as applied to persons with serious mental illnesses.

Sen's Capabilities Approach: Some Axioms and Implications

Given:

- a substantive freedoms approach to human flourishing that places a huge emphasis on *agency* (the exercise of self-determination) and, in consequence, casts a critical eye on development or social assistance programs that target well-being but ignore or impair agency;
- coupled with a sustained concern with *context*: the material goods and social machinery that equips people to *convert* resources and rules into real opportunities;
- a working hypothesis that among the lasting effects of deprivation is its toll on one's "moral self" – specifically, the slowly acquired conviction that limitations are fated if not just, and that hope adjusted downward is the better part of aspiration ventured;
- a specific focus on one's ability to plan a life and participate fully in valued social/civic activities – including a claim to the "social bases of self-respect" that underwrite one's commitment to both planning and participation;
- explicit recognition of the tension between an assured but other-defined well-being and the riskier road to fulfillment that one maps on one's own, if haltingly, through mishaps and instructive failures;
- an implication that fully fledged agency goes beyond the modest sense of intentional action to embrace a *reflective* component – or what might be called "critical agency;"

Therefore:

- any assay of local ledgers of injustice must include both material and symbolic forms of deprivation and devaluation
- assisted development schemes should be judged by how well they enlarge the actual field of valued options in an ordinary life – *and* the process by which they accomplish this.

Added note: Drawing on Sen's work, Appadurai (2004) invites us to re-imagine culture – not simply as providing a storehouse of tradition but as equipping its members to face a future. His concern is with constraints on members' ability to exercise (and thus develop) what he sees as a life-planning (or "navigational") capability. Young people learn about real possibilities in life by trial and error. Sen's locally valued "beings and doings" become real options in one's own life by trying them out and seeing how they fit. (In so doing, the early tracks of life "commitments" may be laid down.) The trick is to minimize the long-term costs of what prove to be poor fits or bad choices. Sometimes the buffers are temporal: horrific summer jobs teach as urgently as they do precisely because one knows they won't last; the risks run are time-limited and subject to self-initiated renewal (after a 9-month period of thinking it over and weighing other options). In contrast: dropping out of high school is difficult to compensate for precisely because the passage is normative and so tightly bound with age-mates and adolescent routine. Household resources and social capital may also play critical roles in salvaging some mistakes; a wasted semester is much tougher to justify when family resources (or financial aid) are in scarce supply. This vision of productive adolescent passage combines hard knocks and soft landings. Brief apprenticeships with bail-out clauses, such ventures are rehearsals for the real thing that both preserve the option of other alternatives and equip one to explore them in a more informed manner.

That last point is worth underscoring with respect to recovery in mental health. It's not just that trial runs or test drives teach one something about how the world works and one's provisional place in it; *they also inform choice*. Over time, the cumulative experience from such ventures equips one with "the kind of judgment that arises only from experience; hunches rather than rules." A sense of both of what's "out there" and what really matters inform (what Appadurai calls) the "capacity to aspire." It's a sense as critically shaped by ruling out options as it is by gaining glimpses of possibilities to be further explored. In ways both unexpected and brusque, even lousy summer jobs can enrich one's own peculiar project of "values clarification."

Rethinking social recovery in schizophrenia: What a capabilities approach might offer

Abstract

Resurgent hopes for recovery from schizophrenia in the late 1980s had less to do with fresh empirical evidence than with focused political agitation. Recovery's promise was transformative: reworking traditional power relationships, conferring distinctive expertise on service users, rewriting the mandate of public mental health systems. Its institutional imprint has been considerably weaker. This article takes sympathetic measure of that outcome and provides an alternative framework for what recovery might mean, one drawn from disability studies and Sen's capabilities approach. By re-enfranchising agency, redressing material and symbolic disadvantage, raising the bar on fundamental entitlements and claiming institutional support for complex competencies, a capabilities approach could convert flaccid doctrine into useful guidelines and tools for public mental health.
Published by Elsevier Ltd.

Keywords: Recovery; Schizophrenia; Capabilities; Disability; Public mental health; USA

Introduction

Ambiguity about core values, operational principles, and organizational goals has its strategic uses, among them the formation of unlikely coalitions in pursuit of structural change. Such amalgams have figured critically in the annals of mental health reform, though the roles of specific groups or external constraints remain disputed and the verdict of history mixed (compare Scull, 1976, with Grob, 1991). Institutional reform inevitably involves a reckoning, a sorting out of competing versions of allegedly shared assumptions, and their selective translation into practice and policy. "Working misunderstandings" can carry a merry band of reformers only so far before political realities step in to call the question and tally the bill.

This article takes stock of the institutional imprint of "recovery" from severe psychiatric disability in US public mental health, and does so from an applied anthropological stance. This may surprise some. Anthropologists are best known for bringing a spoiler's sensibility to their reading of psychiatric procedure, dusting for cultural fingerprints on the suspect premises of clinical practice—like discerning traces of "governmentality" where others see therapy or empowerment (Joseph, 2002; Rose, 1999). A second, lesser-known tradition claims the same ancestry but applies a rather different sensibility. Its proponents (initially Estroff, 1981) tend to portray contemporary community psychiatry as unusually hard repair work in socially suspect precincts (Hopper, 2006; Luhrmann, 2000; Rhodes, 1991, 2004; Robins, 2001; Ware, Lachicotte, Kirschner, Cortes, & Good, 2000), work that has pointedly moral overtones. This inquiry hails from that latter school. It accepts the reality of schizophrenia as ethnographic fact—local, consequential, contested—and asks how its social fortunes may have shifted in response to what looked like an ideological uprising.

Social Recovery in Schizophrenia

The Empirical Record

The enigma of recovery in schizophrenia is partly a confusion of tongues. From the earliest days of clinical tracking, the orthodox view of progressive deterioration was harried by reports (sometimes bewildered) of apparent recovery. Its chief proponent, Emil Kraepelin, was widely cited as documenting a "real improvement" rate of 26%, half of whom showed complete recovery (Hinsie, 1931). Early in 20th century, Eugen Bleuler cautioned that most "end-states" escaped clinical inspection; still, he thought "improvement" to be the modal outcome and favored Kraepelin's phrase "cure with defect" (or "healing with scarring"). Such people could be considered "healthy," if eccentric or moody; but they had purchased provisional stability by "lower[ing] the level of aspirations with regard to their accomplishments and claims on the world" (Bleuler, 1911, p. 163). In the US, Strecker and Willey reported 20% recovery in patients treated in a private hospital. Queried by colleagues about "scarring," they clarified: this rate referred to "adjustment at a social level ... [patients were] getting along quite well in simple life situations." They stressed the capacity of those patients—all of whom were women—to do "important work," child-rearing and household management, in unprotected environments (Strecker & Willey, 1928, pp. 428–430).

Those results were soon favorably cited by a research psychiatrist wryly noting the "established fact" that recovery occurred among patients in "large, over-crowded State hospitals ... [where] no therapeutic measures have been applied, at least wittingly" (Hinsie, 1931, p. 216). Echoing Bleuler, he admitted how little psychiatry knew about recovery outside hospitals; to call it "spontaneous" was simply a "shield" for ignorance. Hinsie's honest appraisal of long-term evaluation was an admission of hitting a brick wall. Fortuitously, field studies of mental illness were just then getting under way in Europe (Hammer & Leacock, 1961). Better understanding of this tantalizing, if still mysterious, prospect of restored functioning would await their results, as well as those of long-term clinical research.

Social recovery's most prominent champion would prove to be Bleuler's son, Manfred, whose magisterial account of the natural history of schizophrenia appeared in 1974. His research took him outside the hospital walls, engaging him in the daily lives of those he treated. In his view, the course of schizophrenia usually tended upwards after 5 years, and potential for improvement was stubbornly apparent in even "very chronic" patients decades after onset. Most did well *without* ongoing medication or social assistance. Still, the therapist was hardly a disinterested bystander: "an open heart and an alert mind," Bleuler counseled, could counter the "resignation and despair" that so often seemed to attend prolonged work with such patients (Bleuler, 1974, p. 253).

Bleuler's enthusiasm was unusual, but his results were not. "Social recovery" proved common enough outside the hospital, when measured by independent living and gainful employment (e.g., Walker and Frost's "social restoration score," 1969). In the 1970s,

Strauss and Carpenter's findings from the WHO International Pilot Study of Schizophrenia (Strauss & Carpenter, 1972, 1974, 1977) put the relative autonomy of distinct domains of functioning on firm empirical footing. Subsequent studies have reinforced the point: whatever their reciprocal interplay might be, the clinical and social courses of schizophrenia need not proceed in lockstep. "Premorbid" competencies are reasonable guides to post-illness performance.

Time, too, has healing power, as Bleuler had shown. Arguably the most persuasive evidence for the long-term prospects of recovery was Harding and colleagues' study of state hospital patients in Vermont (Harding, Brooks, Ashikaga, Strauss, & Breier, 1987a, 1987b). After 36 years in the community, outcome for between one-half and two-thirds of these subjects was "neither downward nor marginal, but an evolution into various degrees of productivity, social involvement, wellness, and competent functioning" (Harding et al., 1987b, p. 730). Even that scrupulous qualifier ("various degrees") can't mask the optimism. And while the yield of later studies has been mixed, by no means have these bracing results—with their promise of "slow, uphill returns to health" (Harding, Zubin, & Strauss, 1992, p. 34)—been overturned.

Such findings resonate with lessons from cross-cultural psychiatric epidemiology (Hopper, 1991, 2003; Kleinman, 1988). Warner's exhaustive appraisal of political economy's role (Warner, 1994) is instructive. The under-appreciated key to this sprawling literature, he argues, is the degree to which social demand accommodates the returning patient and facilitates recovery. Where locally valued positions are available to members impaired by psychiatric disorder, re-integration is assured and the subsequent course of illness more favorable. Scarcity makes collaborative social arrangements likely and these, in turn, can reap therapeutic benefits; chronic sick roles, by contrast, can inadvertently cripple. Opportunities for "appropriate levels of functioning" occur both as a matter of course in traditional subsistence economies and, erratically, in tight labor markets (rebuilding postwar Europe, harvest times in agricultural communities). Where they do, "disability and deterioration" are averted (Warner, 1994, p. 158).

This brief review cannot do justice to the full range of contemporary inquiry or the increasingly sophisticated instruments used to assess disability's impact in everyday life. (Questions of identity, the drag of indwelling stigma, struggles to rebuild a functional self, for example, have not been touched upon.) But it suffices to identify a persisting tension in the enigma of social recovery. On the one hand, psychiatric observers have long noted those adaptive responses, the lowered aspirations and muted claims, which can serve to reconcile the wounded patient to a life of flattened prospects, colorless routine and modest achievement. On the other, the slow crawl of empirical research has underscored the striking difference that social demand, accommodating surrounds, and time can make for enhanced capacity and demonstrated competence. *Some of the confusion surrounding social recovery stems from the fact that both versions of reintegration—"good enough" under ordinary conditions, effectively normal in reach and performance where unusual circumstances obtain—have been marketed as reason for hope.*

The one pays tribute to human resilience; the other, to targeted investments that can substantially enhance such resilience—to undertaking the necessary social work of accommodation to expand real opportunities.

Recovery as Therapeutic Project

"Healing with scarring" has proven a durable trope. Present-day arguments and commentaries have unfolded in a recovery literature of unwieldy breadth (existential dispatch, case history, field report, empirical study), bearing the urgency of an idea whose time has come, the imprint of storied accounts of ordeal, and well-earned skepticism of mental health systems. If a provisional consensus may be hazarded, it would read something like this: recovery is difficult, idiosyncratic, and requires faith—but it is possible (e.g., Deegan, 1988, 2003; Mueser et al., 2002; Ralph, 2000). In making such a case, four themes prevail. Tracing them out yields—if not a formal definition of recovery—then something approximating its meaning in use.

1. *Renewing a sense of possibility*: Serious illness disrupts and unsettles, leaching hope from the future, and installing foreboding in its stead. Stigma, internalized and reinforced by an array of subtle cultural cues, compounds this uncertainty with shame, coupled with fears of distancing and rejection. A first task, then, would seem to be countering that stock of attitudes and beliefs about "craziness" that has been unobtrusively threaded throughout the scaffolding of common sense and conduct of everyday life. A second, hard on its heels, is to take stock of the awful indeterminacy of psychiatric diagnosis, and all that it leaves unsaid. Cure may not apply, but an unordinary life limned with possibility is a reasonable hope. Embodied representatives lend credibility to the claim: people who have themselves gone into maw of psychosis and emerged intact, if not unscathed.[1]

2. *Regaining competencies*: Lingering symptoms or disabilities notwithstanding, effective engagement in culturally valued (or normalized) activities is essential. Chronic sick roles disable by definition and design, encouraging one to find a place in the segregated company of like-damaged others. Contesting membership there, aspiring to more than "programmatic citizenship" (Rowe, 1999), means demonstrating the social skills and presence that mark one as "mainstream" (or fitting in somewhere socially reputable). These involve symptom management, social interaction, remedial schooling or higher education and work in some fashion. For some, acquiring the requisite skills will mean redressing a developmental gap in their biographies, typically at the transition to adulthood, when the tracks of mature social competence are laid down (later onset of schizophrenia tends to be associated with better outcome, attesting in part to being able to build upon established competencies when wrestling with post-illness identity issues).

3. *Reconnecting and finding a place in society*: Social integration may be an elusive target in research and evaluation, but its centrality to recovery is clear. Reconnecting can be tentative and halting; it can be collective and advocacy-oriented; it can be the quiet work of fitting in and getting it together. It may mean taking part in organized efforts to build contrived communities, or setting oneself to the still poorly understood tasks of building family and household. However actualized, it means constructing ways of belonging and reclaiming moral agency (Ware, Hopper, Tugenberg, Dickey, & Fisher, 2007).

4. *Reconciliation work*: The disruptions occasioned by severe disorder wreak havoc with sense of self and career. Repairing this damage requires a good deal of identity work (Snow & Anderson, 1987). This ranges from the delicate, sometimes achingly slow work of rebuilding a functional self—a person apart from the reality of illness—to determined action to deny stigma a destructive power in one's own life. For some, a persisting sense of casualty does daily battle with a struggling one of agency. For others, the transformation is spiritual. Like Jacob, having wrestled nightlong with the angel, the sufferer emerges marked (Jacob limped henceforth) but remade in the process (Clay, 1994).

---

[1] See the website of National Empowerment Center: http://www.power2u. org/recovery.

Equally telling is what's missing from such accounts—structure, first and foremost. Race, gender and class tend to fade away into unexamined background realities, underscoring (intentionally? inadvertently?) the defining centrality of psychiatric disability in these lives. Material deprivation is largely ignored, though poverty and shabby housing bulk large in the lives of many persons with severe mental illness. Vital contextual features—the enabling resources, rules and connections that make prized prospects like a decent job feasible—are either disregarded or casually remarked, as though their provision were unproblematic or of lesser concern to individual reclamation projects.[2] The formal service system comes in for mixed review—maligned by some, thanked by others, with insufficient attention to what (other than attitude) needs to change. Community living is taken as a given, despite the continuing presence of institutional equivalents—great hulking arks of the segregated dispossessed—that have yet to be dismantled. Reformist tools central to the cause of social justice in other walks of American life—litigation[3] and civil rights—are curiously absent here, as though the relevant politics were personal and an organized adversarial posture unnecessary. Nor is there much talk of the moral economy of care, that stock of founding commitments and once-inviolate norms that is easily eroded or remade in an era when "the movements of patients … have become the stuff of which markets are made" (Lewis, Shadish, & Lurigio, 1989, p. 178).

To speak of a "model" of recovery is thus misleading. Movements are not peer-reviewed. Mobilizing committed forces means hoisting rallying cries at odds with one another, tamping down potentially divisive demands, and capitalizing on working misunderstandings. In making the case against therapeutic nihilism, rethinking services, and embracing patients as active agents in their own recuperation, this inclusive approach served well, making common cause of potentially discordant constituencies. But the same medley of affirmation, reckless hope and wide appeal made for later difficulties when converting emancipating creed into actionable policy.

Paradigm Lost? Recovery's Institutional Career to Date

It is not too much to say that in the late 1980s and early 1990s, a nascent social insurrection seemed in the works. Its manifesto—that something resembling a full life after severe mental illness was possible and that public mental health systems should be held accountable to that high standard—fired the imagination of discontented and excluded users (and once-were-users) of public mental health systems. Retribution and reformation seemed credibly in the offing. Those were giddy times, as the welter of what passed for "evidence" in support of the cause of recovery well attests. Case study, demonstration project, empirical research, practice guidelines, memoir and broadsheet—all were pressed into service as claims-making vehicles (Spector & Kitsuse, 1987), circulated as founding texts. So long as the demand was to be taken seriously as a legitimate alternative to business-as-usual, such diversity was welcome; the genre-spanning rhetoric seemed emblematic of a new regime of inclusion.

But the ground shifts and the game changes when prototype goes up against the demands of mass production. The prospect of institutional uptake forced up all those awkward

---

[2]The "few essentials" [sic] listed with brisk efficiency in the recent report of the President's New Freedom Commission on Mental Health (2003, p. 9)—access to health care, work opportunities, affordable housing, and freedom from unjust confinement—appear as mere sidebars, customary provisions to picked up along the way, even as the public system charged with ensuring them is characterized as "in shambles" (Hogan, 2002).

[3]The ADA has not figured prominently in this story. When it does, substantial "justice disparities" appear in its enforcement of claims filed for psychiatric disability (Swanson, Burris, Moss, Ullman, & Ranney, 2006).

questions of specification, fidelity criteria, costs, accountability and regulation that a moral campaign is free to ignore. In the event, a few brave and vital exceptions notwithstanding, system transformation faltered. The hybrid vigor that had sustained a movement failed in substantial measure to inform a program. What had begun variously as a "guiding vision" (Anthony, 1993), an empirical corrective to the "clinician's illusion" of inevitable decline (Harding et al., 1992), a cry of protest (Chamberlin, 1979) and a plea for a "positive culture of healing" (Fisher, 1993), too often devolved in practice into a grab-bag of "assumptions, principles and goals, a set of ideas that were differently interpretable" (Jacobson, 2004). Recovery had become a floating signifier: it all depended, Jacobson shrewdly observed, on the specific problems its various proponents expect it to solve. Wisconsin's (unfinished) story is a case in point.

Recovery and Bureaucracy: One State's Story

In Jacobson's scrupulously detailed account (Jacobson, 2004), Wisconsin committed itself to restructuring its mental health system on what were then vague but enticing principles of recovery in 1996. A remarkable train of events followed: endless rounds of deliberation, argument, planning, design; workgroups, facilitated discussions, draft upon draft of models and guidelines, community meetings and retreats—all pursued in a spirit of inclusiveness and respect. If the recovery movement insisted that experience with the system conferred its own expertise, then a recovery-premised planning process would recognize and build upon that proficiency. This meant that the process would have to rework traditional power relationships that system users had long complained about. Disputes over meaning notwithstanding, participants agreed that recovery had to be installed and tracked at three levels—individual, system and societal.

So what, 8 years and counting, has been the impact on everyday lives and practices? Jacobson's closing field dispatch suggests that progress has been uneven. A "Recovery Workgroup" was reconstituted as a standing advisory board and its hard-won expertise extended. A homegrown model of recovery has been adopted as the official premise of the mental health system. Tools and resources to promote consciousness-raising and self-directed change have been widely disseminated, including a superb workbook and a "guided reflection" exercise that enables agencies to take stock of their own recovery-informed progress. Statewide user advocacy for system-change is thriving and weary champions of recovery now invoke the endorsement of a Presidential Commission. But the "work of specification" *(which* meaning of recovery, geared to what problems, at what levels?), so tricky in the planning phase, has proven harder still in implementation. Demonstration programs are under way in several locales, but their impact will be difficult to assess absent well-positioned research. Financing and reimbursement have been largely shuttered from the contentious recovery debates and "experience as expertise" has had no voice there. The upshot: after nearly a decade of work, wholesale system transformation is still pending. While "change is happening, most of it is still dependent on the work of committed individuals." Recovery remains a cadre enterprise, not yet "institutionalized [as] part of the warp and woof of everyday practice and policy" (Jacobson, 2004, pp. 129–130).

Least well reckoned were the barriers to implementing recovery statewide. Simple inertia translated into routine delay rather than outright opposition. Some providers proclaimed recovery old news and themselves seasoned converts, only to prove holdouts instead, deaf to all the new regime implied about radically restructured treatment relationships. (Local agents of change took this in stride and redeployed to focus on practice and guideline, rather than "attitude change.") Routine policy changes made in other sectors, without knowledge of or concern for principles of recovery, continue to rock settled assumptions and mundane realities mental health partisans. In a world in which services are increasingly provided on a de facto basis—involving venues, actors, rules and considerations unfamiliar with recovery and beholden to other interests—such uncontrolled externalities multiply, introducing further uncertainty. Structurally this means that the pragmatics of reform are inescapably bound up with developments elsewhere. The mental health system's warrant for attending to, let alone orchestrating, such developments is unclear. What was true of recovery narratives (avoidance of rude quotidian realities) is no less true of state plans.

The Politics of Recovery

Reform is hard and the story far from over. Too harsh a judgment of recovery's prospects may be premature. Wisconsin's unfinished project, and other smaller efforts in social experimentation, not only exemplify what can be done but also serve as standing reminders to mental health authorities of just how low their sights are set. Even skeptics are hard put to ignore the real if limited change afoot in some mental health systems and the difference it can make for care options (Floersch, 2002; Jacobson & Curtis, 2000). User-run alternatives and technical assistance, affirmative enterprises, research-based claims of drug-free recovery, quasi-legal measures (advance directives) for safeguarding autonomy in anticipation of future breakdown, gutsy forays into the messy particulars of negotiated treatment, and supported employment should all be inventoried. Weedy thickets of protest, mutual aid, misinformation and solidarity thrive in the still largely unsurveyed provinces of the Internet.

That said, any tour of public mental health services finds much that feels familiar. In well-advertised quarters of system reform, places of business once infiltrated by unruly advocates of a democratized community-based care, the absence of change (or its channeling into safer avenues) is unmistakable (Stocks, 1995). Where confrontation was once recognized as a necessary part of continuing the dialog (Blanch, Fisher, Tucker, Walsh, & Chassman, 1993), a blasé been-there-done-that now prevails. Some states opt for the simulacra of reform: "renaming" old programs suffices to forestall more fundamental questions of power-sharing and responsibility (Jacobson & Curtis 2000, p. 335). Recovery may be the new vernacular, self-help embraced as its "empowering" lay practice, and the message of hope communicated with the anonymous economy of a Hallmark card, but for many (the majority?) persons served by public mental health systems, it remains an irrelevancy. If years of arduous collective work have culminated in a newfound appreciation for self-help, a patchwork of provisional demonstrations, and a slew of promissory slogans, then what, one may be moved to wonder, was all the fuss about? Surely proponents of that long-sought "positive culture of healing" had something more substantial, however inchoate, in mind.

It is difficult to escape the conclusion that operational specificity was unwisely sacrificed in the interest of more efficiently spreading the good news. The movement's watchwords—voice, authenticity, process, settling old scores and filing fresh grievances—proved ill-matched to the grind of institutional sway and regulatory reform. Recovery had merit, morals and the tempered weight of science behind it and so it sashayed into political battle unarmed. An argument for cost-savings was never joined because (one suspects) it could not competently be made. (If the whole point of individualized, needs-and-aspirations-based care is to ratchet up demands as fresh competencies are acquired, it is far from clear that this will be cheaper in the bargain.) Dealing with barriers at street-level bureaucracies was an afterthought (Corrigan et al., 2003). Political timeframes are rudely unaccommodating: state politics are played within close temporal horizons, and the structural reforms implicit in any serious recovery project are substantial and far-reaching. Elections remove critical personnel, realign priorities and leave half-measures to wilt. One administration's bold stroke proves the next one's unwanted legacy. In the process, recovery is easily orphaned.

To say what recovery could mean practically requires an approach that can inform social demands, not dismiss them as foregone accomplishments. It will need to be alert to shaping pressures and possibilities of context even as it recognizes the critical role of advocates. It will have to attend not only to loud requests for "evidence -based" practices but to quiet signs of the demoralizing impact of persistent poverty. It will have to balance claims for agency-enhancing empowerment with demands for system-level reforms. And it should equip us to critically assess that durable tension in recovery's legacy—as evident in patch-worked clinical histories as in rigorous research—the tension between what seemed obscurely possible for the few and what patently sufficed for the many.

Taking Agency Seriously: The Capabilities Approach

An unavoidably moral enterprise, distrustful of experts, concerned with human flourishing, invested in choice but suspicious of plainly self-limiting ones, deeply social in outlook, political by default: these same concerns have driven a parallel movement in global development studies—the capabilities approach. This approach not only ratifies the idea that impairment's standing and impact are socially brokered, but also heeds advocates' calls for respect.

Capabilities emerged as an alternative to utilitarian (resource- or income-based) approaches to human welfare, chiefly through the work of Amartya Sen (Nussbaum, 2000, 2004, 2006; Nussbaum & Sen, 1993; Sen, 1980, 1985, 1992, 1993, 2000). Its originality lies in how it redefines "necessities" and sets the standard by which we measure quality of life or well-being. Instead of satisfaction or utility or some package of "primary goods," Sen proposes that we consider *not* resources but rather *the valued things people are able to do or to be* as a result of having them—the *capabilities* they command. Actual welfare depends less on what I own or have access to than the real opportunities open to me as a result. Because circumstance and need complicate the conversion of goods into opportunities, what people can actually achieve with resources at their disposal will vary with socially recognized diversity, including disability. The nutritional needs of a pregnant woman, like the transportation needs of someone crippled, demand different inputs if equivalent ends (healthy pregnancy, mobility) are to be obtained. Custom complicates matters further: to be a literate women where there are libraries is of little use if gender confines you to the home; casual ridicule on the job can so poison the workplace that even a capable (but visibly "disabled") employee may settle for a disability check instead.

Like poverty, disability can be recast as capabilities deprivation because it interferes with a person's ability to make valued choices and participate fully in society. Social judgments determine whether that deprivation is thought fair, necessary or remediable.Following WHO's lead, interference may be conceived as occurring in two stages (Burchardt, 2004; Mitra, 2006): at the level of the original impairment (here, psychiatric disorder) and at the level of disability (its social reception and consequences). Fully corrective measures must tackle both. Assistive technologies (drugs, rehabilitation, illness management skills—e.g., cognitive techniques to handle voices) can upgrade ability and lower impairment. But success in addressing disability depends upon whether enhanced capacity can then be converted to valued social roles and activities. Training may make someone work-ready, but to convert that into employment requires jobs and willing employers. Social technologies (supported employment, job coaching, affirmative enterprises) can modify environments and ease that opportunity gradient.

Capabilities are substantive freedoms, the potential to do or to be something that is social valued. In practice, they should be distinguished from how they are actually exercised or realized in specific "functionings." This agent-centered approach places a premium on the deliberative process. *What one chooses is less important than the range of valued options actually entertained, developmentally available and socially sanctioned.* In assessing whether capability has expanded, evidence that one can realistically engage in informed and competent consideration of locally valued alternatives is more important than any particular path selected. Such a posture, meant to ensure respect for both cultural context and moral agency, contains an instructive tension. Eying custom critically, it seeks out suppressed discontent and invites people to question received roles and life courses. It prizes choice but makes unexamined commitments problematic.

Taking capabilities seriously means creating imaginative space where other-than-conventionally prescribed possibilities might be glimpsed. Disability offers a test case.

Social Response to Disabling Difference

Disabilities studies (Albrecht, Seelman, & Bury, 2001) begin from the premise that the social meanings and practical impact of "disorders" are selective local readings of and responses to perceived *differences*—differences that are without social import until they are ranked and responded to. (Consider what passes for prized possessions and enviable traits across cultures, classes and castes.)

Disability is one demarcation among many that embodies this social logic. Impairment is converted into (its social phenotype) disability in the same way and with the same apparent "naturalness" (and, in some cases, stigma), as other culturally recognized differences become distinctions of consequence. We may speak of accidents of birth, quirks of fate, or mishaps of nature; but those accidents, quirks and mishaps become real for us only as they are converted into social markers of esteem or disrepute. *Inquiry into the logic of such transformations, the suppressed assumptions about moral worth and limited capacity at stake, links disability studies to the capabilities approach.* Both see this undeclared social conversion process, which transforms injuries of body and mind into locally salient distinctions, as having practical consequences (discrimination) and emotional impact (shame). For both, the indetermi-nacies of that process hold the key to social change.

If disability's social reality—the viable identities and real prospects available to afflicted persons—is determined as much by the rules and resources applied to difference as by any underlying impairment, then restoration and repair become social projects not merely treatment regimens. They require interventions into common meaning-making as well as material provisions of housing and work. Such socio-cultural accommodations enlarge the realm of the possible and transform the meaning of injury.

A capabilities-informed "social recovery" will speak to citizenship as well as health. It will worry about what enables people to thrive, not simply survive. It will explore the tensions between evidence-based prescriptions for restoring well-being and the untidy ambiguities of self-directedness, with its halting, trial-and-error ways. It will critically review past experiences and unexamined assumptions that set the invisible standards against which subjective and objective measures of quality of life are taken. In seeking to come to terms with their own history, ex-patients working together can make recovery a collective project as well as existential ordeal. Institutionally, that project becomes seeing putatively damaged people as preemptively constrained moral agents. The terms and conditions of their release, restoration and livelihood—and the resources needed to assist in that effort—become newly contestable. Recovery asks not what such people should be content with but what they should be capable of, and how that might be best achieved and sustained.

The capabilities approach (CA) provides a robust and dynamic framework for undertaking such rethinking. It supplies a model of human flourishing that encompasses primary goods (material and cultural necessities) as well as more complex competencies (the exercise of practical reason and social connectedness) and representations of worth. Asking how disabling differences translate into durable inequities, it bridges material and socio-cultural registers of disadvantage (Olson, 2001; Robeyns, 2003).

Towards a Capabilities-Informed Agenda

Capabilities rework recovery not from within (where it remains hostage to a rhetoric of suffering), but from without (informed by an idiom of opportunity). *Not healing but equality becomes the operant trope.* This has both participatory and substantive meaning. *How* essential goods and services are distributed can be as consequential as their approximation of equity (Anderson, 1999; Hopper, 2006). This arms us to address both immediate grievances—experiences of humiliation and shame that are central aspects of patienthood's stigma and hierarchy—and long-term prospects for growth and development. Rawls' "social bases of self-respect" is an essential capability, not because people ought to behave decently toward one another but because cultural equivalents of Adam Smith's "linen shirt" (accessories that allow one to appear "creditably" in public without shame) are vital to the social self.[4] Institutionalized disrespect compounds the suffering of those already reeling from psychosis and needs addressing. But for distress to be quelled, capacity instilled, aspiration fueled, real opportunities expanded and the floor of social expectation lifted, more than kindly attitude and respectful posture will be needed. Targeted resources and orchestrated support will necessitate active state involvement.

CA reaches beyond basic needs in prizing agency and deliberation as formative goods. Real opportunities for exercising self-determination and making informed life-changing commitments become paramount. Politically, especially with respect to socially excluded persons, this translates as: "how the realm of the possible is created and how it shapes public decisions about what is desirable" (Weir 1992, p. xiii). How might CA transform our sense of what's possible and re-configure public mental health services?

Linking Capabilities to Recovery

Like recovery, CA is radically underspecified, but not for want of trying. CA is incomplete for reasons of basic principle (Sen, 2004) as well as technical difficulties of operationalizing it in practice (Robeyns, 2006). Any application of capabilities must therefore first define/defend a (full or partial) list of valued functionings (e.g., Nussbaum, 2000), or specify a process for identifying/weighting them (Alkire, 2002), and then devise provisional means for assessing real opportunities for achieving them (capabilities proper). For some purposes, measuring achieved functionings rather than capabilities suffices. (The UN's Human Development Index combines school enrollment, adult literacy, life expectancy

---

[4]Technically, as Nussbaum has recently noted (Nussbaum, 2006, p. 172), this would seem to make them functionings in principle: we do not want to leave open the choice of trading the social bases of self-respect for some other good—of voluntarily enslaving oneself, for example, in exchange for material security. But see comments regarding "dignity of risk" in text.

and per capita GDP.) With respect to persons recovering from psychosis, this incompleteness is both telling and liberating. Because "outcome" expands to include what really matters to people, we need to undertake explorations of the (distinctive?) value palettes of excluded people. At the same time, at least for basic capabilities and using the imperfect tools at our disposal, we need to inventory what actual "valued beings and doings" are open to them. Constructive work of adding fresh voice and perspective proceeds along with documentation of day-to-day realities of disadvantage. Because the lifeways of these people are littered with "programs," we also need to assess the capabilities-enhancing potential of existing interventions.

Social participation is so central to the capabilities enterprise—for setting local priorities and, in the rough-and-tumble dialectic of public discussion, for clarifying valued commitments—that some define core capabilities as those required for responsible citizenship (Anderson, 1999). This is serviceable enough as a starting point for an *inventory of disadvantage* among persons recovering from psychosis. Set aside for the moment the always-arresting condition of "appearing in public without shame" and all that it betokens. We know little enough about the social texture of their everyday lives. How widespread are deficiencies in such elemental competencies and opportunities as functional literacy, access to information, mobility, engagement with others and debate? How often are their faculties of practical reason, for planning a life and making commitments, challenged by something other than a prescription or a program mandate? How commonplace the depredations of ordinary poverty and social isolation?

Exploring the possibly *distinctive value sets* of persons with heavy psychiatric histories is bound to be fraught. The recovery literature bristles with demands for redress of past injuries, injustices and neglect; reparation is a frequent theme. Beyond that, what stands out is the commonplace prayer for home, health, companionship, decent work and the regard of others—with two exceptions. The first is a fierce desire to restructure the contingencies of care for persons in psychiatric treatment; existing initiatives offer some venues for meaningful reform. The second, broached by intimations of the "spiritual," is the transformative power of psychosis itself; this is still largely uncharted territory of unknown promise. Likely a more common complication is the cumulative impact of confinement, steady regimens of surveillance, discrimination and exclusion. This can cripple imagination, investing collective action with like-historied others with potentially redemptive significance.

If persons with histories of psychosis are to participate in public deliberations, undertake the transformative labor of reworking cultural templates of disability, they will need *practice in voice and standing*. (Present-day advocates with their own histories are both exemplary and exceptional in this regard.) Some may require tailored interventions to deal with cognitive impairments. Ex-patients are painfully aware that the real markers of social competence are moral not technical—being recognized as someone who is trustworthy, accountable for her actions, tuned to reciprocity, a person of judgment and good character (Ware et al., 2007). To attain this, both common accoutrements (a job or schooling, decent dwelling, regular interaction, appropriate attire and bearing) and uncommon abilities (the whole repertoire of coping skills and illness-management rehearsed in the recovery literature) are needed. Routine services address few of these well, others unevenly, still others poorly or not at all. Shifting from structured programs to flexibly configured assistance in making a meaningful life that build on extramural collaborations (e.g., supported employment) will require major shifts in approach.

For ex-patients to take the further step, to speak out publicly about the casual slights and unthinking dismissals that veterans of psychosis endure, will require grace and courage—to say nothing of facility with language, self-confidence, humor and presence. Acquiring these will take collective action, training, rehearsal and organization, all of which have been nurtured (often against formidable odds) by organizations of ex-patients. Critical to such efforts is the exemplary power of "others-like-me" who have gone on to well-tempered lives. They should be affirmatively supported.

With respect to formal interventions, a capabilities-informed approach to recovery would stress *enhanced agency*—not public safety, stable placements or reliable program-participation. This means asking under what circumstances exercising reasoned choice should be prized over foreseeable bad consequences in one's life. Can a poor choice, assessed in terms of compromised well-being, be preferred if the foregone benefit could have been won only if imposed? Take social regard. CA endorses Smith's "linen shirt" principle because the esteem of others is essential to achieving self-respect. But so is freedom to put that security at risk (subjecting oneself, say, to ridicule or pity) in pursuit of demanding, potentially destabilizing endeavors. Symptom management is highly valued and avoiding stress is good coping strategy. But electing to try paid work, at risk of upsetting proven routine and established habits, may make sense if potential gains are thought sufficient. (Service-users sometimes call this being accorded "the dignity of risk.") Similarly, court-ordered treatment may circumvent the vicissitudes and uncertainties of negotiated care, but its uneven results are obtained by foreclosing other options. Alternatives to mandated treatment have been shown to be feasible, but require different institutional commitments. Shared decision-making and advance directives can be effective vehicles for enlisting practical reason to manage medications and psychiatric crises (Amering, Stastny, & Hopper, 2005; Hamann, Leucht, & Kissling, 2003), but their practical utility will hinge on coupling formal system endorsement with the necessary front-line resources of time, trained personnel, and logistical support (Thomas, 2003).

Three problems with applying CA should be mentioned. Choice remains problematic— both axiomatic and suspect. Deprivation and disgrace can so corrode one's self worth that aspiration can be distorted, initiative undercut and preferences deformed. Sensitive work will be needed to recover that suppressed sense of injustice and reclaim lost possibility. Second, CA-informed initiatives will not be free-standing or categorically funded. Because they compete with other social investments, what counts as "good enough" in this domain will raise contentious issues of equity. And last, power is both omnipresent and quiet throughout this discussion. CA explicitly avows direct participation in public deliberations about symbolic representations of and material support for excluded people. Abrasive relations with traditional decision-making processes are likely.

Conclusion

Seriously espoused, CA could reclaim recovery's checkered clinical history, reopen old puzzles, and milk their implications for contemporary practice. This means taking on the orphaned "work of specification" and transforming what is now a co-opted, near-toothless gospel of hope into workable guidelines and tools. Affirming human flourishing as the orienting aim of public mental health is foremost. Our metric of progress should be those locally valued commitments people are actually able to make in their everyday lives. A capabilities-informed mental health program endorses reflective deliberation while applying hard-won skepticism to the shibboleth of choice, especially when options are few and the heavy hand of past failure restricts them further. It rejects therapeutic individualism in favor of understanding persons as social beings embedded in networks of distinction and entitlement that reproduce broader material inequities and ratify rank orders of regard. It welcomes procedural fairness, but refuses to allow it to supplant the substantive freedoms available only through the exercise of agency. And it complements the rediscovery of patient power with a durable memory of how critical appropriate rules and resources are to its effective exercise.

In a word, it calls the system's bluff. If recovery is really the watchword of the new public mental health, it will need to contend with unconventional ways and means—both within the system and outside its usual bounds—needed to make it a practical reality. The political-economic task (resources) is difficult enough; the cultural one (real participation), plainly daunting. Implementing CA in practice will mean a willingness to follow the recursive lessons of capabilities through to completion. Recovery on *their* part presumes openness to re-inclusion on *ours*. And that, it seems safe to say, will require not only that we re-evaluate damaged selves but re-examine what it means to hold onto provisionally undamaged ones as well.

Acknowledgments

For critical comments on earlier drafts, I would like to thank Mary Jane Alexander, Barbara Dickey, Dan Fisher, Kris Jones, Sophie Mitra, Beth Shinn, Carole Siegel, Susanna Sussman, Toni Tugenberg, and Norma Ware. This work was supported by NIMH grants MH51359 and MH065247. In memory of Rob Barrett: psychiatrist, anthropologist, stalwart.

References

Albrecht, G. L., Seelman, K. D., & Bury, M. (2001). *Handbook of disabilities studies.* Thousand Oaks: Sage.

Alkire, S. (2002). *Valuing freedoms.* New York: Oxford.

Amering, M., Stastny, P., & Hopper, K. (2005). Psychiatric advance directives: Qualitative study of informed deliberations by mental health service users. *British Journal of Psychiatry, 186,* 247–252.

Anderson, E. S. (1999). What is the point of equality? *Ethics, 109,* 287–337.

Anthony, W. A. (1993). Recovery from mental illness: The guiding vision of the mental health system in the 1990s. *Psychosocial Rehabilitation Journal, 16,* 11.

Blanch, A. K., Fisher, D., Tucker, W., Walsh, D., & Chassman, J. (1993). Consumer-practitioners and psychiatrists share insights about recovery and coping. *Disability Studies Quarterly, 13,* 17–20.

Bleuler, E. (1911). *Dementia praecox, oder Gruppe der Schizo-phrenien.* Leipzig: Deuticke.

Bleuler, M. (1974). The long-term course of the schizophrenic psychoses. *Psychosocial Medicine, 4,* 244–254.

Burchardt, T. (2004). Capabilities and disability: The capabilities framework and the social model of disability. *Disability and Society, 19,* 735–751.

Chamberlin, J. (1979). *On our own.* New York: McGraw-Hill.

Clay, S. (1994). *Conference presentation: The work of recovery: Implications for psychiatry and research,* 17–18 October 1994, Ossining, NY.

Corrigan, P. W., Bodenshausen, G., Markowitz, F., Newman, L., Rasinski, K., & Watson, A. (2003). Demonstrating translational research for mental health services: An example from stigma research. *Mental Health Services Research, 5(2),* 79–88.

Deegan, G. (2003). Discovering recovery. *Psychiatric Rehabilitation Journal, 26(4),* 368–376.

Deegan, P. E. (1988). Recovery: The lived experience of rehabilitation. *Psychosocial Rehabilitation Journal, 11(1),* 11–19.

Estroff, S. (1981). *Making it crazy.* Berkeley: University of California Press.

Fisher, D. B. (1993). *Towards a positive culture of healing, in The DMH core curriculum: Consumer empowerment and recovery, part I.* Boston: Commonwealth of Massachusetts Department of Mental Health.

Floersch, J. E. (2002). *Meds, money, and manners.* New York: Columbia University Press.

Grob, G. G. (1991). *From asylum to community*. Princeton, NJ: Princeton University Press.

Hamann, J., Leucht, S., & Kissling, W. (2003). Shared decision-making in psychiatry. *Acta Psychiatrica Scandinavica, 107*, 403–409.

Hammer, M., & Leacock, E. (1961). Source material on the epidemiology of illness. In J. Zubin (Ed.), *Field studies in the mental disorders* (pp. 418–486). New York: Grune and Stratton.

Harding, C. M., Brooks, G. W., Ashikaga, T., Strauss, J. S., & Breier, A. (1987a). The Vermont longitudinal study of persons with severe mental illness, I: Methodology, study sample, and overall status 32 years later. *American Journal of Psychiatry, 144(6)*, 718–726.

Harding, C. M., Brooks, G. W., Ashikaga, T., Strauss, J. S., & Breier, A. (1987b). The Vermont longitudinal study of persons with severe mental illness, II: Long-term outcome of subjects who retrospectively met DSM-III criteria for schizophrenia. *American Journal of Psychiatry, 144(6)*, 727–735.

Harding, C. M., Zubin, J., & Strauss, J. S. (1992). Chronicity in schizophrenia: Revisited. *British Journal of Psychiatry, 161(Suppl 18)*, 27–37.

Hinsie, L. E. (1931). Criticism of treatment and recovery in schizophrenia. In *Proceedings of the Association for research in nervous and mental disease for 1928. Schizophrenia (dementia praecox)* (pp. 211–223). Baltimore: Williams and Wilkins.

Hogan, M. F. (2002). *Transmittal letter to the President*. Interim report of the President's New Freedom Commission on Mental Health.

Hopper, K. (1991). Some old questions for the new cross-cultural psychiatry. *Medical Anthropology Quarterly, 5*, 299–330.

Hopper, K. (2003). Interrogating culture in the WHO studies of schizophrenia. In R. Barrett, & J. Jenkins (Eds.), *The edge of experience: schizophrenia, culture, and subjectivity*. Cambridge: Cambridge University Press.

Hopper, K. (2006). Redistribution and its discontents. *Human Organization, 65*, 218–226.

Jacobson, N. (2004). *In recovery: The making of mental health policy*. Nashville: Vanderbilt University Press.

Jacobson, N., & Curtis, L. (2000). Recovery as policy in mental health services: Strategies, emerging from the States. *Psychiatric Rehabilitation Journal, 23(4)*, 333–341.

Joseph, M. (2002). *Against the romance of community*. Minneapolis: University of Minnesota Press.

Kleinman, A. (1988). *Rethinking psychiatry*. New York: The Free Press.

Lewis, D., Shadish, W., & Lurigio, A. (1989). Policies of inclusion and the mentally ill: Long-term care in a new environment. *Journal of Social Issues, 45*, 173–186.

Luhrmann, T. M. (2000). *Of two minds*. New York: Knopf.

Mitra, S. (2006). The capability approach and disability. *Journal of Disability Policy Studies, 16*, 236–247.

Mueser, K. T., Corrigan, P. W., Hilton, D. W., Tanzman, B., Schaub, A., Gingerich, S., et al. (2002). Illness management and recovery: A review of the research. *Psychiatric Services, 53(10)*, 1272–1284.

New Freedom Commission on Mental Health. (2003). *Achieving the promise: Transforming mental health care in America*. Final Report, DHHS Pub. No. SMA-03–3832, Rockville, MD.

Nussbaum, M. C. (2000). *Women and human development: The capabilities approach*. New York: Cambridge University Press.

Nussbaum, M. C. (2004). *Hiding from humanity*. Princeton: Princeton University Press.

Nussbaum, M. C. (2006). *Frontiers of justice*. Cambridge:Belknap Press.

Nussbaum, M. C., & Sen, A. (Eds.). (1993). *Quality of life*. New York: Oxford University Press.

Olson, K. (2001). Distributive justice and the politics of difference. *Critical Horizons, 2*, 5–32.

Ralph, R. O. (2000). *Review of recovery literature: A synthesis of a sample of recovery literature*. National Association of State Mental Health Program Directors and the National Technical Assistance Center for State Mental Health Planning.

Rhodes, L. (1991). *Emptying beds: The work of an emergency psychiatric unit*. Berkeley: University of California Press.

Rhodes, L. (2004). *Total confinement: Madness and reason in the maximum security prison.* Berkeley: University of California Press.

Robeyns, I. (2003). Is Nancy Fraser's critique of theories of distributive justice justified? *Constellations, 10,* 538–553.

Robeyns, I. (2006). The capability approach in practice. *Journal of Political Philosophy, 14,* 351–376.

Robins, C. S. (2001). Generating revenues: Fiscal changes in public mental health care and the emergence of moral conflicts among care-givers. *Culture, Medicine and Psychiatry, 25,* 457–466.

Rose, N. (1999). *Governing the soul.* London: Free Association Books.

Rowe, M. (1999). *Crossing the border.* Berkeley: University of California Press.

Scull, A. (1976). *Decarceration.* Englewood Cliffs: Prentice-Hall.

Sen, A. K. (1980). *Equality of what? Tanner lectures on human values.* Salt Lake City: University of Utah Press.

Sen, A. K. (1985). Well-being, agency and freedom. *Journal of Philosophy, 82,* 169–221.

Sen, A. (1992). *Inequality reexamined.* Oxford: Clarendon.

Sen, A. (1993). Capability and well-being. In M. C. Nussbaum, & A. Sen (Eds.), *The quality of life* (pp. 44–55). Oxford: Oxford University Press.

Sen, A. (2000). *Development as freedom.* New York: Anchor.

Sen, A. (2004). Capabilities, lists, and public reason. *Feminist Economics, 10(3),* 77–80.

Snow, D., & Anderson, L. (1987). Identity work among the homeless: The verbal construction and avowal of personal identities. *American Journal of Sociology, 92,* 1336–1371.

Spector, M., & Kitsuse, J. I. (1987). *Constructing social problems.* New York: Aldine de Gruyter.

Stocks, M. L. (1995). In the eye of the beholder. *Psychiatric Rehabilitation Journal, 19,* 89–91.

Strauss, J. S., & Carpenter, W. T. (1972). Prediction of outcome in schizophrenia: I. Characteristics of outcome. *Archives of General Psychiatry, 27,* 739–746.

Strauss, J. S., & Carpenter, W. T. (1974). The prediction of outcome in schizophrenia: II. Relationships between predictor and outcome variables. *Archives of General Psychiatry, 31,* 34–42.

Strauss, J. S., & Carpenter, W. T. (1977). Prediction of outcome in schizophrenia: III. Five-year outcome and its predictors. *Archives of General Psychiatry, 34,* 159–163.

Strecker, E. A., & Willey, C. F. (1928). Prognosis in schizophrenia. In *Proceedings of the association for research in nervous and mental disease for 1925 Schizophrenia (dementia praecox)* (pp. 403–431). New York: P.B. Hoeber.

Swanson, J., Burris, S., Moss, K., Ullman, M., & Ranney, L. M. (2006). Justice disparities. Does the ADA enforcement system treat people with psychiatric disabilities fairly? *Maryland Law Review, 66(1),* 94–139.

Thomas, P. (2003). How should advance statements be implemented? *British Journal of Psychiatry, 182,* 548–549.

Walker, R., & Frost, E. S. (1969). Social recovery index. *American Journal of Psychiatry, 126,* 123–124.

Ware, N., Hopper, K., Tugenberg, T., Dickey, B., & Fisher, D. (2007). Connectedness and citizenship: Redefining social integration. *Psychiatric Services, 58,* 469–174.

Ware, N. C., Lachicotte, W. S., Kirschner, S. R., Cortes, D. E., & Good, B. J. (2000). Clinician experiences of managed mental health care. *Medical Anthropology Quarterly, 14,* 3–27.

Warner, R. (1994). *Recovery from schizophrenia: Psychiatry and political economy.* New York: Routledge and Kegan Paul.

Weir, M. (1992). *Politics and jobs.* Princeton, NJ: Princeton University Press.

43

**Andreasen, N. C. (2007).
DSM and the death of
phenomenology in America:
An example of unintended
consequences.** *Schizophrenia
Bulletin, 33* (1), 108–112

The "unintended consequence" of Nancy Andreasen's article is the radical movement, decades in the making, away from reliance on psychodynamic principles. This movement emerged as a response to the diagnostic imprecision of psychodynamic psychiatry and its shortcomings in evaluating symptoms of psychopathology (see Rosenhan's finding, in this volume, that the poorly faked symptoms of fake patients were still good enough to earn them the most serious of psychiatric diagnoses). The result of an effort to achieve greater precision and diagnostic acuity—the Diagnostic and Statistical Manual of Mental Disorders, Third Edition (DSM-III)—however, has led to what Dr. Andreasen describes as a kind of "cookbook" reliance on the *DSM* system of classification that its creators never intended it to be, and to a decline in effective clinical evaluation in teaching and practice. The atrophy of good clinical sense and expertise based on a general knowledge of psychopathology, she claims, has led to the death of phenomenological analysis and understanding of mental illness. Her call for a return training in "the science and art of psychopathology" (p. 112) is noteworthy for the fact that she was, at the time of the article's publication, president of the American Psychiatric Association.

DSM and the Death of Phenomenology in America: An Example of Unintended Consequences

During the 19th century and early 20th century, American psychiatry shared many intellectual traditions and values with Great Britain and Europe. These include principles derived from the Enlightenment concerning the dignity of the individual and the value of careful observation. During the 20th century, however, American psychiatry began to diverge, initially due to a much stronger emphasis on psychoanalytic principles, particularly in comparison with Great Britain. By the 1960s and 1970s, studies such as the US-UK study and the International Pilot Study of Schizophrenia demonstrated that the psychodynamic emphasis had gone too far, leading to diagnostic imprecision and inadequate evaluation of traditional evaluations of signs and symptoms of psychopathology. *Diagnostic and Statistical Manual of Mental Disorders, Third Edition (DSM-III)* was developed in this context, under the leadership of representatives from institutions that had retained the more traditional British-European approaches (eg, Washington University, Iowa). The goal of *DSM-III* was to create a comprehensive system for diagnosing and evaluating psychiatric patients that would be more reliable, more valid, and more consistent with international approaches. This goal was realized in many respects, but unfortunately it also had many unintended consequences. Although the original creators realized that *DSM* represented a "best effort" rather than a definitive "ground truth," *DSM* began to be given total authority in training programs and health care delivery systems. Since the publication *of DSM-III* in 1980, there has been a steady decline in the teaching of careful clinical evaluation that is targeted to the individual person's problems and social context and that is enriched by a good general knowledge of psychopathology. Students are taught to memorize *DSM* rather than to learn complexities from the great psychopathologists of the past. By 2005, the decline has become so severe that it could be referred to as "the death of phenomenology in the United States."

Key words: DSM, phenomenology, diagnostic criteria, diagnostic reliability, clinical interviews

Introduction

Any discussion of the "death of phenomenology," probably, needs to begin with a definition of what the word "phenomenology" means in any particular discussion. This is especially necessary because meanings of words change over time and within different contexts, and phenomenology has been used in a variety of ways that have generated considerable controversy.[1] The word phenomenon (plural, phenomena) derives from Greek and refers to outward appearances. It was contrasted with lathomenon, which referred to underlying meanings that might lie hidden beneath the surface. The term was subsequently adopted by Kant and Hegel, who contrasted phenomena with noumena; the former retained a meaning similar to the original Greek, while the latter referred to higher realities and meanings. However, the meaning of phenomena shifted with latter philosophers. In Heidigger, Husserl, and Jaspers, phenomena were understood in terms of internal subjective experiences. Because Jaspers was an influential and thoughtful psychiatrist, his definition has had considerable impact on the usage of the term. Other articles in this series will no doubt use the term phenomenology in the Jasperian sense.

However, the term phenomenology has also acquired a meaning in contemporary psychiatry that is different from that used by Jaspers and other philosophers and that is more similar to the original Greek meaning. In many writings in contemporary psychiatry, the term refers to the study of psychopathology, broadly defined, including signs, symptoms, and their underlying thoughts and emotions. When used in this way, phenomenology provides the basis for nosology, or the development of disease definitions, diagnostic categories, or dimensional classifications. In this discussion, the term phenomenology is used in this contemporary psychiatric context.

The Origins of Modern Psychiatry: An International Consensus of Shared Values

Although this article is about contemporary psychiatry, it is helpful to understand when and how modern psychiatry came into existence because it illustrates the importance of principles and values about which an international consensus was achieved during the eighteenth century. Psychiatry is among the oldest of the medical specialties. It began when individuals trained as general physicians developed a special interest in the treatment of the seriously mentally ill. This became a widespread movement throughout Britain, Europe, and the United States through the leadership of individuals such as Chiarugi, Pinel, Rush, or the Tukes. The movement arose from the crucible of the dawn of modern science and the philosophy of the Enlightenment.

The dawn of modern science provided early psychiatrists with a framework for generating and testing ideas about the nature and mechanisms of mental illness. Francis Bacon was among the first to articulate the philosophy that would shape the development and methodology of science for the next few hundred years:

> Man can act and understand no further than he has observed, either in operation or in contemplation, of the method and order of nature.

Novum Organum[2]

Pursuing this guidance, people worked out new ways to know (science = to know) about the world through observation, testing, and empirical proof. For example, one of the founders of modern psychiatry, Philippe Pinel, stated:

> I, therefore, resolved to adopt that method of investigation which has invariably succeeded in all the departments of natural history, viz. To notice successively every fact, without any other object than that of collecting materials for future use; and to endeavor, as far as possible, to divest myself of the influence, both of my own prepossessions and the authority of others.

Treatise on Insanity[3]

Pinel followed those principles faithfully and in the process developed the early principles of epidemiology. He produced case descriptions that are so clear and detailed that his patients can seem to speak in our ears and walk before our eyes. This was phenomenology par excellence, in a prenosological era. As a consequence, the nosology is implicit: the cases are recognizable as classic exemplars of illnesses such as bipolar disorder or paranoid schizophrenia.

The philosophy of the Enlightenment was the second philosophical tradition that shaped the development of modern psychiatry and inspired its early leaders such as Pinel, the Tukes, Rush, or Chiarugi. Its key influence was its emphasis on the dignity of the individual human being and the importance of humanism. There are many famous statements of these principles:

We hold these truths to be self-evident..that all men are created equal..[4]

Know then thyself, presume not God to scan;

The proper study of mankind is man.[5]

In this system of being, there is no creature so wonderful in its nature, and which so much deserves our particular attention, as man, who fills up the middle space between the visible and invisible world..[6]

Guided by these principles, the early psychiatrists attempted to develop therapies that might help to relieve mental pain in as humane and effective a manner as possible. The picture of Pinel freeing the mentally ill from their chains is perhaps the most famous icon of their therapeutic approach. "Moral therapy" was developed in many countries in Europe, in Britain, and in the United States. In an era when no pharmacological treatments were available, it emphasized a variety of psychotherapeutic techniques that included personalizing the care to the individual's needs, using nonintrusive and compassionate approaches, appealing to reason when possible, and giving the patient some responsibility for improving symptoms and behavior.

Because the philosophy of the Enlightenment encouraged the conceptualization of human beings—including those suffering from mental illness—as endowed with reason and individual dignity, the psychiatric writings of this era did not tend to dissociate the psyche or mind from the brain. Instead, they were seen as integrated. For example, the first editor of *The American Journal of Psychiatry,* Amariah Brigham, stated in 1844[7]:

... the brain is the instrument which the mind uses in this life, to manifest itself, and like all other parts of our bodies, is liable to disease, and when diseased, is often incapable of manifesting harmoniously and perfectly the powers of the mind ... it is as if, in some very complicated and delicate instrument, as a watch for instance, some slight alteration of its machinery should disturb, but not stop, its action.

Thus, the gifts of modern science and the philosophy of the Enlightenment to the creation of our specialty of psychiatry included stressing the importance of careful observation in order to understand disease mechanisms and progression, an emphasis on the dignity of the individual, the value of "moral treatment," and the integration of "mind," "spirit," and "brain" rather than a dualistic understanding. This has given psychiatry a firm conceptual and moral grounding that it should strive to maintain.

The Rise Of Psychoanalysis And The Mid-Atlantic Counterrevolution

The ideas of Sigmund Freud, developed in the early- to mid-20th century, offered an interesting alternative approach to many psychiatrists, however. They were embraced in many parts of the world and by many individual psychiatrists. The effect was perhaps most striking in the United States. After World War II, psychoanalysis became the dominant conceptual framework in the United States. For a period of 30–40 years, nearly all the major leaders in American psychiatry embraced psychoanalytic principles and used them to shape psychiatric education and training. This created a new and different zeitgeist. A variety of changes occurred as a result of psychoanalytic dominance.

First, psychoanalysis led to a significant de-emphasis on diagnosis and nosology. As a consequence of work by Kraepelin, Bleuler, and others, a system for diagnosing and classifying psychiatric disorders had been developed in parallel with the development of psychoanalysis and was codified in both the *International Classification of Diseases* and the *Diagnostic and Statistical Manual of Mental Disorders (DSM)* of the American Psychiatric Association. In general, the psychoanalytic movement considered diagnosis and classification to be a fruitless endeavor. Defining the nature and source of intrapsychic conflicts was the goal instead.

Second, psychoanalysis, therefore, also led to a significant de-emphasis on careful observation of signs and symptoms—the "bread and butter" of the early humanistic psychiatrists and the basis for developing a phenomenology. In fact, the psychoanalysts taught that the patient's self-report of both symptoms and other internal experiences should be discounted. The analyst must dig beneath self-report to reach the real truth.

While other countries also had prominent psychoanalysts and psychoanalytic movements, the US acceptance of psychoanalysis was extreme. This distanced most of American psychiatry from Anglo-European traditions and approaches, which continued to teach phenomemology and nosology.

However, a few American institutions maintained ties with Anglo-European psychiatry. The institutions have sometimes been called "the Mid-Atlantics." They included Washington University in St Louis, Johns Hopkins in Baltimore, Iowa Psychiatric Hospital in Iowa City, and New York Psychiatric Institute in New York City.

Despite their small numbers and relative isolation from the rest of American psychiatry, the Mid-Atlantics made some significant contributions to psychiatry during the 1970s. These included the development of the first set of diagnostic criteria,[8] the development of the Research Diagnostic Criteria and Schedule for Affective Disorders and Schizophrenia,[9] the development of other rating scales for psychopathology—eg, the Thought, Language, and Communication and Affect Rating Scales,[10–12] and the highly influential article of Robins and Guze on the validation of psychiatric diagnoses.[13]

In parallel, significant work was occurring in Europe and especially Great Britain, making the 1970s a time of reappraisal. The Present State Examination provided the international community with a structured interview that could be used to conduct a variety of epidemiological diagnostic studies.[14] Foremost among these were the International Pilot Study of Schizophrenia[15] and the US-UK study.[16,17] The results of these 2 major studies suggested that American psychiatrists were overdiagnosing mental illnesses in comparison with the rest of the world and not doing systematic clinical assessments and that their diagnoses and clinical assessments were not reliable.

Adding to the rising tide of criticism from the Mid-Atlantics was the publication in *Science* of *Being Sane in Insane Places.*[18] This article reported that 8 sane "pseudopatients" were admitted to psychiatric hospitals with minimal to questionable psychiatric complaints (eg, hearing a voice saying "thud" on a few occasions); after admission, they denied any symptoms at all, behaved normally, rarely met with staff, and nonetheless remained in the hospital for an average of 19 days and were discharged with a diagnosis of schizophrenia in remission. Clearly American psychiatry was in a troubled state. It was time for a change. The Mid-Atlantics had their opportunity and began their charge.

The Development of *Diagnostic and Statistical Manual of Mental Disorders, Third Edition*: Lofty Goals

The changes that seemed to be obviously needed in the principles and practice of American psychiatry were created by the development and publication of a new *DSM: Diagnostic and Statistical Manual of Mental Disorders, Third Edition (DSM-III)*. Bob Spitzer, then head of Biometrics at New York Psychiatric Institute, was appointed Chair. He assembled a Task Force comprised primarily of Mid-Atlantics. Their work began in the mid-70s and was culminated by the publication of *DSM-III* in 1980. At their first meeting, there was universal consensus among the Task Force members that *Diagnostic and Statistical Manual of Mental Disorders, Second Edition (DSM-II)* should be totally revised. *DSM-III* should be evidence based, use diagnostic criteria instead of general descriptions, and strive for maximal reliability. Principles of validity were also considered important, but much less emphasized; the approach was heavily influenced by the article of Robins and Guze on the validation of schizophrenia.[13] That article suggested that several different methods could be used to determine if a specific psychiatric disorder could be considered valid: familial aggregation, characteristic longitudinal course, response to treatment, and laboratory tests (rarely possible).

The Task Force articulated a group of lofty goals that shaped their efforts:

- To improve communication between clinicians
- To provide reliable diagnoses that would be useful in research
- To enhance teaching: to train psychiatry students in clinical interviewing and differential diagnosis
- To realign American psychiatry with the rest of the world and to be consistent with *International Classification of Diseases, Ninth Revision.*

To achieve these goals, they made major modifications in the old *DSM-II*. An extensive text was written for each of the disorders, expanding the length from 38 pages *of DSM-II to* 295 pages *of DSM-III*. As the writing evolved, Task Force members began to comment to one another that they were writing a new textbook of psychiatry. This new textbook contained a variety of new principles and innovations:

- Atheoretical about etiology (because for most diagnoses etiology is in fact unknown)
- Use of diagnostic criteria
- Dropping of the term "neurosis"
- Provision of a glossary to define the terms used in the criteria
- Multiaxial approach to classification in order to incorporate medical and psychosocial components of a clinical evaluation.

The Task Force members recognized that the increased simplicity and clarity could lead to abuses. Therefore, they filled the introduction with the caveats as follows:

- The problem of using the manual to set policies:
  The use of this manual for non-clinical purposes, such as determination of legal responsibility, competency or insanity, or justification for third-party payment, must be critically examined in each instance with the appropriate institutional context.[19(p12)]

- The risk that *DSM* would be taken as the ultimate authority on diagnosis:
  This final version of DSM-III is only one still frame in the ongoing process of attempting to better understand mental disorders.[19(p12)]

- The lack of adequate validation for the criteria:
  DSM-III provides specific diagnostic criteria as guides for making each diagnosis since such criteria enhance interjudge reliability. It should be understood, however, that for most of the categories the diagnostic criteria are based on clinical judgment, and have not yet been fully validated by data about such important correlates as clinical course, outcome, family history, and treatment response. Undoubtedly, with further study the criteria for many of the categories will be revised.[19(p8)]

- The importance of going beyond *DSM* criteria in history taking:
  Making a DSM-III diagnosis represents an initial step in a comprehensive evaluation leading to the formulation of a treatment plan. Additional information about the individual being evaluated beyond that required to make a DSM-III diagnosis will invariably be necessary.[19p11]

What Went Wrong? The Unintended Consequences

Although the authors of *DSM-III* knew that they were creating a small revolution in American psychiatry, they had no idea that it would become a large one and that it would ultimately change the nature and practice of the field. The American Psychiatric Association, which historically had published *DSM,* was caught completely off guard. Copies sold out immediately, and it took approximately 6 months to catch up with the orders that came flowing in. *DSM* was purchased by psychiatrists, nurses, social workers, lawyers, psychologists—anyone with any connection to psychiatry.

DSM-III and its successors, *Diagnostic and Statistical Manual of Mental Disorders, Revised Third Edition* and *Diagnostic and Statistical Manual of Mental Disorders, Fourth Edition,* became universally and uncritically accepted as the ultimate authority on psychopathology and diagnosis. *DSM* forms the basis for psychiatric teaching to both residents and undergraduates throughout most of the United States.

Knowledge of the criteria is the basis for most exams—even the Board Certification examinations taken after residency. As a consequence, classics in psychopathology are now largely ignored.

The ultimate painful paradox: the study of phenomenology and nosology that was so treasured by the Mid-Atlantics who created *DSM* is no longer seen as important or relevant. Research in psychopathology is a dying (or dead) enterprise.

How and why did this occur? What is wrong with *DSM?*

It is not difficult to come up with a list of obvious problems. First, the criteria include only some characteristic symptoms of a given disorder. They were never intended to provide a comprehensive description. Rather, they were conceived of as "gatekeepers"—the minimum symptoms needed to make a diagnosis. Because *DSM* is often used as a primary textbook or the major diagnostic resource in many clinical and research settings, students typically do not know about other potentially important or interesting signs and symptoms that are not included in *DSM*. Second, *DSM* has had a dehumanizing impact on the practice of psychiatry. History taking—the central evaluation tool in psychiatry—has frequently been reduced to the use of *DSM* checklists. *DSM* discourages clinicians from getting to know the patient as an individual person because of its dryly empirical approach. Third, validity has been sacrificed to achieve reliability. *DSM* diagnoses have given researchers a common nomenclature—but probably the wrong one. Although creating standardized diagnoses that would facilitate research was a major goal, *DSM* diagnoses are not useful for research because of their lack of validity.

These concerns led the author to write several editorials for the *American Journal of Psychiatry* about the current problems that have been created by *DSM*. Here are a few of Cassandra's complaints:

In the United States an older generation of clinical researchers who led the field for many years have died—Eli Robins, Gerry Klerman, George Winokur. Very few younger investigators are emerging to replace them. The word is out—if you want to succeed as a serious scientist, you need to do something relatively basic. Fortunately, the Europeans still have a proud tradition of clinical research and descriptive psychopathology. Someday, in the 21st century, after the human genome and the human brain have been mapped, someone may need to organize a reverse Marshall plan so that the Europeans can save American science by helping us figure out who really has schizophrenia or what schizophrenia really is.[20]

We need to make a serious investment in training a new generation of real experts in the science and art of psychopathology. Otherwise, we high-tech scientists may wake up in 10 years and discover that we face a silent spring. Applying technology without the companionship of wise clinicians with specific expertise in psychopathology will be a lonely, sterile, and perhaps fruitless enterprise.[21]

The creation of an international conference on phenomenology, as summarized in this issue, may help at least a bit to remedy the present situation.

References

1. Andreasen NC. Reply to "Phenomenology or physicialism?" *Schizophr Bull.* 1991;17:187–189.
2. Bacon F. *Novum Organum.* London, UK: W. Pickering; 1850.
3. Pinel P. *A Treatise on Insanity.* London, UK: Messrs Cadell and Davies, Strand; 1806.
4. Jefferson T. *The Declaration of Independence.* 1776.
5. Pope A, American Imprint Collection (Library of Congress). Essay on man, Epistle II. In: Bredvold LI, McKillap AD, Whitney SL, eds. *Eighteenth Century Poetry & Prose.* New York, NY: Ronald Press; 1732–1734:1–2.
6. Addison J, Steele R. *Eighteenth Century Poetry & Prose.* New York, NY: Ronald Press; 1939.
7. Brigham A. Definition of Insanity—nature of the disease. *J Insanity.* 1844;1:97–116.
8. Feighner JP, Robins E, Guze SB, Woodruff RA Jr, Winokur G, Munoz R. Diagnostic criteria for use in psychiatric research. *Arch Gen Psychiatry.* 1972;26:57–63.
9. Endicott J, Spitzer RL. A diagnostic interview: the schedule for affective disorders and schizophrenia. *Arch Gen Psychiatry.* 1978;35:837–844.
10. Andreasen NC. Affective flattening and the criteria for schizophrenia. *Am J Psychiatry.* 1979;136:944–947.
11. Andreasen NC. Thought, language, and communication disorders. I. Clinical assessment, definition of terms, and evaluation of their reliability. *Arch Gen Psychiatry.* 1979;36:1315–1321.
12. Andreasen NC. Thought, language, and communication disorders. II. Diagnostic significance. *Arch Gen Psychiatry.* 1979;36:1325–1330.
13. Robins E, Guze SB. Establishment of diagnostic validity in psychiatric illness: its application to schizophrenia. *Am J Psychiatry.* 1970;126:983–987.
14. Wing JK. A standard form of psychiatric Present State Examinations (PSE) and a method for standardizing the classification of symptoms. In: Hare EH, Wing JK, eds. *Psychiatric Epidemiology.* London, UK: Oxford University Press; 1970.
15. Sartorius N, Shapiro R, Kimura M, Barrett K. WHO international pilot study of schizophrenia. *Psychol Med. 1972;2:* 422–425.
16. Kendell RE. Psychiatric diagnosis in Britain and the United States. *Br J Psychiatry.* 1975;9:453–461.

17. Kendell RE, Cooper JE, Gourlay AJ, Copeland JR, Sharpe L, Gurland BJ. Diagnostic criteria of American and British psychiatrists. *Arch Gen Psychiatry.* 1971;25:123–130.

18. Rosenhan DL. On being sane in insane places. *Science.* 1973;179:250–258.

19. American Psychiatric Association Committee on Nomenclature and Statistics. *Diagnostic and Statistical Manual of Mental Disorders (DSM-III).* Washington, D.C.: American Psychiatric Association; 1980.

20. Andreasen NC. Changing concepts of schizophrenia and the ahistorical fallacy. *Am J Psychiatry.* 1994;151:1405–1407.

21. Andreasen NC. What shape are we in? Gender, psychopathology, and the brain. *Am J Psychiatry.* 1997;154:1637–1639.

Practice and Research Texts

44

Mosher, L. R. (1999). Soteria and other alternatives to acute psychiatric hospitalization: A personal and professional review. *Journal of Nervous and Mental Diseases, 187* (3), 142–149

Mosher, a psychiatrist, is best known for his work and research in the 1970s on the Soteria Project, a community residence with nonprofessional staff that showed remarkable success as a low-cost, noninstitutional alternative to psychiatric hospitalization for acute care of persons with mental illness. Writing 20-plus years later, Mosher reviews the finding of the Soteria Project and its descendants in and outside the United States. The positive findings for these projects have held up, he writes, both as short-term crisis interventions and as aids for longer-term functioning in the community for persons with serious mental illness. Soteria and its subsequent adaptations, he argues, have produced results that entitle them to the status of evidence-based practice. Still, there has been no widespread adoption of these findings on alternatives to psychiatric hospitalization. Mosher gives an engaging personal account of his involvement with Soteria and related projects that he took up on the way to trying to answer a question that emerged for him during the early years of his training as a psychiatrist: "[I]f places called hospitals were not good for disturbed and disturbing behavior, what kinds of social environments were?" [p. 143]

Soteria and Other Alternatives to Acute Psychiatric Hospitalization: A Personal and Professional Review

Abstract

The author reviews the clinical and special social environmental data from the Soteria Project and its direct successors. Two random assignment studies of the Soteria model and its modification for long-term system clients reveal that roughly 85% to 90% of acute and long-term clients deemed in need of acute hospitalization can be returned to the community without use of conventional hospital treatment. Soteria, designed as a drug-free treatment environment, was as successful as anti-psychotic drug treatment in reducing psychotic symptoms in 6 weeks. In its modified form, in facilities called Crossing Place and McAuliffe House where so-called long-term "frequent flyers" were treated, alternative-treated subjects were found to be as clinically improved as hospital-treated patients, at considerably lower cost. Taken as a body of scientific evidence, it is clear that alternatives to acute psychiatric hospitalization are as, or more, effective than traditional hospital care in short-term reduction of psychopathology and longer-term social adjustment. Data from the original drug-free, home-like, nonprofessionally staffed Soteria Project and its Bern, Switzerland, replication indicate that persons without extensive hospitalizations (<30 days) are especially responsive to the positive therapeutic effects of the well-defined, replicable Soteria-type special social environments. Reviews of other studies of diversion of persons deemed in need of hospitalization to "alternative" programs have consistently shown equivalent or better program clinical results, at lower cost, from alternatives. Despite these clinical and cost data, alternatives to psychiatric hospitalization have not been widely implemented, indicative of a remarkable gap between available evidence and clinical practice.
© 1999 Lippincott Williams & Wilkins, Inc.

In 1961, while serving as a medical intern, knowing I was soon to embark on a career as a psychiatrist, I suffered what retrospectively could be labeled an existential crisis. For the first time I experienced the responsibility of caring for persons who would soon die-and I was powerless to do anything about it-except to try to understand their experience of it. They frequently expressed how helpless and depersonalized they felt, "I'm just the one with lung cancer" or "Why can't you do something so I can breathe-I'm drowning" or "All this place has done is to make me into a nobody-you can't do anything for me so you steer clear." For the first time I faced my own mortality and with it the degrading, dehumanizing and helplessness of the process that could accompany it-particularly if I had the misfortune of being in a hospital like the one in which I worked.

Previous intensive psychotherapy as a medical student had obviously not prepared me to face mortality compounded by the degradation ceremonies I presided over within the institution. As a sometime intellectual, I sought help with my conundrum in the library. Rollo May's Existence (1958) was the beginning of a quest for an intellectual foundation for the depth of what I was experiencing personally. With the help of May's book and an existential analytic tutor (Dr. Ludwig Lefebre), I studied the writings of a number of the phenomenologic/existential thinkers (*e.g.*, Allers, 1961; Boss, 1963; Hegel, 1967; Husserl, 1967; Sartre, 1956; Tillich, 1952; and others) in greater depth. I concluded that their open minded, noncategorizing, no preconceptions approach was a breath of fresh air in the era of rationalistic theory driven approaches (such as psychoanalysis) to disturbed and disturbing persons.

So, I brought to my psychiatric residency a phenomenology-based "what you see is what you've got" bias to my interactions with patients and a sensitivity to the issues of a degradation and power—especially as embodied in conventional institutional practices. The good mentors (*e.g.*, Drs. Elvin Semrad and Norman Paul) in my psychiatric training taught me how to listen and attempt to find meaning in the distorted communications of my patients *and their families* (in 1962!) by doing my best to put my feet into their shoes. Harry Stack Sullivan (1962) and the double bind theory (Bateson et al., 1956) provided intellectual support. I also learned how to ask and look for answers to questions of interest from research gods (*e.g., Dr. Martin Orne*). On the other hand, the institution itself gave me master classes in the art of the "total institution" (Goffman, 1961); authoritarianism, the degradation ceremony, the induction and perpetuation of powerlessness, unnecessary dependency, labeling, and the primacy of institutional needs over those of the persons it was ostensibly there to serve-the patients. These institutional lessons were not part of the training program. In fact, my efforts to be helpful to my patients were interrupted by these institutional needs. When brought up they were denied, rationalized, or simply invalidated, "You're just a resident and aren't yet able to understand why these processes are not as you see them." From a series of such experiences, I began to believe that psychiatric hospitals were not usually very good places in which to be insane.

Although the Thorazine assault troops (Smith, Klein, and French's own terminology for its 1956 charge to the company's detail men—see Braden-Johnson [1990]) had already successfully done their job-selling the neuroleptics—I never became a true believer in the "magic bullet" attribution commonly ascribed the neuroleptic drugs. Despite being trained by psychopharmacologic icons (*e.g.*, Dr. Gerald Klerman), I somehow never found a Lazarus among those I treated with the major tranquilizers. Again, my experience led me to question the emerging psychopharmacologic domination of the treatment of very disturbed and disturbing persons. Actually those persons seemed to appreciate my sometimes clumsy attempts to understand them and their lives. Because I hadn't found a large role for drugs in the helping process, I was led to believe more in interpersonal than neuroleptic "cures." I did worry about what went on in the 164 hours a week when my patients were not with me—was the rest of their world trying to understand and relate meaningfully to them?

So, as a career unfolded, the questioning of conventional wisdom remained part of me, albeit not always acted upon in a way that would bring undue attention and consequent retribution. To interests in the meaningfulness of madness, understanding families, and the conduct of research, I added one from my institutional experience; if places called hospitals were not good for disturbed and disturbing behavior, what kinds of social environments were? In 1966–1967, this interest was nourished by R.D. Laing and his colleagues in the Philadelphia Association's Kingsley Hall in London. The deconstruction of madness and the madhouse that took place there generated ideas about how a community-based, supportive, protective, normalizing environment might facilitate reintegration of psychologically disintegrated persons without artificial institutional disruptions of the process.

This, combined with my existential/phenomenologic-interpersonal psychotherapy and anti-neuroleptic drug biases resulted, in 1969–1971, in the design and implementation of the Soteria Research Project. Soteria is a Greek word meaning salvation or deliverance. In addition to my interests, the project included ideas from the era of "moral treatment" in American psychiatry (Bockhoven, 1963), Sullivan's (1962) interpersonal theory and his specially designed milieu for persons with schizophrenia at Sheppard and Enoch Pratt Hospital in the 1920s, labeling theory (Scheff, 1966), intensive individual therapy based on Jungian theory (Perry, 1974) and Freudian psychoanalysis (Fromm-Reichman, 1948; Searles, 1965), the notion of growth from psychosis (Laing, 1967; Menninger, 1959), and examples of community-based treatment such as the Fairweather Lodges (Fairweather et al., 1969).

The Soteria Project (1971–1983)

This project's design was a random assignment, 2-year follow-up study comparing the Soteria method of treatment with "usual" general hospital psychiatric ward interventions for persons *newly diagnosed as having schizophrenia* and deemed in need of hospitalization. It has been extensively reported (see especially Mosher et al., 1978, 1995). In addition to less than 30 days previous hospitalization (*i.e.,* "newly diagnosed"), the Soteria study selected 18- to 30-year-old, unmarried subjects about whom three independent raters could agree met DSM-II criteria for schizophrenia and who were experiencing at least four of seven Bleulerian symptoms of the disorder (Table 44.1). The early onset (18 to 30 years) and marital status criteria were designed to identify a subgroup of persons diagnosed with schizophrenia who were at *statistically* high risk for long-term disability. We believed than an experimental treatment should be provided to those individuals most likely to have high service needs over the long term. All subjects were public sector clients screened at the psychiatric emergency room of a suburban San Francisco Bay Area county hospital.

Basically, the Soteria method can be characterized as the 24 hour a day application of interpersonal phenomenologic interventions by a nonprofessional staff, usually without neuroleptic drug treatment, in the context of a small, homelike, quiet, supportive, protective, and tolerant social environment. The core practice of interpersonal phenomenology focuses on the development of a nonintrusive, noncontrolling but actively empathetic relationship with the psychotic person without having *to do* anything explicitly therapeutic or controlling. In shorthand, it can be characterized as "being with," "standing by attentively," "trying to put your feet into the other person's shoes," or "being an LSD trip guide" (remember, this was the early 1970s in California). The aim is to develop, over time, a shared experience of the meaningfulness of the client's individual social context-current and historical. Note, there were no therapeutic "sessions" at Soteria. However, a great deal of "therapy" took place there as staff worked gently to build bridges, over time, between individuals' emotionally disorganized states to the life events that seemed to have

Table 44.1 The Soteria Project: research admission/selection criteria

1. Diagnosis DSM-II schizophrenia (3 independent clinicians)
2. Deemed in need of hospitalization
3. Four of seven Bleulerian diagnostic symptoms (2 independent clinicians)
4. Not more than one previous hospitalization for 30d or less
5. Age 18–30
6. Marital status: single

precipitated their psychological disintegration. The context within the house was one of positive expectations that reorganization and reintegration would occur as a result of these seemingly minimalist interventions.

The original Soteria House opened in 1971. A replication facility ("Emanon") opened in 1974 in another suburban San Francisco Bay Area city. This was done because clinically we soon saw that the Soteria method "worked." Immediate replication would address the potential criticism that our results were a one-time product of a unique group of persons and expectation effects. The project first published systematic 1-year outcome data in 1974 and 1975 (Mosher and Menn, 1974; Mosher et al., 1975). Despite the publication of consistently positive results (Mosher and Menn, 1978; Matthews et al., 1979) for this subgroup of newly diagnosed psychotic persons from the first cohort of subjects (1971–1976), the Soteria Project ended in 1983. Because of administrative problems and lack of funding, data from the 1976–1983 cohort were not analyzed until 1992. Because of our selection criteria and the suburban location of the intake facilities, both Soteria-treated and control subjects were young (age 21), mostly white (10% minority), relatively well educated (high school graduates) men and women raised in typical lower middle class, blue-collar suburban families.

Results

Cohort I (1971–1976)

Briefly summarized, the significant results from the initial, Soteria House only, cohort were:

Admission Characteristics. Experimental and control subjects were remarkably similar on 10 demographic, 5 psychopathology, 7 prognostic, and 7 psychosocial preadmission (independent) variables.

Six-Week Outcome. In terms of psychopathology, subjects in both groups improved significantly and comparably, despite Soteria subjects not having received neuroleptic drugs. All control patients received adequate anti-psychotic drug treatment in hospital and were discharged on maintenance dosages. More than half stopped medications over the 2-year follow-up period. Three percent of Soteria subjects were maintained on neuroleptics.

Milieu Assessment. Because we conceived the Soteria program as a recovery-facilitating social environment, systematic study and comparison with the CMHC were particularly important. We used Moos' Ward Atmosphere Scale (WAS) and COPES scale for this purpose (Moos, 1974, 1975). The differences between the programs were remarkable in their magnitude and stability over 10 years. COPES data from the experimental replication facility, Emanon, was remarkably similar to its older sibling, Soteria House. Thus, we concluded that the Soteria Project and CMHC environments were, in fact, very different and that the Soteria and Emanon milieus conformed closely to our predictions (Wendt et al., 1983).

Community Adjustment. Two psychopathology, three treatment, and seven psychosocial variables were analyzed. At 2 years postadmission, Soteria-treated subjects from the 1971–1976 cohort were working at significantly higher occupational levels, were significantly more often living independently or with peers, and had fewer readmissions; 57% had never received a single dose of neuroleptic medication during the entire 2-year study period.

Cost. In the first cohort, despite the large differences in lengths of stay during the initial admissions (about 1 month versus 5 months), the cost of the first 6 months of care for both groups was approximately $4000. Costs were similar despite 5-month Soteria and 1-month hospital initial lengths of stay because of Soteria's low per diem cost and extensive use of day care, group, individual, and medication therapy by the discharged hospital control clients (Matthews et al., 1979; Mosher et al., 1978).

Cohort II (1976–1982; includes all Emanon-treated subjects)

Admission, 6-week, and milieu assessments replicated almost exactly the findings of the initial cohort. Nearly 25% of experimental clients in this cohort received some neuroleptic drug treatment during their initial 6 weeks of care. Again, all hospital-treated subjects received anti-psychotic drugs during their index admission episode. In this cohort, half of the experimental and 70% of control subjects received postdischarge maintenance drug treatment. However, in contrast to Cohort I, after 2 years, no significant differences existed between the experimental and control groups in symptom levels, treatment received (including medication and rehospitalization), or global good versus poor outcomes. Consistent with the psychosocial outcomes in Cohort I, Cohort II experimental subjects, as compared with control subjects, were more independent in their living arrangements after 2 years.

Interestingly, independent of treatment group, good or poor outcome is predicted by four measures of preadmission psychosocial competence (Mosher et al., 1992): level of education (higher), precipitating events (present), living situation (independent), and work (successful). Good outcome was narrowly defined as having no more than mild symptoms *and* either living independently or working or going to school at both 1- and 2-year follow-up. (Mosher et al., 1995).

The Second Generation

Although closely involved in the California-based Soteria Project throughout the study's life, I lived in Washington, D.C., while working for the NIMH. In 1972, I became psychiatric consultant to Woodley House, a half-way house founded in Washington, D.C., in 1958. In consultation, staff were often distressed when describing house residents who went into crisis, and there was no option but to hospitalize them. Recovery from such institutionalizations they saw as taking nearly 18 months. So, in 1977, a Soteria-like facility (called "Crossing Place") was opened by Woodley House Programs that differed from its conceptual parent in that it:

1. admitted any nonmedically ill client deemed in need of psychiatric hospitalization regardless of diagnosis, length of illness, severity of psychopathology, or level of functional impairment;
2. was an integral part of the local public community mental health system, which meant that most patients who came to Crossing Place were receiving psychotropic medications; and
3. had an informal length of stay restriction of about 30 days to make it economically appealing.

So, beginning in 1977, a modified Soteria method was applied to a much broader patient base, the so-called "seriously and persistently mentally ill". Although a random assignment study of a Crossing Place model has only recently been published (Fenton et al., 1998), it was clear from early on that the Soteria method "worked" with this nonresearch-criteria-derived heterogeneous client group. Because of its location and "open" admissions Crossing Place clients, as compared with Soteria subjects, were older (37), more nonwhite (70%), multiadmission, long-term system users (averaging 14 years) who were raised in poor urban ghetto families. From the outset, Crossing Place was able to return 90% or more of its 2000 plus (by 1997) admissions directly to the community-completely avoiding hospitalization (Kresky-Wolff et al., 1984). In its more than 20 years of operation, there have been no suicides among clients in residence, and no serious staff injuries have occurred. Although the clients were different, as noted above, the two settings (Soteria and Crossing Place) shared staff selection processes (Hirschfeld et al., 1977; Mosher et al., 1973), philosophy, institutional and social structure characteristics, and the culture of positive expectations.

In 1986 the social environments at Soteria and Crossing Place were compared and contrasted as follows:

In their presentations to the world, Crossing Place is conventional and Soteria unconventional. Despite this major difference, the actual in-house interpersonal interactions are similar in their informality, earthiness, honesty, and lack of professional jargon. These similarities arise partially from the fact that neither program ascribes the usual patient role to the clientele. Crossing Place admits "chronic" patients, and its public funding contains broad length-of-stay standards (1 to 2 months). Soteria's research focus views length of stay as a dependent variable, allowing it to vary according to the clinical needs of the newly diagnosed patients. Hence, the initial focus of the Crossing Place staff is: What do the clients need to accomplish relatively quickly so they can resume living in the community?

This empowering focus on the client's responsibility to accomplish a goal(s) is a technique that Woodley House has used successfully for many years. At Soteria, such questions were not ordinarily raised until the acutely psychotic state had subsided-usually 4 to 6 weeks after entry. This span exceeds the average length of stay at Crossing Place. In part, the shorter average length of stay at Crossing Place is made possible by the almost routine use of neuroleptics to control the most flagrant symptoms of its clientele. At Soteria, neuroleptics were almost never used during the first 6 weeks of a patient's stay. Time constraints also dictate that Crossing Place will have a more formalized social structure than Soteria. Each day there is a morning meeting on "what are you doing to fix your life today" and there are also one or two evening community meetings.

The two Crossing Place consulting psychiatrists each spend an hour a week with the staff members reviewing each client's progress, addressing particularly difficult issues, and helping develop a consensus on initial and revised treatment plans. Soteria had a variety of ad-hoc crisis meetings, but only one regularly scheduled house meeting per week. The role of the consulting psychiatrist was more peripheral at Soteria than at Crossing Place: He was not ordinarily involved in treatment planning and no regular treatment meetings were held.

In summary, compared to Soteria, Crossing Place is more organized, has a tighter structure, and is more oriented toward practical goals. Expectations of Crossing Place staff members are positive but more limited than those of Soteria staff. At Crossing Place, psychosis is frequently not addressed directly by staff members, while at Soteria the client's experience of acute psychosis is often a central subject of interpersonal communication. At Crossing Place, the use of neuroleptics restricts psychotic episodes. The immediate social problems of Crossing Place clients (secondary to being system "veterans" and also because of having come mostly from urban lower social class minority families) must be addressed quickly: no money, no place to live, no one with whom to talk. Basic survival is often the issue. Among the new to the system, young, lower class, suburban, mostly white Soteria clients, these problems were present but much less pressing because basic survival was usually not *yet* an issue.

Crossing Place staff members spend a lot of time keeping other parts of the mental health community involved in the process of addressing client needs. The clients are known to many other players in the system. Just contacting everyone with a role in the life of any given client can be an all-day process for a staff member. In contrast, Soteria clients, being new to the system, had no such cadre of involved mental health workers. While in residence, Crossing Place clients continue their involvement with their other programs if clinically possible. At Soteria, only the project director and house director worked with both the house and the community mental health system. At Crossing Place, all staff members negotiate with the system. Because of the shorter lengths of stay, the focus on immediate practical problem solving, and the absence of clients from the house during the daytime, Crossing Place tends to be less consistently intimate in feeling than Soteria. Although individual relationships between staff members and clients can be very intimate at Crossing Place, especially with returning clients ... it is easier to get in and out of Crossing Place without having a significant relationship (Mosher et al., 1986, pp. 262–264).

A Second-Generation Sibling

In 1990, McAuliffe House, a Crossing Place replication, was established in Montgomery County, Maryland. This county's southern boundary borders Washington, D.C. Crossing Place helped train its staff; for didactic instruction there were numerous articles describing the philosophy, institutional characteristics, social structure, and staff attitudes of Crossing Place and Soteria and a treatment manual from Soteria. My own continuing influence as philosopher/clinician/godfather/supervisor is certain to have made replicability of these special social environments easier. In Montgomery County, it was possible to implement the first random assignment study of a residential alternative to hospitalization that was focused on the seriously mentally ill "frequent flyers" in a living, breathing, never before researched, "public" system of care. Because of this well funded system's early crisis-intervention focus, it hospitalized only about 10% of its more than 1500 long-term clients each year. Again, because of a well-developed crisis system, less than 10% of hospitalizations were involuntary-hence, our voluntary research sample was representative of even the most difficult multi-problem clients. The study *excluded no one* deemed in need of acute hospitalization except those with complicating medical conditions or who were acutely intoxicated. The subjects were as representative of suburban Montgomery County's public clients as Crossing Place's were of urban Washington, D.C.; mid-thirties, poor, 25% minority, long durations of illness, and multiple previous hospitalizations. However, many of the Montgomery County nonminority clients came from well-educated affluent families. The results (Fenton et al., 1998) were not surprising. The alternative and acute general hospital psychiatric wards were clinically equal in effectiveness, but the alternative cost about 40% less. For a system, this means a savings of roughly $19,000 per year for each seriously and persistently mentally ill person who uses acute alternative care exclusively (instead of a hospital). Based on 1993 dollars, total costs for the hospital in this study were about $500 per day (including ancillary costs) and the alternative about $150 (including extramural treatment and ancillary costs).

Important Therapeutic Ingredients

Descriptively, the therapeutic ingredients of these residential alternatives, ones that clearly distinguish them from psychiatric hospitals, in the order they are likely to be experienced by a newly admitted client, are:

1. The setting is indistinguishable from other residences in the community, and it interacts with its community.
2. The facility is small, with space for no more than 10 persons to sleep (6 to 8 clients, 2 staff). It is experienced as home-like. Admission procedures are informal and individualized, based on the client's ability to participate meaningfully.
3. A primary task of the staff is to understand the immediate circumstances and relevant background that precipitated the crisis necessitating admission. It is anticipated this will lead to a relationship based on shared knowledge that will, in turn, enable staff to put themselves into the client's shoes. Thus, they will share the client's perception of their social context and what needs to change to enable them to return to it. The relative paucity of paperwork allows time for the interaction necessary to form a relationship.
4. Within this relationship the client will find staff carrying out multiple roles: companion, advocate, case worker, and therapist-although no therapeutic sessions are held in the house. Staff have the authority to make, in conjunction with the client, and be responsible for, on-the-spot decisions. Staff are mostly in their mid-20s, college graduates, selected on the basis of their interest in working in this special setting with a clientele in psychotic crisis. Most use the work as a transitional step on their way to advanced mental-health-related degrees. They are usually psychologically tough, tolerant, and flexible and come from lower middle class families with a "problem" member (Hirschfeld et al., 1977; Mosher et al., 1973, 1992). In contrast to psychiatric ward staff, they are trained and closely supervised in the adoption and validation of the clients' perceptions. Problem solving and supervision focused on relational difficulties (*e.g.,* "transference" and "counter-transference") that they are experiencing is available from fellow staff, onsite program directors, and the consulting psychiatrists (these last two will be less obvious to clients). Note that the M.D.s are not in charge of the program.
5. Staff is trained to prevent unnecessary dependency and, insofar as possible, maintain autonomous decision making on the part of clients. They also encourage clients to stay in contact with their usual treatment and social networks. Clients frequently remark on how different the experience is from that of a hospitalization. This process may result in clients reporting they feel in control and a sense of security. They also experience a continued connectedness to their usual social environments.
6. Access and departure, both initially and subsequently, is made as easy as possible. Short of official readmission, there is an open social system through which clients can continue their connection to the program in nearly any way they choose; phone-in for support, information or advice, drop-in visits (usually at dinner time), or arranged time with someone with whom they had an especially important relationship. All former clients are invited back to an organized activity one evening a week.

Characteristics of Healing Social Environments

Both clinical descriptive and systematic staff and client perception data (from Moos, 1974, 1975) are available to compare and contrast Soteria, Crossing Place, and McAuliffe House with their respective acute general hospital wards and each other (Mosher, 1992; Mosher et al., 1986, 1995; Wendt et al., 1983).

Clinical characteristics of the hospital comparison wards included in the original Soteria study have been previously described (see Wendt et al., 1983) and are applicable to the hospital psychiatric ward studied in the Montgomery County research. The clinical Soteria-Crossing Place description and "Important Therapeutic Ingredients" explicated earlier are applicable across all three alternative settings. The Moos scale data comparing Soteria with Crossing Place and McAuliffe House are consistent between the three settings and different from the findings from the comparison wards in the general hospitals.

The Moos instrument, the Community-Oriented Program Environment Scales (COPES), is a 100-item true/false measure that yields 10 psychometrically distinct variables that can be grouped into three supraordinate categories: relationship/psychotherapy, treatment, and administration. The patterns of similarities and differences between the two types of alternatives (Soteria vs. Crossing Place and McAuliffe House) have remained constant over many testings, as have the hospital differences and similarities to the two kinds of alternatives. The alternative programs share high scores on all three relationship variables (involvement, spontaneity, and support) and two of four treatment variables-personal problem orientation and staff tolerance of anger. Crossing Place and McAuliffe House, however, differ from Soteria in two of three administrative variables: the second generations are perceived as more organized and exerting more staff control (somewhat similar to the hospital scores) than the parent (Soteria). The differences are to be expected, given the differing nature of the clientele and the much shorter average length of stay (<30 days) in the Soteria offspring.

Other Alternatives to Hospitalization

In the 25 plus years since the Soteria Project's successful implementation, a variety of alternatives to psychiatric hospitalization have been developed in the U.S. Their results (including those of the Soteria Project) have been extensively reviewed by Braun et al., 1981; Kiesler et al., 1982a, 1982b; Straw, 1982; Stroul, 1987. A subset were described in greater detail by Warner (1995).

Each of these reviews found consistently more positive results from descriptive and research data from a variety of alternative interventions as compared with control groups. Straw, for example, found that in 19 of 20 studies he reviewed, alternative treatments were as, or more, effective than hospital care and on the average 43% less expensive. The Soteria study was noted to be the most rigorous available in describing a comprehensive treatment approach to a subgroup of persons labeled as having schizophrenia. It was also noted that, for the most part, the effects of various models of hospitalization had not been subjected to equally serious scientific scrutiny.

Except in California, where there are a dozen, few "true" residential alternatives to acute hospitalization have been developed. Within the public sector, because of cost concerns, there is now a movement to develop "crisis houses." Their extent or success has not been completely described. However, they are not usually viewed or *used* as alternatives to acute psychiatric hospitalization-although this is subject to local variation. It is surprising that managed care, with its focus on reducing use of expensive hospitalization, has neither developed nor promoted the use of these cost-effective alternatives. It is truly notable that nearly all residential alternatives to acute psychiatric hospitalization are in the *public* mental health system. Private insurers and HMOs have been extremely reluctant to pay for care in such facilities (see Mosher, 1983).

THE Fate of Soteria

As a clinical program Soteria closed in 1983. The replication facility, Emanon, had closed in 1980. Despite many publications (37 in all), without an active treatment facility, Soteria disappeared from the consciousness of American psychiatry. Its message was difficult for the field to acknowledge, assimilate, and use. It did not fit into the emerging scientific, descriptive, biomedical character of American psychiatry, and, in fact, called nearly every one of its tenets into question. In particular, it demedicalized, dehospitalized, deprofessionalized, and deneurolepticized what Szasz (1976) has called "psychiatry's sacred cow"-schizophrenia. As far as mainstream American psychiatry is concerned, it is, to this day, an experiment that appears to be the object of studied neglect. Neither of the two recent "comprehensive" literature reviews and treatment recommendations for schizophrenia references the project (Frances et al., 1996; Lehman and Steinwachs, 1998).

There are no new U.S. Soteria replications. It is possible that, if a replication were proposed as research, it might not receive I.R.B. approval for protection of human subjects as it would involve withholding a known effective treatment (neuroleptics) for *a minimum* of 2 weeks.

Surprisingly, Soteria has reemerged in Europe. Dr. Luc Ciompi, professor of social psychiatry in Bern, Switzerland, is primarily responsible for its renaissance. Operating since 1984, Soteria Bern has replicated the original Soteria study findings. That is, roughly two-thirds of newly diagnosed persons with schizophrenia recover with little or no drug treatment in 2 to 12 weeks (Ciompi, 1994, 1997a, 1997b; Ciompi et al., 1992). As original Soteria Project papers diffused to Europe and Ciompi began to publish his results, a number of similar projects were developed. At an October 1997 meeting held in Bern, a Soteria Association was formed, headed by Professor Weiland Machleidt of the Hannover University Medical Faculty. Soteria lives, and thrives, admittedly as variations on the original theme, in Europe.

References

Allers R (1961) *Existentialism and psychiatry*. Springfield, IL: Charles C Thomas.
Bateson G, Jackson DD, Haley J, Weakland J (1956) Toward a theory of schizophrenia. *Behav Sci* 1:251–264.
Bockhoven JS (1963) *Moral treatment in American psychiatry*. New York: Springer.
Boss M (1963) *Psychoanalysis and Daseinanalysis*. New York: Basic Books.
Braden-Johnson A (1990) *Out of bedlam*. New York: Basic Books.
Braun PB, Kochansky G, Shapiro R, Greenberg S, Gudeman JE, Johnson S, Shore MF (1981) Overview: Deinstitutionalization of psychiatric patients: A critical review of outcome studies. *Am J Psychiatry* 138:736–749.
Ciompi L (1994) Affect logic: An integrative model of the psyche and its relations to schizophrenia. *Br J Psychiatry* 164:51–55, 1994.
Ciompi L (1997a) *Non-linear dynamics of complex systems: The chaos theoretical approach to schizophrenia* (pp 18–31). Seattle: Hogrefe & Huber.
Ciompi L (1997b) The concept of affect logic: An integrative psycho-socio-biological approach to understanding and treatment of psychiatry. *Psychiatry* 60:158–170.
Ciompi L, Dawalder HP, Maier CH, Aebi W, Trützsch K, Kupper Z, Rutishauser CH (1992) The pilot project "Soteria Berne" clinical experiences and results. *Br J Psychiatry* 161:145–153.
Fairweather GW, Sanders D, Cressler D, Maynard H (1969) *Community life for the mentally ill: An alternative to institutional care*. Chicago: Aldine.
Fenton W, Mosher L, Herrell J, Blyler C (1998) A randomized trial of general hospital versus residential alternative care for patients with severe and persistent mental illness. *Am J Psychiatry* 155:516–522.
Frances A, Docherty P, Kahn A (1996) Treatment of schizophrenia. *J Clin Psychiatry* 57:1–59.
Fromm-Reichmann F (1948) Notes on the development of treatment of schizophrenics by psychoanalytic psychotherapy. *Psychiatry* 11:263–273.

Goffman E (1961) *Asylums*. Garden City, NY: Anchor.

Hegel G (1967) *The phenomenology of mind*. New York: Harper & Row.

Hirschfeld RM, Matthews SM, Mosher LR, Menn AZ (1977) Being with madness: Personality characteristics of three treatment staffs: *Hosp Community Psychiatry* 28:267–273.

Husserl E (1967) *The Paris lectures*. The Hague: Martinus Nijhoff.

Kiesler CA (1982a) Mental hospitals and alternative care: Noninstitutionalization as potential public policy for mental patients. *Am Psychol* 37:349–360.

Kiesler CA (1982b) Public and professional myths about mental hospitalization: An empirical reassessment of policy-related beliefs. *Am Psychol* 37:1323–1339.

Kresky-Wolff M, Matthews S, Kalibat F, Mosher L (1984) Crossing place: A residential model for crisis intervention. *Hosp Community Psychiatry* 35:72–74.

Laing RD (1967) *The politics of experience*. New York: Ballantine.

Lehman A, Steinwachs DM (1998) Translating research into practice: The schizophrenia patient outcomes research team (PORT) recommendations. *Schizophr Bull* 24:1–11.

May R (1958) *Existence: A new dimension in psychiatry and psychology*. New York: Basic Books.

Matthews SM, Roper MT, Mosher LR, Menn AZ (1979) A non-neuroleptic treatment for schizophrenia: Analysis of the two-year post-discharge risk of relapse. *Schizophr Bull* 5:322–333.

Menninger K (1959) *Psychiatrist's world: The selected papers of Karl Menninger*. New York: Viking.

Moos RH (1974) *Evaluating treatment environments: A social ecological approach*. New York: John Wiley.

Moos RH (1975) *Evaluating correctional and community settings*. New York: John Wiley.

Mosher LR (1983) Alternatives to psychiatric hospitalization: Why so few? *N Engl J Med* 309:1479–148.

Mosher LR (1992) The social environmental treatment of psychosis: Critical Ingredients. In A Wobart, J Culberg (Eds), *Psychotherapy of schizophrenia: Facilitating and obstructive factors* (pp 254–260). Oslo: Scand. Univ. Press.

Mosher LR, Menn AZ (1974) Soteria: An alternative to hospitalization for schizophrenia. In JH Masserman (Ed), *Current psychiatric therapies*. (Vol. XI, pp 287–296). New York: Grune and Stratton.

Mosher LR, Menn AZ, Matthews S (1975) Soteria: Evaluation of a home-based treatment for schizophrenia. *Am J Orthopsychiatry* 45:455–467.

Mosher LR, Menn A (1978) Community residential treatment for schizophrenia: Two-year follow-up. *Hosp Community Psychiatry* 29:715–723.

Mosher LR, Kresky-Wolff M, Matthews S, Menn A (1986) Milieu therapy in the 1980's: A comparison of two residential alternatives to hospitalization. *Bull Menninger Clin* 50:257–268.

Mosher LR, Reifman A, Menn A (1973) Characteristics of non-professionals serving as primary therapists for acute schizophrenics. *Hosp Community Psychiatry* 24:391–396.

Mosher LR, Vallone R, Menn AZ (March 1992) *The Soteria Project: Final progress report; RO1 MH35928, R12 MH20123 and R12 MH25570*. Submitted to the NIMH. (Available from the author).

Mosher LR, Vallone R, Menn AZ (1995) The treatment of acute psychosis without neuroleptics: Six-week psychopathology outcome data from the Soteria project. *Int J Soc Psychiatry* 41:157–173.

Perry JW (1974) *The far side of madness*. Englewood Cliffs, NJ: Prentice Hall.

Sartre JP (1954) *Being and nothingness*. London: Methuen.

Searles HF (1965) *Collected papers on schizophrenia and related subjects*. New York: International Universities Press.

Scheff T (1966) *Being mentally ill*. Chicago: Aldine.

Straw RB (1982) *Meta-analysis of deinstitutionalization* (Doctoral dissertation). Ann Arbor, MI: Northwestern University.

Stroul BA (1987) *Crisis residential services in a community support system*. NIMH Community Support Program: Rockville, MD.

Sullivan HS (1962) *Schizophrenia as a human process*. New York: Norton.

Szasz T (1976) *Schizophrenia: The sacred symbol of psychiatry.* New York: Basic Books.

Tillich P (1952) *The courage to be.* New Haven, CT: Yale University Press.

Warner R (Ed) (1995) *Alternatives to the mental hospital for acute psychiatric treatment.* Washington, DC: American Psychiatric Press.

Wendt RJ, Mosher LR, Matthews SM, Menn AZ (1983) A comparison of two treatment environments for schizophrenia. In JG Gunderson, OA Will, LR Mosher (Eds), *The principles and practices of milieu therapy* (pp 17–33). New York: Jason Aronson.

45

Drake, R. E., Goldman, H. H., Leff, H. S., Lehman, A. F., Dixon, L., Mueser, K. T., & Torrey, W. C. (2001). Implementing evidence-based practices in routine mental health settings. *Psychiatric Services, 52* (2), 179–182

If recovery from and in mental illness is the dominant ideology of public mental health today, then evidence-based practice is the dominant scientific standard in public mental health services. Evidence-based practices, or EBPs—for symptom reduction in schizophrenia, supported employment, and others—have been tested in multiple studies and generally through randomized clinical trials. Drake and his colleagues review the rationale for the dissemination of EBPs, noting the long-time theme in community psychiatry of the failure to disseminate proved and promising practices on a large scale. They discuss the potential shortfalls of EBPs, including, often, their lack of testing with a wide range of ethnic-racial and cultural groups, or with persons with a wide range of psychiatric diagnoses not covered in the research that earned the practice its EBP status. The authors note the limitations of the evidence but propose forging ahead with the dissemination of current EBPs and research for new ones, maintaining clarity about the limitations of the evidence for them, the degree of confidence with which they can be disseminated widely, and the need for further testing and modification for some settings and client groups.

Implementing Evidence-Based Practices in Routine Mental Health Service Settings

The authors describe the rationale for implementing evidence-based practices in routine mental health service settings. Evidence-based practices are interventions for which there is scientific evidence consistently showing that they improve client outcomes. Despite extensive evidence and agreement on effective mental health practices for persons with severe mental illness, research shows that routine mental health programs do not provide evidence-based practices to the great majority of their clients with these illnesses. The authors define the differences between evidence-based practices and related concepts, such as guidelines and algorithms. They discuss common concerns about the use of evidence-based practices, such as whether ethical values have a role in shaping such practices and how to deal with clinical situations for which no scientific evidence exists. *(Psychiatric Services* 52:179–182, 2001)

An important focus of *Psychiatric Services* in 2001 is on the implementation of evidence-based interventions in mental health care. In last month's issue (1), the journal initiated a series of papers on implementing evidence-based practices for the care of persons with severe mental illnesses in routine mental health service settings. Papers in this series will describe the conceptual framework of a national demonstration project, the Evidence-Based Practices Project, which is sponsored by the Robert Wood Johnson Foundation, the Center for Mental Health Services of the Substance Abuse and Mental Health Services Administration, the National Alliance for the Mentally Ill, and several mental health research centers, state mental health authorities, and local mental health programs in New Hampshire, Maryland, Ohio, North Carolina, and Texas.

The goal of the project is to develop standardized guidelines and training materials, in the form of toolkits, and to demonstrate that the toolkits can be used to facilitate the faithful implementation of evidence-based practices and to improve client outcomes in routine mental health service settings.

In this paper we present the concept of evidence-based practices. We describe the background of the movement toward such practices and define evidence-based practices and related concepts. We also discuss common concerns about the use of evidence-based practices in routine mental health service settings.

The Rationale for Evidence-Based Practices

Psychiatric Services' decision to dedicate 2001 to evidence-based practices rests on a series of research findings and philosophical commitments. First, a great deal is now known about efficacious and effective mental health interventions, which we refer to here as evidence-based practices. For example, numerous recent reviews of the research evidence identify a core set of interventions that help persons with severe mental illness attain better outcomes in terms of symptoms, functional status, and quality of life (2–6). The core set includes medications prescribed within specific parameters, training in illness self-management, assertive community treatment, family psychoeducation, supported employment, and integrated treatment for co-occurring substance use disorders (7). In upcoming issues, experts will review research evidence on outcomes, present current knowledge about barriers and strategies related to implementation, and discuss implications.

A second reason for the journal's focus on evidence-based practices is that despite extensive evidence and agreement on effective mental health practices for persons with severe mental illness, research also shows that routine mental health programs do not provide evidence-based practices to the great majority of clients with these illnesses (8). This finding was a major conclusion of the mental health report of the Surgeon General (6). In the most extensive demonstration of this problem, the Schizophrenia Patient Outcome Research Team showed that in two state mental health systems, clients with a diagnosis of schizophrenia were highly unlikely to receive effective services (9). For example, antipsychotic medications were often prescribed at dosages outside the effective range. A minority of clients—often as few as 10 percent—received evidence-based psychosocial services, such as family interventions. Findings from other sources suggest a dearth of evidence-based practices in routine mental health settings (10).

Third, research indicates that offering a service that resembles an evidence-based practice is not sufficient; adherence to specific programmatic standards, often referred to as fidelity of implementation, is necessary to produce expected outcomes (11–13). In other words, if two programs offer a practice of care that is known to be effective, the program with higher fidelity to the defined practice model tends to produce superior outcomes. This critical finding, which contradicts the conventional wisdom that model programs do not transfer and need to be modified extensively to fit local circumstances, suggests that implementation guidelines and toolkits should begin to incorporate manuals and fidelity measures (14).

Fourth, mental health services for persons with severe mental illness should reflect the goals of consumers. People with severe mental illness, like people with other long-term illnesses, want to pursue normal, functional, satisfying lives to the greatest extent possible (15,16). Mental health services therefore should not focus exclusively on traditional outcomes of treatment compliance and prevention of relapses and rehospitalizations. The new paradigm emphasizes helping people attain outcomes such as independence, employment, satisfying relationships, and good quality of life.

Fifth, given that mental health resources are limited, persons with severe mental illness have a right to have access to interventions that are known to be effective and that are delivered in a manner faithful to or consistent with current understandings of the interventions' active ingredients. In other words, to the extent that evidence-based practices exist, they should be the bedrock, the minimum of acceptable offerings, in all mental health settings that provide services for persons with severe mental illness. Additional services may enhance the service offering and may prove to be effective over time, but the basic offering of evidence-based practices should not be displaced by interventions of unknown or lesser effectiveness. Researchers, state mental health directors, consumers, and families support this commitment and have endorsed the urgent need for dissemination and implementation of evidence-based practices (17).

Finally, evidence-based practices do not provide the answers for all persons with mental illness, all outcomes, or all settings. Below we discuss several caveats as well as the judicious and informed use of evidence-based practices. Accurate information about effective practices, including a clear understanding of the limitations of current research and the need for further evidence in many areas, can improve services and outcomes. However, to produce positive changes, the research evidence on effective services and the implementation procedures must be available to all stakeholders in the service system (1).

What are Evidence-Based Practices?

Evidence-based practices are interventions for which there is consistent scientific evidence showing that they improve client outcomes. For example, research shows that using antipsychotic medications within specific dosage ranges and providing education and skill training for family caregivers over several months prevents or delays relapses of schizophrenia (4). The requirements for scientific evidence used by different groups sometimes vary, but in general the highest standard is several randomized clinical trials comparing the practice to alternative practices or to no intervention. When the separate trials are considered together, such as through a meta-analysis, the evidence supports the superiority of the evidence-based practice over the alternatives, including no intervention.

In some situations quasi-experimental studies, with comparison groups that are not assigned by randomization, constitute the best available evidence and consistently support a specific evidence-based practice. Rather than rigid decision rules, which inevitably are more appropriate for some types of interventions than others, we encourage panels of research scientists to review the available controlled studies and to make explicit their criteria for inclusion, the studies reviewed, the review procedures, and the conclusions so that others can examine the same evidence and reasoning.

Open clinical trials, which lack independent comparison groups, provide a significantly lower level of research evidence and are generally not considered to provide sufficiently strong scientific evidence. The lowest level of evidence, which should not be considered research evidence, consists of clinical observations collected as expert opinion. Best practices based on clinical opinions or open clinical trials do not constitute evidence-based practices, because they are not research based, are fraught with potential for error, and are often contradicted by later findings of controlled research.

Some groups, such as the Agency for Healthcare Research and Quality, have identified levels of scientific evidence, which they use to score evidence-based practices. The various practice guidelines developed in the 1990s by the agency—then known as the Agency for Health Care Policy and Research (18)—exemplify this approach by using three levels of evidence: level A refers to good research-based evidence, with some expert opinion. Level B indicates fair research-based evidence, with substantial expert opinion, to support the recommendation. Level C denotes a recommendation based primarily on expert opinion, with minimal research-based evidence.

Although the term evidence-based practice is sometimes used to refer to guidelines that are not based on research, true evidence-based practices are by definition grounded in consistent research evidence that is sufficiently specific to permit the assessment of the quality of the practices rendered as well as the outcomes. For example, supported employment is sufficiently well defined and standardized so that its fidelity can be measured and it can be differentiated from other approaches to vocational rehabilitation (14).

Other guidelines, such as those developed by the American Psychiatric Association (19), are based on a mixture of randomized clinical trials and expert consensus and often lack sufficient specificity to provide tools for judging the quality of interventions. There are also consensus guidelines, such as those developed by the triuniversity consortium (20), that systematically define desired practices through an iterative consensus process among experts. The advantage of the expert consensus approach is that it permits development of guidelines about practices for which no systematic research evidence exists. The major disadvantage is that the expert opinions may reflect current biases in the field rather than demonstrated effectiveness. At the far end of the continuum are guidelines that are written primarily to serve some administrative function and that are supported neither by research evidence nor by expert consensus.

Treatment decisions are typically complex, involving multiple decision steps that depend on the patient's response to treatment at each step. This complexity has led to the development of treatment algorithms that map out a series of decision points based on responses to the previous steps. For example, an algorithm for pharmacologic treatment of a person experiencing acute symptoms of schizophrenia may begin with initiation of an antipsychotic medication within a specific dosage range. If the person fails to respond adequately to the treatment, the algorithm may specify a second option—for example, switching to another class of antipsychotic agent. Failure to respond to the second treatment would lead to a third decision point—for example, initiation of clozapine treatment. Such algorithms may be particularly useful in guiding clinicians through a complex series of treatment decisions.

As with guidelines, algorithms may have varying levels of scientific evidence to support them. A current challenge in algorithm development is that the scientific evidence supporting the successive steps quickly becomes quite thin. Hence even the most evidence-based algorithms typically begin with steps supported by multiple clinical trials and evolve into steps defined through expert consensus. An excellent example of treatment algorithms has been developed in the Texas Medication Algorithm Project (5).

Questions About the Use of Evidence-Based Practices

A number of questions arise in relation to the recent emphasis on evidence-based practices. For example, what is the role of ethical values in shaping practices? What should be done when there are different levels of evidence or changes in evidence? What are the limits of evidence? What should be done in clinical situations for which there is no scientific evidence? We briefly address each of these points below and will do so in greater detail in upcoming issues of the journal.

Values

Mental health services appropriately incorporate humanistic values, ethical principles, and legal standards. For example, addressing adult clients as adults, interacting benignly and respectfully with families, and showing sensitivity with respect to age, sex, race, and cultural background are core values of the health care system (21). Research is not required to support these standards, and nothing about evidence-based practices contravenes the importance of such standards. On the contrary, this discussion assumes that evidence-based practices must incorporate consensual values, ethical principles, and legal standards.

Nature of the Evidence

As noted, research evidence is often complicated, with inconsistent results and differences in the design, quality, and number of studies of any single intervention. Moreover, the evidence evolves rapidly. Thus the need for scientific review is critical and ongoing. For policy purposes, however, the transition from existing practices to evidence-based practices is more clear-cut. Existing practices typically rely on tradition, convenience, clinicians' preferences, political correctness, marketing, and clinical wisdom—none of which is consistently related to improving outcomes. Historically, clinical practice in mental health is often completely unhelpful and sometimes tragically harmful, as in the case of psychosurgery.

The crux of the matter is that precisely because evidence-based practices are grounded in the qualifications imposed by current science, they are standardized, replicable, and effective. A switch to research-based interventions with known effectiveness can dramatically improve outcomes in large practice systems—for example, the overall rate of employment of persons with severe mental illness (22).

Limitations of the Evidence

Research evidence on interventions is often quite specific with respect to population, outcome, and context. For example, research clearly demonstrates that assertive community treatment effectively reduces hospital use for clients with schizophrenia who are unstable, homeless, treatment resistant, or hospital prone, especially in settings in which the alternative services are hospital based or clinic based (23–25). But the evidence is less clear in several areas. Does assertive community treatment improve functional outcomes such as employment? Should clients who are more stable be given assertive community treatment? What about different ethnocultural groups? What about clients with other diagnoses, such as borderline personality disorder, posttraumatic stress disorder, or substance use disorders? Is assertive community treatment needed in settings in which the usual services have incorporated its basic features such as outreach?

The central strategy in defining evidence-based practices is to be straightforward about the limits of the evidence. The provision of evidence-based practices even under circumscribed conditions would be an improvement and would move stakeholders toward awareness of the potential of other evidence-based practices. For example, research indicates that assertive community treatment does not consistently improve vocational outcomes and that supported employment must be a well-integrated component of the intervention to achieve high rates of competitive employment (25). Thus providing assertive community treatment should increase pressure to implement supported employment.

Extensions of the evidence should be careful, logical, and able to be evaluated. Because supported employment improves employment outcomes for white, African-American, and Hispanic-American clients, offering it to other cultural minorities would be a logical decision, unless there are obvious cultural differences in the meaning of work. On the other hand, logic dictates that family psychoeducation may have different meanings and effects in different cultures, and some negative research findings among Hispanic-American families (26) reinforce caution about extending the research on family psychoeducation to other groups (27).

In some situations, essentially no research exists on treatment outcomes, such as treating hepatitis C infection or the sequelae of trauma among people with severe mental illness or evaluating the effects of self-help services. The emphasis on evidence-based practices should create pressure to develop and test these interventions to fill the need for informed rather than expedient public policy. The corpus of evidence-based practices is not static, and outcomes that are valued by consumers and families should influence which interventions are developed and studied.

Conclusions

For each area of evidence-based practices, implementation in routine mental health practice settings is complex and difficult (1). Issues of organizational structure and commitment, resource development, and clarity of roles and responsibilities must be addressed before training can be effective (28). Service boundaries are often involved as well. For example, supported employment involves the interface between clinical and rehabilitative services, and dual diagnosis services highlight differences between the mental health and substance abuse treatment systems. Upcoming articles in *Psychiatric Services* will address implementation barriers and strategies as well as the specific evidence, including boundaries and extensions, for each of several evidence-based practices. Emphasis on evidence-based practices also has implications for public policy, education, research, medical information systems, managed care, liability, and many other topics.

References

1. Torrey WC, Drake RE, Dixon L, et al: Implementing evidence-based practices for persons with severe mental illnesses. Psychiatric Services 52:45–50, 2001
2. Fenton WE, Schooler NR: Editor's introduction: evidence-based psychosocial treatment for schizophrenia. Schizophrenia Bulletin 26: 1–3, 2000
3. Kane JM: Pharmacologic treatment of schizophrenia. Biological Psychiatry 46:1396–1408, 1999
4. Lehman AF, Steinwachs DM, Survey Co-Investigators of the PORT Project: Translating research into practice: the Schizophrenia Patient Outcomes Research Team (PORT) treatment recommendations. Schizophrenia Bulletin 24:1–10,1998
5. Miller AL, Chiles JA, Chiles JK, et al: The Texas Medication Algorithm Project (TMAP) schizophrenia algorithms. Journal of Clinical Psychiatry 60:649–657,1999
6. Mental Health: A Report of the Surgeon General. Washington, DC, Department of Health and Human Services, US Public Health Service, 2000
7. Drake RE, Mueser KT, Torrey WC, et al: Evidence-based treatment of schizophrenia. Current Psychiatry Reports 2:393–397, 2000
8. Leff HS, Mulkern V, Lieberman M, et al: The effects of capitation on service access, adequacy, and appropriateness. Administration and Policy in Mental Health 21:141–160, 1994
9. Lehman AF, Steinwachs DM, Survey Co-Investigators of the PORT Project: Patterns of usual care for schizophrenia: initial results from the schizophrenia Patient Outcomes Research Team (PORT) client survey. Schizophrenia Bulletin 24:11–20,1998
10. Dixon L, Lyles A, Scott J, et al: Services to families of adults with schizophrenia: from treatment recommendations to dissemination. Psychiatric Services 50:233–238, 1999
11. Jerrel JM, Ridgely MS: Impact of robustness of program implementation on outcomes of clients in dual diagnosis programs. Psychiatric Services 50:109–112, 1999
12. McDonnell J, Nofs D, Hardman M, et al: An analysis of the procedural components of supported employment programs associated with employment outcomes. Journal of Applied Behavior Analysis 22:417–428, 1989
13. McHugo GJ, Drake RE, Teague GB, et al: Fidelity to assertive community treatment and client outcomes in the New Hampshire Dual Disorders Study. Psychiatric Services 50:818–824,1999
14. Bond G, Williams J, Evans L, et al: Psychiatric Rehabilitation Fidelity Toolkit. Cambridge, Mass, Evaluation Center@HSRI, 2000
15. Mead S, Copeland ME: What recovery means to us: consumers' perspectives. Community Mental Health Journal 36:315–328, 2000
16. Torrey WC, Wyzik P: The recovery vision as a service improvement guide for community mental health center providers. Community Mental Health Journal 36:209–216, 2000

17. National Institute of Mental Health: Bridging Science and Service. A Report by the National Advisory Mental Health Council's Clinical Treatment and Services Research Workshop. Rockville, MD, National Institute of Mental Health, 1999

18. Depression in Primary Care. AHCPR pub 93-0550. Rockville, Md, Agency for Health Care Policy and Research, 1993

19. American Psychiatric Association: Practice Guidelines for the Treatment of Patients With Schizophrenia. Washington DC, American Psychiatric Press, 1997

20. Frances AJ, Docherty J, Kahn DA: The expert consensus guideline series: Treatment of schizophrenia. Journal of Clinical Psychiatry 57(suppl 12B):1-58, 1996

21. Culver CM, Gert B: Philosophy in Medicine. New York, Oxford Press, 1982

22. Drake RE, Fox T, Leather PK, et al: Regional variation in competitive employment for persons with severe mental illness. Administration and Policy in Mental Health 25:493–504, 1998

23. Burns BJ, Santos AB: Assertive community treatment: an update of randomized trials. Psychiatric Services 46:669–675, 1995

24. Latimer E: Economic impacts of assertive community treatment: a review of the literature. Canadian Journal of Psychiatry 44:443–454, 1999

25. Mueser KT, Bond GR, Drake RE, et al: Models of community care for severe mental illness: a review of research on case management. Schizophrenia Bulletin 24:37–74, 1998

26. Telles C, Kamo M, Mintz J, et al: Immigrant families coping with schizophrenia: behavioral family intervention v case management with a low-income Spanish speaking population. British Journal of Psychiatry 167:473–479,1995

27. Dixon L, Adams C, Lucksted A: Update on family psychoeducation for schizophrenia. Schizophrenia Bulletin 26:5–20, 2000

28. Rapp C, Poertner J: Social Administration: A Client-Centered Approach. White Plains, NY, Longman, 1992

V

Conclusion: Community Psychiatry and the Future

Michael Rowe and Kenneth S. Thompson

We've come a long way. Caution might urge a full stop on the page before this one, for "Community Psychiatry and the Future" could wake avenging angels whose job it is to punish the sin of presumption. The purpose of this chapter, though, is not to predict community psychiatry's future so much as to choose a few of its themes and consider some paths they might take next. What useful or promising elements can the overlapping themes, or domains, of mental illness, psychiatry, practice, funding, policy, community, recovery, and identity offer us? What problematic ones? Throughout, this discussion will attempt to remain grounded in certain processes laid out by Joseph Morrissey and Howard Goldman, and Gerald Grob and Goldman in that historical order over the second and third of our three eras of community psychiatry.

In a 1986 article, Morrissey and Goldman make a claim for the recurrence of reform movements that offer an innovative approach to and a corresponding institutional form of care for mental health treatment, and which exhibit similar patterns of failure. Each of three successive reform cycles—the moral treatment movement with its asylums in the early nineteenth century, the mental hygiene movement with its psychopathic hospitals in the early twentieth century, and the community mental health movement with its community mental health centers in the latter part of the twentieth century—began, they write, with high hopes that early treatment would prevent long-term mental illness. Each made headway for a time and then faltered due to lack of effective treatment technologies and circumstances such as decreased funding and increased demand, and each proved more successful at helping those with mild than with serious and persistent forms of mental illness.[1]

Grob and Goldman, writing in 2006 about the ascending role of the federal government in mental health care after World War II, argue that reform movements in public psychiatry tend toward the radical or incremental. The radical community mental health center movement was born in the 1960s out of the conviction that fundamental change, away from reliance on long-term hospitals and toward providing treatment for persons with mental illness within their home communities, was urgently required. The 1980 National Plan for the Chronically Mentally Ill, which emerged from the wreckage of the community mental health movement, looked, more modestly, to patch together services from currently existing entitlement programs in order to effect incremental change. Incrementalism, Grob and Goldman contend, can be a more effective approach in the United States than radical reform if two conditions are met. First, incrementalism must be guided and backed up by a vision of fundamental reform that, often, is promulgated by a high-level government commission and its report linking vision and goals to incremental objectives and steps, thus constituting a higher-order incrementalism called sequentialism. Second, the implementation of sequential reform requires a hewing to the values of fundamental, or radical, reform throughout, always linking those values to appropriate clinical and systems technologies for achieving them.[2]

The forms and patterns of change these authors have outlined are likely to shape the possibilities that each of this chapter's eight themes will take in the near future. The first three—mental illness, psychiatry, and practice—can be categorized as conceptual and scientific technologies employed in community psychiatry; the middle two—funding and policy—as intervention technologies that are driven, at least partly, by values; and the last three—community, recovery, and identity—as values of community psychiatry.[3] The macro themes of technology and values interact in these second-rank themes. Indeed, traces, if not strong markings, of values, can be seen in technology-driven themes, and of technology in values-driven themes. Mental illness, psychiatry, practice, funding, policy, community, recovery, and identity do lack a certain precision as tools for examining current and future practice in community psychiatry. The mental health workforce, for example, could be linked to psychiatry rather than practice, where it appears in this discussion, and the topic of asylum might fit under psychiatry or practice, rather than community. Law and other regulating institutions of society, which could stand on their own as a ninth theme, take a place under policy here. Culture, race, gender, age, sexuality, class, and poverty deserve more attention than they we give them in the space available here—similarly, politics and economics, Spirituality and the arts, topics that could have a strong impact on community psychiatry of the future, receive no explicit attention (although they do have an association with culture). Still, these eight themes cover a broad swath, aided and guided by the interactions among innovative approaches, institutional forms, and treatment and care technologies that Morrissey and Goldman, and the incrementalism and fundamental reform that Grob and Goldman, elucidate.

1. Mental illness. Conceptions of mental illness change as culture, belief systems, medical knowledge, and other elements in a society change. Mental illness may mean possession in a premodern society and brain disease in a technologically advanced one, even if fears of violent tendencies of persons with mental illness persist in both. In a postmodern world, the place where you are standing changes your perspective on things, and rationality, the standard against which craziness looks crazy, has less foundation. In such a time and setting, then, craziness may look less crazy. Even so, mental illness in contemporary U.S. society represents a lack of control over one's mind and capacities and, thus, one may fear one's very self or another's self witnessing his or her disturbing behavior or seeing the consequences of dysfunction.

The humanistic promise of biological psychiatry is that mental illness, if treated successfully with the technology of medications that target receptors and cells in the brain that have gone awry, will come to be seen as an illness like any other and so lose its stigma. Biological psychiatry, then, is a contemporary response to nature's allocation of mental illness to individuals, and psychiatric medications are its chief products. Social psychiatry looks to nurture, which shows itself in culture, class, material circumstances, stigma, and other factors external to the body, and psychosocial technologies designed to help people compensate for the difficulties these elements, along with their singular disabilities, pose for them, are its chief products. In the near future, the relative importance of nature and nurture and of interventions that correspond to them will depend in part on findings from research and practice and in part on political economics. The pharmaceutical industry with its links to biological and academic psychiatry and the recovery movement with its endorsements at federal and state policy levels have roles to play in both areas, with the pharmaceutical industry playing the strong hand at present, though it is increasingly being challenged in regard to the values of integrity and accountability.

At the margins of present-day community psychiatry, elements are in play that could blur the boundaries between the biological and social. Trauma, resulting from physical, emotional, or sexual abuse of individuals or from large-scale disasters that affect thousands, involves events and actions external to the person, but also has the capacity to affect the brains of affected persons.[4] Environmental approaches to mental health and illness, which in the past referred mainly to the influence of economic and social conditions on health, may come to include scrutiny of the air we breathe and the toxins we ingest. Perhaps there are canaries in the coal mine now who serve as unwilling bearers of these divinations.[5] And if a reinvented form of psychotherapy, narrative medicine,[6] which has found its niche in medicine writ large, makes its way to mental health, it may offer a renewed outlet for those and other voices.

A dual focus on brain and society may lead, finally, to a more synthetic view of mind at the interface of a complex adaptive human system that integrates subjective and objective elements and that is responsive to and shapes both. The social and biological are nested in each other.

2. Psychiatry. Will we call it "community psychiatry" in the future? Many do not call it that now, preferring "public mental health" or "community mental health," and to be sure we have used the term partly as a prod to force the question of psychiatry's contested role in public mental health care. A recovery movement that reached broad consensus on psychiatric medications as one tool in the recovery toolkit might come to have a friendlier relationship with psychiatry, but that discipline's future leadership of public mental health care does not seem assured.

In crafting a vision of itself as a modern, biological, and scientific endeavor, psychiatry has become increasingly decontextualized and ahistorical.[7] "Postpsychiatry," according to U.K. psychiatrists Patrick Bracken and Philip Thomas, whose work hearkens back to that of Franco Basaglia and other radical psychiatrists from the 1970s, positions itself as an alternative to traditional psychiatry. The latter is a child of the enlightenment, they write, built on the triune stool of the primacy of reason and technology as the means for solving human problems, promotion of an orderly society (one that, they note, has led the discipline to collude with the state in coercion of persons with psychiatric disabilities), and mental illness as a disease that afflicts individuals. Postpsychiatry looks to ethics before technology and to a holistic emphasis on social and cultural influences regarding the incidence and outlines of mental illness. It also looks to community leadership for democratic discussion and weighing of different perspectives on responses to mental illness, and supports the primacy of meaning for persons with mental illness over reductionistic explanations for their illnesses.[8] Ronald Diamond and colleagues argue that community psychiatrists have essential roles to play as medical experts and signatories and desirable roles as teachers, scholars, and generalists, along with that of assessing the psychiatric status of new patients.[9] The most obvious medical role for psychiatrists is that of determining the psychopharmacological needs of patients and prescribing medications for them. This is an important function, but a narrow one. A return to phenomenology in psychiatry, as Nancy Andreasen proposes,[10] combined with psychiatrists' medical training and knowledge of the body, could mean a return to the questions of what mental illness is and how to respond to the suffering associated with it. These are questions that practitioners of psychosocial rehabilitation may not be as well equipped, in general, to address as a phenomenologically informed psychiatry, and they still need to be asked. In addition, given the implications of recent research that has demonstrated drastically reduced life expectancies of persons with serious mental illness,[11] psychiatrists may play a new and vital role as both liaisons to and dual practitioners of primary medicine, especially if they will stand at the forefront with others in attending to social inequities in health and health care. Health care reform's impact on community psychiatry, and on the role of psychiatrists, is unclear at this point, although it would seem that, if mental health care is integrated within health care in general, psychiatrists, as physicians, would be in a strong position to lead in terms of both mental health care and the integration of primary and mental health care.

The technology and values of psychiatry are entangled in psychiatry's development as a project of the Enlightenment project, and the tensile strength of each does not necessarily support the other. One strand of psychiatry asks the question, "How do you rid the brain of mental illness?" Another asks, "How do you create circumstances of nonsubjugation to free people from socioeconomic conditions that help create mental illness and that make having it more burdensome?" The first task—ridding the brain of mental illness—involves removing from inside persons a thing that afflicts them. The second—changing external circumstances—involves freeing people from what others do to them because of their mental illnesses.

Looking back to one of psychiatry's founding myths—that of Pinel's single-handedly liberating the insane from their chains at the Bicêtre Hospital—we argue that the chains Pinel broke were not the chains of his patients' mental illness but the chains that society put on them." (We now know that it was his assistant, Poussin, a peer worker, who actually removed the chains.) The questions of ridding the brain of mental illness or ridding society of pestilential living conditions are not fundamentally questions of the technologies of biological and social psychiatry, but political questions. Democracy is challenged at the boundaries it creates when it sets limits on itself and its citizens in terms of gender, race, class, and normality.[12]

3. Practice. A few comments on three forms of the technology of practice—evidence-based practice (EBP), recovery-oriented practice, and prevention of mental illness—will serve to highlight some issues that will be in play over the next few years, if not longer.

EBP—the idea that interventions and approaches proved to be successful through clinical trials should be made widely available to persons with psychiatric disabilities—is an ascendant approach in present-day community mental health care.[12] As noted in the introductory chapter to our "present era" of community psychiatry, EBPs have been criticized for failing to take into account the needs and preferences of a wider range of racial-ethnic, cultural, and diagnostic groups than those on which they were tested. Robert Drake and colleagues argue that this criticism, while holding some water, does not negate the importance of providing evidence-based services to those groups but points instead to the need for additional research on modifications needed to make services as effective for these groups as they proved to be for original research subjects. Another critique of EBPs is that they give short shrift to clients' values and to ethical issues in treatment in general. Proponents, however, can claim that EBP has its own moral imperative—that of bringing effective services to those who have not received them in the past.[13]

Not yet broached directly, although exhaustively researched under the form of systems integration in public mental health, are evidence-based systems of care. And not yet incorporated into EBPs' toolkits is the gestalt, the "itness," of the practice. Take mental health outreach to persons who are homeless, for example. What does it mean when an outreach worker says she makes contact with the core person first, not the prospective patient,[13] when, as happens from time to time, the exterior of that core person does not look or act nice at all, or at least does not until much trust and relationship building has occurred over the course of many months? What kind of person does it take to do such work and stick with it for years? That the person who has the right stuff would likely scoff at the idea of a toolkit to portray her art does not negate the potential importance of having one, but it does suggest that what the toolkit is least likely to capture is the practitioner, the vital spark of the helping relationship, and the gestalt of the practice.

Recovery-oriented practice would ask of EBPs and other approaches, "Does this practice respect and encourage client choice and self-determination?" Recovery-oriented principles such as supporting clients' strengths and partnership in the treatment process, fostering hope, and honoring clients' dignity would seem to be consistent with, or not to contradict, the guiding principles and technology of most present-day mental health interventions. Indeed, many clinicians employ these principles now. Innovations in some psychosocial practices seem to link more directly with a recovery-based approach. The common factor, for example, in both supported employment, where clients are placed in competitive jobs rather than gradually working their way toward it via volunteerism and sheltered work-shops, and supported housing, where people live in their own apartments with their own leases rather than working their way up to them via halfway houses and transitional living programs (as noted in the "present era" chapter) is the notion that persons with mental illness do not need to move through gradually increasing levels of stability, independence and responsibility in order to have what other people have. Work and an apartment of one's own, in fact, may support one's stability, sobriety, and personal growth.

Prevention might be called the stepchild of modern psychiatry,[14] an essential component of the original community mental health movement, but one that has been given short shrift in mental health systems that have focused on the treatment needs of persons already diagnosed. Current efforts in the area of early detection and treatment of serious mental illness before it becomes full-blown psychosis[15] may ultimately fuel greater interest in pre-vention. The technologies of motivational engagement and illness self-management, along with recovery's emphasis on the value of self-determination, may make for some blurring of boundaries between prevention and treatment, since these approaches involve ongoing prevention efforts for persons with psychiatric disabilities.

The concept of social inclusion, recently imported to the United States from Europe, takes a public health approach to mental illness and charges communities and society as a whole with the responsibility of including marginal persons as much, if not more, than it charges marginalized persons with responsibility for finding their niche. Prevention of mental illness is a core value and ingredient of social inclusion, and some work is under way to adapt the European approach for dissemination in the United States.[16]

Looming behind these practices, whether evidence-based, promising, or contested, is the future of the behavioral health workforce. Experts agree that the current workforce is in crisis, with problems recruiting and retaining qualified staff who represent the racial-eth-nic makeup of clientele, a lack of ongoing training, including training in recovery-oriented practice,[17] lack of supervision and paucity of career ladders, and the challenge of meet-ing increased demand for services with fewer resources.[18] Perhaps an expanded National Institutes of Health loan repayment program and a Peace Corps–Americorps style national program to recruit case managers, rehabilitation specialists, social workers, psychologists, and psychiatrists for 2- to 3-year stints could help allay the shortage of person power in behavioral health care and inject new zeal into the work.

4. Funding. Changes in funding and reimbursement for mental health care could have an enormous impact on the quality, accessibility, and equitable distribution of that care. The health care reform has been enacted, but its impact on the accessibility, breadth, and depth of treatment available to persons with mental illness remains to be seen. Currently, some states have in place mental health parity laws, but their application is another mat-ter. Patient co-pays and clinician negotiations with insurers for starting and continuing services can leave the patient in close to the same position of nonparity he or she would have faced before parity. Entry into the system can be a barrier as well, with rejection of applicants who are currently receiving mental health treatment if they are not guaranteed coverage by their employer's contract with the insurer.

Mental health exceptionalism, the carve-out and set-aside of resources to treat persons with serious mental illness as opposed to lumping them in with other health care resources, has been an ongoing theme in community psychiatry. Setting aside funds to serve persons who, otherwise, might lose out to those with less severe and more readily treatable health problems, more money to spend on their problems, and louder voices, is one advantage of mental health exceptionalism. An argument to be made for mainstreaming funds for persons with serious mental illness is that, in theory, mainstreaming funds for these persons will help them to enter the mainstream of society at large. The debate over the two courses will continue, even as exceptionalism has lost some of its hold on mental health policy and funding with the advance of Medicaid and managed care, and exceptionalism and mainstreaming, both, while still in play, may look quite different than they do now with implementation of health care reform.

Funding for innovative services such as reimbursement for peer specialist services through Medicaid waivers (in place in 42 states) is now being engaged. Widespread success, however, could prove to be a double-edged sword. Reimbursement for peer specialist services, for example, gives promise to legitimize an approach that has had limited support in public mental health up to now. Yet that reimbursement mechanism, with its power to define the shape and outcomes of the service it pays for, has the potential to undermine the innovative aspects of it. Development of an evidence base for peer work may serve to moderate this tendency, but dissemination of and funding for effective practices lag years behind demonstration of their effectiveness.

5. Policy. Perhaps no other building block of public services is more subject to reification than the domain of policy. In reification, the meetings, negotiations, advocacy, and compromise that are intrinsic to the policy-making process and the wide range of players from the top on down who participate in it , and the process becomes a thing that someone else—a policy expert—does. In the public mental health field, many tend to think of policy as something that only legislators and experts at state and federal executives devise and negotiate over. Michael Lipsky, however, has demonstrated that "street level bureaucrats"—front-line workers and supervisors—take the guidelines of policy and construct the street-level technology for their approximation, or transformation, at the level of day-to-day practice by juggling formal policy directives with available resources and inexhaustible demands, making do with what they have and have the energy for.[19] Some work has been done in public mental health care regarding the ways in which front-line workers, such as case managers, can push systems of care toward greater integration in addition to coordinating services for individual clients,[20] but street-level explanations have had little influence in our understanding of policy making in mental health care.

Recent scholarship in interpretive policy analysis emphasizes the integral roles of meaning and values in policy making[21] and the ways policy is created through meeting, learning, and creating successive iterations of working documents. Interpretive policy analysis, then, deconstructs policy and reconstitutes it in its practices.[22] Richard Freeman goes so far as to discard the more "traditional alternative" view of multiple levels—high and low, legislative and street level—of policy making and implementation, suggesting instead that policy is taken up, interpreted, translated, and implemented in different sites that provide the opportunities for conducting those activities.

The interpretive approach can inform, for only one example, the work of those engaged in state mental health transformation efforts toward recovery-based systems of care by showing its prime movers that the difficulties of translating recovery-oriented approaches into practice do not always, or only, involve hidebound resistance, co-optation, and watering down of the original pristine approach. Instead, there is also a process of learning and understanding, reshaping, and recreating policy in different sites that provide different opportunities and means for action.[23] Such an understanding can recursively inform strategic planning processes for systems change, staff training, evaluation of fidelity to the original policy or practice, and attempts to learn from and influence these changes as they occur.

Law becomes effective public policy through legislation or judicial decisions, funding that sometimes, but not always, flows from those decisions, and through the criminal justice system. In public mental health, the law has wide-ranging applications and influences, from the criminalization of mental illness to the U.S. Supreme Court's 1999 Olmsted decision, which ruled that unnecessary institutionalization of disabled persons is prohibited by the Americans with Disabilities Act,[24] to involuntary outpatient commitment laws in effect in 43 of the 50 states.[25]

Public and legislative deliberation over changes in law may lead to changes in public policy as well. In 2000, the Connecticut legislature was on the verge of passing an involuntary outpatient commitment law for persons with serious mental illness living in the community who were not engaged in mental health treatment and had histories of violence toward others, or the threat of it. Legislators were swayed by advocates, however, who proposed an alternative, that of peer specialists who would be integrated into community mental health treatment teams in order to engage into treatment persons who would be subject to involuntary outpatient commitment if the law were passed. The initial, 2-year stage of this project produced promising results that appear to have contributed, along with other developments, to the increased use of peer staff in public mental health in Connecticut and have had some impact nationally.[26]

6. Community. A return to the community for persons with psychiatric disabilities has been the dream of community psychiatry for more than forty years. The question, "Can this work?" stood in the wings of the community mental health movement starting in the 1960s. The question, "What have we missed that can make this work?" took center stage in the late 1970s with the community support systems initiative. At that time, economic and ideological factors and structural changes in mental health systems, or nonsystems, of care had shut the door on a return to state hospital systems as the primary locus of public mental health care. "Community integration" (more likely to be called "community inclusion" or social inclusion today) became the working concept starting at the end of the last century, and the question underwent another sea change, becoming, "What kind of life in the community is this that we're trying to help people live?" Norma Ware and colleagues state the problem this way[27]:

> Despite decades of deinstitutionalization and the best efforts of community health services, individuals with psychiatric disabilities living outside the hospital may be described as in the community, but not of it. They may live in neighborhoods alongside people without disabilities. Their residences may resemble those of their neighbors. Yet many people who are psychiatrically disabled lack socially valued activity, adequate income, personal relationships, recognition and respect from others, and a political voice. They remain, in a very real sense, socially excluded.

Another question, returning to a theme in the introduction to this book, is, "What, and whose, community are we talking about?" The long-held notion of community as a place where people meet face to face to conduct their business and social lives with each other is, in good part, a myth. It does not offer a prescription for making it in today's society where, more and more, we need the weak ties of work associates, reference groups, organizations, influences, and networks that span the country if not the globe, as much as we need the strong ties of family, nearby friends, and neighbors.[28] This point does not necessarily scuttle the strong ties version of community for persons with psychiatric disabilities. For persons who have been hospitalized several times for psychiatric problems, are poor, have a thin social network, little work experience, and do not own a computer or know how to use one, building strong ties in their local neighborhood may be a good place for them to start on the way to building some of the weak ones they will need as well. Yet communities may not make this task easy for them, even setting aside the problem of stigma, because the neighborhoods in which these persons can afford to live, and much of the community around them, may be decimated by poverty, crime, a crumbling infrastructure, and high unemployment. A default community in which they may have less trouble making their way, especially if they have co-occurring substance use disorders, is what Kim Hopper and his colleagues describe as the institutional circuit of jail, shelter, and psychiatric hospital.[29] More optimistically, it appears that social interventions that can help people achieve the status and experience of being *of* the community rather than just living *in* it[30] may help to facilitate the development of social groups that simultaneously encourage individual's attempts to make their way in the larger community and become a small community for their members.[31]

One response to the difficulties posed above would be a grand vision and action plan for community psychiatry that fills in the outlines of, yet goes beyond, the community inclusion approach, drawing on social justice theory and advocacy as well as evidence- and recovery-based practices. Another would be to step back and consider whether or not, in Grob and Goldman's formulation, incremental change that draws from such a vision but works toward it via the slower path of sequentialism, is the way to go. Robert Rosenheck posed the twin dilemmas of community psychiatry in a classic article included in the present era. The community mental health movement of the 1960s, borne on a wave of public support for social programs and social justice and of federal leadership to accomplish those objectives, was strong on commitment to radical change, he writes, but weak on the technology needed to carry it out. Under "technology" he includes both the infrastructure that would link the old, hospital-based system of care with an emerging community-based system of care and the knowledge of how to provide community-based individual treatment. Also lacking were a professional orientation to community treatment, the workforce to support it, and, as it would turn out, the resources to implement the new system.

Today, Rosenheck contends, we have the technology in the forms of better organizational linkages and evidence-based practices, but lack public support for community-based systems of care. His proposal for making the best of this quandary is to steer a middle course, but vigorously so. The community psychiatry of the near future, he writes, should bracket the broad social vision that sent its parent onto the rocks and that, in any case, the public has no stomach for. In its place, community psychiatry should target public and legislative support for the effective, but not inexpensive, services it has learned how to deliver, arguing for their cost effectiveness, given their proven results.[32]

This incremental approach to public mental health, which draws on a vision of comprehensive and effective care for the most seriously ill of persons with mental illness, leaves unanswered questions about what its relationship to the recovery and self-help movements would be. These build their own vision of community change that makes room for the full membership of persons with psychiatric disabilities, and that might, or might not, come into conflict with Rosenheck's proposed new era of public mental health care. He does, however, provide a framework for creating systems of care that attend to the needs of persons with serious and persistent psychiatric disabilities, an objective that recovery and self-help advocates do support.

Asylum is rich in history and association with society's power to strike at the bodies and minds of persons. It is both a value and a practice, ordered and honored by God in the Old Testament, then the Church, and then society, dependent on the last for its existence yet inherently a reproach to it. As noted in the commentary to J. K. Wing's classic article on the topic,[33] asylum carries mainly negative associations in mental health care—those of imprisonment, lack of treatment, soul deadening boredom and inactivity, and subhuman conditions in the worst of state hospitals. Another aspect of asylum, which Wing, H. Richard Lamb and Richard Peele, John Talbott, Mona Wasow, and others have argued for, involves rest, refuge, and recuperation from psychosis, difficult life circumstances, and humanistic social and professional responses to the inability to care for oneself at a given point due to the cognitive and functional impacts of mental illness.[34] The availability of these services, Wing argues, is critical for community mental health systems of care. Without it, community care will fail to provide humane and comprehensive care and one day will be just as maligned as the hospital-based system it replaced.

Wing's concept of asylum might be said to emphasize personal vulnerability over society's unwillingness to provide the conditions under which vulnerable persons can survive without sanctuary. Yet he and others argument for asylum maintains a critique of society and its obligations in arguing that asylum is not so much a place or institution but a set of functions, often provided in set-apart places but possible to provide within local communities. Going further, Wing[35] questions the privileged associations of "community" that adhere to places which house people outside institutions, but have little else to recommend them:

> The name "community," in the sense of a small group of people sharing common aims and needs, is much more appropriate to a place that continues the tradition of Tuke's retreat[a] than to the modern localities that are usually given the name.

Others who are not homeless or otherwise living under brutal socioeconomic conditions have their own refuges. For the middle-class, home often is the primary refuge, and a brief summer vacation the secondary. For the better off middle-class, refuge may be a summer home or cottage. For the rich, the very structure of life is that of asylum, and the walls of that structure can only be breached by conscious effort to pay rent to society or by untoward events that topple them from the outside. Coming back to the theme of asylum for persons with mental illness, it is not asylum if you do not choose it.[35]

7. Recovery. Recovery has become an object of controversy and confusion as well as acclaim in the public mental health field, in part because of its growing influence and thus its perceived threat in quarters that have not endorsed it, and in part because recovery tends to be talked about as one thing when it is several. Larry Davidson and colleagues write about three aspects of recovery: improvement in or remission of symptoms and functional impairments, a hopeful and optimistic approach to one's life and psychiatric disability, and mental health practices that are supportive of recovery in the second sense.[36]

Up until the early 1990s, recovery chiefly meant improvement in the social functioning or psychiatric symptoms of people with serious mental illness, particularly those diagnosed with schizophrenia. Researchers such as John Strauss and Courtenay Harding demonstrated that persons with schizophrenia had diverse outcomes that include substantial improvements in function or symptoms, or both, over long periods of time.[37] The World Health Organization's cross-cultural studies of schizophrenia found consistent differences across cultures, with people in developing countries doing better overall than those in industrialized countries, although methodological concerns have been raised about this research.[38]

Over the past decade plus, recovery, more and more, has come to mean that people with mental illness can have a full, rich, and productive life; have friends, jobs, and relationships; and exercise self-determination, managing their own illness with, or sometimes without, the help of clinicians and medications, even if the symptoms and functional constraints associated with their mental illnesses persist. This form of recovery does not deny the reality of recovery as cure, but also does not require it for being "in recovery." Recovery, then, is a process not a thing. As Davidson et al.[39] put it:

> This notion of being in recovery . . . does not have as much to do with a person's level or degree of symptoms, deficits, or pathology as it does with how the person is managing his or her life in the presence of an enduring illness—or perhaps how the person is managing an enduring illness in the context of his or her ongoing life. This form of recovery represents a personal, social, and political reality as much as it does a medical one, as it is significantly impacted by who the person is, the nature and density of his or her support network and milieu, and the rights and responsibilities accorded or denied to the person by virtue of the society in which he or she lives . . .

Recovery in, alongside of, or outside mental illness connects to recovery as a rallying cry and a political movement, a banner around which people can meet, conduct advocacy, and lobby for changes in treatment and engage in stigma busting. Recovery in this sense can be linked to the disability, human, and civil rights movements, although it might be charged with having sidestepped terms, such as "empowerment," that have more collective, politically charged connotations in an individualistically oriented society. On a personal level, participation in the recovery movement can give a sense of solidarity with others, engage people in support of each other's "recovery journeys," and encourage them to tell their story while linking their voice to a collective voice.

Research on recovery as a way of life is still in its infancy. As noted earlier, practices that incorporate principles, such as supporting clients' strengths and full involvement in the treatment process, and that foster hope and human dignity can be said to be recovery oriented, at least in those particulars. Other "do it now, not later" practices—supported housing, supported employment, and motivational engagement, in which motivation is not a thing you have or lack but rather a process that is always present in some changing degree in the person, as well as in others—seem, in theory at least, recovery oriented at their core. In the near future, recovery is likely to be challenged regarding its connection to clinical and functional outcomes, even if it eschews these measures now in defining itself.

New recovery has benefited, however, from its association with old recovery in carrying with it the echoes of the latter's message of improvement in clinical and functional status. "Does new recovery enhance old recovery?" If schizophrenia, for example, has a different course across cultures, then might living a life of recovery in the current sense not facilitate recovery in the old sense? These and other outcome oriented questions are likely to put pressure on new recovery in the future, calling to account its implied or explicit association with old recovery.

A number of research and theoretical efforts intended to push recovery toward surer footing in the everyday lives of people with mental illness are under way. They include interventions and approaches by the names of person-centered treatment planning,[40] social connectedness,[41] social inclusion,[42] capabilities,[43] and citizenship.[44] We can expect more such efforts to ground recovery in the tools, resources, and opportunities that help people make their ways in the world.

8. Identity. Whether in recovery or out of it, subscribing to its principles or not, the person with mental illness knows, perhaps better than most, that sometimes he or she must have to stand naked,[45] bereft of recovery, citizenship, capabilities, empowerment, and self-determination, alone with no one else in sight and left to contemplate the classic questions, "Who am I? Why am I here? Where am I going?" After the initial shock of nakedness wears off, however, the person with mental illness, like others, will probably begin to connect these personal questions to other people who are involved, explicitly or implicitly, with his or her being in the world. A woman with mental illness who concludes that she can claim a measure of courage as a shield against her nakedness traces back that sense of herself to a day when she stood up for a fellow employee at the risk of her own job. A man with mental illness who confesses to himself his fear of heights, thinking that facing his fears will make a shield for him against his nakedness, recalls that he learned his fear frozen halfway up the side of his house on a ladder made by someone else.

Is recovery an end-stage identity? Perhaps so for many, but does one always feel or see oneself to be in recovery? Walking to the store? Making love? "Why not?" a recovery advocate might respond. "Recovery is all about living a life with the joys, headaches, and routines that others have." Yet being in recovery, either in the old sense of cure or remission or the new sense of living a full life, inevitably occurs in relation to one's psychiatric disability. Jenna Howard posits an alternative—an exit from recovery. The recovery identity, she writes, involves a conflict between a temporal, expecting identity—a being on the way to recovery and out of the state one is recovering from—and a permanent accepting identity—a being in mental illness for good and living a life of recovery in relation to it. Yet exit from the recovery identity is possible, she writes, and some are engaged in that process. We need to learn more about how that exit happens, what it is like for people who engage in it, and what it means for recovery as a process and movement.[46]

Howard's theory arguably makes for a better fit with other disorders, such as alcoholism, than with mental illness, since one could argue there is no temporal split in the latter. You may or may not recover from your mental illness in the traditional sense, and you may do that temporarily or permanently. You can, however, have a life regardless of symptom improvement or setbacks, and part of doing so involves overcoming a sense of hopelessness that mental health theories and practice, and society as a whole, too often have conveyed to persons with mental illness. But does this sort of recovery ineluctably bring us back to the sort that means cure?

The discussion here brings us back to the person and society. The "rugged individualist" and "the community" are both great American myths, not so much because the reality of them is different from the rhetoric but because these terms crystallize and organize large hopes, dreams, boasts, and internally structured means of glossing over the cracks in the structure of their own rhetoric. The rugged individualist conquers the wilderness. The community moves in behind him and establishes itself in space and relationships. "Losing one' mind," with its connotation of losing one's self or being, carries a special threat to these foundational myths. The rugged individualist is no doubt brave and probably strong, but he definitely needs to have his wits about him in the wilderness. The threat of mental illness to community may be less pointed, but it is no less potent. In the movie, *It's a Wonderful Life*, George Bailey attempts suicide during the depths of the Great Depression after his bank goes under. His attempt fails and his guardian angel shows him how his life, if not lived, would have impoverished that of his loved ones and others in his hometown of Bedford Falls. But the movie hinges on the implicit notion that George Bailey is a normal guy who fell on hard times, and his guardian angel is a *deus ex machina*, not a *real* hallucination. Can we imagine a George Bailey whose suicide attempt was the last of several, who had been hospitalized a few times, who acts funny, whose skin color is dark, and who has never risen so high in the bank's organizational table as George Bailey? Can we see that person having an impact on the lives of people in his hometown comparable to that of Jimmy Stewart in *It's a Wonderful Life*? Here, the question is not only what our new fictional hero would have to do to survive and prosper in the community, but what a community would look like that made possible affirmative answers to these questions.

At a 2007 seminar on stigma and valued roles of persons with mental illness, a colleague, Patricia Benedict, said, "Accepting someone means accepting their values."[47] As the discussion moved on, we reflected on Benedict's comment: "Acceptance is not tolerance, then. You can tolerate another's presence, recognize or grant her right to be part of the same neighborhood, work place, or block party as yours. But to accept her you have to value her participation and value her as a person even before, and whether or not, she makes her contribution." But then a dialogue between the authors and Benedict suggested itself:

> "If you accept the person with a mental illness, are you accepting her in whole or in part?"
> "In whole, of course."
> "But do you accept the whole person in front of you, or a remembered or possible whole person who's partly concealed under her mental illness?"
> "No, you accept the whole person, period."
> "Well, what if her paranoia drives you up the wall?"
> "That's all right, you don't have to like everything about her to accept and value her."

But there's a twist here. Benedict said "values" plural, not "value," although in talking with her afterward, we learned she meant both. Your personhood, according to her theory, involves certain values and ways of seeing the world that help one to navigate in it, and the experience of difference helps to shape your values. Therefore, accepting the person means accepting that person's values, assuming the fist of them doesn't reach the end of your nose. But could these values threaten the community's, or more benignly, force it to question its values? A like question could be asked regarding other marginalized persons and groups. If the answer is yes, then some part of the future of democratic society and the future of persons with mental illness are not unrelated. The converse of our argument that democracy is challenged when it sets limits based on gender, race, class, and normality is that freeing people from the chains that democracy puts on them makes democracy strong. Doing so, however, involves overcoming the myth that persons with mental illness are not full human beings.

It goes beyond the scope of this concluding chapter to say more than this. The next era of community psychiatry, or whatever name a new generation of practitioners and students give it, may take up some of the questions these themes entail. If so, some of its new classics will be those that either bring together existing thoughts, research, and practice about, or break new ground for, responding to them.

Notes and References

1. Morrissey, J. P., & Goldman, H. H. (1986). Care and treatment of the mentally ill in the United States: Historical developments and reforms. *Annals of the American Academy of Political and Social Science, 484,* 12–27. Howard Goldman gave us helpful comments on a draft this article with reference to his article and his 2006 book with Gerald Grob.
2. Grob, G. N., & Goldman, H. H. (2006). *The dilemma of federal mental health policy: Radical reform or incremental change?* New Brunswick, NJ: Rutgers University Press.
3. We are indebted to Howard Goldman for this classification, which we modified slightly. Of course we are responsible for any mistakes that crept in with this modification, and for our use of the framework.
4. See, for one example among many, Perry, B. D. (2002). Childhood experience and the expression of genetic potential: What childhood neglect tells us about nature and nurture. *Brain and Mind, 3,* 79–100.
5. For a wide-ranging review of environmental influences on health in general, see Kroll Smith, S., Brown, P., & Gunter, V. J., editors. (2000). *Illness and the environment: A reader in contested medicine.* New York: New York University Press.

6. Rita Charon, a physician and leading scholar in this field, writes, "I invented the term 'narrative medicine' to connote a medicine practiced with narrative competence and marked with an understanding of these highly complex narrative situations among doctors, patients, colleagues, and the public." http://litsite.alaska.edu/healing/medicine.html. Accessed March 20, 2008.

7. Thompson, K. S. (1993). Re-inventing progressive psychiatry: The uses of history. *Community Mental Health Journal, 29*(6), 495–508.

8. Bracken, P., & Thomas, P. (2005). *Postpsychiatry: Mental health in a postmodern world.* Oxford: Oxford University Press.

9. Diamond, R., Susser, E., & Stein, L. I. (1992). Essential and nonessential roles for psychiatrists in community mental health centres. *Hospital and Community Psychiatry, 42,* 187–189. See also Rosen, A. (2006). The community psychiatrist of the future. *Current Opinion in Psychiatry, 19.*

10. Andreasen, N. C. (2007). DSM and the death of phenomenology in America: An example of unintended consequences. *Schizophrenia Bulletin, 33*(1), 108–112.

11. U.S. Medical Directors Council of the National Association of State Mental Health Program Directors. (2006). *Morbidity and mortality in people with serious mental illness.* Alexandria, VA: Author.

12. Drake, R. E., Goldman, H. H., Leff, H., et al. (2001). Implementing evidence-based practices in routine mental health service settings. *Psychiatric Services, 52,* 179–182.

13. Rowe, M. (1999). *Crossing the border: Encounters between homeless people and outreach workers.* Berkeley: University of California Press.

14. Larry Davidson, personal communication.

15. See, for example, McGlashan, T. H., & Johannessen, J. O. (1996). Early detection and intervention with schizophrenia: Rationale. *Schizophrenia Bulletin, 22*(2), 201–222.

16. The most recent manifestation of European Union–United States exchange and collaboration on the topic of social inclusion for persons with mental illnesses was the June 12–14, 2008, conference, *Social inclusion and the transformation of mental health services: Transatlantic perspectives,* of the University of Pittsburgh's European Center for Excellence.

17. See Stuart, G., Tondora, J., & Hoge, M. (2004). Evidence-based teaching practice: Implications for behavioral health. *Administration and Policy in Mental Health, 32*(2), 107–130.

18. Hoge, M. A., Morris, J. A., Daniels, A. S., Stuart, G. W., Huey, L. Y., & Adams, N. (2007). *An action plan for behavioral health workforce development: A framework for discussion.* Washington, D.C.: Health and Human Services, Substance Abuse and Mental Health Services Administration.

19. Lipsky, M. (1980). *Street-level bureaucracy: Dilemmas of the individual in public services.* New York: Russell Sage Foundation.

20. Rowe, M., Hoge, M. A., & Fisk, D. (1998). Services for mentally ill homeless persons: Street-level integration. *American Journal of Orthopsychiatry, 68*(3), 490–496.

21. Wagenaar, H. (Forthcoming.) *Interpretation and dialogue in policy analysis.* M. E. Sharpe.

22. Freeman, R. (Forthcoming). Policy opportunities. In Mollica, R., editor. *Project 1 billion: Book of best practices.* Vanderbilt University Press.

23. Freeman, R. (2006). The work the document does: Research, policy and equity in health. *Journal of Health Politics, Policy and Law, 31*(1), 51–70.

24. For a discussion of the mixed story of implementation of the Olmstead ruling, see Mathis, J. (2001). Community integration of individuals with disabilities: An update on *Olmstead* implementation. *Journal of Poverty Law and Policy, November-December,* 395–410.

25. For a thorough review on this topic, see Geller, J. F. (2006). The evolution of outpatient commitment in the USA: From conundrum to quagmire. *International Journal of Law and Psychiatry, 29,* 234–248.

26. Sells, D., Davidson, L., Jewell, C., Falzer, P., & Rowe, M. (2006). The treatment relationship in peer-based and regular case management services for clients with severe mental illness. *Psychiatric Services, 57*(8), 1179–1184.

27. Ware, N. C., Hopper, K., Tugenberg, T., Dickey, B., & Fisher, F. (2007). Connectedness and citizenship: Redefining social integration. *Psychiatric Services, 58,* 469–474.

28. Granovetter, M. (1973). The strength of weak ties. *American Journal of Sociology, 78*(6), 1360–1380.

29. Hopper, K., Jost, J., Hay, T., Welber, S., & Haugland, G. (1997). Homelessness, severe mental illness, and the institutional circuit. *Psychiatric Services, 48*(4), 659–665.

30. Ware et al, *op cit.*

31. See, for example, Rowe, M., Benedict, P., Sells, D., Dinzeo, T., Garvin, C., Schwab, L., Baranoski, M., Girard, V., & Bellamy, C. (2009). Citizenship, community, and recovery: A group- and peer-based intervention for persons with co-occurring disorders and criminal justice histories. *Journal for Groups in Addiction and Recovery, 4*(4), 224–244.

32. Rosenheck, R. (2000). The delivery of mental health services in the 21st century: Bringing the community back in. *Community Mental Health Journal, 36*(1), 107–124.

33. Wing, J. K. (1990). The functions of asylum. *British Journal of Psychiatry, 157,* 822–827.

34. Lamb, H., & Peele, R. (1984). The need for continuing asylum and sanctuary. *Hospital and Community Psychiatry, 35*(8), 798–802; Talbott, J. A. (2004). The need for asylum, not asylums. *Hospital and Community Psychiatry, 55*(10), 1127 [reprint of March 1984 article.]; Wasow, M. (1986). The need for asylum for the chronically mentally ill. *Schizophrenia Bulletin, 12*(2), 162–167.

35. Wing, *op cit,* 825–826.

36. Davidson, L., Drake, R. E., Schmutte, T., Dinzeo, T., & Andres-Hyman, R. (2009). Oil and water or oil and vinegar? Evidence-based medicine meets recovery. *Community Mental Health Journal, 45,* 323–332.

37. Strauss, J. S., Hafez, H., Lieberman, P., & Harding, C. (1985). The course of psychiatric disorder, III: Longitudinal principles. *American Journal of Psychiatry, 142*(3), 289–296; and Harding, C. M., Brooks, G. W., Ashikaga, T., Strauss, J. S., & Brier, A. (1987). The Vermont longitudinal study of persons with severe mental illness, II: Long-term outcome of subjects who retrospectively met DSM-III criteria for schizophrenia. *American Journal of Psychiatry, 144*(6), 727–735.

38. Hopper, K., & Wanderling, J. (2000). Revisiting the developed versus developing country distinction in course and outcome in schizophrenia: Results from ISoS, the WHO Collaborative Follow-up Project. *Schizophrenia Bulletin, 26*(4), 835–846.

39. Davidson et al., *op cit.*

40. Tondora, J., Pocklington, S., Gorges, A., Osher, D., & Davidson, L. (2005). *Implementation of person-centered care and planning. From policy to practice to evaluation. Washington D.C.: Sub*stance Abuse and Mental Health Services Administration.

41. Ware et al., *op cit.*

42. See Morgan, C., Burns, T., Fitzpatrick, R., Pinfold, V., & Priebe, S. (2007). Social Inclusion and mental health: Conceptual and methodological review. *British Journal of Psychiatry, 191,* 477–483.

43. Hopper K. (2007). Rethinking social recovery in schizophrenia: What a capabilities approach might offer. *Social Science and Medicine, 65*(5), 868–879.

44. See Rowe (1999), *op cit*; Rowe, M., & Baranoski, M. (2000). Mental illness, criminality, and citizenship. *Journal of the American Academy of Psychiatry and the Law, 28*(3), 262–264; Rowe, M., Kloos, B., Chinman, M., Davidson, L., & Cross, A. B. (2001). Homelessness, mental illness, and citizenship. *Social Policy and Administration, 35*(1), 14–31; and Rowe et al. (2007). See also Ware et al., *op cit.*

45. This is a paraphrase of a line from the song, "It's alright, ma (I'm only bleeding)." In Dylan, B. (1965). *Bringin' it all back home.* New York: Columbia Records.

46. Howard, J. (2006). Expecting and accepting: The temporal ambiguity of recovery identities. *Social Psychology Quarterly, 69*(4), 307–324.

47. Benedict, P. (2007). Director of the Citizens Project and Leadership Project for the Yale Program for Recovery and Community Health (PRCH), made this comment during a December 2007 PRCH seminar.

Index

Note: Page references followed by "*f*" and "*t*" denote figures and tables, respectively.

Printed in the USA/Agawam, MA
June 5, 2018

676194.016